T0183003

Medical Radiology

Diagnostic Imaging

Series Editors

Hans-Ulrich Kauczor
Paul M. Parizel
Wilfred C. G. Peh

For further volumes:
http://www.springer.com/series/4354

Emilio Quaia

Editor

Imaging of the Liver and Intra-hepatic Biliary Tract

Volume 1: Imaging Techniques and Non-tumoral Pathologies

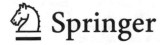 Springer

Editor
Emilio Quaia
Radiology Unit, Department of Medicine - DIMED
University of Padova
Padova, Italy

ISSN 0942-5373   ISSN 2197-4187   (electronic)
Medical Radiology
ISBN 978-3-030-38985-7   ISBN 978-3-030-38983-3   (eBook)
https://doi.org/10.1007/978-3-030-38983-3

© Springer Nature Switzerland AG 2021
This work is subject to copyright. All rights are reserved by the Publisher, whether the whole or part of the material is concerned, specifically the rights of translation, reprinting, reuse of illustrations, recitation, broadcasting, reproduction on microfilms or in any other physical way, and transmission or information storage and retrieval, electronic adaptation, computer software, or by similar or dissimilar methodology now known or hereafter developed.
The use of general descriptive names, registered names, trademarks, service marks, etc. in this publication does not imply, even in the absence of a specific statement, that such names are exempt from the relevant protective laws and regulations and therefore free for general use.
The publisher, the authors, and the editors are safe to assume that the advice and information in this book are believed to be true and accurate at the date of publication. Neither the publisher nor the authors or the editors give a warranty, expressed or implied, with respect to the material contained herein or for any errors or omissions that may have been made. The publisher remains neutral with regard to jurisdictional claims in published maps and institutional affiliations.

This Springer imprint is published by the registered company Springer Nature Switzerland AG
The registered company address is: Gewerbestrasse 11, 6330 Cham, Switzerland

To my beloved Luigi

Contents

Abbreviations

AASLD	American Association for the Study of Liver Diseases
AAST	American Association for Surgery and Trauma
AATD	Alpha-1 antitrypsin deficiency
ABC	Acute bacterial cholangitis
ABCR	α-Fetoprotein Barcelona Clinic Liver Cancer Child-Pugh and Response (score)
ACT	Adoptive cell transfer
ADC	Apparent diffusion coefficient
ADPKD	Autosomal dominant polycystic kidney disease
ADPLD	Autosomal dominant polycystic liver disease
AE	Adverse event
AFP	Alpha-fetoprotein
AGA	American Gastroenterology Association
AGS	Alagille syndrome
AI	Artificial intelligence
AIF	Arterial input function
AIH	Autoimmune hepatitis
AIOM	Italian Association of Medical Oncology
AISF	Italian Association for the Study of the Liver
AKI	Acute kidney injury
AML	Angiomyolipoma
AP	Arterial Phase
APASL	Asian Pacific Association for the Study of the Liver
APHE	Arterial phase hyperenhancement
APS	Arterioportal shunt
APTT	Activated partial thromboplastin time
ARFI	Acoustic radiation force impulse
ARPKD	Autosomal recessive polycystic kidney disease
ART	Assessment for Retreatment with TACE (score)
ASQ	Acoustic structure quantification
AST	Serum aspartate aminotransferase
AUC	Area Under the Curve
AVM	Arteriovenous malformation
BA	Biliary atresia
BASM	Biliary atresia splenic malformation
BCLC	Barcellona Clinic Liver Cancer
BCS	Budd–Chiari syndrome

BD	Bile duct
β-HCA	β-Catenin-mutated type with upregulation of glutamine synthetase hepatocellular adenoma
BF	Blood flow
BH	Biliary hamartomas
BMD	Basis material decomposition
BMI	Body mass index
BRCLM	Breast cancer liver metastases
BSA	Body surface area
BSC	Best supportive care
BV	Blood volume
CAP	Controlled attenuation parameter
CBCTA	Cone-beam computed tomographic angiography
CCC (or CCA)	Cholangiocarcinoma
CDDP	Cisplatin
CDUS	Color Doppler ultrasound
CE	Contrast enhancement
CECT (or CE-CT)	Contrast-enhanced CT
CEMRI (or CE-MRI)	Contrast-enhanced MRI
CEUS	Contrast-enhanced ultrasound
CHA	Common hepatic artery
cHC	Mixed or combined (or biphenotypic) hepatocellular carcinoma and cholangiocarcinoma
CHD	Common hepatic duct
CHF	Congenital hepatic fibrosis
CKD-EPI	Chronic kidney disease epidemiology collaboration
CM	Contrast medium
CMV	Cytomegalovirus
COACH	Cerebellar vermis hypo/aplasia, oligophrenia, ataxia congenital, coloboma, and hepatic fibrosis syndrome
CP	Child-Pugh
CPSS	Congenital portosystemic shunts
CR	Complete response
CRA	Cryoblation
CRC	Colorectal cancer
CRLM	Colorectal cancer liver metastases
CRP	C-reactive protein
CS	Caroli syndrome
CSPH	Clinically significant portal hypertension
CT	Computed tomography
cTACE	Conventional TACE
CTAP	CT arterial portography
CTHA	CT hepatic arteriography
CTP	CT perfusion
CTPI	CT perfusion index
CV	Central vein of the hepatic lobule

DCE	Dynamic contrast enhanced
DCE-US	Dynamic contrast-enhanced ultrasound
DEBIRI	Drug-eluting beads irinotecan-loaded
DEB-TACE	Drug-eluting bead TACE
DECT	Dual-energy CT
DILI	Drug-induced liver injury
DISIDA	Disofenin
DKI	Diffusion kurtosis imaging
dlDECT	Dual-layer detector DECT
DN	Dysplastic nodule
DP	Delayed phase
DSA	Digital subtraction angiography
dsDECT	Dual-Source dual-energy CT
DWI (or DW imaging)	Diffusion-weighted imaging sequence (MRI)
EAP	Early arterial phase
EASL	European Association for the Study of the Liver
ECCM	Extracellular contrast media
ECOG	Eastern Cooperative Oncology Group
EDV	End diastolic velocity
EES	Extravascular-extracellular space
EF	Enhancing fraction
EFSUMB	European Federation of Societies for Ultrasound in Medicine and Biology
EGDS	Esophago-gastro-duodenoscopy
eGFR	Estimated glomerular filtration rate
EHD	Extrahepatic disease
EHE	Epithelioid hemangioendothelioma
EHPVO	Extrahepatic portal vein obstruction
EHS	Extrahepatic spread
EIS	Endoscopic injection sclerotherapy
EMH	Extramedullary hematopoiesis
ENETS	European Neuroendocrine Tumour Society
EOB-DTPA	Ethoxybenzyl diethylenetriamine pentaacetic acid (gadoxetic acid)
EORTC	European Organization for Research and Treatment of Cancer
EPSVS	Extrahepatic portosystemic venous shunt
e-PTFE	Expanded polytetrafluoroethylene
ERCP	Endoscopic retrograde cholangiopancreatography
ESGAR	European Society of Gastrointestinal and Abdominal Radiology
ESMO	European Society for Medical Oncology
EUS	Endoscopic ultrasound
EVL	Endoscopic variceal band ligation
FAST	Focused assessment with sonography in trauma
FBP	Filtered back projection
FDG-PET	Fluorodeoxyglucose-positron emission tomography

FEP	Flow extraction product
FHVP	Free hepatic venous pressure
FLR	Future liver remnant
FNH	Focal nodular hyperplasia
FOLFIRI	Folinic acid–fluorouracicil–irinotecan
FS	Fat saturation
FUDR	Floxuridine
GBCA	Gadolinium-based contrast agents
GDA	Gastroduodenal artery
Gd-BOPTA	Gadobenate dimeglumine
GI	Gastrointestinal
GIST	Gastrointestinal stromal tumor
GRE	Gradient echo (MRI sequence)
GSD	Glycogen storage disease
HA	Hepatic artery
HAI	Hepatic arterial infusion
HAIC	Hepatic arterial infusion chemotherapy
HAP[1]	Hepatic artery pseudoaneurysm
HAP[2]	Hepatoma arterial-embolisation prognostic (score)
HAR	Hepatic artery rupture
HAS	Hepatic artery stenosis
HAT[1]	Hepatic arterial therapy
HAT[2]	Hepatic artery thrombosis
HBCM	Hepatobiliary contrast media
HBP (or HB phase)	Hepatobiliary phase
HCA	Hepatocellular adenoma
HCC	Hepatocellular carcinoma
HCC–CCA (or HCC–CCC, or cHCC–CCA, or cHC)	Mixed hepatocellular carcinoma and cholangiocarcinoma
HE	Hepatic encephalopathy
HFJV	High-Frequency Jet Ventilation
HH	Hepatic hemangioma
H-HCA	Hepatocyte nuclear factor 1-α mutated type
HHT	Hereditary hemorrhagic telangiectasia
HIFU	High-intensity focused ultrasound
HIV	Human immunodeficiency virus
HKLC	Hong Kong Liver Cancer
HL	Hepatolithiasis
HPE	Hepatic portoenterostomy
HPI	Hepatic perfusion index
HPS	Hepatopulmonary syndrome
HRI	Hepatorenal index
HRS	Hepatorenal syndrome
HU	Hounsfield units
HUI	Hepatic uptake index

HV	Hepatic vein
HVPG	Hepatic vein pressure gradient
IAT	Intra-arterial thrombolysis
IBD	Inflammatory bowel disease
ICC	Intrahepatic cholangiocarcinoma
IDA	Iminodiacetic acid
IDR	Iodine delivery rate
IgG4-SC	IgG4-related sclerosing cholangitis
IHBPA	International Hepato-Pancreato-Biliary Association
I-HCA	Inflammatory-type hepatocellular adenoma
IMT	Inflammatory myofibroblastic tumor
INCPH	Idiopathic non-cirrhotic portal hypertension
INR	International normalized ratio
IPMN	Intraductal papillary mucinous neoplasm (of pancreas)
IPNB	Intraductal papillary neoplasm of the bile duct
IPSVS	Intrahepatic portosystemic venous shunt
IPT	Inflammatory pseudotumors
IR	Iterative reconstruction
irAE	Immune-related adverse events
ITT	Intention-to-treat
IVC	Inferior vena cava
IVCM	Intravascular contrast media
IVIM	Intravoxel incoherent motion
KLCSG	Korean Liver Cancer Study Group
LAP	Late arterial phase
LBW	Lean body weight
LCSGJ	Liver Cancer Study Group of Japan
LEHR	Low-energy high-resolution
LFOV	Large field-of-view
LHA	Left hepatic artery
LHD	Left hepatic duct
LHV	Left hepatic vein
LIC	Liver iron concentration
LI-RADS	Liver imaging reporting and data system
LMWH	Low-molecular-weight heparin
LPV	Left portal vein
LRN	Large regenerative nodule
LR-TR	LIRADS Treatment Response
LSA	Laser ablation
LSF	Lung shunt fraction
LT	Liver transplantation
LVD	Liver venous deprivation
MAA	Macroaggregated albumin
M-CCA	Mass-forming cholangiocarcinoma
MCN	Mucinous cystic neoplasm
mCRC	Metastatic colorectal cancer
MDCT	Multi-detector row computed tomography
MDRD	Modification of diet in renal disease

MHV	Middle hepatic vein
MECSE	Multi-echo chemical shift-encoded
MI	Mechanical index
MinIP	Minimum Intensity Projection
MIP	Maximum Intensity Projection
MIRD	Medical Internal Radiation Dosimetry
MMC	Mitomycin
MOLLI	Modified Look-Locker inversion recovery
MPR	Multiplanar Reformatting
MRA	Magnetic resonance angiography
MRCP	Magnetic resonance cholangiopancreatography
MRE	MR elastography
mRECIST	Modified RECIST
MRI (or MR imaging)	Magnetic resonance imaging
MRRT	Management of Radiology Report Templates
MRS	MR spectroscopy
MTT	Mean transit time
MVI	Microvascular invasion
MWA	Microwave ablation
MWI	Microwave irradiation
NAFLD	Nonalcoholic fatty liver disease
NASH	Nonalcoholic steatohepatitis
NBCA	N-butyl-cyanoacrylate
NELM	Neuroendocrine liver metastasis
NET	Neuroendocrine tumour
NET-GEP	Gastroenteropancreatic neuroendocrine tumor
NHFPC-PRCh	National Health and Family Planning Commission of the People's Republic of China
NR	Not reported
NRH	Nodular regenerative hyperplasia
OATP(1) B1 and OATP B3	Organic anionic transport protein B1 and B3
OCP	Oral contraceptive pills
OLTx	Orthotopic liver transplantation
ORR	Objective response rate
OS	Overall survival
PA	Pyogenic abscess
PBC	Primary biliary cirrhosis
PC[1]	Percutaneous cholecystostomy
PC[2]	Prospective cohort (study)
PC-AKI	Postcontrast acute kidney injury
PD	Progressive disease or disease progression
PDFF	Proton density fat fraction
PDUS	Power Doppler ultrasound
PDX	Polydioxanone
PEComa	Perivascular epithelioid cell neoplasm
PEI	Percutaneous ethanol injection

PFS	Progression-free survival
PH	Portal hypertension
PHE	Portosystemic hepatic encephalopathy
PHG	Portal hypertensive gastropathy
PI	Pulsatility index
PNP	Peak negative pressure
PPG	Portal pressure gradient
PPI	Proton pump inhibitor
PR	Partial response
PRS	Post-radioembolisation syndrome
PS[1]	Permeability surface (area product)
PS[2]	Performance status
PSAP	Permeability surface area product
PSC	Primary sclerosing cholangitis
PSV	Peak systolic velocity
PSVS	Portosystemic venous shunt
PT	Prothrombin time
PTA	Percutaneous transluminal angioplasty
PTBD	Percutaneous transhepatic biliary drainage
PTC	Percutaneous transhepatic cholangiography
PTCB	Percutaneous transhepatic cholangio-biopsy
PV	Portal vein
PVA	Polyvinyl alcohol particles
PVE	Portal vein embolization
PVP[1]	Portal venous phase
PVP[2]	Portal venous perfusion
PVS	Portal vein stenosis
PVT	Portal vein thrombosis
PVTT	Portal vein tumour thrombosis (segmental)
QOL	Quality of life
RAHD	Right anterior hepatic duct
RAPV	Right anterior portal vein
RC	Retrospective cohort (study)
RCC	Renal cell carcinoma
RCT(S)	Randomised control trial (study)
RECICL	Response Evaluation Criteria in Cancer of the Liver
RECIST	Response Evaluation Criteria in Solid Tumors
RER	Rough endoplasmic reticulum
RES	Reticuloendothelial system
RFA (or RF ablation)	Radiofrequency ablation
RFS	Recurrence-free survival
RHA	Right hepatic artery
RHD	Right hepatic duct
RHP	Right hepatic vein
RI	Resistive index
RILD	Radiation-induced liver disease
RLE	Relative liver enhancement

RN	Regenerative nodule
RPC	Recurrent pyogenic cholangitis
RPHD	Right posterior hepatic duct
RPPV	Right posterior portal vein
RPV	Right portal vein
rsDECT	Rapid-switching dual energy CT
S	Sinusoids
SAA	Serum amyloid A
SARAH	Strengthening and Stretching for Rheumatoid Arthritis of the Hand
SAT	Systolic acceleration time
SD	Stable disease
SI	Signal intensity
SIR	Signal intensity ratio
SMA	Superior mesenteric artery
SMV	Superior mesenteric vein
SN	Siderotic nodule
SNR	Signal–intensity ratio
SOS	Sinusoidal obstruction syndrome
SPECT	Single-photon emission computed tomography
SPIO	Superparamagnetic iron oxide-based
SR	Structured report
SSC	Secondary sclerosing cholangitis
SSR	Somatostatin receptor
STATE	Selection for transarterial chemoembolisation treatment (score)
SV	Splenic vein
SWE	Shear wave elastography
TACE	Transarterial chemoembolisation
TAE	Transarterial embolisation
TARE	Transarterial radioembolisation
TB	Tuberculosis
TE	Transient elastography (or echo time in MRI)
TFE	Tetrafluoroethylene
THAD	Transient hepatic attenuation differences
THID	Transient hepatic intensity differences
TIC	Time intensity curve
TIPS	Transjugular intrahepatic portosystemic shunt
TLR	Tumour-to-liver ratio
TSE	Turbo spin-echo (MRI sequence)
TSTC	Too small to be characterized (lesions)
TTP	Time to progression
TVDT	Tumor volume doubling time
UCA	Ultrasound contrast agents
UDCA	Ursodeoxycholic acid
UES	Undifferentiated embryonal sarcoma
UNOS	United Network for Organ Sharing

US	Ultrasound
VCs	Vascular complications
VEGF	Vascular endothelial growth factor
VMIs	Virtual monoenergetic images
VNC	Virtual non-contrast
VFA	Variable flip angle
VR	Volume Rendering
WBCT	Whole-body CT trauma
WHVP	Wedged hepatic venous pressure

Part I

Embriology and Normal Radiologic Anatomy

Embryology and Development of the Liver

Lorenzo Ugo and Emilio Quaia

Contents

Abstract

The liver originates from the distal foregut of the embryo from around day 22. Its development takes place in the context of the septum transversum, at the cranial end of the forming abdominal cavity. Both hepatocytes, the main liver constituents, and biliary epithelial cells derive from the endoderm constituting the primitive gut.

L. Ugo · E. Quaia (✉)
Radiology Unit, Department of Medicine - DIMED,
University of Padova, Padova, Italy
e-mail: emilio.quaia@unipd.it

Liver morphogenesis requires interaction with surrounding mesodermal structures, which in turn supply vasculature to the forming organ.

Colonization from mesodermal derived cells provides the liver with a hematopoietic population that serves as the fetus primary source of blood cells from the second month of gestation to the seventh.

During fetal life the liver is the first organ to receive oxygenated blood from the placenta via the left umbilical vein, part of which is diverted to fetal systemic circulation via a shunt provided by the ductus venosum. Both the umbilical vein and ductus venosum will obliterate in extrauterine life.

© Springer Nature Switzerland AG 2021

E. Quaia (ed.), *Imaging of the Liver and Intra-hepatic Biliary Tract*,
Medical Radiology, Diagnostic Imaging, https://doi.org/10.1007/978-3-030-38983-3_1

1   Embryonic Layout at Third Week of Development

Following gastrulation, during the third week after fertilization, the embryo is composed of multiple cavities surrounding the embryo proper, which has the shape of a disc.

Both the dorsal and ventral sides of the embryonic disc face inside two opposing cavities, known, respectively, as the amniotic sac and the yolk sac (also known as umbilical vesicle).

The largest and outermost cavity, which encompasses the embryonic disc, the yolk sac, and the amniotic sac, is called chorionic cavity or extraembryonic coelom.

The core of the embryo development takes place in the embryonic disc, while the other structures mainly have a supporting role to the embryo during pregnancy.

The disc is a trilaminar structure, composed of three layers of cells known as germ layers.

The layer facing the amniotic sac is called ectoderm, the one facing the yolk sac is the endoderm, and the mesoderm is the layer comprised between the two (Fig. 1).

These three distinct lineages of cells will give rise to different tissues and organs. From the ectoderm will mainly develop the epidermis and the nervous tissue; from the mesoderm originate serosae, cardiovascular, connective, and muscular tissues; and from the endoderm the mucosae of the respiratory and the gastrointestinal system. Hepatic development is strictly tied to the development of the gastrointestinal tract, and as such, its main germ layer contributor is the endoderm.

To better understand the adult abdominal cavity conformation, it is now necessary to introduce a slight complication in the trilaminar embryonic layout just described, as from day 17 (Schoenwolf 2015), the lateral portion of the mesodermal layer starts splitting into two parts, one associated with the endoderm (splanchnic mesoderm) and the other with the ectoderm (somatic mesoderm). The space between the splanchnic and somatic mesoderm is in direct continuity with the extraembryonic coelom and will define the space of the abdominal cavity.

2   Embryonic Folding

Despite the fact that at the gastrulation embryonic phase the overall shape of the embryo proper is essentially flat, at this stage all major body axes are already defined. We already talked about a ventral and a dorsal side, but gastrulation also defines the cranio-caudal and latero-lateral axes.

According to those axes, during the fourth week, a period of rapid growth, embryonic folding takes place. Due to the different growth rate between different embryonic structures, as both the amnios and embryonary disc grow faster than the yolk sac, the embryo starts assuming a more tridimensional and complex shape: from a bidimensional disc to a roughly cylindrical shape.

This process involves simultaneous folding around two different axes: the cranio-caudal axis (lateral folding) and the latero-lateral axis (cranio-caudal folding).

Lateral folding results in the development of two lateral body folds, which grow ventrally and then medially, in a hug-like fashion. Folding around the latero-lateral axis results in the development of both the cranial and caudal folds (Figs. 2 and 3).

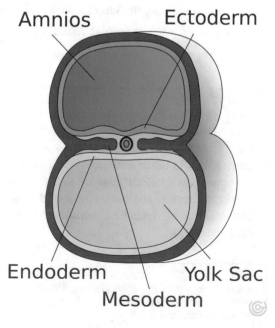

Fig. 1 Axial section of the embryonic disc at trilaminar stage

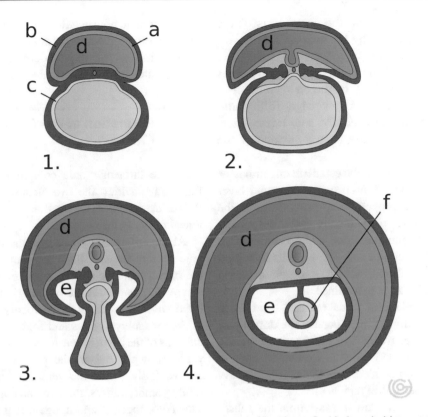

Fig. 2 Lateral folding as seen in the axial plane. Dorsal extremity is up. The ectoderm (**a**) at the periphery of the embryonic disk grows in the ventral direction, enclosing the other embryo structures in a hug-like fashion. From a delamination of the mesodermal layer (**b**), forms the intraembryonic coelom (**e**), which is initially in wide communication with the extraembryonic coelom encompassing the whole embryo. In (*4*) the primitive gut (**f**), lined by cells of the endodermal layer (**c**), is hanging in the intraembryonic coelom by means of a mesodermal dorsal mesentery; the embryo is encircled by the amniotic cavity (**d**). Note that (*4*) corresponds to an axial section slightly off from the craniocaudal embryo midline, where the vitelline duct would be visible

Fig. 3 Craniocaudal folding as seen on the sagittal plane. Cranial extremity is on the left. Heart (*1*), septum transversum, septum transversum (*2*), amniotic sac (*3*), ectoderm (*4*), mesoderm (*5*), yolk sac (*6*), endoderm (*7*). Notice the blind-ended cranial (*8*) and caudal (*9*) extensions of the endoderm, corresponding to the forming primitive gut. Communication between the yolk sac and primitive gut gradually reduces in diameter both on the axial and sagittal planes

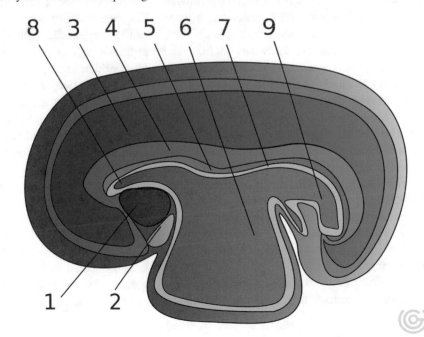

Due to the fact that the dorsal axis of the embryo is stiffened by the concomitant development of the notochord, neural tube, and somites, most of the embryonic folding takes place in the periphery of the embryonic disc. While growing, the outer edge folds onto itself both cranio-caudally and latero-laterally, giving rise to the ventral surface of the embryo.

Folding onto itself, the ectoderm encompasses the other two layer and becomes the outer layer of the embryo proper. As it grows towards the ventral midline, it eventually fuses with itself forming a continuous layer around the embryo with the exception of the umbilical region (Schoenwolf 2015), where a communication with the yolk sac is maintained.

As the endoderm folds ventrally and fuses along the midline, it incorporates the dorsal part of the yolk sac, giving rise cranially and caudally to two blind-ended tubelike structures, both in communication with the bulk of the yolk sac cavity around the central region.

As this connection narrows within the subsequent days, the continuity between the cranial and caudal pockets becomes more obvious and by the end of the sixth week (Schoenwolf 2015) a unitary tubelike structure is defined: the primitive gut.

The cranial, middle, and caudal parts of the primitive gut are named, respectively, foregut, midgut, and hindgut. The connection between midgut and yolk sac becomes a slender duct, called the yolk stalk (also known as vitelline duct or omphalomesenteric duct), which will eventually fully obliterate. The primitive gut is surrounded by the splanchnic mesodermal layer, which accompanies the endoderm during folding. The somatic mesoderm does the same with the ectoderm, of which it lines the inner side while the ectoderm folds inward and forms the anterior embryonic wall. As the embryonic folds fuse along the midline, the space between the splanchnic and the somatic mesoderm, once in communication with the extra-embryonary coelom, gets gradually enclosed forming the intra-embryonary coelom.

Despite the complex tridimensional rearrangement which occurs during embryonic folding, it is interesting to note that the germ layers have the same topologic relation between them as in the embryonic disc, where endoderm and ectoderm are separated by mesoderm interposition.

3 Formation of the Abdominal Cavity

From the intraembryonic coelom will develop four body cavities: the two pleural cavities and the pericardial cavity in the thorax, and the peritoneal cavity in the abdomen.

At the embryonic disc stage, the intraembryonic coelom has the shape of a horseshoe, with the curved part facing up, in the cranial region where the heart starts developing, and the two blind-ended sides along the periphery of the disc.

As the embryo grows and folds, the two caudal ends of the cavity come together medially and ventrally, while the cranial part folds caudally and ventrally. When the ventral midline of the folding embryo fuses, the two ends of the horseshoe come together and merge into a single caudal cavity which surrounds the forming primitive gut.

In the meantime, the embryonic ancestor of the diaphragm, the septum transversum, develops starting from day 22 (Schoenwolf 2015) from the mesoderm in the upper portion of the embryonic disc, just cranially to developing heart. As craniocaudal embryonic folding happens, both the septum transversum and the heart are brought into position to what will become the thoracoabdominal junction, with the septum transversum repositioning just caudally to the heart, on the ventral side of the embryo. The septum transversum will be positioned between the seventh thoracic level anteriorly and the twelfth posteriorly (Schoenwolf 2015).

The intra-embryonary coelom that lies close to the developing heart (first dorsally, and then, following embryonic folding, ventrally), which corresponds to the curved upper part of the coelomic horseshoe, is the primitive pericardial cavity. It is connected to the caudal intra-embryonary coelom via two limbs, the pericardioperitoneal canals. As the septum transversum now divides the ventral thoracoabdominal junction, communication between thoracic and abdominal cavities exists on a somewhat more dorsal plane.

Pericardioperitoneal canals will eventually be obliterated by the growth of the pleuroperitoneal membranes from the dorsal wall, which will fuse ventrally with the septum transversum by the seventh week, finally separating the thoracic from the abdominal cavity; closure of the right and left pleuroperitoneal canal is slightly asynchronous, as the left is bigger and closes later.

4 Dorsal and Ventral Mesentery

When the primitive gut starts taking its shape, it is in broad contact posteriorly with the dorsal body of the embryo.

In the abdominal region however, this posterior area of attachment gradually reduces, and the primitive gut becomes suspended in the abdominal cavity.

Contact with the posterior wall is not completely lost, and is provided by a thin double-layered mesodermal structure, the dorsal mesentery, which is the progenitor of the greater omentum and the mesenteries of the small and large intestine in the fully developed abdomen.

As the coelomic cavity corresponds to the peritoneal space in the adult, the primitive gut is said to be intraperitoneal. Conversely, abdominal structures outside the somatic mesoderm layer are said to be extraperitoneal.

However it is important to note that not all the structures that will originate from the primitive gut will finally be intraperitoneal. Some abdominal organs and some intestinal tracts that develop within the abdominal cavity will later adhere to the walls, effectively obliterating the mesentery and thus becoming secondarily retroperitoneal.

Besides the dorsal mesentery, there is another mesodermic structure which connects the primitive gut to the embryonary body wall: the ventral mesentery.

Unlike its dorsal counterpart, the ventral mesentery does not span the whole abdominal primitive gut, and is limited to the terminal foregut tract, from the distal esophagus to the proximal duodenum. It is a sagittal double-layered membrane (Sadler 2014) which originates from the caudal part of the septum transversum and runs along the midline of the anterior wall of the coelomic cavity to the vitelline duct.

5 Initial Liver Development from the Primitive Gut

The cranial part of the foregut has a thoracic localization and will give rise to the proximal gastrointestinal tract and the respiratory system. Distal foregut, midgut, and hindgut are located in the abdomen.

A useful mnemonic landmark to distinguish abdominal foregut, midgut, and hindgut structures is that they will be vascularized by three different aortic branches: the celiac, superior mesenteric, and inferior mesenteric arteries, respectively. It is important to note that the distinction is not made on the basis of the vasculature alone, as in fact these different tracts are characterized by different gene expression patterns.

From day 22 (Schoenwolf 2015) the endoderm of the distal ventral foregut, in what will be the duodenal tract, starts proliferating and thickens, forming the hepatic plate.

The endoderm shifts from cuboidal to a pseudostratified columnar architecture and the plate gets the shape of a diverticulum which develops in the context of the septum transversum: the hepatic diverticulum or liver bud (Bort et al. 2006; Wells and Melton 1999; Zaret 2001).

Complex interactions between the endodermic liver bud cells and mesodermal cells are necessary for the liver to develop.

Early studies on flies' embryogenesis first shed light over the mechanics of endoderm differentiation, owning it to the influence of the adjacent mesoderm (Immerglück et al. 1990; Panganiban et al. 1990). Transplantation and cell culture studies on animal models then further characterized the initial trigger for foregut differentiation (Douarin 1975; Gualdi et al. 1996).

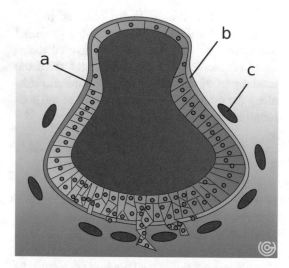

Fig. 4 Septum transversum invasion, as seen from an axial section of the primitive gut in correspondence to the liver bud. Endodermal cells (*a*) proliferate on the ventral side of the gut tube; the basal membrane (*b*) becomes discontinuous allowing for septum transversum invasion. On this side of the gut tube endothelial cells (*c*) are more numerous and interact with endodermal cells

Mesodermal cell of cardiac pertinence has proven to be responsible for the first signalling, namely through FGF mediation, which seems necessary and sufficient to initiate liver development (Jung et al. 1999).

Mesenchymal signalling (mainly through BMP) further guides endodermal cell differentiation, not only implying specific gene expression promotion, but also negative downregulation of alternative pathways that would otherwise lead endodermal differentiation towards organs other than the liver, namely towards pancreatic tissue (Bort et al. 2006; Rossi et al. 2001; Fair et al. 2003).

Liver bud cells are initially separated from the mesoderm by the existence of a laminin-rich basal membrane, which subsequently breaks apart to allow endodermal cells to migrate into the septum transversum mesenchyme (Fig. 4). Mesenchyme invasion seems to require strict interaction between endodermal cells and mesenchymal angioblasts and endothelial cells; in fact, in the regions where the endoderm starts to break into the mesenchyme, early vasculature cells are found in greater numbers (Matsumoto et al. 2001; Margagliotti et al. 2008).

Around day 32 the newly specified hepatic endoderm cells, now called hepatoblasts, grow organized as acini and chords into the mesenchyme of the septum transversum, intercalated by cells of mesodermal descent with a developing vascular differentiation.

In the meantime, the extrahepatic biliary system starts forming in close association to the liver parenchyma. As the liver bud grows, its connection with the foregut narrows, in a structure which will form and the hepatoduodenal ligament and the choledocus. From the middle caudal portion of the stalk connecting the liver bud to the foregut, a secondary ventral outgrowth forms, giving origin to the gallbladder and cystic duct.

6 Liver Parenchyma and Vasculature

To better understand the liver parenchyma layout and the role of this organ in fetal circulation, it is necessary to take a step back and focus on how circulation is developing in the embryo.

Around day 17 (Schoenwolf 2015) hemangioblast starts differentiating in the context of the extraembryonic mesoderm of the yolk sac, giving rise to simple vascular structures, called blood islands (also known as Pander's islands or Wolff's islands) (Sabin 1920). From hemangioblasts originate both hematopoietic progenitors and endothelial precursor cells.

As endothelial cells differentiate from endothelial precursors, vessels start forming de novo in a process known as vasculogenesis. A growing network of vessel invades embryonic tissues and forms the primordial vasculature. In this phase vessel organization is very dynamic, and through angiogenesis the existing vessels are continuously remodelled.

The liver portal system derives from two embryonic venous systems which develop at around week 3: the vitelline veins and the umbilical veins (Fig. 5).

The vitelline veins (also known as omphalomesenteric veins) drain blood from the yolk sac and its main two axes run symmetrically from the yolk stalk to the heart anterolaterally to the primitive gut. In the context of the septum transversum

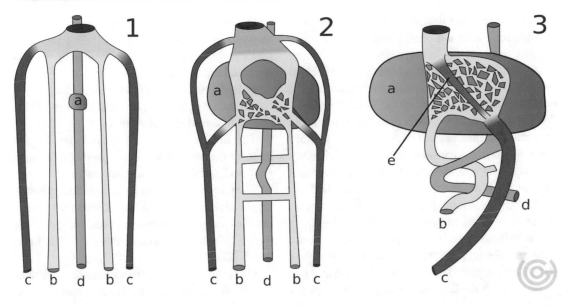

Fig. 5 Development of the portal system. The vitelline veins (**b**) and umbilical veins (**c**) are initially bilateral to the primitive gut (**d**) (*1* and *2*). The liver parenchyma (**a**) develops in close relation to the venous plexuses formed by the vitelline veins; umbilical veins make anastomoses with the vitelline veins, which in turn form a vascular ring around the duodenum (*2*). The proximal end of the umbilical veins obliterates, and the vitelline veins form a vascular ring around the duodenum (*2*). Vascular obliteration results in the sinuous course of the portal vein and the survival of the left umbilical vein (*3*). A shunt develops in the context of the liver vascular plexus, the ductus venosus (**e**)

the right and left vitelline veins develop two venous plexuses that make anastomoses around the midline.

The liver develops at this level, and as endodermal cells interact with angioblasts and endothelial cells, they differentiate into hepatoblasts which grow in chords engulfing the venous plexuses, which will become the hepatic sinusoid system.

More caudally, two more anastomoses are made between the left and right vitelline vessels. One posteriorly to the duodenum and one, the more distal, anteriorly, thus creating a vascular ring.

The cranial segment of the right vitelline vein develops into a big caliber vessel which constitutes the intrahepatic portion of the inferior vena cava. On the other hand the cranial portion of the left vitelline vein obliterates, and its blood is drained into systemic fetal circulation via anastomoses with the right vein in the context of the liver plexus.

In the subhepatic vitelline tract, parts of the vascular ring around the duodenum obliterate, and the result is a vein with a sinuous course,

which runs posteriorly to the proximal duodenum and then crosses anteriorly its distal tract. This vessel corresponds to the portal vein in the developed individual, which is the most conspicuous contributor to adult liver vascularization (Netter and Casasco 1983).

Along with the vitelline veins, the development of the hepatic venous system requires contribution from another vascular axis, the umbilical veins. These two symmetric vessels originate from the placenta and carry oxygenated blood to the embryo via the connecting stalk and then head towards the heart.

They run in the upper abdomen more laterally than the vitelline veins, and undergo extensive remodelling which make them lose the initial symmetric appearance.

Development of the liver is accompanied by obliteration of the left and right proximal portions of the umbilical veins, which initially runs laterally to it. Furthermore on the caudal side, the left umbilical vein prevails over the right one, which disappears.

With the obliteration of the cranial branches, umbilical blood flow towards the heart takes an alternative route in the context of the liver vitel-line plexus, with which the left umbilical vein creates anastomosis in correspondence of a vascular structure known as portal sinus (Mavrides et al. 2001). With the increase of venous input a preferential channel for blood flow is created, the ductus venosus, which effectively bypasses the small-caliber vessels of the plexus. The ductus venosus has a trumpetlike shape and directly connects the portal sinus to the inferior vena cava at its inlet into the heart (Kiserud 2005).

At mid gestation the ductus venosus shunts about 30% of the oxygenated blood coming from the umbilical vein, which is reduced to about 20% at week 30. The significant percentage (from 70% to 80%) of oxygenated blood that has to go through the liver parenchyma before reaching the fetal systemic circulation serves as testimony to the important role of this organ during development.

Interestingly, the entity of the shunting is not fixed but responsive to both passive and active regulatory systems that ensure increased flow towards the inferior vena cava (and thus towards the heart and brain) in case of tendency to hypoxia.

During fetal life, 75% of liver blood inflow comes from the umbilical vein, and 25% from the portal vein (Kiserud 2005).

Both the umbilical vein and ductus venosus are strictly pertinent to intrauterine life, as with the changes occurring to circulation after birth they both obliterate and become, respectively, the ligamentum teres hepatis and the ligamentum venosum.

Liver arterial vessels originate later than the venous system. From week 10 to week 20 arteries start forming from the hilum to the periphery of the organ (Gouysse et al. 2002), in a process which seems to be guided by parallel intrahepatic biliary duct development (Clotman et al. 2003).

The extent of arterial blood supply in the fetus is yet to be determined (Kiserud 2005).

7 Liver Hemopoiesis

Hemopoiesis in the embryo starts in the yolk sac, which continues producing primitive erythrocytes during the first 2 months of development.

During this period, hemopoiesis gradually shifts to other fetal organs, including the liver, which is the main contributor, the spleen, the thymus, and the bone marrow.

Hematopoietic precursors reach the liver in two distinct phases (Dieterlen-Lievre 1975; Dzierzak and Medvinsky 2008).

The first takes place at around day 23 and involves the migration of hematopoietic cell progenitors from the yolk sac mesoderm.

The second phase involves migration of hematopoietic stem cells from the embryonic splanchnic mesoderm of the aorta-gonad-mesonephros region, which starts around day 30 (Tavian and Péault 2005).

From the second month of gestation the liver will be the main fetal source of hematopoiesis, until this role is gradually carried over to the bone marrow, and the liver ceases this function around the seventh month (Sadler 2014).

8 Cell Lineages in the Liver

While hepatocytes represent the most conspicuous cell type in the liver (Si-Tayeb et al. 2010), other cell lineages contribute to the architecture of the organ.

Classical microscopic anatomy distinguishes at least other five distinct components: cholangiocytes, stellate cells, Kupffer cells, pit cells, and endothelial cells.

Cholangiocytes (also known as biliary epithelial cells, BECs) and hepatocytes are strictly related embryologically, as both originate from hepatoblasts.

The development of the intrahepatic bile ducts recognizes five different steps (Lemaigre 2003).

First, as liver vascular system develops, hepatoblasts adjacent to portal vessel start expressing biliary-specific cytokeratins. They then organize into a monolayer of cuboidal cells which surrounds the portal vessel, the so-called ductal plate. In the following step this layer becomes duplicated and subsequently focal dilations appear in its context. The last step involves remodelling of the ductal plate with regression of the nondilated parts, leaving a network of connected tubular structure, which corresponds to the biliary tree.

Hepatocytes on the other hand develop from hepatoblast not in direct contact with the portal vessels.

Stellate cells (also known as perisinuoidal cells or Ito cells) account for (5%–8% of liver cells, Yin et al. 2013) 1.4% of liver cells (Si-Tayeb et al. 2010) and reside in the perisinuoidal space of Disse. Their origin is still unclear, but some authors propose a derivation from the septum transversum (Loo and Wu 2008).

Kupffer cells are macrophage-type cells, located in the liver. Macrophage precursors (fetal macrophages) originate from the yolk sac and then colonize the liver, where they differentiate into adult Kupffer cells (Naito et al. 1997).

Pit cells are lymphoid cells with natural killer (NK) role, specific to the liver. In the adult liver, pit cells are thought to originate from blood NK cells that marginate inside the organ (Luo et al. 2000). In the embryo NK cells are seen in the liver as soon as the sixth week of gestation (Ivarsson et al. 2013).

Finally, as we have already seen, the endothelial cells are of mesodermal descent. Recent genetic studies suggest that at least a part of the liver's vascular system originates from endocardial cells and thus shares origin with coronary arteries (Zhang et al. 2016).

9 Ventral Mesentery and Liver Peritoneum

As the liver grows caudally and bulges in the abdominal cavity, the septum transversum surrounding it anteriorly and posteriorly thins and becomes membranous, giving origin to the ventral mesentery.

The liver separates the ventral mesentery in two parts, one anteriorly, the falciform ligament, between the liver and the anterior wall, and the other posteriorly, the lesser omentum, between the liver on one side and the stomach and duodenum on the other (Fig. 6).

The free end of the falciform ligament contains the umbilical vein during fetal life, which will become the round ligament of the liver (also known as ligamentum teres hepatis) once it is obliterated at birth.

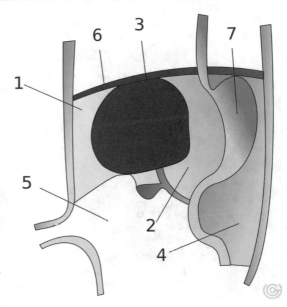

Fig. 6 Development of the liver, gallbladder, and extrahepatic bile duct in the context of the ventral mesentery. Falciform ligament (1), lesser omentum (2), bare area of the liver (3), dorsal mesentery (4), peritoneal cavity (5), diaphragm (6), stomach (7)

The caudal free end of the lesser omentum constitutes the hepatoduodenal ligament, which contains the hepatic triad made up by the hepatic artery, portal vein, and extrahepatic bile duct. The hepatoduodenal ligament will contribute to the delimitation of the Winslow foramen, which connects the omental bursa to the main peritoneal cavity.

The mesoderm of the ventral mesentery will differentiate into a double-layered peritoneal sheath.

The septum transversum mesoderm surrounding the liver will differentiate in both an inner connective tissue capsule (Glisson's capsule) and an external peritoneal single-layered sheath. The liver will thus become an intraperitoneal organ (Yamada 2011).

Not all liver surface will however face inside the peritoneal cavity as the mesoderm covering the liver cranially does not differentiate into peritoneum. The area where the liver contacts the original part of the septum transversum where the diaphragm develops will never be covered by peritoneum and is thus named the bare area of the liver.

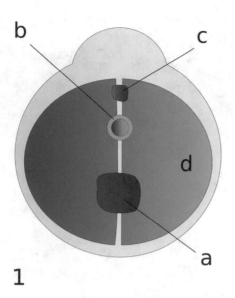

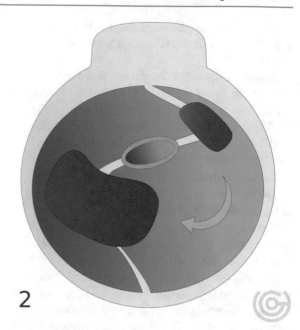

Fig. 7 Effect of gastric rotation in axial view. The liver (*a*) is located in the ventral mesentery anteriorly to the stomach (*b*). The spleen (*c*) develops in the dorsal mesen-tery. Following gastric rotation on the axial plane, the liver shifts from the midline to the right side of the peritoneal cavity (*d*)

The circumference of the bare area of the liver, where the peritoneum reflects against the diaphragm, is called the coronary ligament.

10 Liver Localization Following Intestinal Folding

Liver development takes place around the midline of the embryo, on the ventral side of the foregut, in the context of the septum transversum. Its relative position to the gastrointestinal canal and its final location in the abdomen face relevant changes during the process of gastric rotation.

After week four, the foregut corresponding to the future stomach undergoes important morphology modifications, mainly due to differential growth rate in its different portions.

First it undergoes a 90° axial rotation in the clockwise direction if seen from above, with its left wall rotating anteriorly (Fig. 7). Then as the lesser and bigger curvatures develop, it also undergoes a rotation on the coronal plane in the clockwise direction when seen from the front,

which brings the pylorus, its distal end, upwards and towards the right.

Gastric rotation shifts the ventral mesentery to the right and so consensually does the liver, which locates in the right upper abdominal quadrant (right hypochondrium).

Another result of the axial rotation is the change in orientation of the lesser omentum, the portion of the ventral mesentery which connects the gastric lesser curvature to the hepatic hilum, from the sagittal to the coronal plane.

The continuity between liver, lesser omentum, and stomach on the coronal plane contributes to the delimitation of a recess of the peritoneal cavity behind it, known as lesser sac or omental bursa.

References

Bort R, Signore M, Tremblay K et al (2006) Hex homeo-box gene controls the transition of the endoderm to a pseudostratified, cell emergent epithelium for liver bud development. Dev Biol 290:44 56

Clotman F, Libbrecht L, Gresh L et al (2003) Hepatic artery malformations associated with a primary defect in intrahepatic bile duct development. J Hepatol 39:686–692

Dieterlen-Lievre F (1975) On the origin of haemopoietic stem cells in the avian embryo: an experimental approach. J Embryol Exp Morpholog 33:607–619

Douarin NM (1975) An experimental analysis of liver development. La Medicina Biologica 53:427–455

Dzierzak E, Medvinsky A (2008) The discovery of a source of adult hematopoietic cells in the embryo. Development 135:2343–2346

Fair JH, Cairns BA, Lapaglia M et al (2003) Induction of hepatic differentiation in embryonic stem cells by co-culture with embryonic cardiac mesoderm. Surgery 134:189–196

Gouysse G, Couvelard A, Frachon S et al (2002) Relationship between vascular development and vascular differentiation during liver organogenesis in humans. J Hepatol 37:730–740

Gualdi R, Bossard P, Zheng M et al (1996) Hepatic specification of the gut endoderm in vitro: cell signaling and transcriptional control. Genes Dev 10: 1670–1682

Immerglück K, Lawrence PA, Bienz M (1990) Induction across germ layers in Drosophila mediated by a genetic cascade. Cell 62:261–268

Ivarsson MA, Loh L, Marquardt N et al (2013) Differentiation and functional regulation of human fetal NK cells. J Clin Invest 123:3889–3901

Jung J, Zheng M, Goldfarb M, Zaret KS (1999) Initiation of mammalian liver development from endoderm by fibroblast growth factors. Science 284:1998–2003

Kiserud T (2005) Physiology of the fetal circulation. Semin Fetal Neonatal Med 10:493–503

Lemaigre FP (2003) Development of the biliary tract. Mech Dev 120:81–87

Loo CKC, Wu X-J (2008) Origin of stellate cells from submesothelial cells in a developing human liver. Liver Int 28:1437 1445

Luo D-Z, Vermijlen D, Ahishali B et al (2000) On the cell biology of pit cells, the liver-specific NK cells. World J Gastroenterol 6:1–11

Margagliotti S, Clotman F, Pierreux CE et al (2008) Role of metalloproteinases at the onset of liver development. Develop Growth Differ 50:331–338

Matsumoto K, Yoshitomi H, Rossant J, Zaret KS (2001) Liver organogenesis promoted by endothelial cells prior to vascular function. Science 294:559–563

Mavrides E, Moscoso G, Carvalho JS et al (2001) The anatomy of the umbilical, portal and hepatic venous systems in the human fetus at 14–19 weeks of gestation: anatomy of the ductus venosus. Ultrasound Obstet Gynecol 18:598–604

Naito M, Hasegawa G, Takahashi K (1997) Development, differentiation, and maturation of Kupffer cells. Microsc Res Tech 39:350–364

Netter FH, Casasco E (1983) Embriologia umana ed anomalie congenite: da Atlante di anatomia, fisiopatologia e clinica di Frank H. Netter. Ciba-Geigy edizioni, Origgio

Panganiban GE, Reuter R, Scott MP, Hoffmann FM (1990) A Drosophila growth factor homolog, decapentaplegic, regulates homeotic gene expression within and across germ layers during midgut morphogenesis. Development 110:1041–1050

Rossi JM, Dunn NR, Hogan BL, Zaret KS (2001) Distinct mesodermal signals, including BMPs from the septum transversum mesenchyme, are required in combination for hepatogenesis from the endoderm. Genes Dev 15:1998–2009

Sabin FR (1920) Studies on the origin of blood-vessels and of red blood-corpuscles as seen in the living blastoderm of chicks during the second day of incubation. Carnegie Institution of Washington, Washington, D.C.

Sadler TW (2014) Langman's Medical Embryology, Thirteenth, North American edition. LWW, Philadelphia

Schoenwolf GC (2015) Larsen's human embryology. Churchill Livingstone, Philadelphia, PA

Si-Tayeb K, Lemaigre FP, Duncan SA (2010) Organogenesis and development of the liver. Dev Cell 18:175–189

Tavian M, Péault B (2005) Embryonic development of the human hematopoietic system. Int J Dev Biol 49:243–250

Wells JM, Melton DA (1999) Vertebrate endoderm development. Annu Rev Cell Dev Biol 15:393–410

Yamada DT (2011) Textbook of gastroenterology. Wiley, Hoboken

Yin C, Evason KJ, Asahina K, Stainier DYR (2013) Hepatic stellate cells in liver development, regeneration, and cancer. J Clin Invest 123:1902–1910

Zaret KS (2001) Hepatocyte differentiation: from the endoderm and beyond. Curr Opin Genet Dev 11:568–574

Zhang H, Pu W, Tian X et al (2016) Genetic lineage tracing identifies endocardial origin of liver vasculature. Nat Genet 48:537–543

Liver Anatomy

Lorenzo Ugo, Silvia Brocco, Arcangelo Merola,
Claudia Mescoli, and Emilio Quaia

Contents

L. Ugo · S. Brocco · A. Merola · E. Quaia (✉)
Radiology Unit, Department of Medicine - DIMED,
University of Padova, Padova, Italy
e-mail: emilio.quaia@unipd.it

C. Mescoli
Department of Medicine - DIMED, Pathology and
Cytopathology Unit, University of Padova,
Padova, Italy

Abstract

The liver is an intraperitoneal parenchymal organ located in the upper abdominal cavity, where it is suspended by a series of peritoneal reflections which connect it to adjacent structures and organs.

It has a complex vascular architecture, with one arterial system, fed by the hepatic artery, and two venous systems, the portal vein and the hepatic veins. In addition, the

© Springer Nature Switzerland AG 2021
E. Quaia (ed.), *Imaging of the Liver and Intra-hepatic Biliary Tract*,
Medical Radiology, Diagnostic Imaging, https://doi.org/10.1007/978-3-030-38983-3_2

liver harbours the intrahepatic biliary tract which exits the organ as the common hepatic duct.

According to portal vein anatomy, individual regions of liver parenchyma can be identified, the liver segments, which are characterised by independent portal and arterial blood supply, as well as independent biliary and lymphatic drainage.

Anatomic complexity is further complicated by the existence of common variants regarding vascular and biliary architecture. Less commonly, macroscopic liver morphology or location variants can also occur.

The liver architecture comprises the parenchyma, the connective tissue stroma, the sinusoids and the perisinusoidal spaces. These components have historically been described as anatomical units, the hepatic lobules, or as functional units, the portal lobules.

Liver anatomy may be assessed by ultrasound (US), computed tomography (CT) and magnetic resonance imaging (MRI).

1   Macroscopic Liver Anatomy

1.1   Liver Surface

The liver is the biggest abdominal organ, with a mean weight of 1.5–1.8 kg (Garby et al. 1993; de la Grandmaison et al. 2001; Molina and DiMaio 2012).

It is situated in the upper abdomen, immediately caudally to the diaphragm.

The liver parenchyma is surrounded by an adherent connective tissue layer named Glisson's capsule. It is a dense fibrous sheath with interspersed elastic fibres, in the context of which run nervous fibres and blood and lymphatic vessels (Anastasi 2007).

The liver shape has been described as a partial volume of an ovoid or a wedge, cut by an oblique plane directed cranio-caudally, postero-anteriorly and from left to right.

Its biggest dimension is the transverse diameter, ranging from 20 to 23 cm. Craniocaudally at the midpoint of the right lobe it measures 13–16 cm (Kennedy and Madding 1977). It is important to note however that liver dimensions have high interindividual variability, due to both anatomic variations and pathology.

The most recognisable liver margin is the inferior one, which spans in the upper abdomen from left to right.

We can recognise four faces of the liver: superior, inferior, right and posterior. The first three are continuous one to another, while the inferior face is separated from the superior by the acute inferior margin of the liver.

Traditionally anatomists have described the liver based on its macroscopic surface appearance, and thus established a lobar subdivision according to evident fissures and ligaments. From this morphological standpoint we can distinguish two main lobes, the right and the left one, and two accessory lobes, the caudate and the quadrate lobes (Bismuth 1982).

The anterior face include the falciform ligament which runs on a vertical plane slightly to the right from the abdominal midline (Fig. 1).

The right lobe is typically bigger than the left lobe and occupies the right hypochondrium, while the left lobe usually spans in the anterior portion of the anterior epigastrium and protrudes into the left hypochondrium.

The inferior aspect of the liver is divided into four sectors by several dividing structures which collectively assume the shape of a "H".

The left vertical arm of the H is composed of the round ligament anteriorly and the ligamentum venosum posteriorly. The round ligament terminates at the hepatic hilum, where it reaches the left portal vein (LPV). The ligamentum venosum spans from the LPV to inferior vena cava (IVC).

The horizontal portion of the H corresponds to the liver hilum, which is defined by a transverse fissure known as porta hepatis.

Finally, the vertical right arm of the H is composed of the inferior vena cava posteriorly and the gallbladder fossa (also known as liver bed) (Honda et al. 2008) anteriorly.

Fig. 1 Liver seen from the superior (*1*), posterior (*2*) and anterior (*3*) aspects. The coronary ligament encircles the liver bare area (*a*). On the anterior aspect the falciform ligament may be identified. On the posterior aspect the hepatic artery (*b*), portal vein (*c*) and common bile duct (*d*) can be seen at the liver hilum

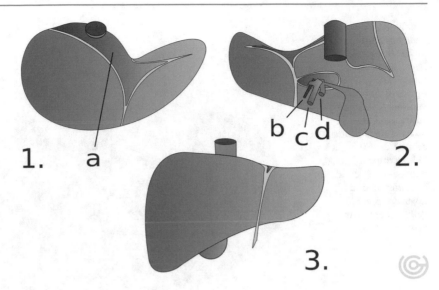

In the region comprised between the two vertical arms of the H, the two accessory lobes are recognisable, the caudate lobe posteriorly and the quadrate lobe anteriorly.

It is important to note that the bed of the gallbladder and IVC are not in close proximity, and thus the right vertical arm of the H is not continuous, with no apparent obvious separation between the right and caudate lobes on the ventral surface; this caudate lobe continuation towards the right is known as caudate process. The medial aspect of the inferior caudate lobe is known as medial papillary process or simply papillary process; it bulges towards the stomach on the left and its appearance may sometimes mimic a porta hepatis lymph node or a pancreatic body lesion (Auh et al. 1984; Donoso et al. 1989).

1.2 Liver Relations with Adjacent Organs

Superiorly the liver is in relation to the inferior face of the diaphragm. Above the diaphragm are the right pleural space, middle and inferior right lung lobes, pericardial space and heart, namely the right ventricle and atrium.

The anterior face of the liver is in relation with the anterior portion of the diaphragm and the anterior abdominal wall.

On the inferior liver face we can identify some impressions on the surface, in the area where it contacts the adjacent abdominal organs (Fig. 2).

On the right lobe there is a posterior triangular impression for the right adrenal gland, a more prominent impression corresponding to the right kidney and a shallower anterior one, pertaining to the hepatic colic flexure.

The duodenum leaves an impression around the mid portion of the lower face, with the pyloric impression in the cranial portion of the quadrate lobe.

The stomach impression occupies the larger part of the inferior portion of the left lobe, with a distinct oesophageal groove in proximity to the fossa for the ductus venosus. The left lobe portion cranial to lesser curvature of the stomach, as it does not receive impression by adjacent organs, slightly bulges backwards and is known as tuber omentale.

On most of its surface, the liver has an intraperitoneal localisation, which means that it is covered by the visceral peritoneum. The exceptions are constituted by the gallbladder fossa, where the liver is in contact with the gallbladder; the liver hilum, where the hepatic triad enters the liver parenchyma; and the liver bare area, where the liver is separated by the diaphragm by loose connective tissue interposition only. Besides the diaphragm, two other important structures make

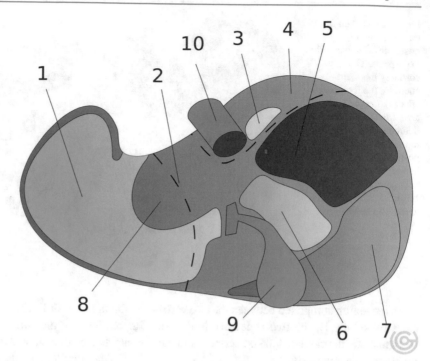

Fig. 2 Impressions of adjacent organs on the posterior aspect of the liver. Stomach impression (*1*), round ligament and ductus venosus (*2*), right adrenal gland impression (*3*), bare area of the liver (*4*), right kidney impression (*5*), duodenal impression (*6*), colic impression (*7*), tuber omentale (*8*), gallbladder (*9*), inferior vena cava (*10*)

contact with the liver in the bare area: the retro-hepatic inferior vena cava (Lowe and D'Angelica 2016) and the right adrenal gland.

The peritoneal space between the liver and the right kidney is known as the hepatorenal recess or Morison's pouch. Being a potential space, under normal circumstances this recess is empty and the right kidney is in close proximity to the liver surface. In the event of intra-abdominal fluid collection (e.g., blood, ascites), the Morison's pouch might expand, and separation between the liver and the right kidney thus becomes apparent. This region is actively assessed in abdominal imaging; as an example scanning of the hepatorenal space constitutes part of the FAST (focused assessment with sonography in trauma), an ultrasound protocol aimed at identification of fluid collection in trauma patients (Scalea et al. 1999).

1.3 Liver Ligaments

The hepatic ligaments are the falciform ligament, the round ligament, the two triangular ligaments, the hepatorenal ligament, the coronary ligament,

the lesser omentum and the ligamentum venosum.

The falciform ligament is located on the anterior surface of the liver. It consists of a double-layered peritoneal sheath with a rounded triangular shape, resembling that of a sickle (hence the name, from "falx, falcis", Latin for sickle). Its anterior side is convex, and inserts onto the anterior abdominal wall cranially from the umbilicus, following the anterior underside of the diaphragm towards IVC.

The inferior side of the falciform ligament is represented by its caudal free edge, where peritoneal reflection occurs. At the free edge corresponds a fibrous string, the round ligament of the liver (also known as teres hepatis ligament), spanning from the umbilicus to the underside of the liver, where an umbilical fissure is identifiable. It corresponds to the obliterated umbilical vein, which in the foetus carries oxygenated blood from the umbilical cord towards the LPV.

The posterior side of the falciform ligament constitutes its hepatic insertion, corresponding to the interlobar fissure.

On the liver surface near IVC, the two peritoneal leaflets of the falciform ligament diverge laterally and posteriorly towards the left and right lobe, respectively; they then abruptly converge towards IVC, identifying with their lateral course two triangularly shaped peritoneal reflections, the left and right triangular ligaments.

Posteriorly to the right triangular ligament, the peritoneal reflection runs towards the anterior surface of the right kidney and the adrenal gland, constituting the hepatorenal ligament.

The whole reflection of the peritoneum around the supero-posterior aspect of the liver effectively encircles the bare area, and is collectively known as the liver coronary ligament.

The lesser omentum is a double-layered peritoneal sheath which spans on the coronal plane from the lesser curvature of the stomach and the proximal duodenum to the liver hilum. It can thus be divided into two parts, the hepatogastric ligament (pars flaccida) and the hepatoduodenal ligament (pars tensa). In the context of the hepatoduodenal ligament runs the hepatic pedicle, made of the hepatic artery, portal vein, common bile duct, nerves and lymphatics.

The ligamentum venosum corresponds to the fibrotic remainder of an obliterated foetal vein, the ductus venosus or Arantius' duct. It spans on the posterior face of the liver from the left portal vein to the inferior vena cava, dividing the left lobe from the caudate lobe. The hepatogastric ligament follows the course of the ligamentum venosum, before its two layers separate to embrace the distal oesophagus (Lowe and D'Angelica 2016).

The liver, the stomach and the connecting lesser omentum form a continuous wall spanning on the coronal plane, which delimits anteriorly a recess of the peritoneal cavity known as lesser sac or omental bursa. The caudal free edge of the lesser omentum, which corresponds to the hepatoduodenal ligament, delimits the passage of communication between the main peritoneal cavity and the omental bursa, known as omental foramen (also known as omental foramen or foramen of Winslow).

1.4 Liver Vascular Systems and Bile Ducts

In the liver we can distinguish three different vascular systems: the arterial system, which supplies arterial blood; the portal venous system, which supplies venous blood to the liver from the guts, the pancreas and the spleen; and the hepatic venous system, which drains venous blood from the liver to the systemic circulation via the inferior vena cava.

Unlike other organs, besides blood circulation the liver also harbours a complex ductal system responsible for bile excretion, the bile ducts.

It is important to consider the arterial, biliary and portal systems together as they are topologically strictly related throughout the liver. They in fact constitute the so-called portal triad, and as such branch together within the parenchyma. The portal triad runs within liver enveloped by a layer of connective tissue which separates it from the surrounding parenchyma, the hepatobiliary sheath. The Glisson's capsule is in continuity with the hepatobiliary sheath at the liver hilum, where the portal triad, here composed by the common hepatic duct, the hepatic artery and portal vein, enters the parenchyma (Yamamoto and Ariizumi 2018). At the hilum the common hepatic duct (CHD) is the rightmost and most anterior of the three structures. The hepatic artery (HA) runs on the left side, while the portal vein runs posteriorly.

From the hilum the portal triad also spans outside of the liver, along the course of the hepatoduodenal ligament.

1.4.1 Hepatic Artery

Around 25% of hepatic blood inflow is arterial (Sureka et al. 2015), and mostly comes from the common hepatic artery (CHA), which is the rightmost of the three terminal branches of the celiac trunk, which in turn is the first major branch of the abdominal aorta. The CHA gives origin to both the right gastric and the gastroduodenal arteries and becomes the hepatic artery proper. It reaches the hepatoduodenal ligament, and heads towards the liver hilum running anteriorly to the portal vein (Draghi et al. 2007).

At the liver hilum, before entering the parenchyma (Aoki et al. 2016), the hepatic artery bifurcates into the right and left hepatic branches.

The right hepatic artery (RHA) is larger than the left, gives off a cystic branch for the gallbladder (Draghi et al. 2007) and bifurcates into anterior and posterior branches just before entering the parenchyma (Aoki et al. 2016). The left branch divides into three vessels for the anterior, posterior and caudate parts of the left lobe.

Hepatic arteries then give off segmental and subsegmental arteries that run and branch in the portal spaces, until they finally merge with liver sinusoids as perilobular arterioles (Draghi et al. 2007).

1.4.2 Bile Ducts

The bile duct system directs bile flow in a hepatofugal direction (that is to say directed away from the liver), from the hepatocytes which produce the bile to the gastrointestinal tract, namely the duodenum. Bile collected by the bile canaliculi converges towards the portal triad, where bile ducts are seen. Smaller bile ducts converge with one another in a rootlike system. We can recognise two main liver ducts, the left hepatic duct (LHD) and the right hepatic duct (RHD). The left collects bile from the individual segments of the left liver (see relevant paragraph), while the right recognises two tributaries, the right posterior hepatic duct (RPHD) and the right anterior hepatic duct (RAHD) (Gazelle et al. 1994).

RHD and LHD converge to form the common hepatic duct (CHD) which exits the liver at the hilum. The common hepatic duct receives the cystic duct, thus becoming the common bile duct (choledochus), which runs along the hepatoduodenal ligament, passes behind the proximal duodenum, crosses the head of the pancreas and reaches the second portion of the duodenum at the major duodenal papilla (ampulla of Vater).

1.4.3 Portal Vein System

As the name implies, the venous portal system revolves around the portal vein (PV) (Fig. 3), which is responsible for around 75% (Sureka et al. 2015) of the liver blood supply.

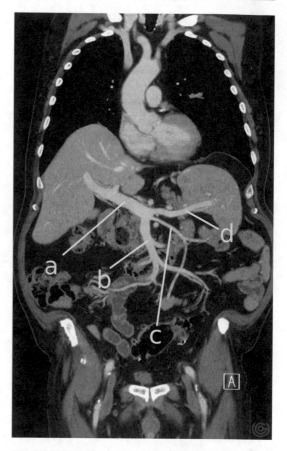

Fig. 3 Portal vein anatomy as seen on elaborated coronal contrast-enhanced CT. Portal vein (*a*), superior mesenteric vein (*b*), inferior mesenteric vein (*c*), splenic vein (*d*). Notice the variant confluence of the inferior mesenteric vein, which normally drains into the splenic vein

It originates at the portal oliva, the confluence between the superior mesenteric vein and the spleno-mesenteric trunk (union of splenic and inferior mesenteric veins), in the retroperitoneum behind the neck of the pancreas around the level of L2 (Gilfillan and Hills 1950). As it travels towards the hepatic hilum passing behind the proximal duodenum, the PV receives smaller venous vessels, namely the left and right gastric veins directly or via the splenic vein (Gilfillan and Hills 1950; Seong et al. 2012), cystic veins and irregular pancreaticoduodenal veins. It is particularly important to remember the connection between the left gastric vein and portal vein, as it can become an important portosystemic shunt in case of portal hypertension, thus feeding the oesophageal varices (Abdel-Misih and Bloomston 2010; Gilfillan and Hills 1950).

The PV is valveless (Abdel-Misih and Bloomston 2010), has a length of around 70 mm (Gilfillan and Hills 1950) and has a maximum diameter just distal to the portal oliva around 10, with 13 mm being commonly considered as the upper limit (Stamm et al. 2016; Weinreb et al. 1982).

It runs in the context of the hepatoduodenal ligament along with the common bile duct and the hepatic artery, both of which are anterior to it.

The PV reaches the hepatic hilum (corresponding to the transverse fissure known as porta hepatis), and then divides into a right portal vein (RPV) and a left portal vein (LPV) for the respective lobes.

In the majority of cases (around 50%), the PV bifurcation occurs outside the Glisson's capsule, that is to say it is extrahepatic. Alternatively it can be intrahepatic (25% of cases) or at the liver capsule (25% of cases) (Madoff et al. 2002).

The LPV has an initial transverse (horizontal) portion and a subsequent umbilical portion (Rex segment (Puppala et al. 2009)) which abruptly bends towards the umbilical fissure, thus entering the parenchyma (Abdel-Misih and Bloomston 2010). The RPV is larger than the LPV (Sureka et al. 2015) and has a shorter extrahepatic course (Abdel-Misih and Bloomston 2010).

From the right portal vein originates the right anterior portal vein (RAPV) for segments S5 and S8, and the right posterior portal vein (RPPV) for segments S6 and S7. The LPV gives off segmental branches for segments S2 and S3, and terminate bifurcating into two branches for S4.

Segment S1 receives portal branches from both the LPV and RPV (Schmidt et al. 2008).

1.4.4   Hepatic Veins

Venous blood of the liver is mainly collected by the hepatic veins, which drain into the IVC in its retrohepatic tract just below the diaphragm; like the PV, hepatic veins are valveless (Porth 2011). We can usually identify three main venous branches: the left, the right and the middle one. Typically the left and middle veins form a short

common tract before reaching the IVC. As opposed to the portal triad, hepatic veins are not encompassed by a surrounding connective tissue sheath, as their tunica adventitia is in direct contact with the liver parenchyma (Clarkson 2013). Segment S1 drains both in the hepatic vein system and directly in the IVC (via the so-called Spieghel veins).

1.4.5   Minor Arterial and Venous Supply of the Liver

It is useful to remember that the liver also receives blood from the systemic circulation by arteries other than the hepatic artery (Prokop et al. 2006) and by venous systems other than the portal vein (Anastasi 2007).

Minor arterial blood supply to the liver (also called extrahepatic collateral blood supply) mainly comes from the right inferior phrenic artery. Other contributors can be the cystic artery, omental arteries, right renal capsular artery, left inferior phrenic artery and right internal mammary artery (Miyayama et al. 2006).

While their interest might be limited in the healthy patient, they can become very relevant in case of certain clinical settings, for example in the embolisation of hepatocellular carcinoma (HCC), where eventual extrahepatic collateral blood supply has to be taken into account (Gwon et al. 2007).

Minor venous systems consist of the parabiliary venous system, cholecystic veins and epigastric-paraumbilical venous system. The parabiliary venous system exists in the context of the hepatoduodenal ligament, and collects blood from the head of the pancreas, the bile duct system and the distal stomach; it usually drains inside the vena porta, but can sometimes enter the liver at the porta hepatis. The cholecystic veins collect blood from the pericholecystic liver parenchyma and might drain into the parabiliary venous system around the porta hepatis or directly into intrahepatic portal veins via the liver bed. The epigastric-paraumbilical system is composed of the superior and inferior veins of Sappey and the vein of Burow that drain venous blood into the liver from body regions in the near vicinity to the falciform ligament.

The importance of these minor venous systems from a radiological standpoint lies in the fact that due to the nonportal nature of their blood supply to the liver, they might be responsible for focal metabolic alteration and subsequent pseudolesion appearance at imaging, which typically occurs near the liver bed (cholecystic veins), on the dorsal aspect of S4 (parabiliary venous system) and near the falciform ligament (epigastric-paraumbilical system).

In addition to that, Sappey's and Burow's veins can also become a path of portosystemic shunt (from the portal venous system to the systemic venous system) in case of portal hypertension (Yoshimitsu et al. 2001).

1.5 Hepatic Lymphatic Drainage

The lymphatic system is fundamental for both interstitial fluid homoeostasis and for immune response surveillance. In fact liver contribution to the lymph production is quite significant, as it can be considered among the most important organs from the quantitative perspective (Tanaka and Iwakiri 2016).

Lymphatic capillaries and vessels exist in the context of the liver parenchyma and are organised into two main drainage axes.

The first one develops along the portal spaces, and drains to the hepatic hilum and greater omentum nodes. The Winslow lymph node, a node in correspondence of the Winslow foramen which is typically bigger and dominant in the area, is part of this system. From these nodes, lymph is drained towards the celiac lymph nodes which in turn drain into the confluence between the main abdominal lymphatic vessels. The confluence might take the shape of a dilated collecting sac, named cisterna chyli, situated in the retroperitoneal space, spanning for around 5–7 cm in a right paramedian position anteriorly to the bodies of the first two lumbar vertebrae and to the right with respect to the abdominal aorta (Standring et al. 2009). From the confluence originates the thoracic duct, which will drain the lymph and chyle in the systemic venous system (namely at the junction between the left subclavian and internal jugular veins).

The second lymphatic drainage axis accompanies the venous drainage of the liver along the hepatic veins. The lymphatic vessels converge towards the inferior vena cava and together with it cross the diaphragm draining into mediastinal lymph node stations.

Lymphatic vessels that accompany portal veins and hepatic veins represent liver's deep lymphatic system.

Lymphatic fluid also flows underneath the Glisson's capsule, constituting the superficial lymphatic system. Depending on its location, this lymph can drain in both aforementioned draining axes. In particular, fluid from the convex liver surface tends to converge cranially along the coronary ligament and to drain into mediastinal lymph nodes. Fluid from the posterior concave surface usually drains towards the liver hilum (Tanaka and Iwakiri 2016).

1.6 Liver Innervation

The hepatic nervous system is composed of a central autonomic component for the liver parenchyma and a peripheral somatosensory component for liver capsule sensitivity.

Liver autonomic system comprises an anterior and a posterior plexus, widely interconnected and branching inside the liver parenchyma, the former following the hepatic artery and the latter following the portal vein and the bile duct. Sympathetic nerves come from the celiac and superior mesenteric ganglia, while parasympathetic fibres originate from the anterior and posterior vagal trunks (Lautt 2009; Standring et al. 2009). The role of these nerves is extremely complex, as they serve as sensory apparatus for a multitude of homeostasis parameters, namely temperature, blood pressure, osmolarity, and ionic and nutrient content of portal blood, as well as regulating liver circulation, bile excretion and hepatocyte metabolism (Jensen et al. 2013).

Glisson's capsule is innervated by fine fibres from the lower intercostal nerves, which provide somatic pain sensitivity, which is prominent on the superior surface and at the bare area of the liver (Standring et al. 2009). Capsule rupture or distension is thus responsible for sharp, well-localised pain.

1.7 Liver Segmentation

While anatomically we distinguish the left and right liver lobes in relation to the falciform ligament course, that does not hold true from a functional and surgical standpoint.

To avoid confusion, we will use the terms right and left liver instead of right and left lobe when referring to functional anatomy (Bismuth 1982).

The left and right liver are separated by Cantlie's line (Fig. 4), a line in the anatomical right lobe spanning from the inferior vena cava (left margin) to the middle of the gallbladder fossa, which is approximately aligned to the course of the middle hepatic vein and is almost vertical (Bismuth 1982).

The Cantlie's line separates the parenchyma in a 60:40 ratio, the bigger portion pertaining to the right liver. Functional hemilivers are more symmetrical than the anatomical counterpart, as the left liver is bigger than the left lobe.

Based on the biliary tree anatomy, each hemiliver can be further divided into two, thus identifying the four corresponding liver sectors: the right posterior, right anterior, left medial and left lat-

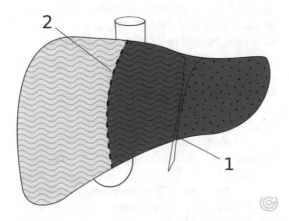

Fig. 4 Liver lobes. (*1*) indicates the falciform ligament. The left liver lobe (violet) is separated by the Cantlie's line (*2*) from the right lobe (yellow)

eral sectors. The right hepatic vein runs between the right posterior and right anterior sector, while the falciform ligament corresponds to the division between the left medial and left lateral sectors. This anatomic division is more popular in the USA, and was first described by Healey and Schroy (Healey and Schroy 1953). Note however that some authors consider a different left liver division, following portal vein second-order division, where the medial and the lateral sectors are divided by the left hepatic vein as opposed to the falciform ligament (Bismuth 1982; Couinaud 1957; Kimura et al. 2015); hereinafter we will adopt this convention.

A further, third-degree subdivision can also be made, following the portal vein third-order ramification, thus identifying the hepatic segments.

The most widely accepted model for liver segmental anatomy was first described by Couinaud (Couinaud 1957), and then popularised by Bismuth (Bismuth 1982; Bismuth et al. 1982; Majno et al. 2014), and is now the most commonly used in Europe. According to these authors, the liver is composed of eight anatomical segments, characterised by independent portal and arterial blood supply, as well as independent biliary and lymphatic drainage. The portal triad runs in the middle of the segments, while hepatic veins run at the periphery.

Each liver sector is divided into two segments, with the exception of the left lateral sector which corresponds to only one segment, segment number two (conventionally noted as S2). Starting from S2, segment numeration proceeds in clockwise order (with the exception of the cranial portion of S4). The left medial sector is divided by the course of the left hepatic vein into S3 on the left and S4 on the right (Bismuth 1982).

The right liver recognises two cranial and two caudal sectors, identified by a horizontal plane corresponding to the portal vein bifurcation. Thus the right anterior sector corresponds to cranial segment S8 and caudal S5, and the right posterior to cranial S7 and caudal S6.

The biggest liver segments are segments S8 and S4 (Murakami and Hata 2002).

S1 has a more peculiar localisation and spans in the posterior aspect of the liver, comprised between the portal vein bifurcation anteriorly and the IVC posteriorly (Majno et al. 2014). It has a different blood supply and venous drainage compared to the other segments as it receives arterial and portal branches from both the right and left divisions of the portal system. Its blood does not only drain in the main hepatic veins but it also has its own hepatic veins which drain directly in the IVC. An interesting and exemplificative consequence of this is that in case of Budd-Chiari syndrome, where venous hepatic outflow is obstructed, in the chronic phase the caudate lobe experiences hypertrophy as it is the only segment with functioning venous drainage (Bismuth 1982).

Finally, a common variation of the aforementioned segmental division involves further bipartition of segment 4 following the horizontal plane of the portal bifurcation in cranial 4a segment and caudal 4b; caution must be taken using this convention in Japan, as there the nomenclature is reversed as S4a and S4b, respectively, correspond to the caudal and cranial portions of S4 (Onishi et al. 2000).

As you may have noted, liver segmentation is not as simple as one might expect, and different authors in the literature have proposed different takes on the subject, sometimes with major differences, and other times with just a subtly different approach. To make things worse, it is sometimes possible to encounter misquotes in the literature which may add to confusion.

Despite all these difficulties, in modern days the most adopted radiological approach to liver segmentation is quite straightforward. It is similar to that suggested by Bismuth, with a slight difference over left liver approach (Fig. 5) (Germain et al. 2014).

S1 is identified at the posterior aspect of the liver; it is delimited on the right by the Cantlie's line, in front by the portal vein bifurcation and on the left by the fissure of the ligamentum venosum.

The remaining liver is divided into eight segments according to three vertical lines and one horizontal line. The vertical lines correspond to the plane of the right hepatic vein, the middle hepatic vein and the left hepatic vein. The horizontal line corresponds to the plane of the portal veins. Four upper segments and four lower seg-

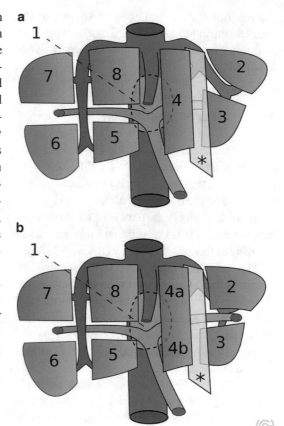

Fig. 5 Liver segmentation according to Bismuth (**a**) and simplified (**b**). Notice the difference in left liver segmental division. The falciform ligament is denoted by the asterisk

ments are thus identified. Going from left to right, the upper segments correspond to S2, S4a, S8 and S7. Again from left to right, the lower segments correspond to S3, S4b, S5 and S6.

1.8 Liver Variants

1.8.1 Intrahepatic Portal Vein Variants

Normal portal vein anatomy implies bifurcation into the left (LPV) and right (RPV) portal veins at the porta hepatis. The right hepatic vein then further bifurcates into the anterior (right anterior portal vein, RAPV) and posterior (RPPV) branches, respectively, for segments S5, S8 and S6, S7. This configuration is encountered in 65–80% of patients (Schmidt et al. 2008).

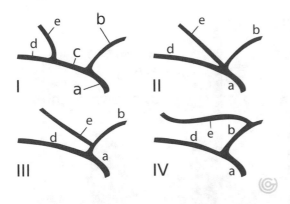

Fig. 6 Portal vein variants according to Cheng. Type I corresponds to normal layout. Portal vein (*a*), left portal vein (*b*), right portal vein (*c*), right posterior portal vein (*d*), right anterior portal vein (*e*)

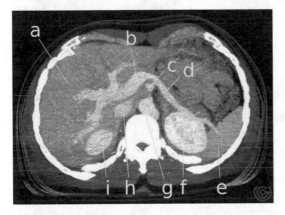

Fig. 7 Maximum intensity projection (MIP) of a contrast-enhanced CT scan at the level of the spleno-portal vein axis, showing variant intrahepatic portal vein trifurcation. Liver (*a*), portal vein (*b*), celiac artery (*c*), splenic vein (*d*), spleen (*e*), right (*i*) and left (*f*) kidney, aorta (*g*), inferior vena cava (*h*)

A well-known classification of portal system variants based on extensive data has been proposed by Cheng (Fig. 6) (Cheng et al. 1996).

Normal anatomy corresponds to Cheng's type I.

The most common variant is the trifurcate variant (type II), in which the portal vein directly gives origin to the left portal vein, RAPV and RPPV (Fig. 6 and Fig. 7). The right portal vein is not present. The second most common variant (type III or "Z anomaly" (Iqbal et al. 2017)) implies direct origin of the RPPV from the main portal vein, which then bifurcates into the LPV and the RAPV. The main portal vein divides into the RPPV and LPV, and the RAPV arises from

the LPV (Fig. 6). Type IV is similar to type III, but the RAPV originates from the distal portion of the LPV (Lee et al. 2013) (Fig. 6). Other variants are possible but very uncommon, collectively accounting for around 2% of cases, including absence of portal vein branching, portal vein duplication (Schmidt et al. 2008), and LPV arising from RAPV. Awareness of portal vein branching pattern is important in planning liver surgery (to ensure that portal perfusion to the future liver remnant is not compromised), liver transplantation (to enable appropriate graft selection), and percutaneous interventional procedures (Carneiro et al. 2019).

Interesting variations are the quadrifurcation and absence of portal vein bifurcation (Schmidt et al. 2008).

The first entails portal vein division into a left portal vein and three right portal branches, respectively, for S6 and S7 and a single branch for S5 and S8 (Madoff et al. 2002).

In the second the horizontal portion (proximal part) of the left hepatic vein is absent, and blood reaches the vertical portion via a transverse vessel departing from S8 and spanning the liver horizontally.

Finally it is interesting to note that patients with variant portal vein configuration tend to have higher percentage of liver biliary system variance (Schmidt et al. 2008).

1.8.2 Hepatic Artery Variants

Normal arterial anatomy is encountered in around 55% of the population, making variants extremely common.

The well-established Michel classification (Fig. 8) differentiates ten layouts (Catalano et al. 2008).

The standard layout (type I) entails right (RHA) and left (LHA) hepatic arteries originating from the common hepatic artery (CHA), branch of the celiac trunk.

The two most common variants with a prevalence of around 10% are type II, where the LHA arises from the left gastric artery, and type III, with origin of the RHA from the superior mesenteric artery.

Type IV represents association of type II and type III, but is more rare.

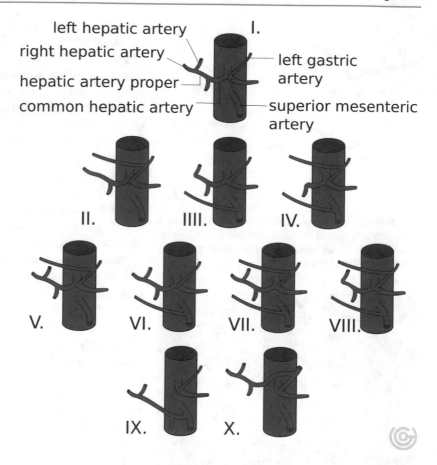

Fig. 8 Michel's classification of hepatic artery variants. Normal (*I*), replaced LHA (*II*), RHA (*III*) or both (*IV*), accessory LHA (*V*), RHA (*VI*) or both (*VII*), accessory LHA and replaced RHA (or vice versa) (*VIII*), replaced CHA originating from superior mesenteric artery (*IX*) or left gastric artery (*X*). See text for description

Other two quite common variants with prevalence higher than 5% are type V, with an accessory LHA from the left gastric artery, and type VI, with an accessory RHA originating from the superior mesenteric artery. Once again, type VII represents presence of both type V and VI variants and is more rare. Variant VIII corresponds to accessory LHA originating from left gastric artery and RHA originating from superior mesenteric artery.

Type IX and type X correspond to a replaced CHA originating, respectively, from the superior mesenteric artery and the left gastric artery.

Finally, in some cases the Michel classification falls short as unclassified variants do exist, namely the origin of the CHA from the abdominal aorta, or the presence of a double-hepatic artery (Covey et al. 2002).

1.8.3 Hepatic Vein Variants

Normal hepatic vein anatomy implies the presence of three main branches, the left, middle and right hepatic veins. The left hepatic vein drains segments S2 and S3. The middle hepatic vein drains segment S4, while S5, S6, S7 and S8 are drained by the right hepatic vein, which is the largest (Germain et al. 2014). In around 60% of the population, the left and middle hepatic veins form a common trunk before reaching the IVC (Catalano et al. 2008).

S1 drains both in the hepatic vein system and directly into the IVC (Murakami and Hata 2002).

Variants are more common in women (Germain et al. 2014).

The most common variant is the presence of an accessory right inferior hepatic vein draining the right posterior liver directly to the vena cava. Less frequently two accessory right hepatic veins can be seen.

Another quite common variant implies direct drainage of the left and middle hepatic veins, without the formation of a common trunk.

Other variants are the absence of the right hepatic vein and the bifurcation of the left or right hepatic veins.

1.8.4 Intrahepatic Bile Duct Variants

The most common intrahepatic bile duct configuration is as follows: the left hepatic duct (LHD) drains the left liver segments and converges with the right hepatic duct (RHD) to form the common hepatic duct (CHD). The RHD is very short and recognises two tributaries, the right posterior hepatic duct (RPHD), which drains segments S7 and S8 and has a more horizontal course, and the right anterior hepatic duct (RAHD), which drains S5 and S8 and is more vertical. The RPHD joins the RAHD posteriorly from the left side (Gazelle et al. 1994).

Bile ducts from S1 can drain to the RHD or the LHD (Healey and Schroy 1953).

Normal intrahepatic bile duct configuration has a prevalence of around 60%, and thus anatomic variants are quite common (Catalano et al. 2008).

Several classification systems have been proposed, namely by Couinaud (1957), Huang et al. (1996), Karakas et al. (2008), Choi (2003), Champetier (1994) and Ohkubo (2004) (Deka et al. 2014).

According to Huang classification (Huang et al. 1996), RHD variants are identified by the A letter and include five types (Fig. 9); higher class number corresponds to rarer variant. A1 refers to the standard configuration. A2 is the most common variant, implying triple confluence between the RPHD, RAHD and LHD. In A3 the RPHD or RAHD joins the LHD, while in A4 and A5, the RPHD joins, respectively, the CHD and the cystic duct.

LHD variants are divided into six classes characterised by the letter B. B1 is standard configuration, with the duct from S2 and S3 forming a common duct which joins the segment from S4. In B2, B3 and B4, the duct from S4 drains, respectively, into the RHD, RAHD and CHD. In B5 S2 and S3 have independent drainage and S2 also collects S4 (Chaib et al. 2014). Finally in B6 S1 drains in the CHD. Again bigger

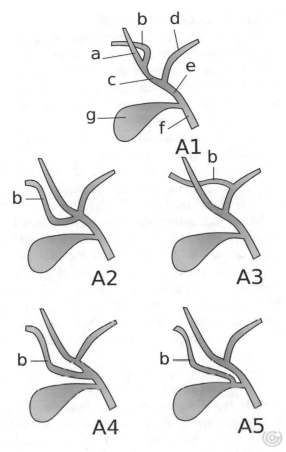

Fig. 9 Right hepatic duct variants according to Huang. Right anterior duct (*a*), right posterior duct (*b*), right hepatic duct (*c*), left hepatic duct (*d*), common hepatic duct (*e*), common bile duct (*f*), gallbladder (*g*). A1 corresponds to normal anatomy

number corresponds to rarer variants, with the exception of B5 and B6.

As from a surgical standpoint if the confluence between RPHD and RAHD is close to the confluence between LHD and RHD it is treated as a triple confluence (A2 variant), Karakas proposed a variation on the Huang classification (Karakas et al. 2008). In his system he divided Huang's A1 into K1 and K2a (the latter indicating a RHD shorter than 1 cm), while variant K2b corresponds to trifurcation. Similarly Karakas divided A3 into K3a and K3b, the latter indicating a confluence between RPHD and LHD >1 cm from CHD origin.

1.8.5 Subvesical Bile Ducts

Also known as Luschka's ducts, the subvesical bile ducts are variant, accessory or aberrant bile ducts that run in close proximity to the gallbladder's bed. Their clinical significance is mainly due to potential damage and subsequent bile leakage after cholecystectomy.

According to Schnelldorfer, four types of subvesical bile ducts can be identified.

Type 1 subvesical bile duct is a bile duct running in close proximity to the gallbladder bed in an otherwise normal anatomy. Type 2 is a supernumerary (accessory) bile duct with a subvesical course. Type 3 identifies bile ducts that directly drain into the gallbladder through the liver bed (hepaticocystic ducts). Type 4 is represented by numerous interconnected small bile ducts in the connective tissue of the gallbladder bed, typically connected to intrahepatic bile ducts but blinded on the opposite side (Schnelldorfer et al. 2012).

1.8.6 Liver Location Variants

Despite being significantly rarer than vascular and biliary variants, macroscopic liver variants are possible, both regarding liver localisation and morphology.

While the liver is usually located directly beneath the diaphragm, the right hepatic flexure of colon might interpose between the two structures, in a variant known as Chilaiditi sign.

While this variant is mostly encountered as an incidental finding, it can sometimes cause abdominal pain and other symptoms, and in this case it is named Chilaiditi syndrome. The presence of interpositio coli has important consequences on liver imaging: on conventional radiographs it has to be distinguished from pneumoperitoneum, and during ultrasound examination the presence of colic air limits the acoustic window for liver insonation.

More drastic liver localisation variation can occur in situs viscerum inversus, where a mirrored liver can be found on the left side of the upper abdomen. The most common situs variation is the situs viscerum inversus totalis, which is a complete mirrored image of the normal anatomy with all the organ on the opposite side when compared to the usual layout; it has an incidence of 1:8000 (Mujo et al. 2015). A rarer variation is the situs inversus with levocardia, where the abdominal organs are mirrored but the heart situs is not.

More complex laterality variations are seen in situs ambiguous or heterotaxy, where an undetermined atrial arrangement is associated with abdominal organ malposition and dysmorphism. Despite the complexity of the matter, classically two types of heterotaxy have been defined, right isomerism (also known as asplenia) and left isomerism (also known as polysplenia). Simplifying, the former indicates that both sides of the body develop as the right side (thus the spleen is absent), while in the latter both sides develop as the left side (thus multiple spleens can be found). The effect of both these variations on the liver is typically a midline localisation (bridging liver) (Applegate et al. 1999). In right isomerism, the inferior vena cava and the abdominal aorta tend to lie on the same side (ipsilateral) with respect to the midline. In left isomerism the intrahepatic inferior vena cava is typically present, but drains towards the heart via the azygos or hemiazygos veins, as the suprarenal IVC is interrupted.

In extremely rare cases, accessory hepatic tissue can be found outside the patient's liver, a condition named ectopic liver. These tissue islands have little or no connection with the liver parenchyma, with subsequent anomalous vascularisation and biliary drainage. They can be located both in the abdomen or in the thorax, the most common site being the gallbladder, and show increased risk of developing HCC (Leone et al. 2004).

1.8.7 Liver Morphology Variants

A relatively common and subtle liver morphology variation entails the presence of accessory liver sulci across the surface of the organ. They typically appear at the right hepatic dome as a result of the presence of muscular bundles of the diaphragm which make an impression on the liver capsule. The possible presence of these variant sulci must be taken into account when evaluating supposedly pathological peripheric liver alterations.

Among liver morphology variations due to defective liver development, three different entities can be identified: agenesis, aplasia and hypoplasia (Fig. 10). Agenesis is referred to as the complete absence of a liver lobe, or part of it. In aplasia, one of the lobes is smaller, and its micro architecture is altered, with few hepatocytes, abnormal vessels, abundant connective tissue and bile ducts. A hypoplastic lobe is a volumetrically small lobe with preserved ultrastructure (Champetier et al. 1985). Before determining the presence of a defective liver variant it is however important to rule out acquired pathological or iatrogenic conditions, which are more common (Caseiro-Alves et al. 2013).

On the other side of the spectrum, some morphology variants involve the presence of superabundant liver parenchyma. This kind of liver variation is not always easily distinguishable from pathological causes of liver enlargement (hepatomegaly).

Riedel's lobe is a morphological variant of the right hepatic lobe (Fig. 11), which is unusually overdeveloped in the craniocaudal dimension,

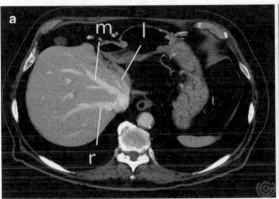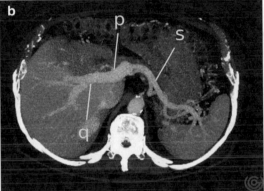

Fig. 10 (**a**, **b**) Hypoplastic left liver lobe as seen on axial CT scan at the level of the hepatic veins confluence (**a**), and axial MIP reconstruction of the portal vein (**b**). Right (*r*), middle (*m*) and left (*l*) hepatic veins, splenic vein (*s*), portal vein (*p*), right branch of the portal vein (*q*). The left hepatic vein is quite small; the left branch of the portal vein is not clearly seen

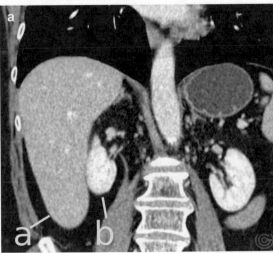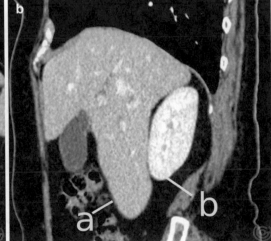

Fig. 11 (**a**, **b**) Riedel lobe as seen in coronal (**a**) and sagittal (**b**) contrast-enhanced CT. Note the liver extending caudally (*a*) below the inferior pole of the right kidney (*b*)

extending inferiorly beyond the limit of the costal cartilage. Its appearances can range from a thin tongue-like projection to a more conspicuous rounded mass. It is not strictly considered an accessory lobe (Yano et al. 2000), though some authors name it as such (Glenisson et al. 2014). Riedel's lobe prevalence in the population is not consistent among different studies, ranging from 3% to 30% (Yano et al. 2000). It is named after the German surgeon Bernhard Moritz Carl Ludwig Riedel (1846–1916) (Riedel 1888).

Finally the beaver tail liver, also known as sliver of liver, is an anatomic liver variant in which the left lobe is particularly developed in the latero-lateral dimension, and thus spans further in the left hypochondrium, making extensive contact with the spleen (Fig. 12). Over this course, the left lobe characteristically curls along the curve of the anterior abdominal wall and seems to embrace the spleen which is deeper and posterior to it.

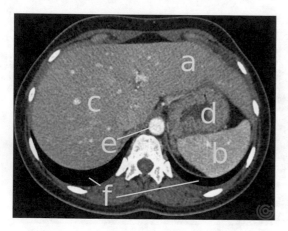

Fig. 12 Beaver tail liver as seen in axial contrast-enhanced CT. Notice the left liver lobe (*a*) reaching the spleen (*b*) on the left side. Right liver lobe (*c*), stomach (*d*), abdominal aorta (*e*), thoracic cavity (*f*)

2 Microscopic Liver Anatomy

2.1 Hepatic Lobule (Classic Lobule)

The anatomical unit of the liver is named hepatic lobule. A normal liver contains about a million hepatic lobules, which measure about 2×0.7 mm.

The hepatic lobule consists of an hexagonal structure composed of plates of hepatocyte that from the periphery converge radially to the centre of the lobule, where the terminal hepatic vein (central vein) is located (Anastasi 2007) (Fig. 13).

2.1.1 Hepatocyte

Hepatocytes constitute 80% of the liver volume. They are polyhedral cells having one, two or

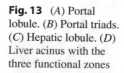

Fig. 13 (*A*) Portal lobule. (*B*) Portal triads. (*C*) Hepatic lobule. (*D*) Liver acinus with the three functional zones

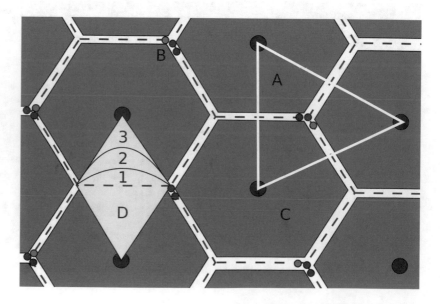

more centrally placed nuclei with well-developed nucleoli. The hepatocytes are relatively long-living cells (lifespan of about 5 months) and are capable of incredible organ regeneration (after surgery, or during chronic hepatic disease) and turnover; hepatocytes share this high proliferative capabilities with cholangiocytes, another cell type constituting the liver. This is due to the presence of stem/progenitor cells in the bile ductules that can migrate and differentiate either as hepatocytes or as cholangiocytes (Ross and Wojciech 2015).

For a simplified representation, we can assume that hepatocytes have four faces: two that face the perisinusoidal spaces, and the other two facing neighbouring cells and forming the bile canaliculi.

The hepatocyte cytoplasm is acidophilic and contains many components as follows:

– **Rough endoplasmic reticulum (RER) (basophilic regions) and free ribosome**

Many enzymes located in the rER can degrade and conjugate toxins and drugs.

After massive administration of drugs, alcohol or chemotherapeutic agents, the volume of ribosomes and function of these enzymes increase with enhanced drug degradation and modification of their pharmacokinetics.

RER also plays an important role in the assembly of lipoproteins (VLDL) (Anastasi 2007).

– **Numerous mitochondria**

The main function of mitochondria is the production of ATP, the most important source of energy for cell metabolism.

– **Golgi complex**

These cytoplasmic components are involved in VLDL synthesis, glycosylation of many proteins and exocrine excretion of bile (Anastasi 2007). They are most abundant near the bile canaliculi.

– **Peroxisomes**

Each hepatocyte contains about 200–300 peroxisomes. They contain many enzymes, namely "oxidases", "catalase" and "alcohol dehydrogenase". Oxidases generate hydrogen peroxide (H_2O_2), a very toxic substance for the cell that is degraded by catalase. This type of reaction is used by hepatocytes in many detoxification processes (e.g. detoxification of alcohol).

Peroxisomes are also involved in gluconeogenesis and metabolism of purine.

– **Deposit of glycogen**
– **Lipid droplets**
– **Lipofuscin pigments within lysosomes**

2.1.2 Biliary Tree

The biliary tree is a system of channels of increasing diameter that flow the bile from the hepatocytes to gallbladder. These channels are lined by cholangiocytes, epithelial cells characterised by the presence of tight junction between adjacent cells and a cilium that can change the flow and composition of bile (Anastasi 2007; Ovalle and Nahirney 2013). Cholangiocytes are small and cuboidal in shape in low-calibre bile ducts, but in larger ducts their volume is increased and their shape changes becoming columnar.

The bile canaliculus is the smallest branch of the biliary tree, which lies in the intercellular space between two adjacent hepatocytes and is formed by the apposition of the two hepatocytes' cell membranes bounded by tight junctions; hepatocytic microvilli protrude into the canalicular lumen.

Bile canaliculi drain into the canals of Hering (Anastasi 2007) which are lined by both hepatocytes and cholangiocytes. They have a contractile activity that allows the flux of bile towards the intrahepatic bile ductule (1–1.5 μm) and the interlobular bile ducts (10–15 μm) which are part of the peripheral portal triad.

Near the canals of Hering there are many cell precursors that during extensive parenchymal damage can migrate and differentiate into hepatocytes and/or cholangiocytes (Overi et al. 2018).

Fig. 14 *CV* central vein with endothelial cells, *S* sinusoid, *BD* bile duct, *PV* portal vein, *HA* hepatic artery

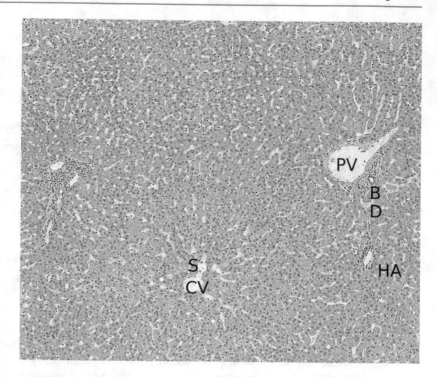

The difference between the canals of Hering and intrahepatic bile ductule lies in the structure of the wall that in the latter is lined completely by cholangiocytes.

As the ducts get larger they gradually acquire connective tissue consisting of elastic fibres and smooth muscle cell.

Intralobular bile ducts join to form interlobular bile ducts, which subsequently merge into the right and left lobar ducts, whose confluence forms the common hepatic duct.

2.1.3 Sinusoid

The sinusoids are vascular canaliculi delimited by plates of hepatocytes. Sinusoids provide the hepatocytes with mixed arterial and portal blood and drain into the central vein (Fig. 14). Sinusoidal blood flows from the periphery to the centre of the liver lobule, in the opposite direction to the bile.

These sinusoids are lined by endothelial cells that have large fenestration (discontinuities of the wall) and lack basal laminae; there is therefore no real barrier between plasma within the sinusoids and the hepatocytes. During cirrhosis the number of fenestration is reduced and a complete basal membrane is formed (a process known as "sinusoidal capillarisation").

The endothelial sinusoidal cells are the most important site for hyaluronic acid degradation; endothelial damage results in increased hyaluronic acid blood content.

The lining of sinusoids contains another type of cells named "Kupffer cell" or "sinusoidal macrophages" that derive from monocytes; they are more numerous near the portal tracts. These cells are interspersed between the sinusoidal endothelial cells without forming junctions with them; their cell processes can span into the sinusoidal lumen and remove many debris from bloodstream (old red cells and cellular fragments) and can response to many types of injury by proliferation and enlargement (activation of macrophages).

Kupffer cells play an important role in the metabolism of iron (Unigastro 2007).

Their most important role is to protect the liver from toxic damage and iron metabolism accumulating ferritin and hemosiderin.

Another cell type that we can find in the sinusoids are "pit cells", large granular lymphocytes which have killer cell activity.

2.1.4 Space of Disse

The "space of Disse" or "perisinusoidal space" is a space between the sinusoidal basal surface of the hepatocytes and the basal surface of the endo-

Fig. 15 Portal triad. *HA* hepatic artery, *BD* bile duct, *PV* portal vein

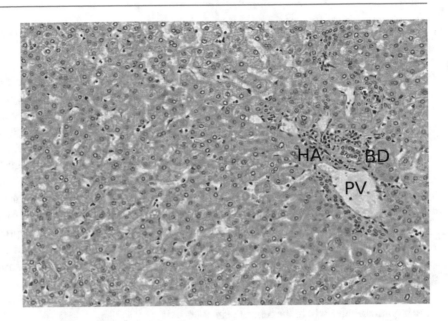

thelium. It is a zone of intercellular exchange between the blood and the hepatocytes and contains small hepatocyte microvilli and other structures like plasma, connective tissue, nerve fibres and perisinusoidal cells as hepatic stellate cells (Ito cells) and pit cells (Anastasi 2007; Gartner 2014). When the liver is compromised, hepatocytes release tumour growth factor β, and in response Ito cells begin to synthesise collagen, leading to fibrosis (Gartner 2014).

The microvilli increase the surface of exchange as much as six times and because there is not a real barrier between plasma and hepatocytes, all the elements produced and excreted in the perisinusoidal space are transferred immediately in the plasma (Ross and Wojciech 2015).

During the foetal period, this space contains "island of blood-forming cells" that can appear again in the adult during periods of chronic anaemia.

2.1.5 Ito Cell

Ito cells (or hepatic stellate cells) are perisinusoidal lipocytes that lie within the hepatic plates between the bases of hepatocytes.

Normally they are in a non-proliferative state and represent the main vitamin A conservation site in the form of retinol ester (within cytoplasmic lipid droplets) and release it as retinol bound to RBP (retinol-binding protein) (Unigastro 2007).

Ito cells are the main responsible for fibrogenesis during many insults under the stimulus of "tumour growth factor beta" produced by hepatocytes (Gartner 2014). The process starts with cell proliferation and migration to the location of damage, increased contractility, differentiation in myofibroblasts and release of type I and type III collagen in the perisinusoidal space; this collagen is continuous with the connective tissue surrounding the central vein and the portal space. During fibrogenesis, Ito cells also lose most of intracellular vitamin A.

Due to this fibrotic tissue production, these cells are the most important cells in certain pathologic conditions such as cirrhosis, chronic inflammation and portal hypertension.

2.1.6 Portal Triad

The portal triad, also known as portal area or portal canal, is the region of connective tissues between hepatic lobules that contain branches of the portal vein, hepatic artery, lymph vessels and bile ducts (Fig. 15); each portal area is surrounded by a plate of modified hepatocytes named limiting plate. The portal areas are located at alternative corners of the classic liver lobule.

The space of Mall is the narrow space that separates the limiting plate from the connective tissue of the portal area. Lymph from the space of Disse crosses the space of Mall and is then collected in the lymph vessels in the portal area. 80% of liver lymph drains in the thoracic duct.

2.1.7 Blood Supply of Liver

The liver has a double blood supply; the hepatic artery provides oxygen-rich blood and supplies 20–30% of the liver's blood (Anastasi 2007).

The portal vein supplies 70–80% of liver's blood; its content includes:

- Nutrients from the alimentary canal
- Endocrine products from the pancreas and enteroendocrine cells of gastrointestinal tract
- Blood cells and blood degradation products from the spleen

Arterial and portal branches run together in the portal area.

Via the hepatic sinusoids, mixed portal and arterial blood flows from the periphery to the centre of the hepatic lobules where the central vein collects it and routes it towards the hepatic vein system.

2.2 Portal Lobule

The portal lobule is the functional unit involved in bile secretion.

It is triangular in shape, with the three vertices positioned at the level of central lobular vein and the central axis corresponding to the interlobular bile duct of the portal triad of the classic lobule (Fig. 13). Bile flows from periphery to the centre of the portal lobule, towards the bile duct.

These portal lobules include portion of three adjacent hepatic lobules.

2.3 Liver Acinus (Acinus of Rappaport)

The liver acinus is the smallest functional unit of the hepatic parenchyma. It is lozenge shaped with the short axis lying along the border between two classic lobules (it contains distributing vessels), and the long axis drawn between the central veins of two contiguous lobules; as such, the liver acinus occupies two triangular portions of two adjacent hepatic lobules (Fig. 13).

The hepatocytes in a single acinus are divided into three concentric elliptical zones on the basis of the proximity to the short axis and therefore to the incoming blood, which reflects three different types of metabolic activity (Ross and Wojciech 2015; Unigastro 2007).

- Zone 1: It is the closest zone to the vessels that supply the hepatocytes with blood from branches of the hepatic artery (HA) and PV and is thus the least susceptible to ischaemia. It is the first zone to show changes after bile obstruction, toxic exposure and regeneration phenomena.
- Zone 2: Intermediate zone.
- Zone 3: Adjacent to the central vein, it represents the central part of the classic lobule; it is thus the most susceptible area to ischaemic damage, and the first to show fat accumulation. It is the last to show changes after toxic substance exposure.

2.4 Liver Functions

The liver is the biggest gland of the human body and plays an important role in many and different functions (Unigastro 2007):

- Biliary secretion and bilirubin metabolism
- Hormones and drug metabolism and detoxification of toxic substances
- Production of many plasma protein
- Lipid and lipoprotein metabolism
- Carbohydrate metabolism
- Urea metabolism
- Blood deposit

2.4.1 Biliary Secretion and Bilirubin Metabolism

Every day the liver produces and secretes 600–1200 mL of bile which is composed of water, bile salts, bile pigments (bilirubin), electrolytes (Na^+, K^+, Ca^{2+}, Mg^{2+}, Cl^-), phospholipid (lecithin) and cholesterol (Gartner 2014; Unigastro 2007).

The bile has two main functions:

- Digestion and absorption of lipid: Bile acids emulsify the big fat particles in little fat particles that are attacked by the pancreatic juice and facilitate transport to the intestinal mucosa.
- Excretion of products that must be eliminated, such as bilirubin (terminal product of haemoglobin catabolism) and excessive amount of cholesterol.

2.4.2 Drug Metabolism and Detoxification of Toxic Substances

Hepatocytes are involved in the metabolism of many substances including drugs, toxics and xenobiotics.

As many of these molecules are hydrophobic, liver metabolism helps the excretion by transforming them into more water-soluble substances.

Metabolism is performed in two phases (Biggio et al. 2011; Ross and Wojciech 2015; Trevor et al. 2015):

– Phase I: It includes oxidation, reduction, hydrolysis and deamination and is performed in the smooth endoplasmic reticulum by cytochrome P450s that are not highly selective in their substrate, so a small number of P450 isoforms can metabolise thousands of drugs. The most important P450 isoforms are CYP3A4/5 and CYP2D6 that are able to metabolise 75% of all drugs.

If after phase I the substances are sufficiently polar they can be excreted; otherwise they must be subjected to phase II metabolism.

It is interesting to note that during phase I oxidation some pharmacologically inactive compounds can be converted into the active form.

– Phase II: The xenobiotic metabolites are conjugated with a polar moiety (glutathione, acetate, glucuronate, sulphate and methyl groups) that augments the molecular weight and renders the compound less active and more polar.

2.4.3 Production of Plasma Protein

Many proteins are produced and metabolised by liver (Ross and Wojciech 2015; Unigastro 2007):

– Albumin: It is involved in plasma volume regulation by maintaining the oncotic pressure (Rugarli 2010).
– Many carrier proteins: Albumin, ceruloplasmin, glycoproteins (haptoglobyn, trasferrin and haemopexin).
– Lipoproteins: Especially VLDL (the most important for the transport of triglycerides from the liver to other tissues).
– α_1-Anti-trypsin, α- and β-globulin (protease inhibitors),

– Intracellular hormones.
– Prothrombin, fibrinogen, coagulation factor (II, VII, IX, X, to maintain homeostasis).

The liver is also responsible for the metabolism of amino acids and the conversion of non-nitrogenous amino acid catabolites to glucose and lipids.

Liver failure has many repercussions on protein metabolism and homeostasis; the most notable are hypoalbuminemia, coagulation abnormalities and sarcopenia (Ruiz-Margáin et al. 2018). In fact during chronic liver failure, the protein deficiency produces an increased metabolic turnover of endogenous proteins (primarily from muscles) with subsequent loss of muscle mass.

2.4.4 Lipid and Lipoprotein Metabolism

The liver is involved in many processes involving lipid metabolism (Greenspan and Baxter 1994):

– Oxidation of the fatty acids for energy production.
– Synthesis of most lipoproteins which are necessary for blood transport of cholesterol and phospholipids.
– Production of cholesterol and phospholipids (Unigastro 2007): Most of the produced cholesterol (80%) is secreted in the bile after being converted into bile salts; the remaining is secreted in the blood, carried by the lipoproteins.
– Conversion of carbohydrates and proteins in lipids.
– Production of biliary acids, which play a crucial role in intestinal fat absorption.

A decrease in serum total cholesterol, LDL, HDL and triglycerides associated with deficiency of fat-soluble vitamin (A, D, E, K) (Tsiaousi et al. 2008) may be found during chronic liver failure (Rugarli 2010).

2.4.5 Carbohydrate Metabolism

The liver plays a very important role in maintaining blood sugar levels and performs numerous tasks in the management of carbohydrate metabolism (Rugarli 2010; Unigastro 2007):

- Glycogen storage: Glucose is accumulated in the liver in the form of glycogen. Excess blood glucose is removed and accumulated in the liver, and when necessary it can be released thanks to the activity of a phosphorylase. This function is important after dietary introduction of carbohydrates (accumulation of glucose) and after many hours of fasting (release of glucose).
- Conversion of galactose and fructose into glucose.
- Gluconeogenesis: When glucose blood levels are low, the liver produces glucose in a process known as gluconeogenesis. Large quantities of amino acids (from proteins) and glycerol (from triglycerides) are used for the production of glucose.
- Production of many intermediate product of the glucose metabolism.

Hypoglycaemia and insulin resistance may be present during chronic liver failure (Johnston and Alberti 1976).

2.4.6 Urea Metabolism

NH_3 (ammonia) is normally produced and absorbed in large part by the intestine and derives from proteins introduced with food. Ammonia is a toxic substance which is normally removed by the liver through the synthesis of urea (Rugarli 2010). During liver failure, the rising of ammonia blood levels and the capability of this substance to pass the blood-brain barrier are responsible for the development of hepatic encephalopathy. Effects of ammonia on the SNC include the following:

- Changes the cell membrane functions with astrocyte swelling.
- Changes the cell metabolism, with increasing the glutamine and GABA production. The latter has an important role as inhibitory neurotransmitter.

2.4.7 Other Metabolic Functions

- Vitamin storage: The most abundant vitamins accumulated in the liver are vitamins A, B_{12} and D (Ross and Wojciech 2015).
- Iron deposit: Most of the iron in our body is located in haemoglobin molecules. The second most important iron source is the liver, which accumulates iron in the form of ferritin (combined with apoferritin) when blood iron levels are high. When the amount of iron in the blood decreases the ferritin is released again from apoferritin.
- Metabolism and storage of folic acid: Patients with liver failure have macrocytic anaemia.
- Production of many coagulation factors (I, II, V, VII, IX, X), some of which are K vitamin dependent (II, VII, IX, X). Haemorrhagic diathesis can arise during liver failure. Sometimes this condition may be due to a biliary salt loss with subsequent reduced vitamin K absorption.

2.4.8 Blood Deposit

Liver is an expandable organ that can store in its vessel a conspicuous amount of blood, which can be introduced into the general circulation in case of need.

Normally the liver contains 450 mL of blood (10% of the total volume of blood). When the pressure of right atrium increases, liver venous drainage is reduced and the blood content can increase up to 1 L.

3 Radiologic Liver Anatomy

3.1 Radiography

The liver is poorly examined by plain x-ray, due to the poor soft-tissue contrast in the upper abdomen.

On abdominal AP x-ray films, the true liver boundaries can sometimes be identified. This is possible in physiologic or para-physiologic (visceral obesity) conditions, when its silhouette is outlined by adjacent fat. Pathologic condition, and in particular the presence of air inside the abdominal cavity (pneumoperitoneum), might also determine a clear outline of the liver. Apparent borders can be identified by liver superposition over gas in adjacent organs, namely the stomach and the colon (Grainger 2001). The inferior border of the liver in particular can be inconsistently identified thanks to the superposition of the gastric, duodenal and colic gas.

The hepatic dome is normally indirectly assessed as it contributes to the convex shape of the right hemidiaphragm on chest X-ray. Pathological processes of the upper abdomen, the pleura or the pulmonary parenchyma may however alter this anatomic landmark, rendering the overall shape of the upper liver unrecognisable or providing false evidence of liver alteration.

Gaseous radiolucency can sometimes be seen between the liver and the diaphragm, in the absence of pneumoperitoneum. This phenomenon is due to air inside the right colic flexure, which has a variant collocation under the right hemidiaphragm, and is known as interpositio coli or Chilaiditi sign. Differential diagnosis between this variant and pneumoperitoneum has to be taken into account; the presence of haustra might suggest the former.

No significant remark can be made about normal liver opacity, whereas some pathologic processes might be evident on X-ray examination (such as presence of air and calcifications) (Cittadini et al. 2008).

3.2 Computed Tomography

Computed tomography (CT) is an X-ray-based tomographic approach which can provide extensive anatomic information about the liver.

Liver CT examination takes place in the context of superior abdominal CT scan or whole-abdomen scans. Thorax scans inevitably include upper liver in the scanning volume due to the overlap of the anterior superior abdominal cavity and the posterior thoracic cavity on the transverse plane.

For the same reason, correct liver imaging should always include scanning of the caudal thorax with a reasonable margin to prevent partial clipping of the hepatic dome.

While modern volumetric CT acquisition allows for multiplanar reformats, the standard reference for liver imaging is the transverse plane. Additional multiplanar reformations might be adopted for particular diagnostic needs. Sagittal and coronal reformats might also prove useful for correct evaluation of the liver dome, where partial volume artefacts are more common.

On unenhanced CT normal liver parenchyma has homogeneous density, which can vary between 55 and 65 HU (Boll and Merkle 2009).

For complete liver CT characterisation, contrast-enhanced CT (CECT) scan is mandatory (Fig. 16); CT contrast media are iodine based and are administered intravenously.

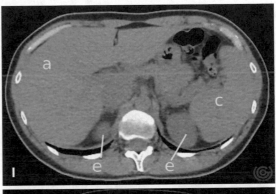

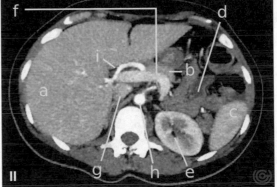

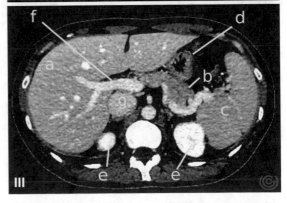

Fig. 16 (**I–III**) Axial CT scan images, showing liver parenchyma appearance in non-enhanced scan (**I**), late arterial (**II**) and portal venous phases (**III**). Non-enhanced and portal venous phases belong to the same patient. The arterial phase shows the enhanced hepatic artery entering the liver. Liver (*a*), pancreas (*b*), spleen (*c*), stomach (*d*), kidney (*e*), portal vein (*f*), inferior vena cava (*g*), abdominal aorta (*h*), hepatic artery (*i*)

CECT is a dynamicscan, as liver parenchyma contrast changes throughout time according to the time from contrast bolus injection.

Since liver scanning takes a finite amount of time and every scan increases the radiation dose delivered to the patient, only few selected phases of bolus dynamic are typically documented.

We can thus distinguish a non-enhanced phase, an early arterial phase, a late arterial phase, a portal venous phase and an equilibrium phase. Not all phases are always documented; selected phases are typically chosen according to the diagnostic setting.

In arterial phase (15–20 s after contrast injection initiation, p.i.), the contrast media is still confined in the arterial system; the HA is clearly seen; liver parenchyma is not enhanced. In the late arterial phase (25–35 s p.i.) (DeMaio 2010), structures getting blood from arterial circulation become enhanced; normal liver parenchyma does not show strong enhancement as the HA only provides 25% of liver blood inflow (Sureka et al. 2015) and initial enhancement of the PV is seen in this phase (Prokop et al. 2006). In the portal venous phase (60–70 s p.i.) the PV and hepatic parenchyma show maximum enhancement; hepatic veins show initial enhancement. In the equilibrium phase (2–3 min p.i.) contrast enhancement is less prominent than in the venous portal phase and minimal difference is seen between contrast enhancement of different vascular structures and the parenchyma.

As morphological and vascular landmarks are clearly seen on contrast - enhanced CT scans, the segmental anatomy of the organ can be easily defined (Fig. 17).

3.3 Ultrasound

The liver is typically scanned in the context of an abdominal or upper abdominal US examination. In the adult, it requires the adoption of a convex transducers, with frequency ranging from 3.5 to 5 MHz. In children or in case the area of interest is particularly superficial, a higher frequency linear transducer (7.5–10 MHz) might be used (Berzigotti and Piscaglia 2011).

Normal liver US does not involve contrast media administration. In selected diagnostic settings however, the usage of intravenously administered echogenic agents might prove useful (CEUS, contrast-enhanced ultrasound, see relevant chapter).

CEUS is a dynamic exam, during which the operator can observe the progression of the echogenic bolus in the liver circulatory system and assess contrastographic behaviour of a particular area of interest. Important differences between contrast-enhanced CT and CEUS are that CEUS grants the possibility of continuous real-time scanning of bolus progression, typically limited to a single or few target areas, while CT provides imaging of few selected, brief time frames (ideally instantaneous) in a panoramic fashion.

Normal localisation of the liver is in the right hypochondrium, epigastrium and part of the left hypochondrium. Under free breathing, the biggest sonographic window is typically identified in the epigastrium, between the costal cartilages, where the middle part of the liver parenchyma is seen (Fig. 18). Under this condition, both the left and right lobes are typically partially covered by the ribcage.

Inspiratory breath-hold forces diaphragm contraction and caudalisation, which brings the liver downwards and exposes more parenchyma to probe insonation below the costochondral arches.

Besides the thoracic cage, another factor to be taken into consideration as a possible obstacle to proper insonation is the presence of bowel and gastric gas which might hinder hepatic evaluation due to acoustic shadowing. In these cases, patient mobilisation and gradual probe compression might prove useful to displace the interfering viscera.

Nevertheless, unfavourable patient anatomy, abundant gastrointestinal gas, scarce collaboration or pathology may force the operator to prefer an intercostal sonographic window.

Finally, sonographic assessment might prove limited especially on the deepest part of the organ in case of voluminous patients (e.g. obesity, ascites), as the US beam might get too attenuated for producing diagnostic image quality. The same concept applies to extensive alterations of liver parenchyma which might determine early

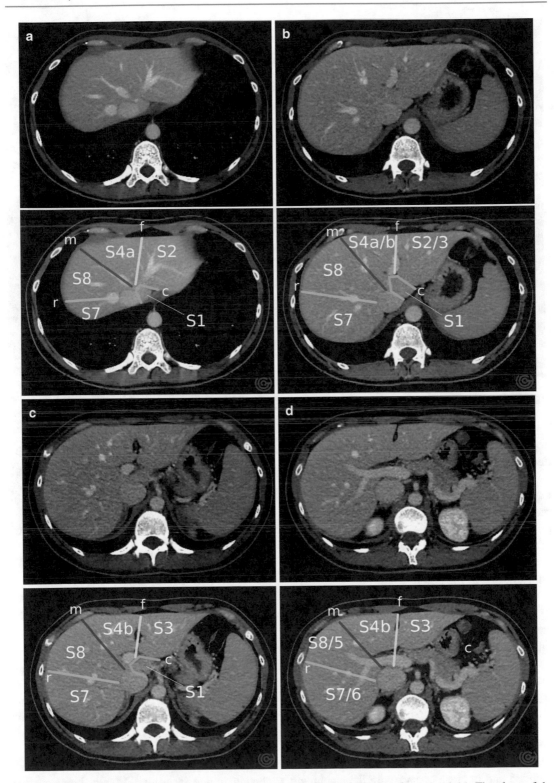

Fig. 17 (**a**–**e**) Liver segments seen on axial contrast-enhanced CT from cranial (**a**) to caudal (**e**). On annotated images: lines spanning on the plane of the right hepatic vein (*r*), the middle hepatic vein (*m*), the falciform liga-ment (*f*) and the limits of segment 1 (*c*). The plane of the portal vein branches delimits the upper from the lower segments

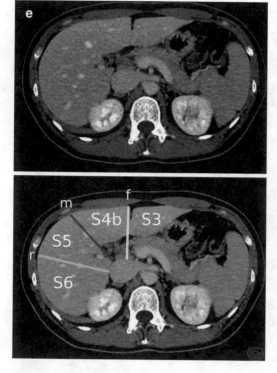

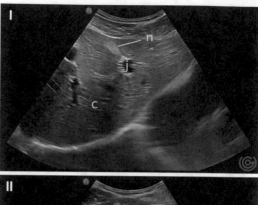

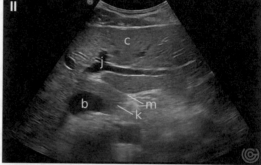

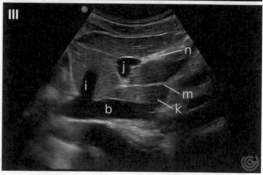

Fig. 17 (continued)

degradation of the US beam and thus hide the deepest structures (such as in liver steatosis).

An important landmark that should be explored during US liver examination is the recess of Morison (Fig. 19), located between the posterior face of the liver and the anterior aspect of the right kidney. It is a peritoneal recess which is typically empty, with the two organs strictly adjacent one to the other.

The presence of material in the peritoneal cavity, namely ascites or a haematic collection, might cause distension of the Morison pouch and separation between the liver and the right kidney.

Liver parenchyma typically has homogeneous intermediate echogenicity, similar to that of the adjacent right kidney, which is usually used as a reference.

Liver contour is smooth. The inferior and left liver margin should be acute, with the left usually being more acute. The right hepatic cupola is rounded and in close contact with the diaphragm. Immediately cranially to it, a strongly hyperechoic interface is seen, due to the air content of the lung. Because of the reflective nature of this type of interface, reflection artefacts of liver structures inside the

Fig. 18 (**I–III**) Ligamentum venosum and round ligament of the liver as seen on ultrasound on axial (**I** and **II**) and sagittal (**III**) scanning planes. Liver parenchyma (*c*), vena cava (*b*), left hepatic vein (*i*), left portal vein (*j*), segment S1 (*k*), fissure for ligamentum venosum (*m*), round ligament (*n*)

thoracic cavity are typical of this area. Loss of air-tissue interface constitutes an important sign of pathology, namely the presence of pleural effusion.

The left liver lobe is in contact cranially with the left hemidiaphragm; above it the pericardium, heart and heart chambers are easily seen.

Liver craniocaudal diameter at the right midclavicular line is around 14 cm, being mainly influenced by body mass index (BMI) and height (Kratzer et al. 2003).

Vessel and bile ducts are distributed inside the parenchyma and appear as elongated anechoic

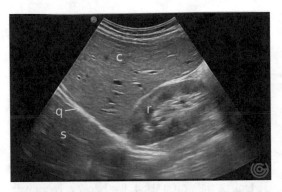

Fig. 19 Morison pouch on ultrasound on the sagittal plane. Liver parenchyma (*c*), right kidney (*r*), diaphragm (*q*), right thoracic cavity (*s*). Liver and kidney parenchyma have the same echogenicity; under normal circumstances the space between the two organs is a virtual peritoneal recess. Notice the presence of spurious echoes inside the thoracic cavity due to mirroring effect of liver structures caused by the diaphragm

Fig. 20 (**I–III**) Longitudinal view of the portal vein on ultrasound from left (**I**) to right (**III**). Portal vein (**a**), inferior vena cava (**b**), liver (**c**), pancreas head (**d**), aorta (**e**), pancreas body (**f**), splenic vein (**g**)

structures. Their calibre is not homogeneous throughout the organ, and the smallest peripheral branches are not resolved by US. The constituents of the portal triad (arteries, portal veins and bile ducts) widen towards the hepatic hilum, while hepatic veins widen towards the subdiaphragmatic inferior vena cava.

At the liver hilum we can recognise the hepatic pedicle entering the parenchyma. The pedicle runs in the context of the hepatoduodenal ligament and is made up by the common bile duct, the hepatic artery proper and the portal vein (Fig. 20), which is the most conspicuous of the three.

Normal PV diameter at this level is inferior to 13 mm (Berzigotti and Piscaglia 2011). Doppler imaging shows hepatopetal blood flow, a phasic, gently undulating spectral waveform, with a

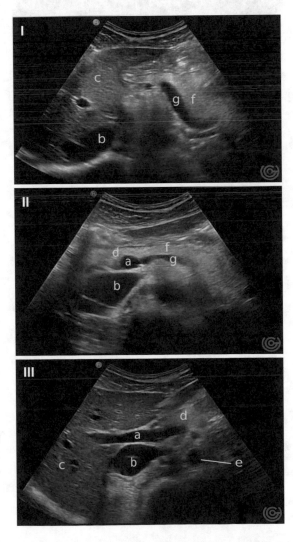

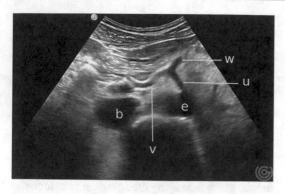

Fig. 21 Axial view at the level of the celiac trunk. Aorta (*e*), celiac trunk (*u*), common hepatic artery (*v*), splenic artery (*w*), inferior vena cava (*b*)

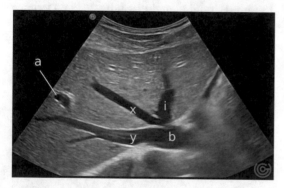

Fig. 22 Axial view of the liver at the level of the hepatic vein confluence. Inferior vena cava (*b*), left (*i*), middle (*x*) and right (*y*) hepatic veins, branch of the right portal vein (*a*). The left and middle hepatic veins form a common trunk before reaching the IVC. Notice the different echogenicity of the vessel walls: the portal branch is strongly echogenic due to the hepatobiliary sheath, while the hepatic veins show echogenic walls only when perpendicularly insonated (as in *y*)

mean velocity between 16 and 40 cm/s (McNaughton and Abu-Yousef 2011).

The origin of the common hepatic artery (CHA) from the celiac trunk is typically easily identified, due to the unmistakable shape of the celiac trifurcation (Fig. 21). Upon Doppler examination, blood flow in the HA is pulsatile, and hepatopetal throughout the cardiac cycle, with a spectral waveform typical of a low-resistance artery. Normal RI ranges between 0.55 and 0.7 (McNaughton and Abu-Yousef 2011).

Glisson's capsule branching inside the liver parenchyma, the hepatobiliary sheath, is clearly visible on US as a hyperechoic layer surrounding the portal triad. This finding might however become less prominent in cases where background liver

echogenicity is augmented such as in steatosis (Gluskin 2017).

The hepatic vein confluence into the vena cava can be easily seen just below the diaphragm. On the axial plane they can be seen radiating from the vena cava in a spoke-wheel configuration (Fig. 22). They are quite large vessels, with a mean diameter around 15 mm (Draghi et al. 2007), gradually tapering towards the periphery.

Unlike the portal triad, the hepatic veins lack any hyperechoic external sheath, and no clear hyperechoic delimitation from the surrounding parenchyma is seen. Occasionally however, hepatic vein wall might be seen as a thin hyperechoic layer when it lays perfectly perpendicular to the incoming ultrasound waves.

On Doppler US, hepatic vein flow is typically tri- or quadri-phasic, predominantly antegrade (hepatofugal) (McNaughton and Abu-Yousef 2011).

3.4 Magnetic Resonance Imaging

In many instances, magnetic resonance represents the best performing radiology imaging technique for liver evaluation and lesion characterisation.

Current standards for liver imaging require adoption of magnetic fields upwards of 1.5 T.

The multiplanar and multiparametric capabilities of MRI provide exhaustive information on both morphology and tissue characteristics. A notable advantage against CT is represented by the fact that thanks to the non-ionising properties of MRI, additional sequences do not increase the radiation dose to the patient.

Like CT, liver MRI can benefit from the adoption of intravenous contrast media, which in the case of MRI are typically gadolinium based. Dynamic contrast enhancement protocol is thus possible, depicting arterial, venous and late phases.

Additionally, some MRI gadolinium-based agents (namely Gd-BOPTA and Gd-EOB-DTPA) benefit from a specific late hepatocyte and biliary phase, which adds important functional and morphology information besides classical contrast dynamic shared with non-hepatospecific contrast agents (Fig. 23).

Interference of the nearby stomach and duodenum in obtaining clear depiction of liver

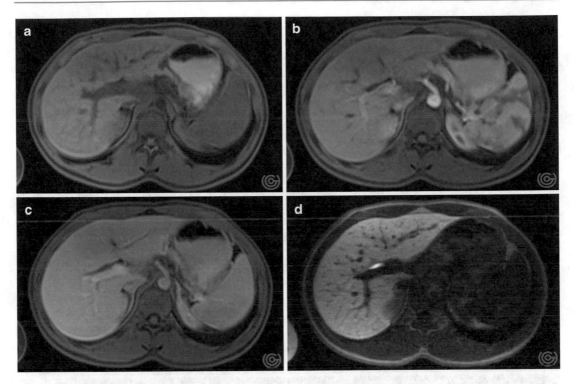

Fig. 23 Contrast enhanced MRI in the axial plane: T1W sequences with fat saturation in pre-contrastographic (**a**), arterial (**b**), portal venous (**c**) and hepatobiliary (**d**) phases. Notice the liver contrast enhancement as opposed to adjacent structures in the hepatobiliary phase; the strongly hyperintense signal at the liver hilum corresponds to the common hepatic duct

structures in certain sequences, namely the one aimed at depicting the biliary ducts, can be reduced by administering negative oral contrast media to reduce the signal from gastrointestinal content (e.g. superparamagnetic contrast agents).

Different clinical settings and pathologies call for different imaging protocols. We can however distinguish some sequences that are typically found in a liver MRI study: spoiled GE T1-weighted sequences with fat suppression before and after e.v. contrast media administration (dynamic), in-phase and opposed-phase T1-weighted, T2-weighted with and without fat suppression, and diffusion-weighted sequences (Fig. 24). In addition, the assessment of the intrahepatic and extrahepatic biliary duct tree benefits from specific MR cholangiopancreatographic (MRCP) sequences.

Fast sequences, breath-hold acquisition and respiratory triggering are used to reduce motion artefacts, which are mainly due to diaphragm excursion.

The favourite imaging plane for liver parenchyma evaluation is the axial plane, while MRCP sequences are typically assessed on the coronal plane.

Liver MRI is however a highly adaptable exam, where both sequences and imaging planes can be tailored to meet particular diagnostic needs.

In in-phase T1-w images, liver parenchyma signal is hypointense to fat tissue, but slightly more intense than the kidney, spleen and skeletal muscles.

Normal liver parenchyma in opposed-phase T1-w images shows analogous characteristics as the in-phase sequence, with the exception of the presence of solid black lines where an interface between water- and fat-rich tissues exists, such as around the capsule of the liver (Merkle and Nelson 2006).

In T2-w images liver is even more hypointense when compared to fat tissue, while it has signal similar to that of skeletal muscle; kidneys and the spleen are more hyperintense than the liver in this sequence. On fat-suppressed sequences, as the name implies, basic T1-w and T2-w signal characteristics are maintained, while fat tissue signal is minimised.

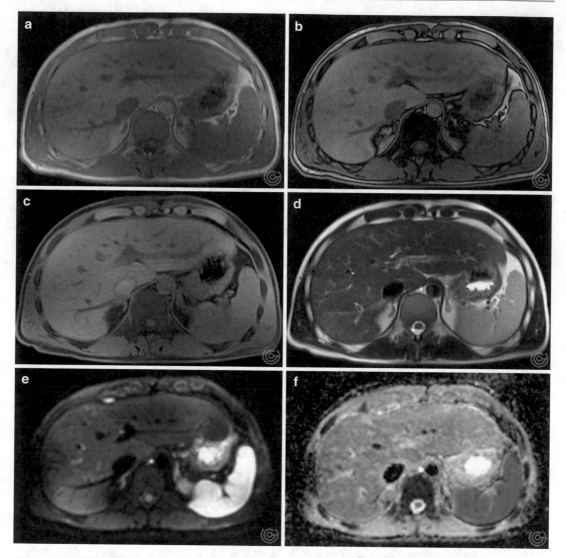

Fig. 24 Liver appearance in the axial plane in different MRI sequences. T1 weighted (**a**), opposed-phase T1 weighted (**b**), T1 weighted with fat saturation (**c**), T2 weighted (**d**), Diffusion Weighted Imaging with high b value (**e**), Apparent Diffusion Coefficient Map (**f**)

Diffusion-weighted MRI sequences provide a means to assess the diffusivity of water molecules inside the liver parenchyma, a characteristic that may be altered in various conditions and pathologies. Normal apparent diffusion coefficient (ADC) values for liver parenchyma vary between 0.7 and 1.30 (Taouli and Koh 2010).

Finally MRCP sequences are particular T2W sequences where the only retained signal comes from stationary fluid; as the name suggests they are mainly used to assess both intra- and extrahepatic bile ducts and pancreatic ducts, of which they provide a high-contrast anatomic depiction (Fig. 25).

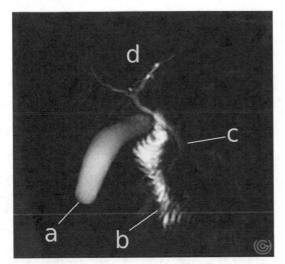

Fig. 25 Magnetic resonance cholangio-pancreatography: MIP reconstruction on the coronal plane. Gallbladder (*a*), duodenum (*b*), common bile duct (*c*), intrahepatic biliary tree (*d*). The common bile duct and the duodenum are partly superimposed in this reconstruction

References

Abdel-Misih SRZ, Bloomston M (2010) Liver anatomy. Surg Clin North Am 90:643–653

Anastasi G (2007) Trattato di anatomia umana (Edi. Ermes)

Aoki S, Mizuma M, Hayashi H, Nakagawa K, Morikawa T, Motoi F, Naitoh T, Egawa S, Unno M (2016) Surgical anatomy of the right hepatic artery in Rouviere's sulcus evaluated by preoperative multidetector-row CT images. BMC Surg 16:40

Applegate KE, Goske MJ, Pierce G, Murphy D (1999) Situs revisited: imaging of the heterotaxy syndrome. Radiogr Rev Publ Radiol Soc N Am Inc 19:837–852; discussion 853–854

Auh YH, Rosen A, Rubenstein WA, Engel IA, Whalen JP, Kazam E (1984) CT of the papillary process of the caudate lobe of the liver. AJR Am J Roentgenol 142:535–538

Berzigotti A, Piscaglia F (2011) Ultrasound in portal hypertension—part 1. Ultraschall. Med Stuttg Ger 1980(32):548–568; quiz 569–571

Biggio G, Riccardi C, Cuomo V, Rossi F (2011) Farmacologia: principi di base e applicazioni terapeutiche. Minerva medica, Torino

Bismuth H (1982) Surgical anatomy and anatomical surgery of the liver. World J Surg 6:3–9

Bismuth H, Houssin D, Castaing D (1982) Major and minor segmentectomies "réglées" in liver surgery. World J Surg 6:10–24

Boll DT, Merkle EM (2009) Diffuse liver disease: strategies for hepatic CT and MR imaging. Radiogr Publ Radiol Soc N Am Inc 29:1591–1614

Carneiro C, Brito J, Bilreiro C, Barros M, Bahia C, Santiago I, Caseiro-Alves F (2019) All about portal vein: a pictorial display to anatomy, variants and physiopathology. Insights into Imaging 10(1)

Caseiro-Alves F, Seco M, Bernardes A (2013) Liver anatomy, congenital anomalies, and normal variants. In: Hamm B, Ros PR (eds) Abdominal imaging. Springer, Berlin, Heidelberg, pp 983–1000

Catalano OA, Singh AH, Uppot RN, Hahn PF, Ferrone CR, Sahani DV (2008) Vascular and biliary variants in the liver: implications for liver surgery. Radiogr Rev Publ Radiol Soc N Am Inc 28:359–378

Chaib E, Kanas AF, Galvão FHF, D'Albuquerque LAC (2014) Bile duct confluence: anatomic variations and its classification. Surg Radiol Anat SRA 36: 105–109

Champetier J (1994) Les voies biliaires. In: Chevrel JP, (ed). Anatomie Clinique, Le tronc. Springer, Paris. p. 416–417

Champetier J, Yver R, Létoublon C, Vigneau B (1985) A general review of anomalies of hepatic morphology and their clinical implications. Anat Clin 7:285–299

Cheng YF, Huang TL, Lee TY, Chen TY, Chen CL (1996) Variation of the intrahepatic portal vein; angiographic demonstration and application in living-related hepatic transplantation. Transplant Proc 28:1667–1668

Choi JW, Kim TK, Kim KW, Kim AY, Kim PN, Ha HK, Lee M-G (2003) Anatomic variation in intrahepatic bile ducts: an analysis of intraoperative cholangiograms in 300 consecutive donors for living donor liver transplantation. Korean J Radiol 4:85–90

Cittadini G, Sardanelli F, Cittadini G, Mariani G (2008) Diagnostica per immagini e radioterapia. ECIG, Genova

Clarkson A (2013) A text-book of histology: descriptive and practical. For the Use of Students (Butterworth-Heinemann)

Couinaud C (1957) Le foie; études anatomiques et chirurgicales. Masson, Paris

Covey AM, Brody LA, Maluccio MA, Getrajdman GI, Brown KT (2002) Variant hepatic arterial anatomy revisited: digital subtraction angiography performed in 600 patients. Radiology 224:542–547

de la Grandmaison GL, Clairand I, Durigon M (2001) Organ weight in 684 adult autopsies: new tables for a Caucasoid population. Forensic Sci Int 119:149–154

Deka P, Islam M, Jindal D, Kumar N, Arora A, Negi SS (2014) Analysis of biliary anatomy according to different classification systems. Indian J Gastroenterol 33:23–30

DeMaio DN (2010) Mosby's exam review for computed tomography—E-book (Elsevier health sciences)

Donoso L, Martínez-Noguera A, Zidan A, Lora F (1989) Papillary process of the caudate lobe of the liver: sonographic appearance. Radiology 173:631–633

Draghi F, Rapaccini GL, Fachinetti C, de Matthaeis N, Battaglia S, Abbattista T, Busilacchi P (2007) Ultrasound examination of the liver: Normal vascular anatomy. J Ultrasound 10:5–11

Garby L, Lammert O, Kock KF, Thobo-Carlsen B (1993) Weights of brain, heart, liver, kidneys, and spleen in healthy and apparently healthy adult Danish subjects. Am J Hum Biol 5:291–296

Gartner LP (2014) BRS cell biology and histology 7Ed (Wolters Kluwer)

Gazelle GS, Lee MJ, Mueller PR (1994) Cholangiographic segmental anatomy of the liver. Radiogr Rev Publ Radiol Soc N Am Inc 14:1005–1013

Germain T, Favelier S, Cercueil J-P, Denys A, Krausé D, Guiu B (2014) Liver segmentation: practical tips. Diagn Interv Imaging 95:1003–1016

Gilfillan RS, Hills HL (1950) Anatomic study of the portal vein and its main branches. Arch Surg Chic Ill 61:449–461

Glenisson M, Salloum C, Lim C, Lacaze L, Malek A, Enriquez A, Compagnon P, Laurent A, Azoulay D (2014) Accessory liver lobes: anatomical description and clinical implications. J Visc Surg 151:451–455

Gluskin JS (2017) Chapter 15: Ultrasound of the liver, biliary tract, and pancreas. In Blumgart's Surgery of the Liver, Biliary Tract and Pancreas, 2-Volume Set (Sixth Edition), WR Jarnagin, ed. (Philadelphia: content repository only!), pp 245–275.e4

Grainger RG (2001) Grainger & Allison's diagnostic radiology: a textbook of medical imaging (London [etc.]: Churchill Livingstone)

Greenspan FS, Baxter JD (1994) Basic and clinical endocrinology. Prentice-Hall, Englewood Cliffs, NJ

Gwon DI, Ko G-Y, Yoon H-K, Sung K-B, Lee JM, Ryu SJ, Seo MH, Shim J-C, Lee GJ, Kim HK (2007) Inferior phrenic artery: anatomy, variations, pathologic conditions, and interventional management. Radiogr Rev Publ Radiol Soc N Am Inc 27:687–705

Healey JE, Schroy PC (1953) Anatomy of the biliary ducts within the human liver; analysis of the prevailing pattern of branchings and the major variations of the biliary ducts. AMA Arch Surg 66:599–616

Honda G, Iwanaga T, Kurata M (2008) Dissection of the gallbladder from the liver bed during laparoscopic cholecystectomy for acute or subacute cholecystitis. J Hepato-Biliary-Pancreat Surg 15:293–296

Huang TL, Cheng YF, Chen CL, Chen TY, Lee TY (1996) Variants of the bile ducts: clinical application in the potential donor of living-related hepatic transplantation. Transplant Proc 28:1669–1670

Iqbal S, Iqbal R, Iqbal F (2017) Surgical implications of portal vein variations and liver segmentations: a recent update. J Clin Diagn Res 11:AE01–AE05

Jensen KJ, Alpini G, Glaser S (2013) Hepatic nervous system and neurobiology of the liver. Compr Physiol 3:655–665

Johnston DG, Alberti KG (1976) Carbohydrate metabolism in liver disease. Clin Endocrinol Metab 5:675–702

Karakas HM, Celik T, Alicioglu B (2008) Bile duct anatomy of the Anatolian Caucasian population: Huang classification revisited. Surg Radiol Anat SRA 30:539–545

Kennedy PA, Madding GF (1977) Surgical anatomy of the liver. Surg Clin North Am 57:233–244

Kimura W, Fukumoto T, Watanabe T, Hirai I (2015) Variations in portal and hepatic vein branching of the liver. Yamagata Med J 33:115–121

Kratzer W, Fritz V, Mason RA, Haenle MM, Kaechele V, Roemerstein Study Group (2003) Factors affecting liver size: a sonographic survey of 2080 subjects. J Ultrasound Med 22:1155–1161

Lautt WW (2009) Hepatic circulation: physiology and pathophysiology, vol 1. Morgan & Claypool Life Sciences, San Rafael, CA, p 1

Lee SY, Cherqui D, Kluger MD (2013) Extended right hepatectomy in a liver with a non-bifurcating portal vein: the hanging maneuver protects the portal system in the presence of anomalies. J Gastrointest Surg 17:1494–1499

Leone N, De Paolis P, Carrera M, Carucci P, Musso A, David E, Brunello F, Fronda GR, Rizzetto M (2004) Ectopic liver and hepatocarcinogenesis: report of three cases with four years' follow-up. Eur J Gastroenterol Hepatol 16:731–735

Lowe MC, D'Angelica MI (2016) Anatomy of hepatic resectional surgery. Surg Clin North Am 96:183–195

Madoff DC, Hicks ME, Vauthey J-N, Charnsangavej C, Morello FA, Ahrar K, Wallace MJ, Gupta S (2002) Transhepatic portal vein embolization: anatomy, indications, and technical considerations. Radiogr Rev Publ Radiol Soc N Am Inc 22:1063–1076

Majno P, Mentha G, Toso C, Morel P, Peitgen HO, Fasel JHD (2014) Anatomy of the liver: an outline with three levels of complexity—a further step towards tailored territorial liver resections. J Hepatol 60:654–662

McNaughton DA, Abu-Yousef MM (2011) Doppler US of the liver made simple. Radiogr Rev Publ Radiol Soc N Am Inc 31:161–188

Merkle EM, Nelson RC (2006) Dual gradient-echo in-phase and opposed-phase hepatic MR imaging: a useful tool for evaluating more than fatty infiltration or fatty sparing. Radiogr Rev Publ Radiol Soc N Am Inc 26:1409–1418

Miyayama S, Matsui O, Taki K, Minami T, Ryu Y, Ito C, Nakamura K, Inoue D, Notsumata K, Toya D et al (2006) Extrahepatic blood supply to hepatocellular carcinoma: angiographic demonstration and transcatheter arterial chemoembolization. Cardiovasc Intervent Radiol 29:39–48

Molina DK, DiMaio VJM (2012) Normal organ weights in men: part II-the brain, lungs, liver, spleen, and kidneys. Am J Forensic Med Pathol 33:368–372

Mujo T, Finnegan T, Joshi J, Wilcoxen KA, Reed JC (2015) Situs ambiguous, levocardia, right sided stomach, obstructing duodenal web, and intestinal nonrotation: a case report. J Radiol Case Rep 9:16–23

Murakami G, Hata F (2002) Human liver caudate lobe and liver segment. Anat Sci Int 77:211–224

Ohkubo M, Nagino M, Kamiya J, Yuasa N, Oda K, Arai T, Nishio H, Nimura Y (2004) Surgical anatomy of the bile ducts at the hepatic hilum as applied to living donor liver transplantation. Ann Surg 239:82–86

Onishi H, Kawarada Y, Das BC, Nakano K, Gadzijev EM, Ravnik D, Isaji S (2000) Surgical anatomy of the medial segment (S4) of the liver with special reference to bile ducts and vessels. Hepato-Gastroenterology 47:143–150

Ovalle WK, Nahirney PC (2013) Netter's histology flash cards, updated edition (Saunders)

Overi D, Carpino G, Cardinale V, Franchitto A, Safarikia S, Onori P, Alvaro D, Gaudio E (2018) Contribution of resident stem cells to liver and biliary tree regeneration in human diseases. Int J Mol Sci 19:2917

Porth C (2011) Essentials of pathophysiology: concepts of altered health states. Lippincott Williams & Wilkins, Philadelphia

Prokop M, Galanski M, Bonomo L (2006) Tomografia computerizzata. Spirale e multistrato. Elsevier, Mailand

Puppala S, Patel J, Woodley H, Alizai NK, Kessel D (2009) Preoperative imaging of left portal vein at the rex recess for rex shunt formation using wedged hepatic vein carbon dioxide portography. J Pediatr Surg 44:2043–2047

Riedel I (1888) Über den zungenformigen Fortsatz des rechten Leberlappens und seine pathognostische Bedeutung für die Erkrankung der Gallenblase nebst Bemerkungen über Gallensteinoperationen. Berl Klin Wochenschr 29.577–581

Ross MH, Wojciech PM (2015) Histology: a text and atlas: with correlated cell and molecular biology. Lippincott Williams & Wilkins, Philadelphia

Rugarli C (2010) Medicina interna sistematica. Elsevier, Milano

Ruiz-Margáin A, Méndez-Guerrero O, Román-Calleja BM, González-Rodríguez S, Fernández-Del-Rivero G, Rodríguez-Córdova PA, Torre A, Macías-Rodríguez RU (2018) Dietary management and supplementation with branched-chain amino acids in cirrhosis of the liver. Rev Gastroenterol Mex 83:424–433

Scalea TM, Rodriguez A, Chiu WC, Brenneman FD, Fallon WF, Kato K, McKenney MG, Nerlich ML, Ochsner MG, Yoshii H (1999) Focused assessment with sonography for trauma (FAST): results from an international consensus conference. J Trauma 46:466–472

Schmidt S, Demartines N, Soler L, Schnyder P, Denys A (2008) Portal vein normal anatomy and variants: implication for liver surgery and portal vein embolization. Semin Interv Radiol 25:86–91

Schnelldorfer T, Sarr MG, Adams DB (2012) What is the duct of Luschka?—a systematic review. J Gastrointest Surg 16:656–662

Seong NJ, Chung JW, Kim H-C, Park JH, Jae HJ, An SB, Cho BH (2012) Right gastric venous drainage: angiographic analysis in 100 patients. Korean J Radiol 13:53–60

Stamm ER, Meier JM, Pokharel SS, Clark T, Glueck DH, Lind KE, Roberts KM (2016) Normal main portal vein diameter measured on CT is larger than the widely referenced upper limit of 13 mm. Abdom Radiol N Y 41:1931–1936

Standring S, Barni T, Billi A (2009) Anatomia del Gray. Le basi anatomiche per la pratica clinica. Elsevier, Milano

Sureka B, Patidar Y, Bansal K, Rajesh S, Agrawal N, Arora A (2015) Portal vein variations in 1000 patients: surgical and radiological importance. Br J Radiol 88:20150326

Tanaka M, Iwakiri Y (2016) The hepatic lymphatic vascular system: structure, function, markers, and lymphangiogenesis. Cell Mol Gastroenterol Hepatol 2:733–749

Taouli B, Koh D-M (2010) Diffusion-weighted MR imaging of the liver. Radiology 254:47–66

Trevor AJ, Katzung BG, Knuidering-Hall M (2015) Katzung & Trevor's pharmacology examination and board Review, 11th edition. McGraw-Hill Education/Medical, New York Chicago San Francisco Athens London Madrid Mexico City Milan New Delhi Singapore Sydney Toronto

Tsiaousi ET, Hatzitolios AI, Trygonis SK, Savopoulos CG (2008) Malnutrition in end stage liver disease: recommendations and nutritional support. J Gastroenterol Hepatol 23:527–533

Unigastro (2007) Manuale di gastroenterologia. Editrice Gastroenterologica Italiana, Roma

Weinreb J, Kumari S, Phillips G, Pochaczevsky R (1982) Portal vein measurements by real-time sonography. AJR Am J Roentgenol 139:497–499

Yamamoto M, Ariizumi S-I (2018) Glissonean pedicle approach in liver surgery. Ann Gastroenterol Surg 2:124–128

Yano K, Ohtsubo M, Mizota T, Kato H, Hayashida Y, Morita S, Furukawa R, Hayakawa A (2000) Riedel's lobe of the liver evaluated by multiple imaging modalities. Intern Med Tokyo Jpn 39:136–138

Yoshimitsu K, Honda H, Kuroiwa T, Irie H, Aibe H, Shinozaki K, Masuda K (2001) Unusual hemodynamics and pseudolesions of the noncirrhotic liver at CT. Radiogr Rev Publ Radiol Soc N Am Inc 21 Spec No:S81–S96

Part II

Imaging and Interventional Modalities

Ultrasound of the Liver

Vasileios Rafailidis and Paul S. Sidhu

Contents

Abstract

Ultrasound (US) represents the first-line imaging modality for initial diagnostic assessment of liver pathology and in many cases the optimal modality for serial follow-up. US not only offers anatomic information with excellent spatial resolution in the near and mid field with grayscale imaging, but also provides the possibility to assess physiologic information about hepatic vasculature, making use of Doppler US techniques. Doppler US techniques are capable of subjectively visualizing blood flow with color and also quantifying

V. Rafailidis · P. S. Sidhu (✉)
Department of Radiology, King's College Hospital,
King's College London, London, UK
e-mail: paulsidhu@nhs.net

© Springer Nature Switzerland AG 2021
E. Quaia (ed.), *Imaging of the Liver and Intra-hepatic Biliary Tract*,
Medical Radiology, Diagnostic Imaging, https://doi.org/10.1007/978-3-030-38983-3_3

flow characteristics using spectral analysis. The role of US in the evaluation of liver disease has been further augmented with the introduction of new technologies: contrast-enhanced ultrasound (CEUS) and elastography. Although aspects of these new techniques are still under development, promising results have been reported, placing them at the center of modern ultrasonographic assessment of liver pathology. As with every imaging modality, the physician performing the examination needs to be aware of the basic physical and technical principles of the technique, not only for better understanding of the technique's parameters and capability to improve image quality by adjusting scanning parameters but also for prompt identification of artifacts and hence avoidance of misdiagnosis. A better understanding of the technique will lead to optimal image quality and better diagnostic confidence, for the benefit of the patient.

1 Introduction

The terms "ultrasound" and "ultrasonography" (US) are usually interchangeably used to describe the same imaging technique. Nevertheless, and as Prof David Cosgrove has once eloquently pointed out, these terms are actually different, with the first describing the sound waves used to acquire images of the human body while the second referring to the imaging technique as an entirety making use of these sound waves to produce images (Cosgrove 2017).

Even with impressive advances in the fields of abdominal computed tomography (CT) and magnetic resonance imaging (MRI), US remains the first-line imaging modality for the patient presenting with abdominal symptoms or laboratory findings suggestive of liver disease, while in certain cases it is the only modality needed to establish the diagnosis and follow-up the patient. Well-known advantages of this modality include low cost, good patient tolerability, widespread availability, absence of adverse effects on the patient with potential to be performed anywhere

from the patient's bedside to the emergency department, and the operating room. In addition, US has the advantage of providing a range of information related to anatomy (grayscale) and physiology of liver (color Doppler, pulsed-wave Doppler interrogation). The information provided by US has been developed by the incorporation of new US techniques including contrast-enhanced ultrasound (CEUS) and elastography, justifying the term "multi-parametric ultrasound" or MPUS (Sidhu 2015).

Modern US devices have predefined settings for various scanning conditions and target organs, including liver in average-sized or obese patients. Nonetheless, it is essential for a physician who routinely performs US examinations to be familiar with the technical principles of the imaging modality. This is invaluable in difficult scanning conditions, when adjusting a particular variable will improve image quality, and for early recognition of artifactual findings. US technology has shown rapid advances, especially with the introduction of contrast-enhanced ultrasound (CEUS) and elastography, as well as encouraging results but many aspects are still under development, with a promising future. It is crucial for the physician involved in these fields to be aware of the basic principles of these new technologies.

In this chapter, we discuss the basic principles associated with ultrasonographic techniques. Both conventional techniques such as grayscale and color Doppler technique and more recently developed techniques like CEUS and elastography are presented in terms of technical foundation.

1.1 About Ultrasound Wave Production and Propagation

The creation of an image with US is achieved through the interaction of US waves with biologic tissues and materials. The transducer represents the most important part acting as both the generator and transmitter of the US wave and the receiver of waves reflected by the body tissues. With increased rate at which transducers emit and receive US waves, the image produced is virtually real time (typical frame rates are 12–30/s).

Ultrasound waves constitute mechanical pressure waves of alternating compression and refraction which need a material to be propagated through. Ultrasound waves used for diagnostic applications lie in the range of million cycles per second frequency (MHz), usually between 2.5 and 18 MHz, depending on the targeted application. This range of frequencies is much higher than the audible range of frequencies (20–20,000 Hz). If plotted, an US wave is a sinusoidal curve, where the Y-axis represents pressure and the X-axis indicates time, with alternating positive and negative peaks (representing compression and rarefaction, respectively). Four principle characteristics govern an US wave: (a) **wavelength** (λ) being defined as the distance in meters between two corresponding points of adjacent curves of the sinusoidal curve, (b) **period** (T) representing the amount of time needed for a single cycle to be completed, (c) **frequency** (f) being the number of cycles per unit of time, and (d) **amplitude** which is the amount of pressure found between the line of zero and a maximum (positive or negative) peak. Frequency and period are associated with the equation $f = 1/T$ or $T = 1/f$ (Merritt 2018; Fulgham 2013).

The US transducer is an electronic device where US waves are generated and emitted. US waves are produced according to the **piezoelectric effect**. An alternating current is applied to piezoelectric crystals within the transducer, allowing them to alternatively expand and contract. This continuous change in the crystal's shape is responsible for the production of US waves (Mason 1981). Ultrasound waves can travel through solid or liquid materials but not air; the existence of a "coupling medium" is needed between the transducer and the skin of the patient, usually with a gel. US waves emitted by the transducer travel the transducer's direction (**longitudinal waves**) and are at least partially reflected in the contrary direction (back towards the transducer). **Transverse** waves are generated when US wave encounters tissues and travels on a direction perpendicular to that of the original beam. Longitudinal waves are exploited for the grayscale and Doppler techniques, while the transverse waves are used in shear wave elastog-

raphy. The **velocity** (v) of the US beam is proportional to tissue stiffness and density but also depends on the beam's characteristics based on the equation $v = f\lambda$. The velocity of US inside the body may vary slightly with the different tissues, but it is generally regarded as a constant: 1540 m/s. The display of tissues exhibiting significantly different values of velocity may lead to artifacts as the device considers that they travel with the average velocity. As a result, the visualization of structures deeper than they really are is called the **misregistration** artifact. Wavelength (λ) is a key factor of spatial resolution and as previously shown is inversely related to frequency ($\lambda = v/f$). As a consequence, as the frequency drops from 10 to 1 MHz, the wavelength increases from 0.15 to 1.5 mm. For this reason different frequency transducers are selected for abdominal (lower frequencies) and superficial applications (higher frequencies). When the US waves reflected (or echoes) by the tissues reach the transducer, the piezoelectric effect is again used and these waves are converted to electricity, which in turn is used to generate the image displayed on the screen (Merritt 2018; Fulgham 2013).

With this "bidirectional" nature of the piezoelectric effect, the transducer acts both as a sender and as a receiver of ultrasound waves. In the majority of US modes, 2–4 ultrasound waves are successively emitted at a time (forming an ultrasonographic **pulse**). Once the pulse leaves the transducer, the latter then remains silent in order to receive the reflected waves. In fact, the transducer acts as a receiver for more than 99% of an US examination time. The frequency with which pulses are emitted constitutes an essential parameter of US imaging, the **pulse repetition frequency** (PRF). Given that the velocity of US inside the body is assumed to be constant, the US device has the opportunity to time each pulse from transmission to reception and thus calculate the distance of any object reflecting the waves. This method of distance calculation is called the **echo ranging** and this mode of US function is termed the **pulsed-wave US**.

For an US wave to be reflected, a reflecting interface must be encountered within the tissues examined. The term "reflecting interface" or "acoustic interface" describes the junction surface of two materials or tissues with different acoustic impedance. Such interfaces reflect variable proportions of an US pulse (the **backscatter**) and generate variable intensities on grayscale imaging. If a wave travels through a perfectly homogeneous material containing no interfaces (or reflectors), then this material appears **anechoic** or cystic. The acoustic impedance (Z) of a particular tissue is calculated by the eq. $Z = \rho v$, where ρ is the density of the medium and v the velocity of sound. The higher the difference in acoustic impedance in two tissues forming an interface, the higher the backscatter (for example in a junction of muscle and bone) and the brighter the pixel on screen. In interfaces with lower difference of acoustic impedance, only a small part of the beam is reflected backwards and a lot of sound energy continues forward.

Tissues cause a series of alterations in the emitted US wave including loss of energy, change of direction, and change of frequency. The term **attenuation** is used to describe the loss of kinetic energy of an US wave interacting with tissues. Different types of tissue cause different attenuations to the US beam. For example, muscle causes higher attenuation compared with water and thus US waves travel easier through water than muscle. Attenuation occurs with three mechanisms: absorption, scattering, and reflection. **Absorption** occurs when the mechanical kinetic energy carried with US waves is converted to heat within the tissue. The higher the wave's frequency, the more rapidly the wave is attenuated, which is another reason why low frequencies travel deeper inside the body and are used in liver US. Compensation for the attenuation exhibited by US waves reaching deeper parts of liver can be achieved with increasing gain settings and by using a lower frequency. **Refraction** is the interaction of an US wave with an acoustic interface, which it hits at an angle different than 90°, with part of the wave being reflected backwards at an identical angle and part being transmitted through the interface and at a different angle. Refraction is minimal when the insonation angle is 90° and then the risk for artifacts is minimal. Regarding

reflection, two types of reflectors exist: the specular and the diffuse reflectors. **Specular reflectors** are large and smooth interfaces reflecting echoes to the transducer like a mirror but only when hit by the US beam in a 90° angle (**angle of insonation**). Examples of specular reflectors are the vascular wall and the diaphragm. **Diffuse reflectors** are much more widespread inside the body and are small interfaces with dimension smaller than the US wave's wavelength, thus scattering echoes towards every direction (and not exclusively back towards the transducer). This type of reflectors account for the echogenicity pattern encountered within the parenchyma of solid organs (liver, spleen, and kidney) (Merritt 2018; Fulgham 2013).

1.2 Artifacts Associated with Ultrasound

The interaction of tissue with the ultrasonic waves results in changes in the wave's characteristics, which are predefined and, in some cases, assumed as constants by the US device for the purpose of forming the image. When some of the assumptions made by the device are significantly different from what happens to the wave, then artifacts occur.

The "**increased through transmission**" occurs when the US wave traverses a fluid-filled cystic structure, causing only minimal attenuation. Consequently, echoes returning from the tissues lying deeper to a cyst have greater amplitude than those returning from the adjacent hepatic parenchyma. This artifact is useful in confirming the cystic nature of a liver lesion and can be mitigated with adjusting time-gain compensation. The term "**acoustic shadowing**" refers to the strong attenuation of US wave reaching a strongly reflecting and absorbing acoustic interface, deep to which an anechoic shadow will appear. This is the case with calcifications of the liver parenchyma and gallstones. Since information lying behind the reflecting surface is lost, a spherical structure (gallstone) may appear crescent shaped and accurate measurements may not be possible. Changing the direction of the transducer and thus angle of insonation may enable visualization of part of the hidden area. This problem can be mitigated by **spatial compounding**, another useful technique, where several overlapping scans are acquired of the same object but from different viewing angles. This technique results in improved image quality and better contrast-to-noise ratio and reduces the extent of acoustic shadowing (completely eliminating it for small-sized and fine calcifications). The **edging artifact** occurs when sound waves are reflected away of the transducer by a curved surface due to the insonation angle used. As a result, information is lost along a line lying behind the rounded surface. In liver imaging, this artifact can be found in the upper pole of the right kidney causing a deep-situated linear shadow. When an ultrasound wave is "trapped," bouncing back and forth between at least two reflective interfaces, the **reverberation artifact** is created. The first echo reflected by the interface creates a bright area of pixels. The successive echoes arrive with a delay (interpreted by the device as deeper in location)

but also attenuated due to longer transmission through tissue (and thus visualized with lesser brightness). As a result, the reverberation artifact is visualized by a number of successive echoes lying in increasing depth and with decreasing brightness. Changing the transducer's position or angle of insonation may alleviate this artifact. A special form of reverberation is the so-called comet-tail artifact which occurs when the US beam hits a small but highly reflective object. This artifact appears as a triangular echogenic tail situated deep to a hyperechoic focus and is characteristically associated with gallbladder adenomyomatosis where cholesterol crystals deposited within the Rokitansky-Aschoff sinuses are responsible for the generation of this artifact. Except for adenomyomatosis, the "comet-tail artifact" has also been associated with other benign conditions of the gallbladder such as chronic cholecystitis, xanthogranulomatous cholecystitis, and cholesterolosis (Fig. 1) (Oh et al. 2018). The **refraction artifact** is caused by the refraction of the ultrasonographic beam and leads

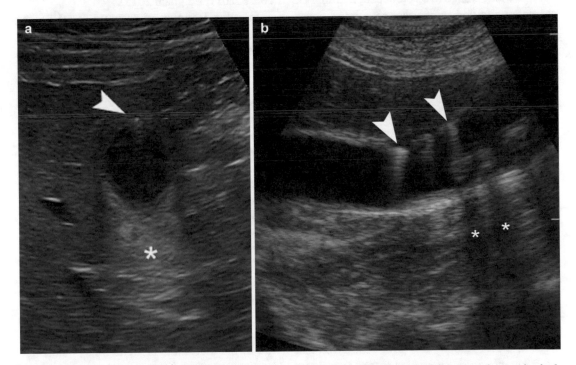

Fig. 1 Examples of the comet-tail artifact (arrowheads) in two cases of gallbladder adenomyomatosis. Note the increased through transmission of the ultrasound beam deep to the gallbladder (asterisk in **a**) and acoustic shadowing caused by gallstones (asterisks in **b**)

to the false visualization of an object at a location different from the true. If part of the beam is oriented perpendicular to the object and a different part detects it after being refracted, then two images of the same object will be displayed (Merritt 2018; Fulgham 2013).

1.3 Grayscale Imaging

The signals received by the US device can be visualized in a number of ways. **A-mode**, the first technique introduced, is derived from amplitude and this technique simply produces a line representing the amplitude of the returning echoes in relation to time (and thus distance). In the **M-mode** (motion Mode) technique, the device displays the amplitude of returning echoes over time and thus visualizes moving reflectors. The mainstay of liver US is real-time grayscale **B-mode** (brightness mode or simply grayscale) technique. In this technique every pixel's brightness represents the amplitude of reflected signals. For a B-mode image to be produced, multiple US pulses are emitted in adjacent scan lines, covering the full length of the transducer's surface and producing a two-dimensional image. The higher the brightness on grayscale technique, the stronger the reflectivity of the underlying structure and current US devices may attribute up to 256 different shades of gray to tissue. The image is refreshed with a frame rate ranging from 15 to 40 frames/s, hence creating a real-time sense.

1.4 Doppler US

Doppler US enables visualization and quantification of blood flow in real time. The **Doppler effect** (named after the Austrian mathematician and physicist Christian Andreas Doppler) constitutes the basic principle governing Doppler technique. According to this effect, the frequency of the sound wave reflected by a moving object depends on its velocity and direction. Given that the frequency initially emitted by the transducer is known and defined at the beginning of the examination, the **shift in frequency** (Δf) caused

by a moving particle depends on the particle's velocity. If the reflector is static, the returning frequency is the same with the emitted and thus the Δf is zero. If the reflector travels towards the transducer, the frequency reflected is higher, whereas the opposite happens when the reflector travels away of the transducer. This frequency shift can be readily detected and measured by the transducer. However, it is dependent on the angle created by the directions of the transducer and the moving object (**the Doppler angle or θ**). When the two directions are identical ($\theta = 0°$), the Doppler frequency shift is maximal, while it is zero when the transducer is oriented perpendicular to the moving particle ($\theta = 90°$). As a result, the accuracy of Δf measurement and thus velocity estimation strongly depends on the Doppler angle. The equation attributed to Δf is $\Delta F = F_R - F_T = (2 \times v \times \cos\theta)/C$ where F_R is the reflected frequency, F_T the transmitted frequency, v the blood velocity, C the speed of sound in soft tissue (1540 m/s), and θ the Doppler angle of insonation (Merritt 2018; McNaughton and Abu-Yousef 2011; Fulgham 2013).

In **color Doppler ultrasound (CDUS)**, the frequency shifts detected within the imaging plane are visualized on a color map inside a box placed in the area of interest. The speed of blood flow is represented by the color's brightness while different colors are used to demonstrate the blood flow's direction. As a general principle, blue codes motion away from the transducer, while red demonstrates motion towards the transducer and the brighter the color, the greater the velocity. In liver imaging, this can be demonstrated in CDUS of portal vein and hepatic artery. Under normal conditions, these should have the same color, although the latter exhibits pulsatility. In portal hypertension though, retrograde flow may be recorded in the portal vein. Accurate investigation of blood flow characteristics requires proper angle of insonation; it is essential that the Doppler angle is ≤60°. This can be achieved either by manually changing the position of the transducer or by digitally "steering" the direction of the US pulse and thus achieving a correct Doppler angle (McNaughton and Abu-Yousef 2011).

In **power Doppler ultrasound (PDUS)**, the US device examines only the amplitude of frequency shift and attributes a color. Even though this mode does not provide information about velocity or flow direction, it is independent to the Doppler angle in comparison with CDUS. The main advantage of PDUS is the improved sensitivity to the detection of blood flow, even slow flow (Rubin et al. 1994).

Color Doppler ultrasound with spectral display (also referred to as pulsed-wave Doppler technique, spectral Doppler, spectral analysis, color duplex or triplex scan) is the mode combining the color information provided by CDUS with the display of a waveform characterizing a specific area of interrogation. This mode is valuable in assessing portal vein and hepatic artery hemodynamics. The term pulsed-wave Doppler has been described in contrast to the continuous-wave Doppler, which is a non-imaging technique employing two transducers continuously emitting and receiving US waves (one exclusively emitting and one receiving). The main disadvantage of continuous-wave Doppler is that it lacks discrimination of motion originating from different depths and cannot detect the source of a signal. **Hemodynamic parameters** usually assessed with spectral analysis include the peak systolic velocity (PSV), end diastolic velocity (EDV), pulsatility index (PI), and resistive index (RI). The RI is defined by the equation (PSV-EDV)/PSV and the PI (PSV-EDV)/mean velocity. It should be noted that the PI of the portal vein is calculated differently, with the simple ratio of EDV/PSV (McNaughton and Abu-Yousef 2011; Merritt 2018; Fulgham 2013).

CDUS is valuable in liver imaging as it is used for evaluation of native liver blood vessels, transjugular intrahepatic portosystemic shunts (TIPS), and vasculature of the transplanted liver. Physicians performing US of the liver should be familiarized with normal and abnormal waveforms encountered in liver normal and abnormal vasculature. Fortunately, normal waveforms in liver have typical appearances and most liver conditions cause only a few characteristic waveform patterns. When it comes to the assessment of hepatic vessel waveforms the following terms

can be used: (a) **pulsatile** flow referring to a waveform with abrupt increase of velocity in systole and gradual decrease in diastole, (b) **phasic** flow which shows gradual alterations (increases and decreases) in blood velocity, (c) **non-phasic** when there is a continuous flow with more or less a constant velocity, and (d) **aphasic** when there is no flow. Pulsatile flow is typical for arteries or abnormal veins, phasic flow is observed in normal veins, non-phasic flow is seen in abnormal veins, and aphasic flow is seen in occluded vessels (McNaughton and Abu-Yousef 2011).

Three vascular structures should be examined in a Doppler examination of the liver: the portal vein, the hepatic artery, and the hepatic veins. The location of each vessel (being systemic arterial, venous, or portal venous) and the pressure alterations generated by the heart create the characteristic waveforms recorded in each case.

The **hepatic artery** (Fig. 2) is normally a low-resistance artery with a pulsatile arterial waveform, characterized by an RI normally ranging from 0.55 to 0.7, but may be normal at 0.81 (McNaughton and Abu-Yousef 2011). Values outside this range should be interpreted as abnormal, suggestive of disease. In general, a very low RI of the hepatic artery may be the result of either proximal stenosis (e.g., arterial anastomosis in a liver transplantation or atherosclerosis of native hepatic artery) or vascular shunting in severe cirrhosis with portal hypertension, trauma, or Osler-Weber-Rendu syndrome. A high RI cannot be readily interpreted as this is nonspecific and found in many conditions including the postprandial state, advanced age, distal microvascular disease, chronic hepatocellular disease, hepatic venous congestion, cold ischemia posttransplantation, and any stage of transplant rejection. Furthermore cirrhosis affects the arteries of the liver in a complicated way, with unpredictable measured RI. Consequently, the RI of the hepatic artery cannot be used alone to diagnose or grade cirrhosis. Doppler spectral broadening is a normal finding when interrogating the hepatic artery due to the small diameter of this vessel and the "dragging" effect the wall exerts on the peripherally moving red blood cells, moving with a slower velocity. The **tardus-parvus** waveform

Fig. 2 Normal
waveform recorded in
the hepatic artery

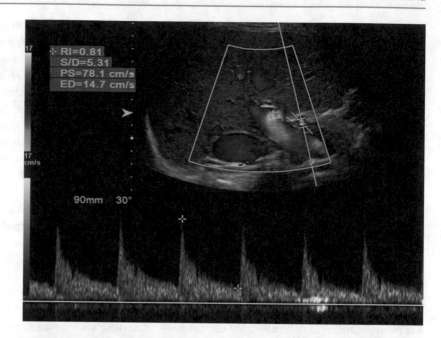

Fig. 3 Normal
waveform recorded in
the portal vein

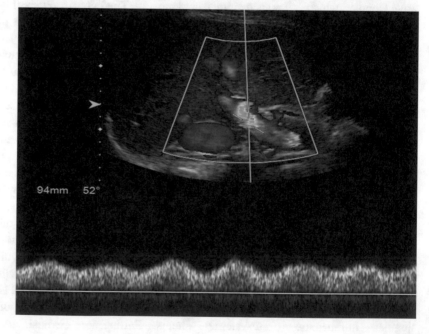

is characterized by a low RI and subjectively a prolonged and low peak during systole, seen in the hepatic artery when a more proximal part of the vessel is stenotic (McNaughton and Abu-Yousef 2011).

The **portal vein** (Fig. 3) exhibits a waveform which is always antegrade (or hepatopetal) and phasic (with one phase towards the liver) with gentle undulations of the velocity recorded. The velocity of the portal vein is relatively low (16–40 cm/s) and the PI (defined as PSV/EDV in the case of the portal vein) should be higher than 0.5. Retrograde flow in the portal vein is an abnormal finding, termed hepatofugal. Causes of pulsatility in the portal vein include tricuspid regurgitation, right-sided chronic heart failure, cirrhosis with arterio-portal shunting, and hereditary hemor-rhagic telangiectasia. Portal vein Doppler inter-rogation that should point towards portal hypertension includes low portal vein velocity (<16 cm/s), hepatofugal flow, open portosystemic shunts (umbilical vein), and increased diameter of the portal vein. Absent flow is recorded in cases of stagnant flow due to severe portal hyper-tension, or portal vein thrombosis (either bland or malignant thrombus) causing complete occlusion of the lumen. Some blood flow signals will be appreciable in case of incomplete thrombosis. Clues for differential diagnosis of bland and malignant portal vein thrombosis can be found in Table 1.

The hepatic vein (Fig. 4) shows an antegrade flow (towards the cardiac chambers), with phasic alterations of the waveform and two or three dis-tinct phases (changes in flow direction above and below the baseline) making the waveform resem-ble the letter "W." These changes in flow direc-tion are caused by the pressure alteration within the cardiac chambers during systole and diastole. Pulsatile flow can be encountered in the hepatic veins in case of tricuspid regurgitation, or right-sided chronic heart failure. Decreased phasicity in the hepatic veins can be seen in hepatic vein thrombosis (Budd-Chiari syndrome) and hepatic veno-occlusive disease or obstruction of the hepatic veins of any cause. No flow (aphasic

Table 1 US findings helping differentiate bland and malignant portal vein thrombosis

Parameter	Bland thrombus	Neoplastic thrombus	Comment
Echogenicity	Echogenic	Echogenic\nPresence of adjacent liver mass	May be anechoic if acute
Portal vein diameter	Increased if acute thrombosis	Usually enlarged but may be normal	Unreliable criterion
Color Doppler	No blood flow signals	In some cases color signals within the thrombus	
Spectral analysis	No flow recorded	Arterial (pulsatile) waveform	
Collateral vessels	Seen in chronic occlusion	Less frequently seen	Also termed "cavernous transformation" and takes months to years to develop

Fig. 4 Normal waveform recorded in the hepatic vein

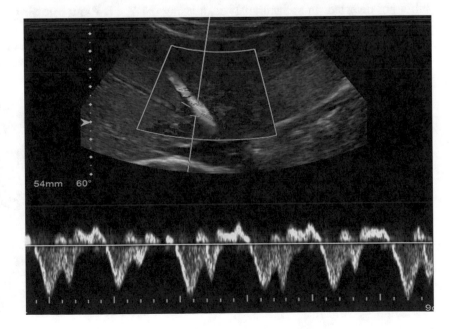

waveform) is seen in thrombosis, although Budd-Chiari syndrome may also present with partial (incomplete) obstruction and reduced phasicity or turbulence at the point of stenosis (McNaughton and Abu-Yousef 2011).

1.5 Artifacts Associated with Doppler US

The **twinkle artifact** (Fig. 5) is a characteristic artifact occurring when an US pulse encounters a highly reflective surface and the color Doppler mode is active. The distortion of the US wave returning to the transducer is interpreted by the device as motion deep to the reflecting surface. In liver US, the twinkle artifact can be appreciated with gallstones or hepatic parenchyma calcifications, although not every calcification causes this type of artifact.

Aliasing is another crucial artifact commonly encountered with CDUS and spectral analysis. It is caused by a low frequency of successive pulse generation (insufficient PRF) which fails to detect blood movement with high velocity. As a rule of thumb, aliasing happens when the PRF is less than twice the shifted Doppler frequency. Aliasing appears on CDUS as turbulence (color mosaic) in the area containing the frequency shifts not detected. In spectral analysis, aliasing appears with truncation of the PSV and projection of this frequency shifts below the baseline. Aliasing phenomenon can be readily addressed

by the following ways: (a) increasing the PRF, (b) increasing the Doppler angle of insonation, (c) decreasing the frequency of the emitted US wave, or (d) digitally lowering the baseline of the displayed waveform. **Blooming artifact** (or color bleed artifact) occurs when color blood flow signal is falsely visualized outside the vascular lumen and specifically extending outside the true boundaries of blood vessels. It is usually caused by inappropriately high color gain and may hide a hepatic artery lying adjacent to the portal vein (Merritt 2018; Fulgham 2013).

1.6 Tissue Harmonic Imaging

Tissues in the human body may reflect the emitted US wave in a nonlinear pattern, thus producing frequencies different from those emitted, which are called the harmonics and are characterized by greater frequency (double, triple of fundamental, etc.), lower amplitude, and less noise. As a result, if the transducer and the device are adjusted to selectively display harmonic frequencies, it is possible to achieve less artifacts and improved resolution and image quality (Merritt 2018; Fulgham 2013).

1.7 B-Flow Imaging

B-Flow™ (GE Healthcare) is a blood flow visualization technique marketed by a specific manu-

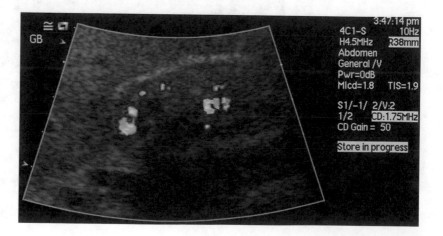

Fig. 5 Twinkle artifact observed on a color Doppler image of a gallbladder containing gallstones

facturer which has the capability to display blood flow echoes in grayscale mode as a non-Doppler technique. The intensity of grayscale echoes depends on the reflector (red blood cells) speed and dynamics. Beyond visualizing blood flow with improved sensitivity and in real time, B-Flow is able to digitally suppress static tissue and noise in order to improve image quality. Compared with conventional color Doppler technique, B-Flow is independent of Doppler angle and overwriting artifact and achieves higher frame rate and spatial resolution. Doppler technique applies a high-pass filter in order to suppress frequency shifts of low amplitude which are caused by physiologic movements of the imaged tissue. Although this improves image quality, it also leads to obliteration of Doppler shifts generated by slowly flowing blood and as a consequence limits the technique's sensitivity. This is not applicable to B-Flow technique which can adequately depict slow flow within a partially thrombosed portal vein or hepatic artery (Wachsberg 2007). The technique's inherent advantages also render it valuable for evaluation of transjugular intrahepatic portosystemic shunt (TIPS) function where conventional color Doppler technique may provide misleading findings because of its inherent limitations and artifacts.

2 CEUS

2.1 Introduction

The introduction of microbubbles as ultrasonographic contrast agents has rendered contrast-enhanced ultrasound (CEUS) a valuable complementary ultrasonographic technique for the evaluation of hepatic parenchyma microvasculature, with contrast agents and contrast-specific imaging modes widely available (Claudon et al. 2008). The interaction of the ultrasound beam with microbubbles and the post-processing of the US device allows the CEUS examination to depict micro- and macro-vascularity accurately.

CEUS offers the possibility to assess the perfusion pattern of a focal liver lesion in all vascular phases including the arterial, venous, and delayed phase. Although this can also be achieved with computed tomography (CT) and magnetic resonance (MR) imaging, CEUS is superior with real-time assessment of vascularity, potential of continuous scanning for >3 min, not feasible with CT where the evaluation is limited in three or four acquisitions and MR where more images can be obtained but only slower real-time scanning is possible. The CEUS real-time capability is particularly valuable for evaluation of early arterial enhancement. A limitation of CEUS is that it can only assess a single lesion during the examination compared with the global imaging of CT and MR (Claudon et al. 2013).

2.2 Physical Principles of CEUS

The advantages of CEUS stem from the characteristics of the ultrasonographic contrast agents (UCA). These agents consist of microbubbles with a mean diameter of 2.5 μm (99% measure <11 μm). This is slightly smaller or equal to that of a red blood cell and hence the microbubble cannot traverse the vascular endothelium, ensuring that the microbubble is strictly a blood pool contrast agent, a valuable intravascular "tracer," accounting for the excellent contrast resolution between static tissue and micro- and macro-vasculature (Cosgrove and Harvey 2009), and remains intravascular throughout the examination. Contrast agents used in CT and MR imaging diffuse into the interstitium which may obscure "washout" from a tumor in the portal and late venous phase (Wilson et al. 2007).

2.3 Nonlinear Imaging

Contrast-specific US imaging techniques, a prerequisite for a CEUS examination, cancel the linear US signals originating from static tissue and exploit the nonlinear US signals originating from the microbubbles. This produces images exclusively visualizing the microbubbles (Claudon et al. 2008). Static tissues tend to reflect the ultrasound beam and receive the reflected sound wave at the same frequency as that initially emitted. Microbubbles demonstrate a nonlinear response through two mechanisms, (a) perform a stable nonlinear oscillation at low acoustic pressure and (b) perform a more intense oscillation in multiple axes, and are disrupted with higher acoustic pressures resulting in a nonlinear response including a range of different frequencies. When exposed to the US beam, microbubbles act as resonant scatterers, oscillating in a nonlinear pattern, and produce harmonic frequencies, increasing the backscatter signal by up to 30 dB. Currently, low acoustic pressure constitutes the standard method of imaging with CEUS. Although static tissues primarily generate linear signals, nonlinear harmonic signals may also be produced following distortion of US beam during propagation. These nonlinear harmonic signals are adverse, interfering with signals produced by microbubbles, and influence the image quality. These signals tend to increase with increasing mechanical index (MI), which is an indicator of acoustic pressure. The MI represents an estimation of the maximum amplitude of the pressure pulse exerted on tissues and thus the acoustic pressure of the ultrasound beam or the power of the system. The MI can be calculated as the PNP (peak negative pressure of the ultrasound beam in MPa and derated for modeled attenuation) divided by the squared root of F_c (central frequency of the ultrasound wave in MHz) (Claudon et al. 2013). Given that microbubbles are disrupted by high-MI US beams and static tissues respond nonlinearly, CEUS currently is performed using the low-MI technique. An MI value can be generally characterized as low when lower than 0.3, although currently available US devices can achieve MI as low as 0.05. If cancellation of static tissue signals is successfully performed, the initial image prior to the administration of microbubbles should be completely black. Nonetheless, heavily reflecting structures such as large blood vessels and diaphragm are still visible due to incomplete cancellation. Although this is inadvertent, it can be useful for orientation. Dual-display imaging is also useful in this respect with a low-MI gray-scale image being displayed in one half of the image and the CEUS image being displayed in the other half. Although the low-MI grayscale image lacks the quality of normal MI grayscale image, it is sufficient for orientation purposes (Claudon et al. 2013).

2.4 Harmonic Imaging

In the early clinical applications of CEUS development, microbubbles were visualized using the conventional grayscale imaging or color Doppler technique and the increase of blood echogenicity or color signals caused were interpreted. This technique was not able to evaluate the tissue perfusion and microvascularity, and was essentially a "Doppler rescue" tool. When microbubbles oscillate in a nonlinear fashion, they tend to expand more than they contract, resulting in ultrasound reflection of both the fundamental (emitted) frequency and additional subharmonic frequencies (higher and lower). These frequencies can be successfully detected and visualized using harmonic ultrasound imaging. With the introduction of pulse-inversion harmonic imaging, exploitation of the different frequencies generated by the microbubbles and static tissues achieves exclusive visualization of the microbubble, suppressing signals from tissue. The transducer emits a sequence of two pulses in rapid succession, which are identical in frequency and amplitude but the second is 180° out of phase compared to the first (an inverted copy of the first). As a consequence, static tissues reflect the same frequencies which are cancelled but when these two pulses hit microbubbles, the generated harmonic frequencies are added to produce a strong harmonic signal detectable by the transducer. Pulse-inversion technique is the basis of most contrast-specific methods used currently (Fig. 6). Amplitude and phase modulation CEUS technique represents another technique, a variation of the pulse-inversion technique, where the transducer emits a series of pulses with different strengths, with linearly reflected signals from static tissues cancelled while signals generated by the microbubbles are selectively visualized

Pulse-inversion imaging

Low MI Imaging

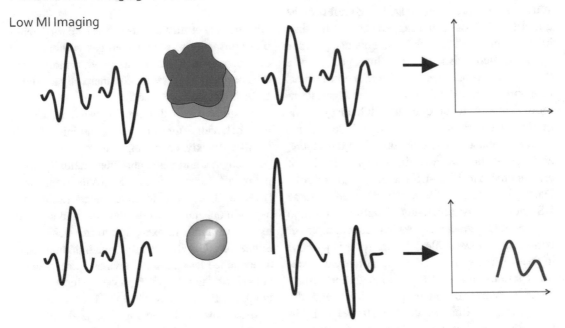

Fig. 6 Diagrammatic representation of low MI, pulse inversion CEUS technique. Two US pulses equal in amplitude but with 180° difference in phase are initially emitted (left hand of the image). Static tissue (orange color) reflects the same pulses which are thus cancelled (right hand of the image). Microbubbles (blue color) generate harmonic frequencies which can thus be selectively detected by the transducer

(Eckersley et al. 2005; Piscaglia et al. 2012; Forsberg et al. 1994; Dietrich et al. 2011; Forsberg et al. 2007; Forsberg et al. 1996). In temporal maximum intensity projection imaging (MIP), similarly to CT, the ultrasound scanner records bright echoes for a selected time period and aggregates them to produce detailed images of the macro- and microvasculature. This type of imaging starts with a high-MI flash which disrupts all the microbubbles and erases the image. Every microbubble appearing in-plane after that point is recorded and its signal added to the image.

CEUS with low-MI technique can adequately assess lesions lying up to 12–15 cm in depth, depending on machine's capabilities, patient body habitus, and underlying liver parenchyma (cirrhosis or fatty infiltration). Increasing MI, lowering emitted frequency, or using lower frequency transducers are beneficial in cases of deep lesions, although at the expense of increased microbubble disruption, especially in the near field. In general, the amplitude or power modulation technique offers better depth penetration but lower spatial resolution as compared to pulse-inversion technique (Dietrich et al. 2018). The reflected signal's intensity depends on two factors: (a) the concentration of microbubbles in the scanned area and (b) the frequency of the ultrasound beam. One useful coincidence is that commercially marketed UCA has a frequency of optimal oscillation at approximately 3 MHz, a frequency commonly used in abdominal examinations including the liver. This is the reason why only a small dose of microbubbles can achieve such an intense enhancement of the liver and an optimal signal-to-noise ratio. As with the propagation of ultrasound in other tissues, the interface formed by the microbubble's surface and the surrounding aqueous medium functions as a reflector of the ultrasound beam. This reflection results in the enhancement of blood echogenicity and the improved contrast between the blood and surrounding tissues.

The term dynamic contrast-enhanced ultrasound (also abbreviated as DCE-US) refers to the quantification of enhancement using the time intensity curve (TIC) analysis. This analysis can be performed either after a bolus injection of a dose of microbubbles or with the intravenous infusion of microbubbles and the disruption-replenishment technique. In TIC analysis the quantitative parameters assessed include the time to peak enhancement duration of enhancement, and wash-in and washout times. Quantification of enhancement in DCE-US needs specialized software which can be found incorporated in some US devices. Alternatively, VueBox® (Bracco Suisse SA, Suisse) represents an example of commercially available software for this purpose in the off-line setting. DCE-US primary applications include the evaluation of a tumor's treatment response in oncologic patients and the evaluation of inflammation in bowel wall in patients with inflammatory bowel disease (Dietrich et al. 2018; Lassau et al. 2011; Tranquart et al. 2012; Hudson et al. 2009).

2.5 US Contrast Agents

Ultrasound contrast agents (UCA) are microbubbles consisting of a contained gas within a shell of either protein (albumin) or phospholipid. A summary of the currently commercially available UCA is detailed in Table 2.

Despite small differences between UCAs, their behavior after intravenous administration is similar, quickly enhancing the arteries, hepatic parenchyma, and veins and then gradually dissipating after some minutes. SonoVue®/Lumason® (Bracco SpA) is able to enhance tissues for 3–8 min depending on the duration and continuity of scanning. An exception to this behavior is Sonazoid® (GE Healthcare), which demonstrates an extended late phase, known as "post-vascular phase" or "the Kupffer phase." This phase is unique in that it starts when the UCA disappears from the vascular bed and is visualized within the hepatic and splenic parenchyma, having been phagocytosed by Kupffer cells (Strobel et al. 2005; Dietrich et al. 2018).

Table 2 Currently commercially available UCA

Agent	Company	Outer shell	Inner gas	Approved indications	Countries licensed
SonoVue®/ Lumason®	Bracco Imaging SpA, Milan, Italy	Lipid	Sulfur hexafluoride	Left ventricle opacification/ endocardial border definition in echocardiography Diagnostic assessment of macrovasculature including extracranial carotid and peripheral arteries Diagnostic assessment of microvasculature in liver and breast lesions (also for pediatric use in liver assessment) US of the excretory urinary tract in pediatric patients for detection of vesicoureteral reflux	EU, Norway, Switzerland, China, Singapore, Hong Kong, South Korea, Iceland, India USA (Lumason®)
Sonazoid®	GE Healthcare	Lipid	Perflubutane	Liver Breast	Japan, South Korea, Norway
Definity®/ Luminity®	Lantheus Medical Imaging	Lipid	Perflutren	Left ventricle opacification/ endocardial border definition in echocardiography Liver Kidney Diagnostic assessment of vessels	USA, Canada, Europe, Australia, parts of Asia
Optison®	GE Healthcare	Albumin	Perflutren	Left ventricle opacification/ endocardial border definition in echocardiography	USA, Europe

2.6 Tips for Reporting and Performing CEUS

When reporting a CEUS examination of the liver, it is important to comment on the degree of enhancement and the timing (phase) of enhancement. The terms "hyperenhancing," "isoenhancing," and "hypoenhancing" can be used to describe a lesion with higher, equal, or lower enhancement compared with adjacent liver parenchyma, respectively. The term "non-enhancing" can be attributed to a lesion that exhibits no enhancement such as a simple cyst. A description of the enhancement pattern should be made for all phases of enhancement (arterial, portal venous, and late phases). If the agent Sonazoid® is used a description should also be included for the postvascular phase. The term "wash-in" refers to the period starting from the arrival of microbubbles in the field of examination and lasts up to the time point of maximum enhancement of the lesion under examination. The term "wash-in" can be used both in qualitative characterization of enhancement in routine reports and in quantitative analysis of enhancement using specialized software. "Peak enhancement" refers to the maximum enhancement observed and "washout phase" corresponds to the period of gradually decreasing enhancement starting right after the point of peak enhancement. The pattern of enhancement should be characterized in terms of timing (as quick or slow) and in terms of quality (homogenous or heterogeneous and centripetal or centrifugal) (Fig. 7).

Prior to the administration of microbubbles it is crucial to decide which is the best position of

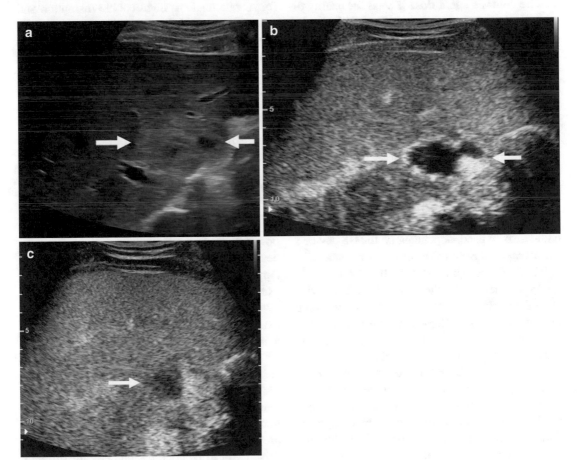

Fig. 7 Liver hemangioma (arrows) appearing hyperechoic on grayscale US (**a**) and demonstrating early peripheral nodular enhancement on CEUS (**b**) and gradual centripetal filling over time (**c**)

the patient both for patient convenience and for optimal lesion visualization. Secondly, it is important to decide whether the lesion should be scanned on a transverse or longitudinal plane given the displacement of the lesion with respiratory movements. Quiet breathing or suspension in neutral position may be a better choice compared with full inspiration when it comes to CEUS examination.

An adequately sized intravenous **catheter** (usually 20 gauge) should be placed, usually in an antecubital vein, in order to minimize microbubble disruption during administration. Central lines and port systems can also be used if there is no filter but careful evaluation is required as the contrast arrival time will be shortened (Eisenbrey et al. 2015). The agent should be administered at 1–2 mL/s and followed by 10 mL saline flush.

The contrast agent **dose** is vital for quality of examination. A lower dose will result in inadequate enhancement of organs in the late phase and nondiagnostic examinations for the assessment of washout. Excessively high doses of microbubbles will result in artifacts such as acoustic shadowing and signal saturation hindering quantification. A second dose of UCA can be administered if needed, for instance if more than one focal liver lesion needs to be characterized. In this case, a period of 10–15 min is needed for the disappearance of the initial dose of microbubbles. For SonoVue®/Lumason® 2.4 mL (half the commercially available vial) although 1.2 mL could also be used, depending on the US device's sensitivity. For Sonazoid® the recommended dose is 0.015 mL/kg (approximately 0.5–1 mL).

As a general rule, the **focus** of the US device should be placed just deep to the lesion being investigated in order to achieve uniform acoustic field, improved sensitivity to microbubbles, and lower disruption rate (Dietrich et al. 2018).

The **gain** is adjusted in order to achieve optimal image quality; this should be set slightly above the noise threshold, so that the image prior to the administration of microbubbles appears dark with only minimal noise. Setting the gain too low would cause not detecting some microbubble signals while setting it too high would lead to signal saturation and thus nonvisualization of part of the microbubbles due to

clipping of echoes above certain amplitude (Dietrich et al. 2018).

The **dynamic range** (also known as compression) of the US device corresponds to the range of different signal intensities that can be displayed. In other words, a wide dynamic range results in more gray levels being visualized and hence better differentiation of different degrees of enhancement. A small dynamic range is adequate if very low signal is expected but a wide dynamic range should be opted for in case of quantification analysis, in order to avoid signal saturation (Dietrich et al. 2018).

The **frame rate** is important as some highly vascularized lesions may exhibit a wash-in rate of only a second, and an adequately high frame rate (at least 15 frames/s) should be set prior to the administration of UCA. However, increased frame rate leads to microbubble disruption and cannot be applied for the entire duration of the examination. As a consequence, a high frame rate can be used in the first part of the examination (evaluation of arterial phase) and then the frame rate can be lowered in the rest of the examination to prevent disruption of microbubbles and achieve longer enhancement time (Dietrich et al. 2018; Greis 2014).

2.7 Artifacts in CEUS

CEUS has some artifacts which may lead to diagnostic errors and misinterpretation, with awareness of these artifacts allowing avoidance. Appropriate setting of the US device prior to the examination is crucial to avoid these artifacts. Two major sources of artifacts during CEUS examinations are inappropriately high MI and gain (Claudon et al. 2013; Dietrich et al. 2011).

The nonlinear propagation artifact or pseudoenhancement occurs when the ultrasound wave traverses an area with high concentration of microbubbles and exhibits nonlinear propagation. This effect generates echoes similar to those produced by microbubbles. Differentiation of these two can be done by realizing the different nature of artifactual echoes, or by identifying those bright areas in the low-MI grayscale image. This artifact can be mitigated if a lower dose of

UCA is used or by avoiding scanning on a plane with a vascular structure lying above the target lesion (Dietrich et al. 2018; Fetzer et al. 2018).

The use of an inappropriately high MI may result in disruption of the microbubble shell. After the shell's destruction, the contained gas diffuses and as a result the UCA no longer reflects the ultrasound wave. This can be caused by continuous and prolonged scanning, as well as a high-MI pulse, perceived as a loss of enhancement over time or at depth of the examined field. This loss of enhancement can be misinterpreted as washout of a malignant tumor, especially if identified in a limited part of the examined field of view. Disruption of microbubbles could also be caused by changing the contrast-specific (low-MI) mode used in a regular (high-MI) grayscale technique for any reason. Normally, once the UCA is administered no changes in the scanning protocol should be made. Care should be taken to minimize disruption of microbubbles by the use an MI as low as possible and tailoring the scanning protocol. An accepted manner to scan a CEUS examination of the liver would be to continuously record a cine loop from the time of injection and up to 60 s (thus recording the complete arterial phase). After this point static images or short cine loops can be recorded with an interval of 30–60 s, in order to thoroughly examine the washout pattern without microbubble disruption (Dietrich et al. 2018). Disruption of microbubbles is prominent in the upper part of the US image (the near field), so loss of enhancement in this area should be expected without optimal scanning conditions. This manifests as a linear area of no (or reduced) enhancement when swiping through the hepatic parenchyma in an area that was previously scanned in a continuous fashion. This results from holding the transducer in the same plane for several minutes, causing focal disruption of microbubbles. Microbubbles in adjacent areas are not insonated and are preserved. If a swiping maneuver is performed for detection of additional washed-out lesions after the initial part of the examination, the area initially scanned will appear hypoechoic (Fetzer et al. 2018).

Aggregation of microbubbles or use of an excessive dose of microbubbles can cause excessive scattering of ultrasound wave and thus acoustic shadowing and obscuration of the far-field area. Consequently the dose of the UCA should be adapted to the patient's body habitus, transducer, frequency used, and clinical indication (Dietrich et al. 2018).

2.8 Safety Profile of UCA

UCAs are safe, and the reported incidence of side effects is low. These agents have no side effects on the liver and kidneys, and are not excreted via the renal pathway, requiring no laboratory test to be performed prior to administration. The incidence of severe hypersensitivity events is lower compared with contrast agents used in CT and comparable with MR agents. In CEUS abdominal applications, life-threatening anaphylactoid reactions have been reported in 0.001% of cases, while no death was recorded in more than 23,000 patients. Allergic reactions with a potential to cause death have been encountered in less than 0.002% of examinations performed (Piscaglia and Bolondi 2006; ter Haar 2009). A series of studies on the safety of UCA with data on more than 6000 patients have shown that headache, nausea, chest pain, and discomfort are the most common adverse reactions encountered, all with frequency of $\leq 2.1\%$. In the majority of cases, adverse reactions resolve spontaneously within a short time interval with no need for treatment. The overall reported mortality rate associated with SonoVue® (Bracco SpA) is low, at 14 deaths in 2,447,083 patients exposed to this agent (0.0006%, the mortality for iodinated contrast is approximately 0.001%), all with an underlying medical condition reported to have played a role in the adverse outcome. The safety of UCA has also been demonstrated in studies with large series of patients examined for cardiologic applications of CEUS (Appis et al. 2015). Deaths in critically ill patients undergoing contrast echocardiographic examinations have been reported but no evidence of causal relationship with microbubbles has been documented (Main et al. 2009).

SonoVue® was initially contraindicated in patients with known right-to-left shunts, unstable coronary syndromes, congestive heart failure, severe pulmonary hypertension, and pregnancy or breast-feeding. Nonetheless, in June 2014 the decision was made to remove the contraindication for patients with recent acute coronary syndrome or clinically unstable ischemic heart disease (Appis et al. 2015). Notwithstanding the excellent safety profile reported for UCA, resuscitation facilities and trained personnel should be readily available in US departments where CEUS is performed.

In theory, it is possible that the interaction of ultrasound beam and microbubbles could generate bio-effects. No clinical evidence is available for any negative effects on the human liver. Studies performed in vitro have shown sonoporation, hemolysis, and cellular death occurring as a consequence of these effects. Experiments in small animal models have shown that disruption on a microvascular level is possible when UCAs are exposed to an ultrasound beam (Skyba et al. 1998). Low MI should be used for CEUS examinations of the liver to prevent these theoretical risks and care should be taken to weigh benefits and risks when using high-MI technique. UCAs should not be administered 24 h prior to a session of extracorporeal shock wave therapy.

CEUS is performed off-label in the pediatric population and in a series of applications apart from liver in the adult population (Sidhu et al. 2018). Nevertheless, the Food and Drug Administration (FDA) has approved the use of Lumason® (equivalent of SonoVue® for USA, Bracco, SpA) for pediatric liver imaging and characterization of focal liver lesion (Sidhu et al. 2018; Lumason 2017).

3 Elastography

3.1 Introduction to Technical Basis of Elastography

In general, the stiffness of any tissue can be measured using some form of elastography, which can be considered a form of digital palpation. A variety of terms can be found in the literature and awareness of the basic terms is desirable. There are elastographic methods using imaging techniques (primarily US and currently MR) and non-imaging techniques. Elastographic techniques not relying on imaging which take measurements of a defined region are usually referred to as "**point elastographic methods.**" The term "**elastometry**" is attributed to the measurement of a characteristic of elasticity of tissue, which can be based both on imaging and non-imaging techniques. The term "**elastogram**" refers to any image presenting information related to any elastic property of tissue (Dietrich et al. 2017). As an umbrella definition, "**elastography**" is a technique which measures and displays the biomechanical properties of tissue related to the elastic restoring forces acting against shear deformation caused by an applied force. This definition can be applied to any form of elastography (Dietrich et al. 2017; Sigrist et al. 2017).

The elastic modulus is a property of materials (or tissues) which describes their stiffness and can be defined as the ratio of the stress and strain (stress/strain) and the corresponding curve calculated during elastic deformation of the tissue. As a result, the higher the elastic modulus, the stiffer the tissue and vice versa. Depending on the variables placed in the elastic modulus equation and the method of deformation, three moduli can be calculated: (a) the elastic modulus or Young's modulus (ratio of longitudinal stress to strain), (b) the shear modulus, and (c) the bulk modulus, with the first being the most commonly used in applications of elastography. All forms of elastography consist of three basic steps: (a) application of stress to tissue, (b) tissue response (strain) measurement, and (c) estimation of parameters (Jeong et al. 2014; Nowicki and Dobruch-Sobczak 2016).

Elastographic techniques can be broadly classified into two categories: (a) displacement or strain elastographic imaging and (b) shear wave elastography (SWE). With liver applications, shear wave speed elastographic techniques are the most commonly used, followed by displacement and strain imaging for focal liver lesions (Dietrich et al. 2017). In SE there is a quasi-static mechanically induced applied force which can be originated either actively and externally from pressure applied to the transducer during the measurement or passively from internal physiological movements such as pulsation of heart and blood vessels or respiratory movements. These forces cause axial displacement of the tissues under the transducer, which can be measured and converted to strain or strain rate. The methods for measuring displacement include speckle tracking using radiofrequency backscatter or Doppler processing. Being qualitative in nature, this technique produces color maps refreshed at the same rate with US frame rate. Although qualitative, this technique can provide quantitative data when the strain of an area is divided by a reference area (usually subcutaneous fat or adjacent normal parenchyma) in order to calculate a ratio. However, these methods are still currently under development and are not recommended for clinical practice, especially in liver imaging. Strain elastography works better with superficial structures such as breast and thyroid (Sigrist et al. 2017; Dietrich et al. 2017).

In acoustic radiation force impulse imaging (ARFI), there is an ultrasound-induced and focused dynamic radiation force impulse (lasting for only 0.1–0.5 ms) applied at a certain depth which measures displacement and provides qualitative data about a predefined area in a single image. The displacement of tissue is propagated in the longitudinal direction (parallel to US beam) and can be measured (Dietrich et al. 2017; Sigrist et al. 2017).

The main SWE techniques include transient elastography (TE), point SWE (pSWE or ARFI quantification), and two-dimensional and three-dimensional SWE (2D-SWE and 3D-SWE). In all techniques the US transducer applies a perpendicular stress force on the target tissue to cause "shear" or change of tissue initial shape. Once the tissue is displaced, transversely propagating ultrasound waves appear, travelling at very low velocity. These transverse waves are termed "the shear waves" and constitute the basis of SWE. The tissue response to the applied force can be measured by the machine by successively obtaining and comparing images with the reference image. Depending on the specific elastographic technique the M-mode or the Doppler technique can be used to measure the Young's modulus or the velocity of a shear wave, respectively (Jeong et al. 2014). In TE which was the first commercially available technique and the most widely validated, a mechanically induced impulse produced by an external mechanical vibrator causes the production of shear waves and then quantitative data of this wave's speed can be obtained in a single measurement by a transducer. This technique is designed only for liver elasticity measurement and is used by non-imaging specialists. Similarly, with pSWE or ARFI quantification, the ultrasonographic transducer produces a focused high-intensity radiation force impulse at a predefined depth which produces quantitative measurements of shear wave speed in a single measurement. In this method grayscale US images are used only for orientation and selection of area of measurement, while no elastogram is produced. In 2D-SWE and 3D-SWE, radiation forces emitted by the transducer produce shear waves whose speed can be quantified over a predefined area. Color maps (elastograms) containing this information can be produced and measurements (including statistical variables such as mean and standard deviation) can be performed based on regions of interest (ROI) defined by the physician performing the examination. The results of this technique are expressed either in m/s (for actual shear wave speed measurements) or in kPa (for the Young's modulus E as converted by speed measurements).

A difference between pSWE and 2D-SWE is that with pSWE the reading is provided following a single-shot emission and is available instantaneously, whereas in 2D-SWE scanning is continuous for 4–5 s, until a stable SWE image is acquired, so that the physician can choose an adequate ROI and obtain the measurement. In 2D-SWE information regarding the quality of estimations is available and pixels containing inaccurate measurements can be discarded, avoiding false measurements. Variations exist among different manufacturers regarding the technique's principles and visualization of measurement quality. The Young's modulus (E) is measured in kPa and can be calculated with the equation $E = 3\rho c_s^2$, where c_s represents the speed of shear waves and ρ the tissue density. It is generally preferred to rely on measurements of speed rather than Young's modulus for several reasons. Firstly, since the equation of the Young's modulus needs many assumptions which are not always met, it can lack validity. For this reason, the Food and Drug Administration has only approved systems presenting measurements of shear wave speed. Secondly, confusion can occur in the literature as the elastic modulus of a tissue can be estimated using both the shear modulus (G) and the Young's modulus (E). Although both variables are measured in kPa, they are not directly comparable as a conversion is needed using the equation $E = 3G$ (Dietrich et al. 2017; Sigrist et al. 2017). An overview of elastographic techniques can be found in Fig. 8 and a comparative presentation of them in Table 3. Manufacturers offering the various elastographic techniques in commercially available systems can be found in Table 4. Examples of elastographic techniques can be found in Fig. 9.

3.2 Tips for SWE of Liver

Shear wave elastography can be used to investigate the degree of fibrosis and indirectly portal hypertension. Patients should be examined in the supine position with their right arm extended, with the transducer placed in an intercostal space, to visualize the right liver lobe. Any areas of artifact, large blood vessels, the liver capsule, and the gallbladder should be avoided. Optimal quality measurements in pSWE and 2D-SWE are produced when the ROI is placed at least 1–2 cm and up to 6 cm deep to the liver capsule. SWE measurements are better when performed with the patient holding their breath in a neutral position for a few seconds, as deep inspiration affects measurements. The right liver lobe is used as measurements are significantly higher and more variable in the left liver lobe (Horster et al. 2010; Karlas et al. 2011). Fasting for at least 2 h and a 10-min rest period are recommended prior to SWE examination. The studies on normal values of various techniques have been summarized (Dong et al. 2017) as have cutoff values of SWE

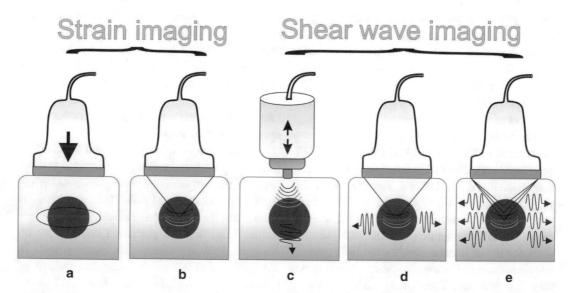

Fig. 8 Overview of US elastographic techniques. The measured physical quantity differs between techniques. The displacement caused by external or physiologic internal compression is measured in strain imaging (**a**). In ARFI (**b**) the displacement caused by an ARFI is measured. The speed of shear waves generated perpendicular to the direction of US beam is measured in SWE (**c–e**). A mechanical vibrating device compresses the tissue and shear waves are produced in TE (**c**). Shear waves produced by an ARFI can be measured in one focus (pSWE-D) (**d**) or an area (2D-SWE-E) (**e**)

Table 3 Comparative presentation of shear wave elastography (SWE) methods for evaluation of hepatic parenchyma

Transient elastography (TE)	Point-SWE (pSWE)	2D-SWE
Dynamic stress caused by an external mechanical vibrator	Dynamic stress by ARFI in the direction of US beam in a **single** focal location	Dynamic stress induced by ARFI in the direction of US beam and in **multiple** focal zones
The stiffness is estimated along an US A-line Shear waves are measured parallel to excitation The region is fixed and cannot be adjusted by the user	Shear waves are generated and measured perpendicular to the plane of excitation	Shear waves are generated and measured perpendicular to ARFI application Multiple focal zones are examined in a rapid succession, allowing for real-time monitoring of shear waves in two dimensions
An US transducer is used to calculate both C_s and E (quantitative analysis)	Both C_s and E can be reported (quantitative analysis)	Both C_s and E can be reported (quantitative analysis)
Nor grayscale image is provided nor elastogram	Grayscale image used for orientation and selection of an appropriate point for measurement of elasticity No elastogram is produced	Grayscale image used for orientation and selection of an appropriate ROI for measurement of elasticity Color elastogram is produced in real time and is superimposed on grayscale image. This is used to place a ROI for measurement of elasticity

C_s speed of shear waves, E Young's modulus, US ultrasound, $ARFI$ acoustic radiation force impulse, ROI region of interest, SWE shear wave elastography, TE transient elastography

Table 4 Manufacturers offering the various elastographic modes in commercially available systems

Elastographic technique	Manufacturers and systems
SE	Esaote, GE, Hitachi Aloka, Philips, Samsung Medison, Siemens, Toshiba, Ultrasonix, Mindray Zonare
ARFI	Siemens (Virtual Touch® Imaging VTI/ARFI)
TE	Echosens (FibroScan®)
pSWE	Siemens (Virtual Touch® Quantification (VTQ/ARFI) Philips (ElastPQ®), Hitachi Aloka, Esaote
2D-SWE	SuperSonic Imagine, Philips, Toshiba, GE, Siemens, Mindray Zonare
Combination of TE and 2D-SWE	GE

(pSWE, 2D-SWE, etc.) in liver disease. The exact range of normal values of SWE measurements varies among different manufacturers, techniques, and even models of the same manufacturer so the relative literature should be consulted (Dietrich et al. 2017).

Liver stiffness assessed with SWE reflects liver fibrosis. Nevertheless, a number of physiologic and pathological confounding factors exist, influencing the measurements. Food ingestion increases measurements for more than 2 h. Diseases affecting SWE measurements include hepatic inflammation, obstructive cholestasis, hepatic congestion, amyloidosis, lymphoma, and extramedullary hemopoiesis. As a consequence, laboratory examinations should be taken into consideration and SWE measurements should not be performed if AST and/or ALT are increased >x5 the normal limits (Dietrich et al. 2017).

It is generally recommended that ten valid measurements of **pSWE** are obtained and the median is reported. If the mean and standard deviations are used, a low standard deviation shows good quality of measurements. pSWE is characterized by excellent intra- and interobserver reproducibility for evaluation of liver stiffness in healthy subjects and patients with chronic liver disease (Dietrich et al. 2017; Fang et al. 2018; Fang et al. 2017).

In **2D-SWE** it is important to have homogeneous color filling in the color map obtained during the examination. As with pSWE, in 2D-SWE the color box should be placed at least 2 cm deep to the liver capsule. The ROI for measurement

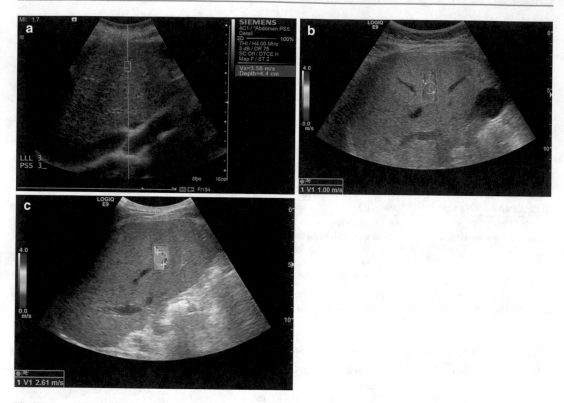

Fig. 9 Example of ARFI® (Siemens) pSWE in a case of cirrhosis (**a**), a 2D-SWE (by GE) in a normal volunteer (**b**), and in a case of cirrhosis (**c**)

should be placed in the middle line of the elasto-gram (not on the edges) and over a homoge-neously isoechoic part of the liver, containing no nodule, blood vessel, or any artifact. With 2D-SWE there is no agreement as to objective quality criteria for measurements. For the Logiq E9 device (GE Healthcare, USA), the manufac-turer recommends that an IQR/M value lower than 30% should be calculated for measurements with outliers being excluded from analysis for the benefit of measurement consistency and hence accuracy. The stability of consecutive elasto-grams during scanning with 2D-SWE is another indicator of quality. As with pSWE, it is essential that physicians starting to apply this technique should follow the manufacturer's advice on qual-ity control of measurements. Regarding reporting 2D-SWE results, 3–15 measurements have been suggested in the literature; 3 measurements appear sufficient for adequate assessment of liver fibrosis and portal hypertension. Both mean and median value can theoretically be used for report-ing results but since median and interquartile range (IQR) are more appropriate for non-normally distributed data, these may be prefera-ble. Excellent intra-observer agreement has been reported for 2D-SWE measurements both in healthy subjects and in patients with liver dis-ease. Factors hindering appropriate examination and leading to failure include obesity, poor breath hold, large amounts of ascites, pulsatility induced by the heart, poor ultrasound window, an exami-nation depth of less than 4 cm, and technical arti-facts (Dietrich et al. 2017).

As a general rule, SWE measurements cannot be compared between different US systems, manufacturers, and techniques since different acquisition techniques and parameters apply and two different variables may be measured: shear wave speed (measured in m/s) or Young's modu-lus (measured in kPa). Factors known to affect the variability of measurements include the depth of measurement, transducer frequency, position of the transducer in subcostal or intercostal approach, operator experience, and patient characteristics.

3.3 Technical Comments on US of Liver Transplantations

Liver transplantation is a valuable method of treatment for end-stage liver disease and different types of liver transplantation exist including (a) whole-liver transplantation from a cadaveric donor, (b) split-liver transplantation where a liver from a cadaveric donor is divided and transplanted to two recipients, and (c) living donor liver transplantation where usually a relative of the recipient provides a section of his/her liver. US plays a pivotal role in detecting and following up complications in the early and late postoperative period. A list of the complications encountered post-liver transplantation can be found in Table 5. Radiologists scanning liver transplants need to be aware of normal findings in order to avoid misdiagnosis (Crossin et al. 2003).

In an attempt to achieve sufficient liver volume for an average-sized adult, the right lobe (segments 5–8) is most commonly implanted in the recipient with segments 4–8 only being required for larger recipients. The transplanted liver has the potential to augment in volume during the weeks following the operation, reaching its normal capacity. Knowledge of the various surgical techniques is essential for adequate US examination of the transplanted liver. During liver transplantation, one biliary anastomosis and four vascular anastomoses need to be performed. (a) **Choledocho-choledochostomy** is the end-to-end anastomosis performed between the donor's common bile duct and the recipient's common hepatic duct. During this technique, the sphincter of Oddi is successfully preserved, thus preventing the reflux of enteric fluids into the biliary tree. When the recipient's common hepatic duct is abnormal though, it is resected and a **choledochojejunostomy** is preferred, albeit a higher risk for complications such as bleeding, leakage, or breakdown of the anastomosis and infection. Resection of the gallbladder is routinely performed in all liver transplants. (b) The anastomosis between the donor's and the recipient's **hepatic arteries** is a "fish-mouth" anastomosis performed between the donor's common hepatic and splenic artery branches (or alternatively the celiac axis) and the recipient's

Table 5 A summary of complications post-liver transplantation

Category of complications		Complications
Vascular	Hepatic artery	• Thrombosis • Stenosis • Pseudoaneurysm
	Portal vein	• Thrombosis • Stenosis
	Inferior vena cava	• Thrombosis • Stenosis
Biliary ducts		• Leak and perihepatic fluid collection formation (biloma) • Stricture • Stones/sludge • Dysfunction of the sphincter of Oddi • Recurrence of disease
Liver parenchyma	Neoplastic conditions	• Recurrence of neoplasia • Posttransplantation lymphoproliferative disorder
	Parenchymal conditions	• Infarct • Abscess • Biloma • Conditions preexisting in donor liver (hemangioma, cyst, etc.) • Metastasis
Perihepatic space		• Fluid collection (bile, blood, pus, lymph, or ascites) • Ascites
Right adrenal gland		• Hemorrhagic and enlarged due to venous ischemia

right and left hepatic artery bifurcation (or the gastroduodenal/proper hepatic artery bifurcation). In patients with dual vascular supply of the native liver, the larger artery is chosen during the surgery, while in case of severe stenosis of the hepatic artery or coeliac axis, a graft (the donor iliac artery) is used to connect the aorta with the hepatic arteries. (c) The **portal vein** anastomosis is an end-to-end anastomosis, although a venous graft may be used to connect the superior mesenteric or splenic vein with the donor portal vein in case of thrombosis. (d) The **supra- and infrahepatic vena cava** anastomoses are typically performed with an end-to-end pattern although end-to-side or side-to-side patterns may be opted for depending on surgical conditions (Crossin et al. 2003).

A liver transplant should be routinely examined with grayscale for evaluation of parenchyma and biliary tree and Doppler techniques for evaluation of the vasculature. CEUS has been shown to improve the diagnostic accuracy for detection of liver transplantation complications such as hepatic artery stenosis and thrombosis, portal vein stenosis and thrombosis, biliary strictures at the anastomotic site, and biliary-arterial fistulas. Microbubbles can be administered both intravenously and intra-cavitary through percutaneous catheter tubes of the biliary tree (Clevert et al. 2009; Ren et al. 2016; Berry and Sidhu 2004; Daneshi et al. 2014; Crossin et al. 2003; Rafailidis et al. 2018). The transplanted liver parenchyma appears homogeneous on grayscale or mildly heterogeneous in texture. The intrahepatic bile ducts should exhibit no dilatation. Free fluid can be observed intra-abdominally or in the perihepatic space during the first week and up to 10 days after the operation. In patients where a T tube is placed within the biliary tree, the extrahepatic biliary ducts may appear thick walled. The surgical staples appear as echogenic spots, possibly causing mild acoustic shadowing. Vascular complications can be firstly appreciated on grayscale technique but confirmation with Doppler technique is a prerequisite for diagnosis. On spectral analysis, all vascular structures demonstrate waveforms similar to those of the native liver (Crossin et al. 2003). If findings suggestive of complications (stenosis or thrombosis) are demonstrated, an angiographic method such as MDCTA should be performed for confirmation.

References

Appis AW, Tracy MJ, Feinstein SB (2015) Update on the safety and efficacy of commercial ultrasound contrast agents in cardiac applications. Echo Res Pract 2:R55–R62

Berry JD, Sidhu PS (2004) Microbubble contrast-enhanced ultrasound in liver transplantation. Eur Radiol 14:P96–P103

Claudon M, Cosgrove D, Albrecht T et al (2008) Guidelines and good clinical practice recommendations for contrast enhanced ultrasound (CEUS)—update 2008. Ultraschall Med 29:28–44

Claudon M, Dietrich CF, Choi BI et al (2013) Guidelines and good clinical practice recommendations for contrast enhanced ultrasound (CEUS) in the liver—update 2012: a WFUMB-EFSUMB initiative in cooperation with representatives of AFSUMB, AIUM, ASUM, FLAUS and ICUS. Ultraschall Med 34:11–29

Clevert DA, Stickel M, Minaifar N et al (2009) Contrast-enhanced ultrasound in liver transplant: first results and potential for complications in the postoperative period. Clin Hemorheol Microcirc 43:83–94

Cosgrove DO (2017) Evolution of ultrasonography since the 1970s. Ultrasound Med Biol 43:2741–2742

Cosgrove D, Harvey C (2009) Clinical uses of microbubbles in diagnosis and treatment. Med Biol Eng Comput 47:813–826

Crossin JD, Muradali D, Wilson SR (2003) US of liver transplants: normal and abnormal. Radiographics 23:1093–1114

Daneshi M, Rajayogeswaran B, Peddu P, Sidhu PS (2014) Demonstration of an occult biliary-arterial fistula using percutaneous contrast-enhanced ultrasound cholangiography in a transplanted liver. J Clin Ultrasound 42:108–111

Dietrich CF, Ignee A, Hocke M, Schreiber-Dietrich D, Greis C (2011) Pitfalls and artefacts using contrast enhanced ultrasound. Z Gastroenterol 49:350–356

Dietrich CF, Bamber J, Berzigotti A et al (2017) EFSUMB Guidelines and Recommendations on the Clinical Use of Liver Ultrasound Elastography, Update 2017 (Long Version). Ultraschall Med 38:e16–e47

Dietrich CF, Averkiou M, Nielsen MB et al (2018) How to perform contrast-enhanced ultrasound (CEUS). Ultrasound Int Open 4:E2–E15

Dong Y, Sirli R, Ferraioli G et al (2017) Shear wave elastography of the liver—review on normal values. Z Gastroenterol 55:153–166

Eckersley RJ, Chin CT, Burns PN (2005) Optimising phase and amplitude modulation schemes for imaging microbubble contrast agents at low acoustic power. Ultrasound Med Biol 31:213–219

Eisenbrey JR, Daecher A, Kramer MR, Forsberg F (2015) Effects of needle and catheter size on commercially available ultrasound contrast agents. J Ultrasound Med 34:1961–1968

Fang C, Konstantatou E, Romanos O, Yusuf GT, Quinlan DJ, Sidhu PS (2017) Reproducibility of 2-dimensional shear wave elastography assessment of the liver: a direct comparison with point shear wave elastography in healthy volunteers. J Ultrasound Med 36:1563–1569

Fang C, Jaffer OS, Yusuf GT et al (2018) Reducing the number of measurements in liver point shear-wave elastography: factors that influence the number and reliability of measurements in assessment of liver fibrosis in clinical practice. Radiology 287:844–852

Fetzer DT, Rafailidis V, Peterson C, Grant EG, Sidhu P, Barr RG (2018) Artifacts in contrast-enhanced ultrasound: a pictorial essay. Abdom Radiol (NY) 43:977–997

Forsberg F, Liu JB, Burns PN, Merton DA, Goldberg BB (1994) Artifacts in ultrasonic contrast agent studies. J Ultrasound Med 13:357–365

Forsberg F, Goldberg BB, Liu JB, Merton DA, Rawool NM (1996) On the feasibility of real-time, in vivo harmonic imaging with proteinaceous microspheres. J Ultrasound Med 15:853 860. quiz 861-852

Forsberg F, Piccoli CW, Merton DA, Palazzo JJ, Hall AL (2007) Breast lesions: imaging with contrast-enhanced subharmonic US—initial experience. Radiology 244:718–726

Fulgham PF (2013) Physical principles of ultrasound. In: Fulgham PF, Gilbert BR (eds) Practical urological ultrasound. Humana Press, Totowa, NJ, pp 9–26

Greis C (2014) Technical aspects of contrast-enhanced ultrasound (CEUS) examinations: tips and tricks. Clin Hemorheol Microcirc 58:89–95

Horster S, Mandel P, Zachoval R, Clevert DA (2010) Comparing acoustic radiation force impulse imaging to transient elastography to assess liver stiffness in healthy volunteers with and without Valsalva manoeuvre. Clin Hemorheol Microcirc 46:159–168

Hudson JM, Karshafian R, Burns PN (2009) Quantification of flow using ultrasound and microbubbles: a disruption replenishment model based on physical principles. Ultrasound Med Biol 35:2007–2020

Jeong WK, Lim HK, Lee HK, Jo JM, Kim Y (2014) Principles and clinical application of ultrasound elastography for diffuse liver disease. Ultrasonography 33:149–160

Karlas T, Pfrepper C, Wiegand J et al (2011) Acoustic radiation force impulse imaging (ARFI) for non-invasive detection of liver fibrosis: examination standards and evaluation of interlobe differences in healthy subjects and chronic liver disease. Scand J Gastroenterol 46:1458–1467

Lassau N, Chami L, Chebil M et al (2011) Dynamic contrast-enhanced ultrasonography (DCE-US) and anti-angiogenic treatments. Discov Med 11:18–24

Lumason (2017). https://imaging.bracco.com/sites/brac-coimaging.com/files/technica_sheet_pdf/us-en-2017-01-04-spc-lumason.pdf

Main ML, Goldman JH, Grayburn PA (2009) Ultrasound contrast agents: balancing safety versus efficacy. Expert Opin Drug Saf 8:49–56

Mason WP (1981) Piezoelectricity, its history and applications. J Acoust Soc Am 70:1561–1566

McNaughton DA, Abu-Yousef MM (2011) Doppler US of the liver made simple. Radiographics 31:161–188

Merritt CRB (2018) Chapter 1: Physics of ultrasound. In: Rumack CM, Levine D (eds) Diagnostic ultrasound, 5th edn. Elsevier, Amsterdam, pp 1–33

Nowicki A, Dobruch-Sobczak K (2016) Introduction to ultrasound elastography. J Ultrason 16:113–124

Oh SH, Han HY, Kim HJ (2018) Comet tail artifact on ultrasonography: is it a reliable finding of benign gallbladder diseases? Ultrasonography 38:221–230

Piscaglia F, Bolondi L (2006) The safety of SonoVue in abdominal applications: retrospective analysis of 23188 investigations. Ultrasound Med Biol 32:1369–1375

Piscaglia F, Nolsoe C, Dietrich CF et al (2012) The EFSUMB Guidelines and Recommendations on the Clinical Practice of Contrast Enhanced Ultrasound (CEUS): update 2011 on non-hepatic applications. Ultraschall Med 33:33–59

Rafailidis V, Fang C, Yusuf GT, Huang DY, Sidhu PS (2018) Contrast-enhanced ultrasound (CEUS) of the abdominal vasculature. Abdom Radiol (NY) 43:934–947

Ren J, Wu T, Zheng B-W, Tan Y-Y, Zheng R-Q, Chen G-H (2016) Application of contrast-enhanced ultrasound after liver transplantation: Current status and perspectives. World J Gastroenterol 22:1607–1616

Rubin JM, Bude RO, Carson PL, Bree RL, Adler RS (1994) Power Doppler US: a potentially useful alternative to mean frequency-based color Doppler US. Radiology 190:853–856

Sidhu PS (2015) Multiparametric ultrasound (MPUS) imaging: terminology describing the many aspects of ultrasonography. Ultraschall Med 36:315–317

Sidhu PS, Cantisani V, Dietrich CF et al (2018) The EFSUMB Guidelines and Recommendations for the Clinical Practice of Contrast-Enhanced Ultrasound (CEUS) in Non-Hepatic Applications: Update 2017 (Short Version). Ultraschall Med 39:154–180

Sigrist RMS, Liau J, Kaffas AE, Chammas MC, Willmann JK (2017) Ultrasound elastography: review of techniques and clinical applications. Theranostics 7:1303–1329

Skyba DM, Price RJ, Linka AZ, Skalak TC, Kaul S (1998) Direct in vivo visualization of intravascular destruction of microbubbles by ultrasound and its local effects on tissue. Circulation 98:290–293

Strobel D, Kleinecke C, Hansler J et al (2005) Contrast-enhanced sonography for the characterisation of hepatocellular carcinomas—correlation with histological differentiation. Ultraschall Med 26:270–276 ter Haar G (2009) Safety and bio-effects of ultrasound contrast agents. Med Biol Eng Comput 47:893–900

Tranquart F, Mercier L, Frinking P, Gaud E, Arditi M (2012) Perfusion quantification in contrast-enhanced ultrasound (CEUS)—ready for research projects and routine clinical use. Ultraschall Med 33:S31–S38

Wachsberg RH (2007) B-flow imaging of the hepatic vasculature: correlation with color Doppler sonography. AJR Am J Roentgenol 188:W522–W533

Wilson SR, Kim TK, Jang HJ, Burns PN (2007) Enhancement patterns of focal liver masses: discordance between contrast-enhanced sonography and contrast-enhanced CT and MRI. AJR Am J Roentgenol 189:W7–w12

Computed Tomography of the Liver

Domenico De Santis, Federica Landolfi,
Marta Zerunian, Damiano Caruso,
and Andrea Laghi

Contents

D. De Santis · F. Landolfi · M. Zerunian · D. Caruso
A. Laghi (✉)
Department of Surgical and Medical Sciences and
Translational Medicine, School of Medicine and
Psychology, "Sapienza"—University of Rome,
Sant'Andrea University Hospital, Rome, Italy
e-mail: andrea.laghi@uniroma1.it

© Springer Nature Switzerland AG 2021
E. Quaia (ed.), *Imaging of the Liver and Intra-hepatic Biliary Tract*,
Medical Radiology, Diagnostic Imaging, https://doi.org/10.1007/978-3-030-38983-3_4

Abstract

Multidetector Computed Tomography (CT) plays a pivotal role in the evaluation of liver pathologies due to its fast acquisition time, thinner image thickness and narrow collimation, resulting in high temporal and spatial resolution, fundamental to detect subtle liver lesions and to optimize radiation exposure.

State-of-the-art liver imaging requires proper patient preparation, the implementation of optimized contrast dye injection strategies, and a thorough CT scanner configuration.

A multiphasic CT examination is mandatory to maximize diagnostic performances in terms of lesion identification and is the current choice in daily clinical practice. In the other hand, functional imaging, such as CT perfusion, provides quantitative parameters that improve diagnostic capabilities in selected cases. Operators needs to know different imaging reconstruction strategies and master all the available post-processing techniques, in order to select the best option in every clinical scenario. Over the last decades, Dualenergy CT has further expanded the diagnostic possibilities in liver imaging and is currently widely implemented in multiple Institutions worldwide. Eventually, photon-counting CT is the very latest technical advancement in CT imaging and is at the forefront of scientific research, bearing the potential to revolutionize liver imaging.

1   Introduction

Multiphasic computed tomography (CT) is one of the leading imaging techniques in the evaluation of liver diseases. Since its introduction in the 1970s, multiple technical improvements have expanded its clinical capabilities to the point that CT currently plays a pivotal role in the diagnosis and management of liver diseases, both in emergency and in elective clinical scenarios. This chapter provides a technical overview on multiphasic liver CT, including patient preparation, contrast media administration techniques, CT technical parameters, current technology, and future perspectives.

2   Patient Preparation

No specific patient preparation is recommended, but fasting for at least 6 h prior to the examination in case of intravenous contrast medium (CM) administration is required.

Positive oral CM is not deemed necessary for abdominopelvic CT scan: neutral contrast agent, as water, may be used as equally effective with a dose of 500–600 mL (Lee et al. 2013, 2016).

As general recommendation to a CT scan, it is advisable to remove any clothes and, if possible, any metallic item which can produce artifacts, reducing diagnostic performance of the examination (Barrett and Keat 2004).

A proper peripheral intravenous access must be placed to ensure high-quality angiographic and parenchymal studies. Choosing the most appropriate vascular access allows to avoid complications such as extravasation of CM: the preferred route is the antecubital or forearm area. However, central lines such as peripherally inserted central catheters or port-a-cath devices might be used, as long as long they are marked as "power injectable," not exceeding the maximum flow rate printed on the catheter itself (Williamson and McKinney 2001).

Patients who undergo CT scan with intravenous administration of iodinated CM must be screened to estimate the risk of renal and nonrenal adverse reactions.

2.1   Renal Adverse Reactions

Renal adverse effects consist of renal function deterioration in a short time window after intravascular administration of iodinated CM (van der

Molen et al. 2018a). Until a few years ago any decrease in renal function occurring after CM administration used to be considered as contrast-induced nephropathy in the absence of an alternative etiology. However, a high rate of fluctuation in kidney function occurs even in patients without exposure to iodinated CM (Bruce et al. 2009), making it challenging to determine whether or not CM is the actual determinant of renal function deterioration. Postcontrast acute kidney injury (PC-AKI) is defined as an increase in serum creatinine (sCr) ≥ 0.3 mg/dL (or ≥ 26.5 µmol/L), or sCr ≥ 1.5–1.9 times baseline, within 48–72 h of intravascular administration of CM (Thomas et al. 2015; Ad-Hoc Working Group of E et al. 2012). The most important risk factors for PC-AKI are impaired renal function (eGFR less than 30 mL/min/1.73 m^2 before CM intravenous administration), dehydration, and repeated CM administration within a short interval (48–72 h) (van der Molen et al. 2018a). Other possible predisposing factors may be identified in old age, female gender, low BMI, cardiovascular diseases, and metabolic factors (Moos et al. 2013; Kanbay et al. 2017; Kwasa et al. 2014).

Patient's serum creatinine level is necessary to derive the estimated glomerular filtration rate (eGFR) by applying the modification of diet in renal disease (MDRD) equation or the chronic kidney disease epidemiology collaboration (CKD-EPI) equation. The latter formula is recommended since it allows a more accurate categorization of patients at lower risk of chronic kidney disease into higher eGFR categories (van der Molen et al. 2018a). Each patient eGFR should be estimated before the CT examination in order to safely inject CM.

Details about PC-AKI and its medical management go beyond the purpose of this chapter. However, it is worth to mention that oral hydration alone does not prevent PC-AKI and that modern nonionic iodinated CM can also be safely administered to patients with hematologic disorders with normal renal function (van der Molen et al. 2018b). As a general rule, the incidence of PC-AKI is related to the dose of CM and therefore it is recommended to use the lowest dose of contrast medium to obtain a diagnostic examination (Stacul et al. 2011).

3 Contrast Media Administration

The CM intensifies the attenuation differences between healthy liver parenchyma and focal liver lesions, improving lesions' conspicuity and detectability. A multiphasic approach is mandatory to correctly identify and characterize focal liver lesions.

Liver contrast enhancement (CE) results from distribution of CM into the extravascular interstitial space and is related to *iodine concentration* and *iodine delivery rate* (IDR—mg of iodine entering the circulation per second, which depends on flow rate) and amount of injected CM. The quality of liver enhancement during the arterial phase is strictly dependent on the injection rate, while parenchymal enhancement during portal venous phase and delayed phase is determined by the total dose of iodine administered and is less dependent on the injection rate, due to CM recirculation phenomenon (Bae 2010). The optimal flow rate for a proper CE of liver parenchyma should be 3–4 mL/s or higher, allowing for an optimal temporal separation between pure arterial and portal venous phase. Injection rates of 5–10 mL/s are generally reserved to CT perfusion studies (Laghi 2007).

Highly concentrated CM (350, 370, and 400 mgL/mL) allows to reach adequate IDRs even when a low flow rate is mandatory due to small-caliber i.v. access. When highly concentrated CM, even if in a small volume, is administered at a fixed injection rate, a fast delivery of iodine mass per unit time occurs, resulting in an earlier and greater arterial peak enhancement even if shorter in duration: the magnitude of overall hepatic enhancement is not substantially affected during venous and delayed phases, but the detection of hypervascular lesions is improved (Awai et al. 2002).

A parenchymal enhancement of 50 HU is required for diagnostic purposes and it has been demonstrated that the iodine load required to reach such enhancement is slightly higher than 500 mgL/kg (Heiken et al. 1995). Therefore, patient's size plays a fundamental role in contrast enhancement and has to be considered when performing a contrast-enhanced CT scan. Although

total body weight is the most widely used parameter in clinical practice, it must be considered that body fat contributes minimally in dispersing
• CM. Therefore, the risk of adjusting the amount of iodine load for the body weight, using a 1:1 linear scale, is an overestimation of the required amount of CM in obese patients. It has been established that lean body weight (LBW) is a more accurate method to estimate the iodine dose required to obtain a congruous liver enhancement (Kondo et al. 2010). LBW can be estimated by Boer formula (Boer 1984):

$$LBW_{male}^{Boer} = (0.407 \bullet W) + (0.267 \bullet H) - 19.2$$

$$LBW_{female}^{Boer} = (0.252 \bullet W) + (0.473 \bullet H) - 48.3$$

where W represents the patient weight in kilograms and H the patient height in meters, or by James formula (James et al. 1976), as follows:

$$LBW_{male}^{James} = (1.10 \bullet W) - 128 \bullet \left[\frac{W^2}{(100 \bullet H)^2} \right]$$

$$LBW_{female}^{James} = (1.07 \bullet W) - 148 \bullet \left[\frac{W^2}{(100 \bullet H)^2} \right]$$

where W represents the patient weight in kilograms and H the patient height in meters.

While both formulas provide equal results in the vast majority of patients, Boer formula better estimates the LBW in obese patients, and therefore it is one of the first choices in such subpopulation (Caruso et al. 2018).

Additional patient-related parameters affecting contrast enhancement include cardiac output, age, gender, venous access, and some pathologic hepatic conditions such as hepatomegaly and/or diffuse parenchymal diseases such as cirrhosis, which may be associated with decreased hepatic enhancement because of reduced portal venous perfusion related to fibrosis and increased hepatic resistance (Bae 2010).

A saline chaser (up to 50 mL) should follow the CM injection to improve bolus geometry and avoid the waste of a certain volume of CM that, otherwise, would remain in "dead spaces" such as the injector tubing, the peripheral veins, the right heart, or the pulmonary circulation. The bolus chaser also increases hydration and washes

out any residual CM which may obstruct the i.v. access, especially in case of central venous access.

Scanning the liver at predetermined time points and employing fixed scan delay without taking into account specific patient and/or CM characteristics should be avoided (Laghi 2007). It is strongly preferable to employ precise methods to monitor CM arrival time and accurately calculate the scan delay, such as test bolus and bolus tracking:

• *Test bolus* consists of injecting a small bolus (10–20 mL) of CM before injecting the full amount of CM, after placing a region of interest (ROI) in a target district, generally at the starting level of the diagnostic sca. Sequential monitoring images are acquired, obtaining a time-enhancement curve of contrast enhancement within the ROI. The interval time needed to determine the peak of contrast enhancement is used to estimate scan delays for full-bolus diagnostic CT.

• *Bolus tracking* method consists of the injection of full diagnostic bolus of CM, administered without performing any prior test, while scanning a single level in upper abdomen with a ROI placed in aorta, generally at the level of celiac axis during a pre-contrast acquisition. Low-radiation-dose sequential images are acquired every 1–3 s providing a time-attenuation curve which maps the arrival time of contrast material; when a predetermined threshold (generally around 150–180 HU) has been reached, the diagnostic scan is triggered. An additional delay, called diagnostic delay, corresponding to the interval time running from the trigger to scan initiation, must be added.

4 MDCT: Technical Parameters

Since its advent, multi-detector CT represented a dramatic technical advance over single-detector scanners. Its rapid volume coverage speed and faster acquisition time, combined with thinner image thickness and narrow collimation, result in time-efficient image acquisition of large body volumes and, therefore, in high temporal and spatial resolution.

Thin sections minimize partial-volume artifacts but also increase image noise and decrease length of coverage (Hu et al. 2000). A reduced coverage can be counteracted by increasing the pitch, defined as the ratio between the distance of the CT table per 360° gantry rotation and the X-ray beam collimation width. A pitch ≤1 is generally considered adequate in liver imaging (Laghi 2007).

Tube potential (kVp) and tube current (mAs) are the two main parameters affecting radiation exposure. A kVp reduction improves tissue contrast, but also increases image noise: in standard liver imaging a tube potential of 120 kVp is usually preferred, reserving 140 kVp for obese patients.

Automated tube voltage and tube current modulation systems have been introduced with the aim to optimize the radiation exposure. Depending on the attenuation differences of the various anatomic regions obtained during the scout scan, such systems automatically module kVp and mAs throughout the diagnostic scan to achieve a predefined level of image noise, reducing radiation exposure (Spearman et al. 2016).

5 Multiphasic Approach

Liver parenchyma ought to be studied before and after i.v. CM administration, by adopting proper delayed scan times in order to obtain arterial phase, portal-venous phase, and delayed phase, chosen on a case-by-case basis, aiming at tailoring the scan protocol to each patient and clinical scenario.

5.1 Unenhanced Phase

Although its utility is sometimes debated, the unenhanced phase still plays an important role in liver imaging. In fact, in several clinical scenarios, it proves to be a very helpful tool in the characterization of focal lesions such as focal hemorrhage, fat, or calcifications, which are easily recognized before contrast enhancement

(Casillas et al. 2000; Patnana et al. 2018; Pickhardt et al. 2012). Additionally, an unenhanced phase should be performed in the evaluation of every cirrhotic liver and during follow-up of oncologic patients, in which noncontrast images may reveal a useful tool to differentiate benign from malignant focal liver lesions (Federle and Blachar 2001). CT scans acquired prior to CM injection are also extremely important in monitoring patients who underwent hepatic chemoembolization, demonstrating in detail the distribution of chemoembolization material (Johnson and Fishman 2013).

5.2 Contrast-Enhanced Phases

Liver has a unique dual circulatory dynamic: approximately 75–80% of the hepatic blood flow is supplied by the portal venous system, whereas the remaining 20–25% comes from the hepatic artery. Inherent consequences reflect in both normal and pathologic vasculature of liver parenchyma and focal lesions, respectively.

Hepatic arterial phase (AP) depicts liver parenchyma at the time CM reaches the aorta and the hepatic arteries, before it circulates through the spleen and the mesentery opacifying the portal venous system, generally 30–40 s later (Federle and Blachar 2001).

In a proper AP liver parenchyma is minimally enhanced and hepatic arteries display a conspicuous opacification. No enhancement of the hepatic veins should be obtained, whereas just some enhancement of the portal vein should be accomplished. AP can be subdivided into an *early arterial phase (EAP)* and a *late arterial phase (LAP)*, during which the hepatic enhancement predominantly reflects the arterial inflow through the hepatic arteries and an initial, thus relatively minor, tranche of splanchnic venous inflow through the portal vein (Foley 2002).

EAP starts approximately 25 s after initiating contrast injection, and lasts approximately 8–10 s. Therefore, to obtain a proper EAP by means of bolus tracking technique, a diagnostic delay ≤6 s should be selected (Laghi 2007; Foley 2002). Acquiring such phase should be reserved to cases in which CT angiography would be of proven benefit by providing a tool for therapy planning. The most frequent indications to perform an EAP are:

- Defining arterial anatomy and anomalies, such as arterial stenosis, aberrant or replaced hepatic arteries
- Preoperative imaging in patients who are candidates for surgical hepatic resection and/or percutaneous ablation therapy

LAP occurs 35–45 s after initiating CM injection and has a temporal window of approximately 8–10 s. Therefore, to obtain a proper LAP by means of bolus tracking technique, a diagnostic delay of approximately 20 s should be selected (Laghi 2007; Foley 2002).

Hypervascular liver lesions, either benign or malignant, receive nearly all their blood supply from prominent neovasculature arising from the hepatic artery. Thus, they are best demonstrated during the LAP, in which they receive all their functional blood flow through the hepatic artery, virtually without any dilution from the unenhanced portal vein flow, enhancing to a greater degree than liver parenchyma (Foley 2002). Additionally, in clinical scenarios of portal hypertension, such as in liver cirrhosis, portal venous inflow is reduced, further increasing hypervascular lesion conspicuity during LAP images.

Right after the arterial circulation, the contrast-enhanced blood flows through the spleen, gut, and mesentery until it opacifies the portal vein. A dataset acquired at this time point is defined *portal venous phase (PVP)* and yields the maximal liver parenchymal enhancement. PVP occurs 60–80 s after initiating CM injection and is the most widely used acquisition phase in routine abdominal imaging, both in general-purpose abdominal CT scans and in oncologic settings (Foley 2002).

An adequate PVP shows homogeneous liver enhancement with a conspicuous opacification of hepatic veins and portal vein, which appear hyperdense compared to liver parenchyma (Federle and Blachar 2001). Such phase maximizes the detectability of hypovascular lesions,

due to the combination of minimal arterial hepatic flow supplying these lesions and the significant enhancement of liver parenchyma (Soyer et al. 2004). On the contrary, hypervascular liver lesions may not be detectable on PVP since they enhance to the same degree of surrounding parenchyma.

Delayed phase (DP) occurs subsequently to PVP, begins 100–120 s after CM injection, and is characterized by gradual CM distribution in the hepatic interstitial spaces. Consequently, attenuation differences between focal liver lesions and liver parenchyma are minimized (Federle and Blachar 2001). Main indications for performing a DP are the investigation of hepatocellular carcinoma (Furlan et al. 2011), cholangiocarcinoma, and detection of liver metastases (Kanematsu et al. 2006). In clinical routine it is also useful to characterize cavernous hemangiomas, identified by the typical centripetal enhancement pattern (Kim et al. 2001). Figure 1 provides an overview of the different phases routinely acquired in liver imaging.

More delayed CT image set may be additionally acquired 10–15 min after CM injection only with specific indications, generally including suspected cholangiocarcinoma, primary sclerosing cholangitis, or any focal hepatic mass associated with intrahepatic bile duct obstruction: in such cases, in fact, it has been established that the presence of a large component of fibrosis causes a very characteristic prolonged stromal enhancement (Federle and Blachar 2001).

6 CT Perfusion

CT liver perfusion (CTP) is a promising functional imaging technique that aims to provide information about regional and global liver microcirculation and to improve the evaluation of hepatic parenchyma through the possibility of an early characterization of focal liver lesions (Meijerink et al. 2008). Perfusion imaging quantifies the transport of blood to a unit volume of tissue, per unit of time, through dynamic CT acquisitions, by repeatedly scanning the liver multiple times at short time intervals, during and after CM injection.

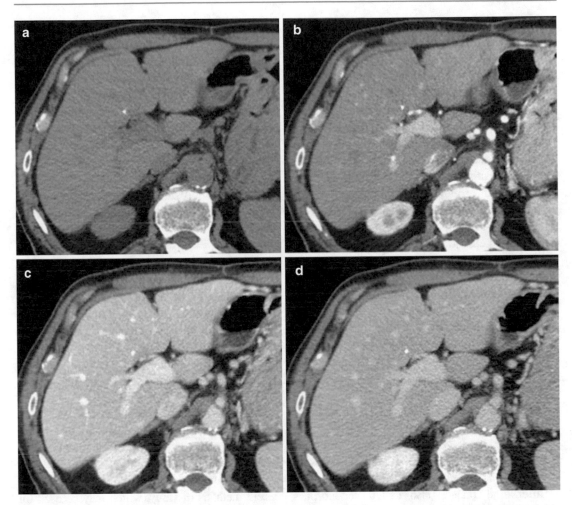

Fig. 1 Multiphasic liver CT examination. (**a**) Unenhanced phase demonstrates slightly higher parenchymal density than the portal venous system. A microcalcification is also easily identifiable. During late hepatic arterial phase (**b**) the aorta and the hepatic artery are the vessel characterized by the highest attenuation values, while portal vein and liver parenchyma enhance to a lesser degree. Subsequent portal venous phase (**c**) maximizes portal vein attenuation and liver enhancement, while the hepatic artery density is reduced. During delayed phase (**d**) the contrast medium is distributed in the hepatic interstitial spaces, and thus the attenuation differences between vessels and liver parenchyma are reduced

The basic principle of CTP is based on tissue attenuation changes, expressed in HU, which are directly proportional to the local concentration of CM within the tissue's microvasculature and interstitial space, as a function of time: the increase and subsequent decrease of CM concentration provide quantitative information about blood flow characteristics and allow quantification of the tissue vascularity (Sahani 2012).

Conventional CT can only achieve a qualitative assessment of contrast enhancement, since any time point during arterial, portal, and delayed phases represents a mixed result of entering and exiting of CM; CTP overcomes such limitations by allowing quantitative measurements (Kartalis et al. 2017).

The proper CTP protocol consists of a precontrast image acquisition, required to identify the optimal scan coverage, followed by dynamic sequential CT scanning of same volume, over time, after intravenous injection of CM (Kambadakone and Sahani 2009). The sequential dynamic image acquisition is necessary to obtain a time-attenuation curve (TAC), corresponding to the arterial input function, which enables the evaluation of blood flow and its possible alterations. The TAC of the tissue being analyzed is compared to the time-intensity curve of a ROI placed into the lumen of the vessel supplying the tissue of interest. Because of dual circulatory liver dynamic, two different ROIs should be placed in the portal vein and in the abdominal aorta, respectively. This particular approach allows the estimation of both intravascular and extravascular properties. A single-input model assuming only a unique vascular supply has been proposed; however, it has not been validated because the separation of arterial and portal blood supply is an important information for characterization of focal lesions, enabling an early detection of alterations in liver perfusion (Kim et al. 2014).

After CM injection, it is possible to identify two different phases: *perfusion phase* and *interstitial phase* (Kartalis et al. 2017; Kambadakone and Sahani 2009):

- Perfusion phase (also called first-pass phase) is an intravascular phase study during which iodine is largely contained within the lumen of the vessels. It lasts approximately 40–60 s and it is mainly determined by the blood flow.
- Interstitial phase (also called second-pass phase or delayed phase) is an extravascular phase during which iodine passes into the extravascular-extracellular compartment. It lasts approximately 2–10 m and it is mostly influenced by CM passive diffusion, largely depending on the blood volume and the permeability of the capillaries to CM.

To achieve precise time-intensity curves CT scans are acquired without any table feed, during a scan time of 55 s with a gantry rotation time of 0.5 s. During first-pass phase one image/s is obtained, whereas a lower temporal resolution can be applied during the second-pass phase, allowing one image every 10 s (Sahani 2012).

A small volume of high-concentrated CM (30–60 mL followed by a 50 mL saline flush) has to be injected at >4–5 mL/s to obtain a short and sharp bolus. A tube voltage of 80–100 kVp with

a tube current of 50–120 mAs may be employed to perform CTP, in order to maximize iodine conspicuity. A 5 mm image reconstruction thickness is usually suggested (Kim et al. 2014).

To avoid errors in the calculation of perfusion values, it is important to prevent beam-hardening artifacts performing CTP in areas without any metallic device and try to reduce motion and respiratory artifacts giving proper instruction to the patient regarding breath-holding.

CTP-acquired sets of images may be evaluated with three different methods (Kartalis et al. 2017):

1. Qualitative analysis, based on visual evaluation of TAC shape, morphology, and color-coded perfusion maps
2. Semiquantitative analysis, based on measurement of TAC peak enhancement times and peak attenuation values
3. Quantitative analysis, based on the application of kinetic models

Only the latter method allows the calculation of various perfusion parameters in the tissues being analyzed and it is, therefore, the more precise and recommended.

CTP quantitative analysis includes three different methods of study, which may be used for quantification of tissue perfusion and/or permeability (Sahani 2012; Kim et al. 2014):

- *Model-free maximum slope method*: Both hepatic arterial and portal perfusion are calculated (in mL/min/100 mL) using the time to peak splenic enhancement, which is considered as a time point indicating the end of arterial phase and the beginning of the portal venous phase of liver perfusion and, thus, used to separate HAP from PVP.

This method is very often used for the quantification of liver perfusion parameters, although it takes into consideration only the first-pass phase of the liver TAC. It assumes that there is no venous outflow (to achieve a condition of no venous outflow a very high injection rate of 15–20 mL/s should be employed, which is not technically feasible in routine clinical practice) (Kim et al. 2014) and parameters such as blood volume, mean transit time (MTT), or capillary permeability surface product may not be calculated.

- *Compartment model-based method:* This analytical method is subdivided into two different mathematical modeling, usually indicated as "single compartment" and "dual compartment," respectively. The *single compartmental model* considers CM as confined in only one compartment, represented by both intravascular and extravascular spaces, freely communicating through sinusoid fenestrae. It is based on Fick's principles and estimates perfusion parameters from the maximal slope or from the peak height of the liver time-intensity curve normalized to the arterial input function. Parameters calculated by this analytical methods are (1) blood flow (BF, expressed as mL/min/100 mL) indicating volume flow rate of blood through liver vasculature; (2) blood volume (BV, expressed in units of mL/100 mL) representing the volume of blood flowing in the vasculature; and (3) MTT, indicating the average time it takes the blood to pass from the arterial to the venous flow.

The *dual (or two)-compartment model* assumes that CM is distributed between vascular and interstitial space considered as two separated compartments, allowing the evaluation of capillary permeability and the estimation of second-pass phase-related parameters, such as permeability surface area product (PSAP) and flow extraction product (FEP). PSAP is the result of permeability per total surface area of capillary endothelium in a unit mass of tissue (measured as mL/min/100 mL), whereas FEP is the result of blood flow per extraction fraction (EF, measured as mL/min/100 mL), with the latter representing the amount of CM passing in the extravascular space in a single passage through the vasculature.

- *Distributed parameter model-based method:* This analytical method assumes that there is a concentration gradient from the arterial inlet and the venous outlet at capillary level and a backward flux from the extravascular-extracellular compartment to the intravascular compartment. The parameters calculated by using a distributed model-based method are blood flow, blood volume, MTT, and permeability.

Even a combination of all these methods may be used.

Through the analysis of these quantitative parameters, functional information reflecting blood flow status is captured: because many liver diseases may affect the dual blood supply in a predictable way, CTP can be useful for diagnosis, risk stratification, and therapeutic monitoring of many pathologic processes (Fig. 2).

Allowing an estimation of angiogenesis, CTP may provide information regarding differential diagnosis between benign and malignant lesions: increased hepatic arterial blood flow and decreased portal venous flow, frequently observed in cirrhosis and liver tumors, both primary and metastatic, may be easily assessed (Ippolito et al. 2012; Guyennon et al. 2010).

CTP may also allow the prediction of prognosis based on tumor vascularity, reflecting tumor neoangiogenesis, that is known to be related to tumor aggressiveness (Garcia-Figueiras et al. 2013). Additionally, it may predict early response to oncologic therapy and monitor patients during treatment, especially assessing tumor response to antiangiogenic therapy which often induces disease stabilization, rather than changing tumor size, detectable by CTP much earlier than conventional morphologic imaging (Jiang et al. 2013).

Promising results have been accomplished also using CTP for early identification of tumor recurrence and for assessment of vascular layout after interventional procedures (Weidekamm et al. 2005; Choi et al. 2010).

Recent technical advances are addressing CTP's major limitations of high radiation exposure and motion artifacts, mainly by implementing low-tube-voltage techniques, iterative reconstruction algorithms, and motion correction tools of image registration software (Ng et al. 2011).

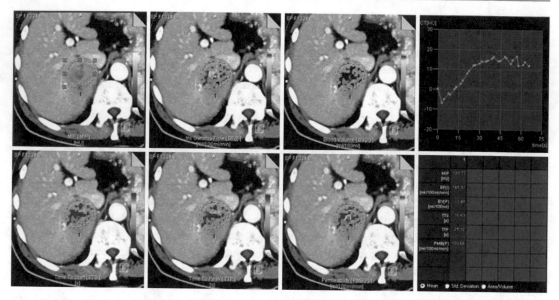

Fig. 2 Liver CT perfusion of a hepatocellular carcinoma. A region of interest is placed within the liver lesion and different parameters (blood flow, blood volume, time to start, time to peak, and permeability) are visually dis-played on color-coded maps and precisely quantified (lower right). Time-attenuation curve (upper right) is eventually generated to depict variations of perfusion parameter as function of time

CTP still presents some limitations such as limited accessibility to perfusion software and lack of standardization in methods. However, these still unsolved problems are being addressed in the last few years.

7 Image Reconstruction

Over the years, different reconstruction algorithms have been developed to determine voxel attenuation values from raw and projection data. To date, reconstruction algorithms may be divided into two major categories:

- *Analytical algorithms*, with filtered back projection (FBP) being the most representative
- *Iterative algorithms*, such as statistical based and model-based reconstruction

7.1 Filtered Back Projection

It has been the standard CT reconstruction method for many years, due to its computational stability and short reconstruction time. FBP is a simple analytic method which ensures an ade-quate image quality by transforming intensity values transmitted at the detector in attenuation values in the projection domain. The latter are then filtered, using different reconstruction algorithms termed "kernels," to exploit peculiar image characteristics. Each kernel, in fact, has its trade-off between spatial resolution and noise: depending on the specific clinical application, a sharper or a smoother kernel may be used to obtain images with higher spatial resolution and increased image noise (e.g., to evaluate lung parenchyma) or images with lower noise and reduced spatial resolution, as recommended for imaging the liver and other soft tissues. Eventually, filtered projection data are back projected in the image domain (Geyer et al. 2015).

Various FBP-type algorithms were developed for different generations of CT scanners; however, all these approaches are based on simplifications such as the pencil-beam geometry of the X-ray and the intensity measurement performer only on a point located at the detector cell center, which affect the robustness.

Additionally, image acquired in specific clinical scenarios (reduced tube output or CT imaging of obese patients) may be affected by consistent image noise, due to the small number of photons reaching the detectors. The result is increased image noise and blooming artifacts, which interfere with structure delineation and impair detectability of low-contrast lesions (Geyer et al. 2015; Fleischmann and Boas 2011).

7.2 Iterative Reconstruction

Iterative reconstruction (IR) was firstly introduced in 1970 and was originally implemented as reconstruction method in first cross-sectional images. However, due to lack of computational power and large amount of data in CT imaging, it was not clinically applicable for routine examinations. Recently, the advances of computational power and the greater attention given to radiation exposure have driven the renaissance of IR approach and the development of a variety of specific algorithms (Willemink and Noel 2018).

IR algorithms rely on a multistep image processing. First, an initial image estimation is created from the projection data, and the second step consists of the generation a new simulated image via a forward projection. Subsequently, the two images are compared, and in case of discrepancy, the first image is updated, through cyclic iterations, according to preselected objective parameters inherent in the algorithm.

Iterations may take place in the projection domain, in the image domain, or in both spaces, and these corrections are repeated until only minimal differences between the two datasets are found. Eventually, the final image is generated, characterized by both noise and artifact reduction and improved contrast and spatial resolution. Although the precise mechanism of each reconstruction algorithm is vendor specific and proprietary, IR algorithms may be classified into statistical based IR and model-based IR, depending on the models underlying the algorithm employed during the reconstruction process (Patino et al. 2015). However, irrespective of the algorithm being used, all IR techniques enable artifact reduction and, moreover, radiation dose savings without an excessive increase of image noise, which represents the main limitation of FBP in achieving diagnostic examinations at low radiation exposure. When applied in clinical practice, IR ensures high image quality and consistent dose reduction compared with FBP, down to 75% in selected clinical scenarios (Fig. 3) (Geyer et al. 2015; Willemink et al. 2013).

IR techniques have demonstrated their benefits also in liver imaging by improving lesion conspicuity and reducing image noise (Marin et al. 2010; Lv et al. 2015; Yu et al. 2013). Additionally, achieving dose reductions without affecting image quality may result to be particularly useful also in hepatic perfusion imaging, which traditionally requires high radiation doses. One of the limitations affecting IR is the generation of "plastic" or "blotchy" datasets, due to image oversmoothing. To mitigate this effect, hybrid reconstruction algorithms, combining FBP and IR, have been developed (Geyer et al. 2015).

In the last few years the scientific community has been working on applying artificial intelligence (AI) to improve CT images' reconstruction process, mostly employing neural networks, aiming at further optimizing image quality and reducing both radiation exposure and reconstruction time. Even though AI is not yet available for clinical implementation, it is expected to play an important role in IR in the foreseeable future (Litjens et al. 2017; Wang and Summers 2012).

8 Post-processing Techniques

The term "post-processing" refers to a specific procedure which enables to display CT images with characteristics—such as orientation and/or thickness viewing—different from those shown in the original presentation. Most common post-processing techniques include:

- Multiplanar reformatting (MPR)
- Maximum intensity projection (MIP)
- Minimum intensity projection (MinIP)
- Volume rendering (VR)

Each of these tools yields different insights into patients' anatomy and shows its peculiar strengths and limitations which impact clinical applications.

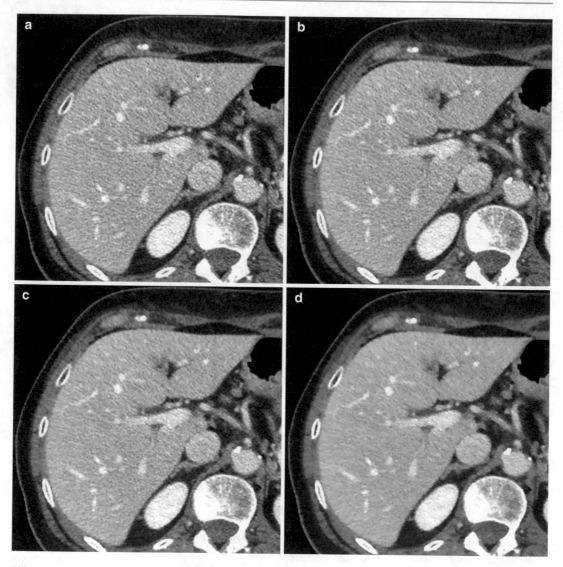

Fig. 3 (**a**) Shows a CT image reconstructed using filtered back-projection algorithm. Modern iterative reconstruction algorithms can be applied with low strength (**b**), medium strength (**c**), or high strength (**d**). Increasing levels of strength indicate a greater noise removal. The choice of the appropriate strength level depends on the clinical purpose and the optimal trade-off between dose reduction and image quality improvement. Despite less noisy, high strength levels (**d**) may result in "plastic" appearance

8.1 Multiplanar Reformatting (MPR)

It refers to planar cross sections oriented through planes other than the axial one, such as coronal and sagittal ones (Fig. 4). For non-orthogonal structures being imaged, oblique planes can also be derived. MPR utility in liver imaging has been especially established in lesion detection in difficult locations, such as subcapsular ones, and/or in heterogeneous parenchyma, such as occurs in cirrhotic liver. MPRs are also useful in the assessment of lesion-enhancing patterns and in the evaluation of tumor vascularity, for either vascular displacement, encasement, invasion, or

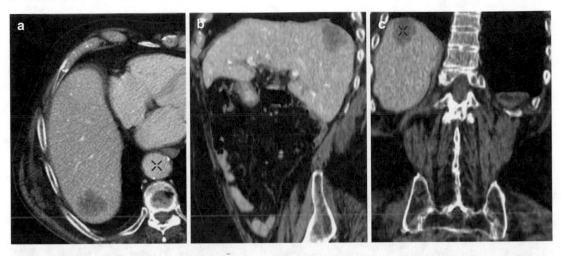

Fig. 4 Multiplanar reformatting images of the liver. Axial image (**a**) shows a hypovascular liver lesion located in the VII segment. Sagittal (**b**) and coronal (**c**) reformats allow for a more precise anatomical assessment especially in cases of subcapsular lesions

neoangiogenesis. Additionally, MPR reformatting may play an important role in preoperative planning, before hepatic surgery (Kamel et al. 2003).

8.2 Maximum Intensity Projection (MIP)

It employs parallel-viewing rays traced from the expected position of the operator and projected through the CT volume: only the highest density voxels detected along the ray path are depicted to be displayed along a predefined axis of the image, generating MIP images. MIP post-processing allows structures that are not in the same plane to be visualized along their entire length, such as occurs in hepatic arteries, providing also useful information about tumor vascularity, feeding vessels, and draining veins (Fig. 5). In general terms, MIP images are useful for depiction of vascular anatomy, providing CT angiography images useful in both preoperative planning of interventional procedures (i.e., chemoembolization) and postoperative evaluation of vascular complications (i.e., after liver transplantation), resulting as a valid tool also in focal lesion characterization due to increased conspicuity (Johnson and Fishman 2018).

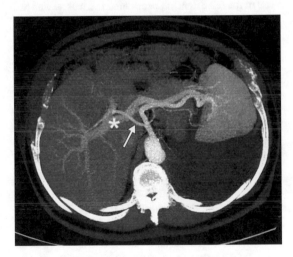

Fig. 5 Maximum intensity projection on the axial plane at the level of the hepatic hilum allows to depict on a single image the course of the hepatic artery (arrow) and the portal vein (asterisk) along with its intrahepatic branches

8.3 Minimum Intensity Projection (MinIP)

Conversely to MIP, only the lowest attenuation values detected along the ray path in each view are depicted to generate MinIP images. It is very useful in displaying structures with lower attenuation values such as the bile ducts and the hepatic biliary tree, showing more evident margins (Fig. 6) (Maher et al. 2004).

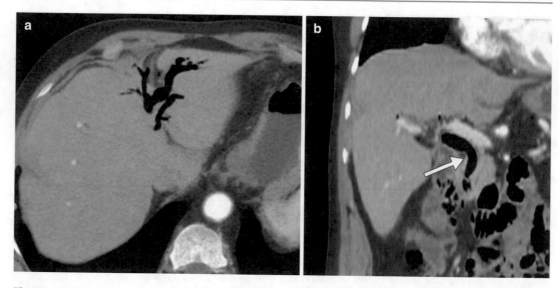

Fig. 6 Minimum intensity projection on the axial plane (**a**) and coronal plane (**b**) provides a comprehensive overview of the full extent of pneumobilia in a patient who had undergone endoscopic retrograde cholangiopancreatography. Pneumobilia involves the common bile duct and the intrahepatic ducts of liver segments II and IV

8.4 Volume Rendering (VR)

It produces 3D images, which can depict an entire organ or volume of interest in a single image. It consists of interpolating all data from scanned volume to provide realistic visualizations of objects, presented from multiple-view angles and freely rotating around an arbitrary point or plane of interest. All voxel values are assigned a color and an opacity level (from 0% to 100%) which may be interactively adjusted to alter the display in real time, possibly enhancing the visualization of particular structures within the imaged volume (Fig. 7) (Maher et al. 2004; Furlow 2014). VR enables the depiction of both hepatic arterial and venous anatomy with an optimal visualization of vascular details and potential anatomical variants, even better than angiography; moreover, it can provide a detailed overview of the liver architecture as well as orientation and characterization features of contingent masses. Moreover, VR reformatting may allow calculation of precise hepatic volumetry, which represents a clinical need in case of surgical planning for both liver transplantation and atypical resections, to evaluate remnant liver volume. Completely manual, semiautomatic, and completely automatic software are available to calculate liver volume,

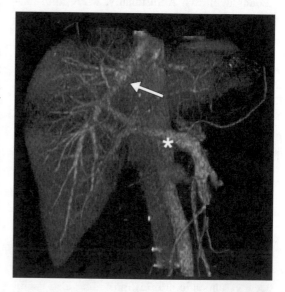

Fig. 7 Three-dimensional volume rendering of the liver on the axial plane provides a comprehensive overview of parenchyma and vessels, such as the portal vein (asterisk) and the hepatic veins (arrow)

allowing a complete assessment in a single study, obviating other radiological procedures (Cai et al. 2016; Lodewick et al. 2016).

Post-processing reformatting enables faster and more efficient interpretation of CT images and, with increasing computer processing power, accuracy, specificity, and post-processing speed are expected to further improve.

9 Dual-Energy CT: Basic Principles and Technical Parameters

Dual-energy CT (DECT), also referred to as *spectral CT,* relies on a simultaneous acquisition of two datasets at different X-ray tube energy levels: a low-energy image dataset, acquired at 70–80 kVp, and a high-energy image dataset, typically acquired at 140–150 kVp. Various DECT techniques have been implemented, exploiting different methods to generate the two energy spectra:

- **Dual-Source DECT (dsDECT):** A single gantry is equipped with two independent X-ray tubes operating at two different potentials, with two corresponding opposite detector rows.
  Low-energy tube commonly operates at 80 kV, and high-energy tube operates at 140 kV. Depending on the scanner, other voltage settings such as 70, 90, and 100 kVp for low-energy tube and 150 kVp for high-energy tube are possible, especially in second- and third-generation dsDECT scanners (Siegel et al. 2016; McCollough et al. 2015; Flohr et al. 2006; Johnson et al. 2007). Disadvantages of such technology are the smaller field of view of the high energy, which may reduce the capability of evaluation of peripherally located abdominal structures in larger patients and the possibility of reduced material decomposition accuracy in rapidly moving structures (Forghani et al. 2017a).
- **Rapid-switching DECT (rsDECT):** The gantry is equipped with a single X-ray tube, performing multiple rapid alternations between high kVp and low kVp during a single gantry rotation. Such technology has a shorter temporal offset compared to dsDECT, leading to reduced beam-hardening artifacts and improved material decomposition accuracy. However, to adapt the two scan acquisitions at each position, rsDECT gantry rotation time is slower than in dsDECT, which might result in higher motion artifacts and nullify the short temporal offset (Furlow 2015).
- **Dual-layer detector DECT (dlDECT):** A combination of a single X-ray source, operating at a single tube potential, and a "sandwich" detector. The innermost layer of the detector is composed by a yttrium-based scintillator absorbing low-energy photons selectively, whereas the outermost detector consists of $Gd_2O_2S_2$ and absorbs high-energy photons (Siegel et al. 2016; McCollough et al. 2015). Spectral separation is limited because it occurs at the level of the detectors. Additionally, this design does not permit alterations of the spectra at the source. However, it ensures excellent temporal and spatial registration. More disadvantages are related to cross-scatter photons: low-energy photons may hit the outermost layer and vice versa, resulting in a contamination of datasets between the two detector layers (Forghani et al. 2017a).
- **Twin-beam DECT:** A combination of a single source and a single detector in which a split filter, consisting of gold, capable to decrease X-ray photon energy, and tin, capable to increase X-ray photon energy, is applied right after the X-ray source to obtain spectral separation. The resultant X-ray beam is split along the z-axis in a low-energy half and a high-energy half (Forghani et al. 2017a; Goo and Goo 2017).
  Advantages of this design include full FOV, relative hardware ease, and lower cost.
  Among the disadvantages, the need of a helical scan, to avoid a different portion of the patient being irradiated by the low- and high-energy spectra, must be considered. Additionally, the central part of the beam is composed by a mixed energy spectrum, disabling material discrimination from that portion of the data. Eventually, cross-scatter photons from one side of the beam may contaminate data at the other side of the beam (Forghani et al. 2017a).
- **Sequential DECT:** Two spiral or sequential scans are sequentially acquired at two different X-ray beams. This DECT design was the first one ever experimented, and may be performed in both volume and helical modes. In volume

mode, consecutive scans of the anatomic section are obtained using two single-rotation acquisitions, performed with different milliamperage settings for each kVp; however, this method was significantly affected by long interscan delay. The helical mode consists of consecutive scans of the entire volume obtained switching the tube potential at each anatomic section level (McCollough et al. 2015). The time delay between the two scans is relatively long and the temporal skew between the acquisitions is a significant disadvantage which may impair temporal registration, especially in moving organs or during contrast opacification. Furthermore, spectral data may be significantly distorted by any patient motion between the different acquisitions (Siegel et al. 2016; Forghani et al. 2017a).

10 Dual-Energy CT: Post-processing

10.1 Blended Images

Typically, the two image datasets acquired at high and low energy levels are by default blended together to generate images resembling conventional 120 kVp CT datasets, which radiologists are familiar with in clinical practice (Forghani et al. 2017b).

Blended images may be derived from linear blending algorithms with different proportion of low- and high-energy data in order to exploit different material characteristics: shifting blending ratio toward lower energies results in images with increased iodine signal but noisier, whereas moving blending ratio toward higher energies results in less image noise, as well as reduced iodine attenuation (Fig. 8) (Scholtz et al. 2015; Tawfik et al. 2012; Yu et al. 2012). Nonlinear blending algorithms may selectively combine information from both datasets with different weighting factors, improving contrast resolution and tissue characterization (Bongers et al. 2016).

10.2 Basis Material Decomposition

My means of basis material decomposition (BMD) the chemical composition of different materials is obtained by quantifying the X-ray attenuation measured at different X-ray energies.

SECT can differentiate tissues only on the basis of their attenuation coefficient (HU). However, HU shows consistent overlap between tissues and materials characterized by very different chemical composition. On the contrary, DECT uses the unique linear attenuation coefficients (μ) obtained by imaging at two different energies, and by modeling the energy

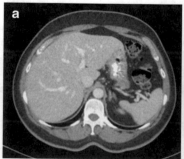 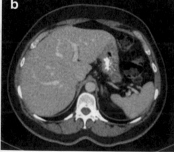 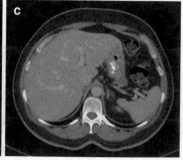

Fig. 8 Blended images generated by third-generation dual-energy dual-source CT scanner. Data from low-kVp tube and high-kVp tube are merged together to generate datasets resembling conventional 120 kVp images radiologist are accustomed to. (**a**) Depicts an image generated by a linear mixing of 90% data from low-kVp tube and 10% data from high-kVp tube. (**b**) Was generated by a blend of 60% data from low-kVp tube and 40% data from high-kVp tube, while (**c**) derives blending 30% data from low-kVp tube and 70% data from high-kVp tube. The higher the contribution of low-kVp tube data in the genesis of the image, the higher the image contrast and beam-hardening effect. The blending ratio can be freely modified by the operator based on the specific diagnostic task. Image courtesy of Dr. Moritz H. Albrecht—University Hospital Frankfurt

dependence of the photon on material mass density (ρ) and atomic number (Z), material-specific information may be obtained, providing diagnostic capabilities far beyond conventional CT (Silva et al. 2011; Marin et al. 2014).

Two different approaches are used, depending on the employed DECT technology:

- *Two-material decomposition*, used in single-source DECT
- *Three-material decomposition*, used in dual-source DECT

The first approach uses a specific algorithm applied in the projection space domain, before images are reconstructed from the low- and high-energy datasets: two selected materials having different atomic numbers and mass attenuation coefficients, most commonly including water and iodine, are used to obtain two sets of images. Consequently, all human tissues are expressed as function of the chosen basis pair. The second approach uses a different algorithm applied in the image space domain, after imaging reconstruction, and is based on the decomposition of three primary elements, generally iodine, soft tissue, and fat (Siegel et al. 2016). Precisely identifying iodine-containing pixels allows to generate a

selective iodine material density display and subtract them from enhanced image, generating a virtual unenhanced display which corresponds to water material density image (Silva et al. 2011). Material decomposition can also be used in liver imaging to assess liver fat quantification (Hyodo et al. 2017).

10.3 Iodine Maps

Material decomposition allows quantifying the iodine content of a single pixel, expressed as mg/mL, with the consequent generation of selective images, representing iodine content in tissues. Such iodine-specific DECT datasets are named *iodine maps* and consist of images generated by assigning a color to the voxels containing iodine. They can be overlaid to standard grayscale images, allowing both qualitative assessment of iodine presence and quantitative measurement of the amount of iodine within a region of interest (Fig. 9) (Foley et al. 2016). Quantitative assessments and selective visualization of iodine CM permit to improve the conspicuity of iodine uptake and, thus, of lesion characterization (Siegel et al. 2016; Krauss 2018; Muenzel et al. 2017a).

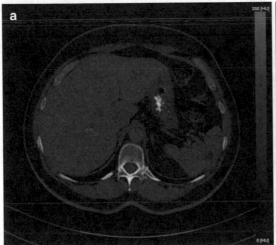 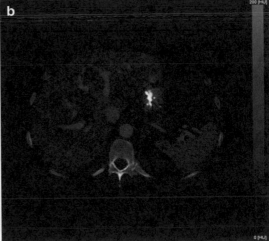

Fig. 9 Iodine map encodes the iodine distribution in each CT voxel and can be superimposed onto conventional CT dataset, with different percentages, resulting in a color-coded iodine overlay image (**a**: 50% superimposition; **b**: 100% superimposition). Red pixels reflect the presence of iodine, while the intensity of the color correlates with the amount of iodine. Image courtesy of Dr. Moritz H. Albrecht—University Hospital Frankfurt

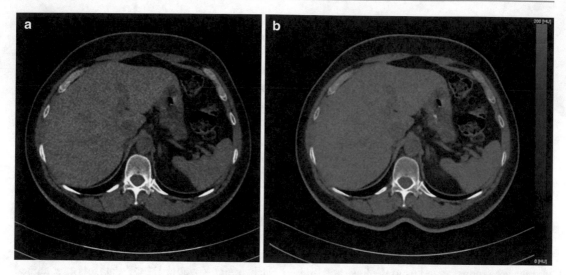

Fig. 10 Virtual non-contrast image (**a**) has comparable image quality of corresponding true non-contrast dataset (**b**), potentially allowing for a significant radiation dose saving by avoiding the need of a pre-contrast scan. Image courtesy of Dr. Moritz H. Albrecht—University Hospital Frankfurt

10.4 Virtual Non-contrast Images

The precise quantification of iodine distribution allows also the virtual removal of the iodine component from the CT number in each image voxel, produced by subtracting the iodine map from the enhanced DECT image (Kartalis et al. 2017; Goo and Goo 2017). The resultant virtual non-contrast (VNC) images have nowadays comparable image quality to true unenhanced datasets (Fig. 10). They allow substantial radiation dose and scanning time reduction by replacing true unenhanced images (Sauter et al. 2018). However, when assessing liver lesions after transarterial chemoembolization with lipiodol as a drug delivery system, true unenhanced images may be required for diagnostic purposes, since VNC alone might erroneously suggest enhancement and presence of viable tumor (Flemming et al. 2016).

10.5 Virtual Monoenergetic Images

X-ray beam used in conventional single-energy CT is polyenergetic, meaning it is composed by a broad spectrum of photons at different energy levels. DECT allows to generate virtual monoenergetic images (VMIs), which are particularly useful in reducing beam-hardening artifacts and increasing iodine attenuation.

VMIs are created in the projection domain or in the image domain, depending on the DECT technology (Yu et al. 2012). Low-keV VMIs, approximating the iodine K-edge (33.2 keV), are characterized by high contrast resolution. On the other hand, they are also intrinsically noisy. Conversely, high-keV VMIs are characterized by less image noise and reduced beam-hardening artifacts; nevertheless, they have low contrast resolution. It has been demonstrated that 60–75 keV VMIs may be considered equivalent to conventional 120 kVp SECT (Siegel et al. 2016) (Fig. 11).

Additionally, VMI may improve tissue characterization through the evaluation of the "spectral attenuation curves" generated by graphically plotting the attenuation values of a material as a function of energy, for every monochromatic energy of the spectrum. For example, iodine is known to show an attenuation peak at lower energies: only structures significantly enhancing after CM administration demonstrate sharp, sloping curves at lower kiloelectron-volt values, whereas structures not showing consistent CM

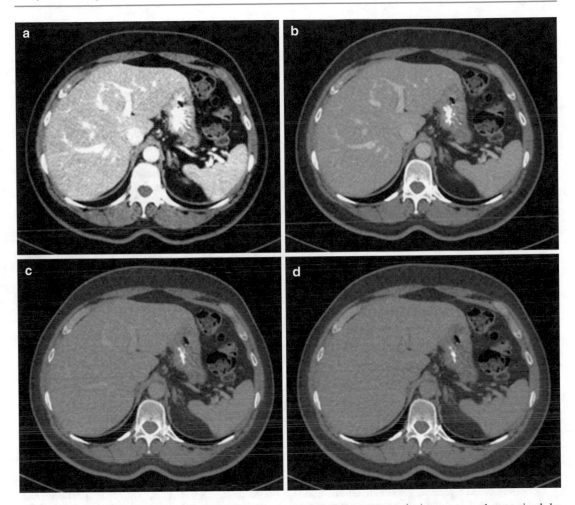

Fig. 11 Virtual monoenergetic images generated at (**a**) 40 keV, (**b**) 70 keV, (**c**) 100 keV, and (**d**) 130 keV. Low-keV monoenergetic images maximize iodine attenuation but are affected by relatively high image noise. Conversely, high-keV monoenergetic images are characterized by lower vascular contrast but reduce calcium blooming and beam-hardening artifacts. Image courtesy of Dr. Moritz H. Albrecht—University Hospital Frankfurt

enhancement display a relatively flatter kiloelectron-volt curve (Agrawal et al. 2014).

11 Future Perspective: Photon-Counting CT

CT scanners currently used in clinical practice are equipped with energy-integrating detectors. Such detector technology operates with a two-step process: the first step consists of absorbing the X-rays and converting them in visible light, which in turn is converted into electric signal by a photodiode. The amplitude of the electric signal is proportional to the total amount of energy that reaches the detectors.

Conversely, photon-counting detectors directly convert X-ray photons in electric signal, without the need of generating visible light. The height of the electrical pulses generated by each photon is proportional to the individual photon energy. The number of pulses exceeding a certain energy (set as threshold) contributes to the genesis of the image, while pulses below the energy threshold are considered as electronic noise and hence excluded from photon counts. Main advantages over photon-counting detectors over energy-integrating detectors are noise reduction and consequent increased signal-to-noise ratio and increased spatial resolution.

More importantly, photon-counting detectors also differentiate multiple contrast agents (such as gadolinium and iodine); such characteristics might result in a single-acquisition multiphasic examination by injecting multiple contrast media at specific time points and then scanning the patient just once, reconstructing arterial and portal venous phase in post-processing. The implementation of this technology would be beneficial in terms of radiation dose savings and small lesion characterization, due to the perfect anatomic match of the different reconstructed phases. Photon-counting CT scanners (Muenzel et al. 2017b; Willemink et al. 2018) for humans are currently available only for research use. Manufacturers and researchers are actively working to optimize such CT systems and implement photon-counting CT in clinical practice in the foreseeable future.

References

Ad-Hoc Working Group of E, et al (2012) A European Renal Best Practice (ERBP) position statement on the Kidney Disease Improving Global Outcomes (KDIGO) clinical practice guidelines on acute kidney injury: part 1: definitions, conservative management and contrast-induced nephropathy. Nephrol Dial Transplant 27(12):4263–4272

Agrawal MD et al (2014) Oncologic applications of dual-energy CT in the abdomen. Radiographics 34(3):589–612

Awai K et al (2002) Aortic and hepatic enhancement and tumor-to-liver contrast: analysis of the effect of different concentrations of contrast material at multidetector row helical CT. Radiology 224(3):757–763

Bae KT (2010) Intravenous contrast medium administration and scan timing at CT: considerations and approaches. Radiology 256(1):32–61

Barrett JF, Keat N (2004) Artifacts in CT: recognition and avoidance. Radiographics 24(6):1679–1691

Boer P (1984) Estimated lean body mass as an index for normalization of body fluid volumes in humans. Am J Phys 247(4 Pt 2):F632–F636

Bongers MN et al (2016) Frequency selective non-linear blending to improve image quality in liver CT. RöFo 188(12):1163–1168

Bruce RJ et al (2009) Background fluctuation of kidney function versus contrast-induced nephrotoxicity. AJR Am J Roentgenol 192(3):711–718

Cai W et al (2016) Comparison of liver volumetry on contrast-enhanced CT images: one semiautomatic and two automatic approaches. J Appl Clin Med Phys 17(6):118–127

Caruso D et al (2018) Lean body weight-tailored iodinated contrast injection in obese patient: Boer versus James formula. Biomed Res Int 2018:8521893

Casillas VJ et al (2000) Imaging of nontraumatic hemorrhagic hepatic lesions. Radiographics 20(2):367–378

Choi SH et al (2010) The role of perfusion CT as a follow-up modality after transcatheter arterial chemoembolization: an experimental study in a rabbit model. Investig Radiol 45(7):427–436

Federle MP, Blachar A (2001) CT evaluation of the liver: principles and techniques. Semin Liver Dis 21(2):135–145

Fleischmann D, Boas FE (2011) Computed tomography--old ideas and new technology. Eur Radiol 21(3):510–517

Flemming BP, De Cecco CN, Hardie AD (2016) Limitation of virtual noncontrast images in evaluation of a liver lesion status post-transarterial chemoembolization. J Comput Assist Tomogr 40(4):557–559

Flohr TG et al (2006) First performance evaluation of a dual-source CT (DSCT) system. Eur Radiol 16(2):256–268

Foley WD (2002) Special focus session: multidetector CT: abdominal visceral imaging. Radiographics 22(3):701–719

Foley WD et al (2016) White Paper of the Society of Computed Body Tomography and Magnetic Resonance on Dual-Energy CT, Part 2: Radiation Dose and Iodine Sensitivity. J Comput Assist Tomogr 40(6):846–850

Forghani R, De Man B, Gupta R (2017a) Dual-energy computed tomography: physical principles, approaches to scanning, usage, and implementation: part 1. Neuroimaging Clin N Am 27(3):371–384

Forghani R, De Man B, Gupta R (2017b) Dual-energy computed tomography: physical principles, approaches to scanning, usage, and implementation: part 2. Neuroimaging Clin N Am 27(3):385–400

Furlan A et al (2011) Hepatocellular carcinoma in cirrhotic patients at multidetector CT: hepatic venous phase versus delayed phase for the detection of tumour washout. Br J Radiol 84(1001):403–412

Furlow B (2014) CT image visualization: a conceptual introduction. Radiol Technol 86(2):187CT–204CT; quiz 205CT–207CT

Furlow B (2015) Dual-energy computed tomography. Radiol Technol 86(3):301ct–321ct; quiz322ct–325ct

Garcia-Figueiras R et al (2013) CT perfusion in oncologic imaging: a useful tool? AJR Am J Roentgenol 200(1):8–19

Geyer LL et al (2015) State of the art: iterative CT reconstruction techniques. Radiology 276(2):339–357

Goo HW, Goo JM (2017) Dual-energy CT: new horizon in medical imaging. Korean J Radiol 18(4):555–569

Guyennon A et al (2010) Perfusion characterization of liver metastases from endocrine tumors: computed tomography perfusion. World J Radiol 2(11):449–454

Heiken JP et al (1995) Dynamic incremental CT: effect of volume and concentration of contrast material and patient weight on hepatic enhancement. Radiology 195(2):353–357

Hu H et al (2000) Four multidetector-row helical CT: image quality and volume coverage speed. Radiology 215(1):55–62

Hyodo T et al (2017) Multimaterial decomposition algorithm for the quantification of liver fat content by using fast-kilovolt-peak switching dual-energy CT: clinical evaluation. Radiology 283(1):108–118

Ippolito D et al (2012) Quantitative assessment of tumour associated neovascularisation in patients with liver cirrhosis and hepatocellular carcinoma: role of dynamic-CT perfusion imaging. Eur Radiol 22(4):803–811

James WPT, Waterlow JC, DHSS/MRC Group on Obesity Research (1976) Research on obesity: a report of the DHSS/MRC group, vol ix. H.M.S.O., London, p 94

Jiang T, Zhu AX, Sahani DV (2013) Established and novel imaging biomarkers for assessing response to therapy in hepatocellular carcinoma. J Hepatol 58(1):169–177

Johnson PT, Fishman EK (2013) Routine use of precontrast and delayed acquisitions in abdominal CT: time for change. Abdom Imaging 38(2):215–223

Johnson PT, Fishman EK (2018) Enhancing Image Quality in the Era of Radiation Dose Reduction: Postprocessing Techniques for Body CT. J Am Coll Radiol 15(3 Pt A):486–488

Johnson TR et al (2007) Material differentiation by dual energy CT: initial experience. Eur Radiol 17(6):1510–1517

Kambadakone AR, Sahani DV (2009) Body perfusion CT: technique, clinical applications, and advances. Radiol Clin N Am 47(1):161–178

Kamel IR, Georgiades C, Fishman EK (2003) Incremental value of advanced image processing of multislice computed tomography data in the evaluation of hypervascular liver lesions. J Comput Assist Tomogr 27(4):652–656

Kanbay M et al (2017) Serum uric acid and risk for acute kidney injury following contrast. Angiology 68(2):132–144

Kanematsu M et al (2006) Imaging liver metastases: review and update. Eur J Radiol 58(2):217–228

Kartalis N, Brehmer K, Loizou L (2017) Multi-detector CT: liver protocol and recent developments. Eur J Radiol 97:101–109

Kim T et al (2001) Discrimination of small hepatic hemangiomas from hypervascular malignant tumors smaller than 3 cm with three-phase helical CT. Radiology 219(3):699–706

Kim SH, Kamaya A, Willmann JK (2014) CT perfusion of the liver: principles and applications in oncology. Radiology 272(2):322–344

Kondo H et al (2010) Body size indexes for optimizing iodine dose for aortic and hepatic enhancement at multidetector CT: comparison of total body weight, lean body weight, and blood volume. Radiology 254(1):163–169

Krauss B (2018) Dual-energy computed tomography: technology and challenges. Radiol Clin N Am 56(4):497–506

Kwasa EA, Vinayak S, Armstrong R (2014) The role of inflammation in contrast-induced nephropathy. Br J Radiol 87(1041):20130738

Laghi A (2007) Multidetector CT (64 slices) of the liver: examination techniques. Eur Radiol 17(3):675–683

Lee CH et al (2013) Use of positive oral contrast agents in abdominopelvic computed tomography for blunt abdominal injury: meta-analysis and systematic review. Eur Radiol 23(9):2513–2521

Lee CH et al (2016) Water as neutral oral contrast agent in abdominopelvic CT: comparing effectiveness with Gastrografin in the same patient. Med J Malaysia 71(6):322–327

Litjens G et al (2017) A survey on deep learning in medical image analysis. Med Image Anal 42:60–88

Lodewick TM et al (2016) Fast and accurate liver volumetry prior to hepatectomy. HPB (Oxford) 18(9):764–772

Lv P et al (2015) Combined use of automatic tube voltage selection and current modulation with iterative reconstruction for CT evaluation of small Hypervascular hepatocellular carcinomas: effect on lesion conspicuity and image quality. Korean J Radiol 16(3):531–540

Maher MM et al (2004) Techniques, clinical applications and limitations of 3D reconstruction in CT of the abdomen. Korean J Radiol 5(1):55–67

Marin D et al (2010) Low-tube-voltage, high-tube-current multidetector abdominal CT: improved image quality and decreased radiation dose with adaptive statistical iterative reconstruction algorithm--initial clinical experience. Radiology 254(1):145–153

Marin D et al (2014) State of the art: dual-energy CT of the abdomen. Radiology 271(2):327–342

McCollough CH et al (2015) Dual- and multi-energy CT: principles, technical approaches, and clinical applications. Radiology 276(3):637–653

Meijerink MR et al (2008) Total-liver-volume perfusion CT using 3-D image fusion to improve detection and characterization of liver metastases. Eur Radiol 18(10):2345–2354

Moos SI et al (2013) Contrast induced nephropathy in patients undergoing intravenous (IV) contrast enhanced computed tomography (CECT) and the relationship with risk factors: a meta-analysis. Eur J Radiol 82(9):e387–e399

Muenzel D et al (2017a) Material density iodine images in dual-energy CT: detection and characterization of hypervascular liver lesions compared to magnetic resonance imaging. Eur J Radiol 95:300–306

Muenzel D et al (2017b) Simultaneous dual-contrast multi-phase liver imaging using spectral photon-counting computed tomography: a proof-of-concept study. Eur Radiol Exp 1(1):25

Ng CS et al (2011) Reproducibility of CT perfusion parameters in liver tumors and normal liver. Radiology 260(3):762–770

Patino M et al (2015) Iterative reconstruction techniques in abdominopelvic CT: technical concepts and clinical implementation. AJR Am J Roentgenol 205(1):W19–W31

Patnana M et al (2018) Liver calcifications and calcified liver masses: pattern recognition approach on CT. AJR Am J Roentgenol 211(1):76–86

Pickhardt PJ et al (2012) Specificity of unenhanced CT for non-invasive diagnosis of hepatic steatosis: implications for the investigation of the natural history of incidental steatosis. Eur Radiol 22(5):1075–1082

Sahani D (2012) Perfusion CT: an overview of technique and clinical applications. http://cds.ismrm.org/protected/10MProceedings/files/Tues%20E09_02%Sahani.pdf

Sauter AP et al (2018) Dual-layer spectral computed tomography: virtual non-contrast in comparison to true non-contrast images. Eur J Radiol 104:108–114

Scholtz JE et al (2015) Non-linear image blending improves visualization of head and neck primary squamous cell carcinoma compared to linear blending in dual-energy CT. Clin Radiol 70(2):168–175

Siegel MJ et al (2016) White Paper of the Society of Computed Body Tomography and Magnetic Resonance on Dual-Energy CT, Part 1: Technology and Terminology. J Comput Assist Tomogr 40(6):841–845

Silva AC et al (2011) Dual-energy (spectral) CT: applications in abdominal imaging. Radiographics 31(4):1031–1046. discussion 1047-50

Soyer P et al (2004) Detection of hypovascular hepatic metastases at triple-phase helical CT: sensitivity of phases and comparison with surgical and histopathologic findings. Radiology 231(2):413–420

Spearman JV et al (2016) Effect of automated attenuation-based tube voltage selection on radiation dose at CT: an observational study on a global scale. Radiology 279(1):167–174

Stacul F et al (2011) Contrast induced nephropathy: updated ESUR contrast media safety committee guidelines. Eur Radiol 21(12):2527–2541

Tawfik AM et al (2012) Dual-energy CT of head and neck cancer: average weighting of low- and high-voltage acquisitions to improve lesion delineation and image quality-initial clinical experience. Investig Radiol 47(5):306–311

Thomas ME et al (2015) The definition of acute kidney injury and its use in practice. Kidney Int 87(1):62–73

van der Molen AJ et al (2018a) Post-contrast acute kidney injury—part 1: definition, clinical features, incidence, role of contrast medium and risk factors: recommendations for updated ESUR contrast medium safety committee guidelines. Eur Radiol 28(7):2845–2855

van der Molen AJ et al (2018b) Post-contrast acute kidney injury. Part 2: risk stratification, role of hydration and other prophylactic measures, patients taking metformin and chronic dialysis patients: recommendations for updated ESUR contrast medium safety committee guidelines. Eur Radiol 28(7):2856–2869

Wang S, Summers RM (2012) Machine learning and radiology. Med Image Anal 16(5):933–951

Weidekamm C et al (2005) Effects of TIPS on liver perfusion measured by dynamic CT. AJR Am J Roentgenol 184(2):505–510

Willemink MJ, Noel PB (2018) The evolution of image reconstruction for CT-from filtered back projection to artificial intelligence. Eur Radiol

Willemink MJ et al (2013) Iterative reconstruction techniques for computed tomography part 2: initial results in dose reduction and image quality. Eur Radiol 23(6):1632–1642

Willemink MJ et al (2018) Photon-counting CT: technical principles and clinical prospects. Radiology 289(2):293–312

Williamson EE, McKinney JM (2001) Assessing the adequacy of peripherally inserted central catheters for power injection of intravenous contrast agents for CT. J Comput Assist Tomogr 25(6):932–937

Yu L, Leng S, McCollough CH (2012) Dual-energy CT-based monochromatic imaging. AJR Am J Roentgenol 199(5 Suppl):S9–S15

Yu MH et al (2013) Low tube voltage intermediate tube current liver MDCT: sinogram-affirmed iterative reconstruction algorithm for detection of hypervascular hepatocellular carcinoma. AJR Am J Roentgenol 201(1):23–32

Magnetic Resonance Imaging of the Liver: Technical Considerations

António Pedro Pissarra, Raquel Madaleno, Manuela França, and Filipe Caseiro-Alves

Contents

Abstract

Magnetic resonance imaging (MRI) is one the leading imaging modalities to evaluate liver diseases, with an active role both on focal liver lesions and diffuse parenchymal evaluation.

A. P. Pissarra · R. Madaleno
Imaging Department, University Center Hospital of Coimbra (CHUC), Coimbra, Portugal

M. França
Imaging Department, Centro Hospitalar Universitário do Porto, Porto, Portugal

F. Caseiro-Alves (✉)
Imaging Department, University Center Hospital of Coimbra (CHUC), Coimbra, Portugal

Faculty of Medicine, University of Coimbra, Coimbra, Portugal
e-mail: lcalves@fmed.uc.pt

Despite its diagnostic capabilities, MR imaging is far more difficult to manage than computed tomography (CT). The aim of the current chapter is to review the protocols for liver imaging using standard technical specifications able to provide reproducible image quality, and to review advanced applications encompassing quantification issues, allowing therapeutical monitoring and disease follow-up. The chapter also adresses strategies to derive functional information, especially using diffusion-weighted imaging and dedicated liver specific contrast agents. Its scope is to allow the reader an in-depth vision of modern MR of the liver from a clinical point of view, proposing imaging protocols effective at 1.5 and 3T magnets.

© Springer Nature Switzerland AG 2021
E. Quaia (ed.), *Imaging of the Liver and Intra-hepatic Biliary Tract*,
Medical Radiology, Diagnostic Imaging, https://doi.org/10.1007/978-3-030-38983-3_5

1 Introduction

Magnetic resonance imaging (MRI) actually plays an important role in the detection and characterization of focal liver lesions as well as evaluation of diffuse hepatic diseases, proving to be more efficient than computed tomography (CT).

This imaging modality enables a comprehensive assessment of tissue characteristics through its multiparametric capabilities, providing accurate qualitative and quantitative data (Donato et al. 2017; Guglielmo et al. 2014; Van Beers et al. 2015). To fully harness the potentialities of MRI in liver study, it is important to optimize parameters in order to reduce artifacts and improve imaging interpretation, selecting the adequate contrast agent for each clinical situation (Bitar et al. 2006; Donato et al. 2017; Guglielmo et al. 2014). The aim of this chapter is to review basic and advanced protocols needed to produce a diagnostic MR study of the liver.

2 Standard Liver Protocols

2.1 Basic Sequences

Sequences applied in liver MRI can be divided into two main groups: fast or turbo spin echo (or FSE, characterized by multiple "refocusing pulses" of 180° after the initial 90° radiofrequency (Rf) pulse) and gradient echo (or GRE, where the phase coherence after the initial 90° pulse is regained by the inverted rephasing lobe of the frequency-encoding gradient) (Pooley 2005). For FSE moderately T2-weighted (−w) imaging with TE of 60–120 ms (ideally 80–100 ms) or heavily T2-w sequences (SSFSE or HASTE) using a longer TE in the range of 160 ms (ideally 180–200 ms) may contribute to differentiate cysts and hemangiomas from other solid liver tumors (Fig. 1). Since gradient echo sequences (GRE) are highly sensitive to susceptibility artifacts, induced by the presence of iron,

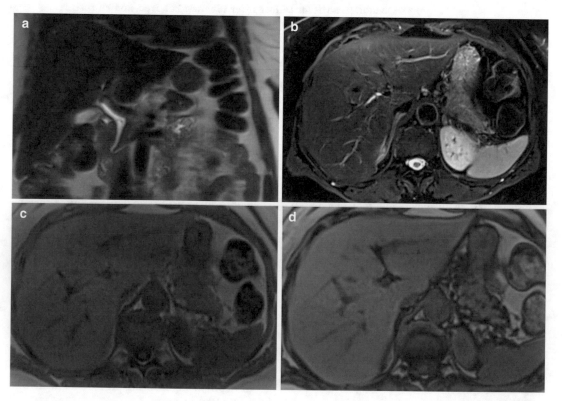

Fig. 1 Mandatory pre-contrast sequences in a liver MRI study. (**a**) HASTE sequence in the coronal plane. (**b**) T2 sequence with fat suppression in the axial plane. (**c**, **d**) T1 GRE in and out of phase

calcium, air, or metal (Donato et al. 2017), they can be applied to disclose individual proton species, such as detection of microscopic fat (in focal liver lesions such as hepatocellular adenomas or diffusely in liver steatosis) using opposed-phase images (Fig. 1). The TE in opposed phase should be lower than in-phase (usually 2.3 ms and 4.6 at 1.5T, respectively), and as low as possible in order to reduce the T2* decay. Short time inversion recovery sequences (STIR) are an alternative to FSE T2-w FS sequences. With this type of sequence focal liver lesions display higher contrast-to-noise ratio (CNR) due to the profound fat signal suppression but unfortunately spatial resolution is hampered making it seldom used in liver MR protocols. For contrast-enhanced imaging, 3D GRE T1-w fat-saturated sequences are usually applied, and allow obtaining high SNR, spatial resolution, and image detail when compared with 2D techniques (Guglielmo et al. 2014; Matos et al. 2015).

2.2 Specified Techniques to Optimize Liver MRI Study

2.2.1 Modified Dixon Technique

Modified Dixon technique is based on the principle of chemical shift between water and fat protons, which difference is directly proportional to the intensity of the static magnetic field. With this technique, it is possible to null more homogeneously the fatty components without the use of additional fat-selective gradient pulses. With this approach, four sequences can be simultaneously acquired within the same breath-hold, in-phase, opposed-phase, water-only, and fat-only images, contributing to increase image quality and reduce the overall scan time (Pokharel et al. 2013).

2.2.2 Free-Breathing Sequences: Multiphasic Liver Imaging and Compressed Sensing

Dynamic contrast-enhanced MR of the liver (DE-MR) is acquired during a single breath-hold typically of 15–20 s, using 3D GRE T1-w gradient-echo fat-suppressed sequences (Kaltenbach et al. 2017). In the last decade, free-breathing sequences have been developed using a combination of central k-space sampling (keyhole technique) with radial acquisition of the k-space data. This modification makes the acquisition less sensitive to respiratory artifacts since acquisition of the relevant k-space to provide image contrast is performed first reducing motion-related artifacts.

Late arterial phase acquisition—corresponding to the best hypervascular tumor-related enhancement—is critical for detection of small hypervascular lesions, namely hepatocellular carcinoma, in order to increase sensitivity. However, obtaining this phase may be technically challenging because it depends on many variables: patient's cardiac output, type of contrast agent, rate of contrast injection, and imaging protocol (Clarke et al. 2015). Using the keyhole strategy, it is possible to obtain several phases of liver enhancement in the same breath-hold period (Chandarana et al. 2013). As such, it is possible to obtain three or more sets of images (each for 4–5 s) within the same breath-hold period of 15–20 s. Adding the multicoil compressed sensing reconstruction technique with the highly accelerated free-breathing volumetric dynamic MRI technique with radial sparse parallel MRI (acronyms: GRASP from Siemens manufacturer and Hypersense from General Electric) instead of one, several phases can be acquired (10–20) of the whole liver in a free-breathing mode (Fig. 2).

2.3 Diffusion-Weighted Imaging (DWI)

This technique has been increasingly applied to liver MRI and has revealed itself as an integral part of state-of-the-art MR liver studies, increasing clinical confidence and reducing false positives. DW-MRI is based on the physical process of random movement of water molecules in the extracellular and intravascular spaces, which is not entirely free since it depends on physical interactions with biological barriers like cell membranes, macromolecules, and flow within tubular structures (like vessels and ducts) (Lewis et al. 2014; Matos et al. 2015). Tissues with dif-

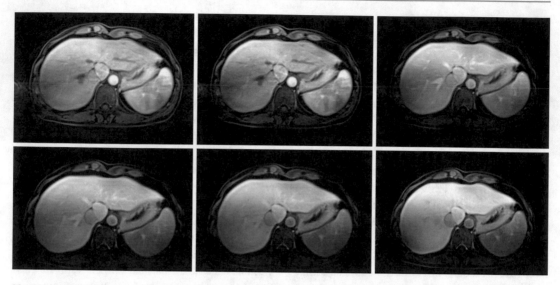

Fig. 2 Dynamic contrast-enhanced 3D GRE using the free-breathing multiarterial compressed sense technique. More than 15 phases of free-breathing liver images are obtained increasing the diagnostic capabilities of CE-MRI. To note the enhancing nodule at segment 1, taking up Gd-EOB-DTPA in the transitional phase (last image)

ferent cellularity allow different degrees of water proton mobility and consequently DWI derives image contrast from these differences. Different series of DW images are generally acquired (two or more) through modification of the gradient strength and magnitude, referred to as b-value. At a b-value of 0 s/mm^2 no diffusion gradient is applied and consequently no diffusion information is retrieved, giving similar information as T2-w FS sequences. In images obtained with a low b-value ($b < 100$ s/mm^2) rapid movement of water molecules inside the vessels translates into marked signal attenuation of these structures, resulting in a "black blood" effect improving conspicuity for lesions located near the dark vessels. At higher b-value images (b 500–1000 s/mm^2), water movement restriction in highly cellular tissues translates into persistent bright appearance, with greater SNR and CNR and less artifacts (Fig. 3) (Chilla et al. 2015; Lewis et al. 2014).

The interpretation of DW images can be done visually but also quantitatively, through the apparent diffusion coefficient (ADC) map (Boyle et al. 2006). The ADC map reflects the intrinsic tissue properties and is the graphical representation of the ratio of DW signal intensities.

2.4 Contrast Agents

T1-w two- (2D) or three-dimensional (3D) gradient echo (GRE) sequences with fat suppression (or nulling) are the sequences of choice in dynamic liver MRI (Huh et al. 2015; LeBedis et al. 2012; Thian et al. 2013). These sequences offer a very good temporal resolution being obtained during a single breath-hold, with suitable spatial resolution and signal-to-noise ratio (Huh et al. 2015; Thian et al. 2013). TR and TE should be as short as possible since a short TR reduces acquisition time and increases T1 weighting, while short TE reduces susceptibility artifacts. Tipically, the flip angle varies from 10° to 15°. Fat suppression is essential since it minimizes abdominal wall artifacts by suppressing subcutaneous fat. Some of the most employed 3D GRE sequences in liver examination are VIBE (Volumetric Interpolated Breath-Hold Examination; Siemens Healthcare, Erlangen, Germany), LAVA (Liver Acquisition Volume Acceleration; GE Healthcare, Milwaukee, WI, USA), and eTHRIVE (enhanced T1-high-resolution isotropic volume excitation; Philips

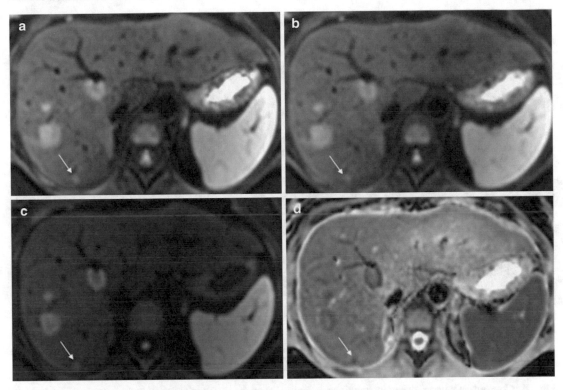

Fig. 3 Diffusion-weighted imaging obtained with b-values of 50 (**a**), 100 (**b**), and 800 s/mm² (**c**) showing restricted diffusion of metastases in the right liver lobe. (**d**) Corresponding ADC map depicting lower ADC values. Note the sub-centimeter subcapsular lesion (arrow), easily detected with DWI

Healthcare, Best, The Netherlands) (Huh et al. 2015, Thian et al. 2013).

There are three major types of MRI contrast agents, according to its biodistribution: (1) non-specific extracellular gadolinium agents, (2) hepatobiliary-specific agents, and (3) blood pool agents (Bashir 2014; LeBedis et al. 2012). Extracellular Gd chelates remain the most commonly used, with wide applicability in liver and other organ imaging. They are the best documented and those who have the longest clinical experience (LeBedis et al. 2012; O'Neill et al. 2015). Currently, with the generalized use of macrocyclic agents instead of those with a linear configuration, no additional cases of nephrogenic systemic fibrosis (NSF) are being reported. This is due to the stability of the Gd molecule of macrocyclic agents avoiding decomplexation of the metal from the chelating agent DTPA. Dynamic contrast-enhanced imaging is performed in order to encompass the late arterial, portal venous, and interstitial or delayed phases (Fig. 4). To achieve the most effective late arterial phase, the peak of the contrast bolus and the acquisition of the central lines of *k*-space, which encode tissue contrast, should be synchronized. An individual, tailored, acquisition delay is preferred than a fixed delay, either using a test bolus or bolus-tracking techniques (Bashir 2014; LeBedis et al. 2012; Wile and Leyendecker 2010). Typically, the late arterial phase (occurring 30–40 s after the beginning of the contrast injection) is recognized by excellent arterial enhancement, enhancement of the main portal vein, and absence of contrast in the hepatic veins.

Hepatobiliary-specific agents are multiphasic agents that combine extracellular and hepatocyte-selective properties. After reaching the hepatic sinusoids, these agents are transported across the functioning hepatocytes via membrane receptors at the sinusoidal pole of the hepatocytes and are eliminated via the biliary tract, by transporting polypeptides located at the biliary pole of the

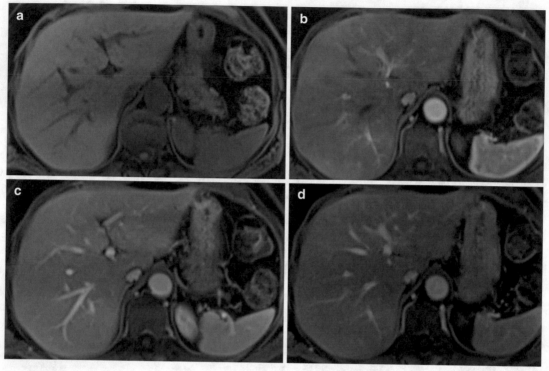

Fig. 4 Contrast-enhanced dynamic multiphase liver study. (**a**) Plain 3D T1 GRE with the Dixon technique water images. (**b**) Arterial phase acquired 35 s after intra- venous contrast injection. Portal venous (**c**) and late inter- stitial (**d**) phases, obtained, respectively, 70 s and 5 min after contrast administration

hepatocyte. Currently, two Gd-based hepatobiliary-specific agents are available in the majority of countries: gadobenate dimeglumine (Gd-BOPTA, MultiHance®, Bracco Imaging, Milan, Italy) and gadoxetic acid (Gd-EOB-DTPA, Primovist®, Bayer Schering Pharma AG, Berlin, Germany) (Donato et al. 2017).

Gd-BOPTA-recommended dose is 0.1 mmol/ kg administered in a bolus injection (2 mL/s). Only 5% of the contrast is cleared by the biliary tract, with the remaining being eliminated by renal excretion. The hepatobiliary phase is achieved 1–2 h following contrast injection (LeBedis et al. 2012). It has a better dynamic phase imaging compared to Gd-EOB-DTPA and extracellular agents. Gd-EOB-DTPA-recommended dose is 0.025 mmol/kg and about 50% is excreted by the biliary system. The patient can be scanned only once with a waiting time to allow for hepatocyte uptake around 10–20 min after injection depending on the baseline liver function (Fig. 5). Increasing the flip angle to

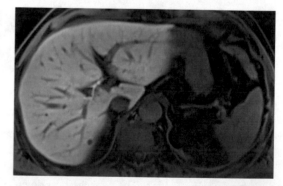

Fig. 5 Hepatobiliary phase 20 min after intravenous administration of the hepatobiliary contrast Gd-EOB-DTPA. Vivid enhancement of the right hepatic duct in a patient with normal liver function and biliary excretion of the contrast media

30–35° in the hepatobiliary phase acquisition improves CNR of liver lesions by increasing the signal of the enhanced liver and biliary tract and decreases the signal intensity of non-enhancing structures (Guglielmo et al. 2014; Thian et al. 2013).

3   Liver MRI at 1.5T and 3T

Scanners operating at a 3T magnetic field are being used more and more frequently in clinical practice over the last decade. The stronger static magnetic 3T field (when compared to 1.5T) translates into increased SNR, and spatial and temporal resolution (Chang et al. 2008). T1 relaxation time of a proton refers to the time necessary for its return to the original energy state after excitation by the RF pulse. T1 values depend on the proton microenvironment (decreasing with greater structural organization) and the static magnetic field strength (increasing in stronger fields, being therefore longer at 3T when compared to 1.5T) (Chang et al. 2008). In-phase and out-phase sequences at 3T imaging suffer modifications, since the precession frequencies of water and fat protons are reduced to half of the values found at 1.5T. At 3T the shortest out-phase and in-phase TEs are 1.15 ms and 2.3 ms, respectively (Chang et al. 2008; Ramalho et al. 2007).

Although liver tissue T1 relaxation times substantially increase at 3T, the higher magnetic field strength results in minimal changes for T1 gadolinium-shortening effects, leading to higher liver-to-lesion contrast, which can be used to improve contrast resolution; use of thinner slices; or reduced scan time, which is important in uncooperative patients (Chang et al. 2008; Huh et al. 2015).

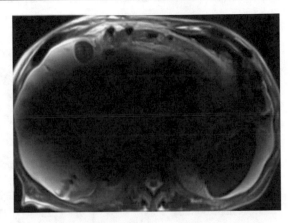

Fig. 6 Dielectric artifact observed at a 3T MR study in a patient with ascites, rendering the study unreadable

Performing exams with a stronger magnetic field has some disadvantages, resulting from a greater radiofrequency power transmission to the patient (especially in T2-w TSE sequences due to the larger number of RF pulses) resulting in high SAR values (Girometti 2015). The so-called standing wave or dielectric artifact is also more common at 3T imaging, occurring in patients with large abdominal diameters (such as obese or when ascites is present), that exceeds the RF pulse wavelength, resulting in heterogeneous deposition of energies and large variations in signal intensities (Fig. 6) (Chang et al. 2008; Girometti 2015; Huh et al. 2015).

Protocols for 1.5T and 3T liver MRI exams are hereby presented below:

Sequence	Plane	TR (ms)	TE (ms)	Flip angle	Fat saturation	Matrix	FOV (mm)	No. of slices	Slice thickness (mm)
HASTE	Coronal	900	77	150°	None	256 × 243	400	40	5
HASTE	Axial	900	77	150°	None	256 × 218	400	44	5
T2 TSE FS	Axial	1550	93	150°	Fat sat	384 × 269	380	20	8
T1 GRE in and out of phase	Axial	100	2.27 5.19	70°	None	256 × 192	380	20	8
Diffusion	Axial	2300	70	90°	Fat sat	160 × 120	450	20	8
T1 3D GRE VIBE	Axial	4.88	2.38	10°	Fat sat	256 × 205	380	60	3
T1 3D GRE VIBE hepatobiliary	Axial	4.88	2.38	30°	Fat sat	256 × 205	380	60	3

Liver MRI protocol for 1.5T

Sequence	Plane	TR (ms)	TE (ms)	Flip angle	Fat saturation	Matrix	FOV (mm)	No. of slices	Slice thickness (mm)
HASTE	Coronal	2500	121	119°	None	384 × 326	380	32	5
HASTE	Axial	2500	117	158°	None	320 × 304	400	40	4
T2 TSE FS	Axial	3000	94	84°	SPAIR	384 × 314	380	40	4
T1 GRE VIBE in and out of phase	Axial	4.39	1.37 2.81	9°	None	320 × 240	370	64	3
Diffusion (b 50,100 e 800)	Axial	4600	43	90°	SPAIR	134 × 134	380	35	5
T1 3D GRE VIBE DIXON	Axial	4	1.31 2.54	9°	DIXON	320 × 320	370	80	2.5
T1 3D GRE VIBE DIXON hepatobiliary	Axial	4	1.31 2.54	9° (DIXON) 30° (VIBE)	DIXON	320 × 320	370	80	2.5

Liver MRI protocol for 3T

4 Quantitative MR for Diffuse Liver Diseases: Fat, Iron, and Fibrosis

4.1 MR Techniques for Quantification of Hepatic Fat (Proton Density Fat Fraction)

4.1.1 MR Spectroscopy

Both fat and water contain protons that process at a characteristic frequency. The intensity of its signal is proportional to the amount of those protons, or proton density (PD). MR spectroscopy is a technique that measures the amplitude of each peak in the frequency spectrum. Therefore, in a fat-water admixture such as a fatty liver, knowing a priori the resonance frequencies of fat and water protons, their concentrations can be measured directly from their spectral signal (Yokoo and Browning 2014). Hepatic fat (triglyceride) signal has multiple frequency components, the dominant one being located at a frequency shift of 420 Hz (1.46 ppm) relative to water peak, on 3T magnetic field. Fat proton density results from the sum of these diverse multiple fat peaks, and proton density fat fraction can be determined by measuring the sum of the fat peaks and the water peak. MRS is an accurate and reproducible method for quantification of proton density fat fraction (PDFF), being considered the imaging gold standard for hepatic fat quantification

(Reeder et al. 2011). However, it is time consuming, it needs dedicated software tools, it is limited to a small sampling volume (1 to 2 cm voxel), and it is only available in specialized hospital or research centers (Reeder et al. 2011; Yokoo and Browning 2014).

4.1.2 Multi-echo Chemical Shift-Encoded Sequences

In the last decade, advanced multi-echo chemical shift-encoded (MECSE) GRE MR sequences have emerged as an accurate tool for PDFF quantification (Reeder et al. 2011) (Fig. 7; see also chapter "Liver Steatosis and NAFLD", Figs. 12–15). These sequences, performed with more than 3 echoes (usually between 6 and 12), take advantage of the chemical shift of water and fat protons, separating the fat and water signal intensities and allowing to quantify fat fraction. For precise fat quantification, these sequences must be corrected for the main confounding factors such as the T1 and T2* relaxation effects and the fat spectral complexity (Reeder et al. 2011, 2012; Yokoo and Browning 2014). The effect of T2* relaxation between different echoes may confound PDFF quantification, particularly when there is concomitant iron deposition in the liver parenchyma, but also in normal livers. By using more than three echoes, the signal-fitting model of the multiple echoes allows to quantify fat and also to estimate the T2* relaxation. The T2*

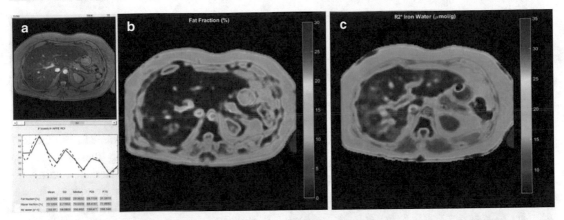

Fig. 7 Hepatic fat and iron quantification using a MECSE MR sequence. Hepatic fat (PDFF, %) and iron (R2*, s⁻¹) can be measured with ROIs placed in the liver parenchyma (**a**), or in PDFF and R2* parametric maps (**b, c**). In this patient with nonalcoholic fatty liver disease, there is severe steatosis (PDFF 30%) and also mild elevation of R2* (150 s⁻¹) indicating coexistent iron deposition

estimation will be used to correct the effect of T2* relaxation on PDFF quantification and, furthermore, because liver T2* is related to the amount of iron deposition, it can also be used for simultaneous quantification of iron deposits (Donato et al. 2017; França et al. 2017; Reeder et al. 2011, 2012; Yokoo and Browning 2014). Fat protons have a shorter T1 relaxation time than water protons. Therefore, a significant bias in fat fraction estimation will occur if the acquisition is T1 weighted. The T1 relaxation effect can thus be minimized using a low flip angle (<10°) (Liu et al. 2007). Finally, the fitting model should also incorporate the multiple frequencies of fat spectrum to take into account the spectral complexity that results from multiple proton resonance frequencies of triglycerides (Reeder et al. 2011, 2012, Yokoo and Browning 2014).

Quantification of PDFF can be performed using in-house advanced methods or commercially available sequences, in both 1.5-T and 3.0-T MR equipment. Fat measurements can be presented in parametric maps, demonstrating the hepatic PDFF values, pixel by pixel, with the advantage to demonstrate the distribution of fat throughout the liver parenchyma. MECSE-MR imaging sequences are accurate for quantification of hepatic steatosis (França et al. 2017; Idilman et al. 2013; Tang et al. 2013) and a recent meta-analysis from the RSNA Quantitative Imaging

Biomarker Alliance PDFF Committee has demonstrated that MR imaging PDFF measurements, when compared with MR spectroscopy, have an excellent linearity, bias, and precision across different manufacturers, field strengths, and reconstruction methods (Yokoo et al. 2018).

4.2 MR Techniques for Quantification of Hepatic Iron Overload

MR imaging is sensitive to the presence of iron due to its paramagnetic effect on the neighborhood protons, increasing the T2* signal decay. The T2* signal decay is, therefore, proportional to the amount of iron concentration. There are two methods to quantify liver iron concentration (LIC): the signal-intensity ration (SIR) and relaxometry methods.

4.2.1 Signal Intensity Ratio Methods

The most widely used method for quantification of LIC is a SIR method that requires five different IP GRE sequences and compares the signal intensity between the liver and a non-overloaded reference tissue (paraspinal muscles) (Gandon et al. 2004), using an algorithm available on a free website, and it was calibrated for 1.5-T and, more recently, for 3.0-T (Paisant et al. 2017). However,

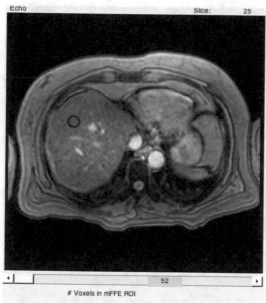

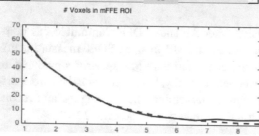

Fig. 8 R2* relaxometry for hepatic iron quantification, using a multi-echo GRE sequence with 12 TEs. The plot of mean SI within a circular ROI is modeled as a function of TE, as a bi-exponential decay curve. The estimated R2* is 530 s⁻¹, corresponding to LIC of 86 μmol/g dry liver

Hepatic T2 and T2* (or R2, R2*) are closely related to LIC, and several papers calibrated relaxometry measurements against liver biopsies, to generate empirical calibration curves between MR measurements and LIC (mg Fe/g or μmol Fe/g) (Garbowski et al. 2014; Hankins et al. 2009; Henninger et al. 2015; St Pierre 2005; Wood 2005). LIC can be estimated from the R2* or T2* measurements, using these calibration curves, as long as they are calculated with validated acquisition and analysis protocols.

The most used R2 relaxometry method (St Pierre 2005) is available as a commercial service (FerriScan®) and requires five T2-weighted sequences, acquired during free breathing, and images are forwarded for centralized image data analysis and quantification. These SE techniques are less sensitive to external magnetic inhomogeneities; however they are more prone to artifacts, since they require longer acquisition time than R2* techniques (Sirlin and Reeder 2010).

On the other hand, R2* relaxometry methods are performed with GRE multi-echo sequences, during one or two breath-hold acquisitions (Garbowski et al. 2014; Hankins et al. 2009; Henninger et al. 2015; Wood 2005). T2* or R2* measurements are then calculated using commercial post-processing software or in-house-developed software (Fig. 8). For precise quantification, even in heavily overloaded livers, the first echo should be as short as possible (less than 1 ms) and the echo spacing should be short enough (1 ms or less) (Yokoo and Browning 2014).

Furthermore, as mentioned above, the MECSE MR sequences that are used for PDFF quantification can also be used for simultaneous R2* estimation and LIC quantification (see Fig. 6; chapter "Liver Steatosis and NAFLD", Figs. 12–15) (França et al. 2017; Martí-Bonmatí et al. 2011; Sirlin and Reeder 2010; Yokoo and Browning 2014).

Although MR imaging is being widely used for LIC quantification, there is still a lack of standardization and consensus across different methods, mainly because relaxation rates are dependent on imaging acquisition parameters and magnetic field strengths (Yokoo and Browning 2014).

these measurements can be biased by coexisting hepatic steatosis and/or muscle fatty infiltration and overestimated iron overload (Castiella et al. 2010). Consequently, this algorithm was recently modified, and now it uses a SIR method for heavy overloads and relaxometry for low or moderate overloads.

4.2.2 Relaxometry

Relaxometry methods use a series of images acquired with increasing TE, with a SE or a multi-echo GRE sequence. The liver signal intensity is modeled as a function of TE, using a mono-exponential or bi-exponential decay model, calculating the signal decay constants (T2 or T2*) or the signal decay rates (R2 or R2*, which is the inverse of T2 or T2*) (Fig. 8).

4.3 MR Advanced Techniques for Quantifying Hepatic Fibrosis

Imaging evaluation of hepatic fibrosis is widely performed with ultrasound-based methods, such as transient elastography or shear wave elastography. Nevertheless, MR techniques have the advantage to analyze a larger volume of liver parenchyma and to allow deeper penetration into tissues. Therefore, MR imaging techniques allow assessing the whole liver and, moreover, provide morphologic information and are not limited by obesity or ascites. Furthermore, evaluation of liver fibrosis can be performed as a part of a tailored liver evaluation, together with quantification of liver steatosis and iron overload.

4.3.1 MR Elastography

MR elastography (MRE) is an advanced MR imaging technique that quantifies the liver stiffness, measuring the speed of shear waves propagating through the liver. For this technique, a dedicated hardware is required, an acoustic driver system that is located outside the magnet, coupled to a passive driver that is placed overlying the liver, which is used to induce the shear waves (Venkatesh et al. 2013). A phase-contrast MR sequence with motion-encoding gradients detects the shear waves, which are converted in quantitative maps (elastograms) of tissue stiffness (measured in kPa). MRE can be implemented on most conventional MR system, using modified GRE, SE, or echo-planar imaging sequences (Venkatesh et al. 2013), and the propagating waves in the liver are usually well tolerated.

The mechanical properties are not dependent on magnetic field strength and MRE measurements can be performed in 1.5T–7T equipment (Venkatesh et al. 2013). Liver stiffness increases with the progression of liver fibrosis and several studies demonstrated that MRE has a high sensitivity and specificity for diagnosing and staging liver fibrosis, in patients with chronic liver diseases from different etiologies (Godfrey et al. 2013; Singh et al. 2015a, b). Furthermore, MRE is robust across different MR manufacturers, field strengths, and pulse sequences (Petitclerc et al. 2016; Yin et al. 2016).

MRE performance is not significantly affected by gadolinium administration (Hallinan et al. 2015), neither by obesity nor by ascites (Petitclerc et al. 2016). Nevertheless, liver stiffness measurements can be confounded by liver inflammation and moderate-to-severe iron overload (Horowitz et al. 2017; Petitclerc et al. 2016; Venkatesh et al. 2013). Modified SE MRE sequences provide higher SNR images and are advantageous in patients with iron-overloaded livers, in whom the conventional GRE MRE failed due to low liver signal intensity (Mariappan et al. 2016; Wagner et al. 2016).

4.3.2 T1 Mapping

Measuring the liver T1 relaxation time (T1 rho) may provide information about the tissue composition, as T1 relaxation increases with higher fibrosis stages (Petitclerc et al. 2016).

A single breath-hold shortened modified look-locker inversion recovery (shMOLLI) sequence is acquired to obtain T1 relaxation time maps of the liver (Banerjee et al. 2014; Donato et al. 2017). This technique has the advantage of requiring neither contrast agent nor additional hardware. Nevertheless, contradictory results were reported about the role of T1 relaxation for staging hepatic fibrosis, and more investigational and clinical studies are still required (Petitclerc et al. 2016).

References

Banerjee R, Pavlides M, Tunnicliffe EM et al (2014) Multiparametric magnetic resonance for the non-invasive diagnosis of liver disease. J Hepatol 60(1):69–77

Bashir MR (2014) Magnetic resonance contrast agents for liver imaging. Magn Reson Imaging Clin N Am 22(3):283–293

Bitar R, Leung G, Perng R et al (2006) MR pulse sequences: what every radiologist wants to know but is afraid to ask. Radiographics 26:513–537

Boyle GE, Ahern M, Cooke J et al (2006) An interactive taxonomy of MR imaging sequences. Radiographics 26:e24

Castiella A, Alústiza JM, Emparanza JI et al (2010) Liver iron concentration quantification by MRI: are recommended protocols accurate enough for clinical practice? Eur Radiol 21(1):137–141

Chandarana H, Feng L, Block TK et al (2013) Free-breathing contrast-enhanced multiphase MRI of the liver using a combination of compressed sensing, parallel imaging and golden-angle radial sampling. Investig Radiol 48:1

Chang KJ, Kamel IR, Macura KJ et al (2008) 3.0-T MR imaging of the abdomen: comparison with 1.5T. Radiographics 28:1983–1998

Chilla GS, Tan CH, Xu C et al (2015) Diffusion weighted magnetic resonance imaging and its recent trend - a survey. Quant Imaging Med Surg 5:407–422

Clarke SE, Saranathan M, Rettmann DW et al (2015) High resolution multi-arterial phase MRI improves lesion contrast in chronic liver disease. Clin Invest Med 38(3):E90–E99

Donato H, França M, Candelária I et al (2017) Liver MRI: from basic protocol to advanced techniques. Eur J Radiol 93:30–39

França M, Alberich-Bayarri A, Martí-Bonmatí L et al (2017) Accurate simultaneous quantification of liver steatosis and iron overload in diffuse liver diseases with MRI. Abdom Radiol 24:1–10

Gandon Y, Olivié D, Guyader D et al (2004) Non-invasive assessment of hepatic iron stores by MRI. Lancet 363(9406):357–362

Garbowski MW, Carpenter J-P, Smith G et al (2014) Biopsy-based calibration of T2* magnetic resonance for estimation of liver iron concentration and comparison with R2 FerriScan. J Cardiovasc Magn Reson 16(1):1–11

Girometti R (2015) 3.0 Tesla magnetic resonance imaging: a new standard in liver imaging? World J Hepatol 7(15):1894–1898

Godfrey EM, Mannelli L, Griffin N et al (2013) Magnetic resonance elastography in the diagnosis of hepatic fibrosis. Semin Ultras CT MRI 34(1):81–88

Guglielmo FF, Mitchell DG, Roth CG et al (2014) Hepatic MR imaging techniques, optimization, and artifacts. Magn Reson Imaging Clin N Am 22:263–282

Hallinan JTPD, Alsaif HS, Wee A et al (2015) Magnetic resonance elastography of liver: influence of intravenous gadolinium administration on measured liver stiffness. Abdom Imaging 40(4):783–788

Hankins JS, McCarville MB, Loeffler RB et al (2009) R2* magnetic resonance imaging of the liver in patients with iron overload. Blood 113(20):4853–4855

Henninger B, Zoller H, Rauch S et al (2015) R2* relaxometry for the quantification of hepatic Iron overload: biopsy-based calibration and comparison with the literature. Fortschr Röntgenstr 187(06):472–479

Horowitz JM, Venkatesh SK, Ehman RL et al (2017) Evaluation of hepatic fibrosis: a review from the society of abdominal radiology disease focus panel. Abdom Radiol 13:1–17

Huh J, Kim SY, Yeh BM et al (2015) Troubleshooting arterial-phase MR images of gadoxetate disodium-enhanced liver. Korean J Radiol 16(6): 1207–1215

Idilman IS, Aniktar H, Idilman R et al (2013) Hepatic steatosis: quantification by proton density fat frac-tion with MR imaging versus liver biopsy. Radiology 267(3):767–775

Kaltenbach B, Roman A, Polkowski C et al (2017) Free-breathing dynamic liver examination using radial 3D T1-weighted gradient echo sequence with moderate undersampling for patients with limited breath-holding capacity. Eur J Radiol 86:26–32

LeBedis C, Luna A, Soto JA (2012) Use of magnetic resonance imaging contrast agents in the liver and biliary tract. Magn Reson Imaging Clin N Am 20:715–737

Lewis S, Dyvorne H, Cui Y et al (2014) Diffusion-weighted imaging of the liver: techniques and applications. Magn Reson Imaging Clin N Am 22(3):373–395

Liu C-Y, McKenzie CA, Yu H et al (2007) Fat quantification with IDEAL gradient echo imaging: correction of bias from T1 and noise. Magn Reson Med 58(2):354–364

Mariappan YK, Dzyubak B, Glaser KJ et al (2016) Application of modified spin-echo-based sequences for hepatic MR elastography: evaluation, comparison with the conventional gradient-echo sequence, and preliminary clinical experience. Radiology 10:160153

Martí-Bonmatí L, Alberich-Bayarri A, Sánchez-González J (2011) Overload hepatitides: quanti-qualitative analysis. Abdom Imaging 37(2):180–187

Matos A, Velloni F, Ramalho M et al (2015) Focal liver lesions: practical magnetic resonance imaging approach. World J Hepatol 7(16):1987–2008

O'Neill EK, Cogley JR, Miller FH (2015) The ins and outs of liver imaging. Clin Liver Dis 19:99–121

Paisant A, Boulic A, Bardou-Jacquet E et al (2017) Assessment of liver iron overload by 3 T MRI. Abdom Radiol 20:1–8

Petitclerc L, Sebastiani G, Gilbert G et al (2016) Liver fibrosis: review of current imaging and MRI quantification techniques. J Magn Reson Imaging 45(5):1276–1295

Pokharel S, Katarzyma M, Ihab K et al (2013) Current MR imaging lipid detection techniques for diagnosis of lesions in the abdomen and pelvis. Radiographics 33:681–702

Pooley RA (2005) AAPM/RSNA physics tutorial for residents: fundamental physics of MR imaging. Radiographics 25:1087–1099

Ramalho M, Altun E, Herédia V, Zapparoli M et al (2007) Liver MR imaging: 1.5T versus 3T. Magn Reson Imaging Clin N Am 15:321–347

Reeder SB, Cruite I, Hamilton G et al (2011) Quantitative assessment of liver fat with magnetic resonance imaging and spectroscopy. J Magn Reson Imaging 34(4):spcone–spcone

Reeder SB, Hu HH, Sirlin CB (2012) Proton density fat-fraction: a standardized MR-based biomarker of tissue fat concentration. J Magn Reson Imaging 36(5):1011–1014

Singh S, Venkatesh SK, Loomba R et al (2015a) Magnetic resonance elastography for staging liver fibrosis in non-alcoholic fatty liver disease: a diagnostic accuracy systematic review and individual participant data pooled analysis. Eur Radiol 26(5):1431–1440

Singh S, Venkatesh SK, Wang Z et al (2015b) Diagnostic performance of magnetic resonance elastography in staging liver fibrosis: a systematic review and meta-analysis of individual participant data. Clin Gastroenterol Hepatol 13(3):440–446

Sirlin CB, Reeder SB (2010) Magnetic resonance imaging quantification of liver iron. Magn Reson Imaging Clin N Am 18(3):359–381

St Pierre TG (2005) Noninvasive measurement and imaging of liver iron concentrations using proton magnetic resonance. Blood 105(2):855–861

Tang A, Tan J, Sun M et al (2013) Nonalcoholic fatty liver disease: MR imaging of liver proton density fat fraction to assess hepatic steatosis. Radiology 267(2):422–431

Thian YL, Riddell AM, Koh D (2013) Liver-specific agents for contrast-enhanced MRI: role in oncological imaging. Cancer Imaging 13(4):567–579

Van Beers BE, Daire J-L, Garteiser P (2015) New imaging techniques for liver diseases. J Hepatol 62:690–700

Venkatesh SK, Yin M, Ehman RL (2013) Magnetic resonance elastography of liver: technique, analysis, and clinical applications. J Magn Reson Imaging 37(3):544–555

Wagner M, Besa C, Bou Ayache J et al (2016) Magnetic resonance elastography of the liver: qualitative and quantitative comparison of gradient echo and spin echo echoplanar imaging sequences. Investig Radiol 51(9):575–581

Wile GE, Leyendecker JR (2010) Magnetic resonance imaging of the liver: sequence optimization and artifacts. Magn Reson Imaging Clin N Am 18: 525–547

Wood JC (2005) MRI R2 and R2* mapping accurately estimates hepatic iron concentration in transfusion-dependent thalassemia and sickle cell disease patients. Blood 106(4):1460–1465

Yin M, Glaser KJ, Talwalkar JA et al (2016) Hepatic MR elastography: clinical performance in a series of 1377 consecutive examinations. Radiology 278(1): 114–124

Yokoo T, Browning JD (2014) Fat and iron quantification in the liver: past, present, and future. Top Magn Reson Imaging 23(2):73–94

Yokoo T, Serai SD, Pirasteh A et al (2018) Linearity, bias, and precision of hepatic proton density fat fraction measurements by using MR imaging: a meta-analysis. Radiology 286(2):486–498

Nuclear Medicine of Hepatobiliary System (SPECT and PET)

Pietro Zucchetta and Diego Cecchin

Contents

Abstract

Nuclear medicine techniques allow the functional evaluation of the liver and the biliary system. Biliary scintigraphy using technetiated iminodiacetic acid (IDA) derivatives explores the biliary excretion from the uptake at the vascular pole of the hepatocyte to the bile excretion in the intestinal lumen. Positron Emission Tomography (PET), either in a PET/CT scanner or in a PET/MR tomograph, relies on 18F-fluoro-deoxy-glucose (18F-FDG) or labelled choline to detect more aggressive and less aggressive hepato-cellular carcinomas (HCC) respectively. Neuroendocrine tumors arising in the gastroenteric tract or in the pancreas (NET-GEP) are best evaluated by DOTA compounds (DOTATOC, DOTANOC, and DOTANOE), labelled with 68Ga. They share a high affinity for the SSR-2, which is widely expressed in NET-GEP and represents an excellent opportunity for the evaluation of the primary tumor and the metastatic disease, including the liver.

1 Introduction

The liver is divided into two lobes (right and left lobe) and is characterized by a double blood supply (hepatic artery arising from the celiac trunk and portal vein, draining the GI tract) mixing at the capillary level in the hepatic sinusoids.

Functional liver anatomy is segmental, based on the distribution of arterial, portal, and biliary system (left lobe: S2, S3; right lobe: S4, S5, S6, S7, S8; S1 is functionally independent).

1.1 Biliary Scintigraphy

Biliary scintigraphy allows the evaluation of the hepatocyte function (radiopharmaceutical uptake

P. Zucchetta (✉) · D. Cecchin
Nuclear Medicine Department,
Padua University Hospital, Padua, Italy
e-mail: pietro.zucchetta@unipd.it;
diego.cecchin@unipd.it

© Springer Nature Switzerland AG 2021
E. Quaia (ed.), *Imaging of the Liver and Intra-hepatic Biliary Tract*,
Medical Radiology, Diagnostic Imaging, https://doi.org/10.1007/978-3-030-38983-3_6

at the vascular pole of the hepatocyte) and of the bile excretion.

1.1.1 Radiopharmaceuticals

The radiopharmaceuticals used for the hepatic-biliary scintigraphy are derivatives of the imino-diacetic acid (IDA). They are labelled with ^{99m}Tc and are taken up from the bloodstream, after intravenous injection, from the vascular pole of the hepatocyte, sharing the transporter with endogenous bilirubin. The most frequently used molecules are disofenin (DISIDA) and mebro-fenin (bromide) (Figs. 1 and 2).

The excretion at the biliary pole is fast, because these compounds are not conjugated with glucuronic acid, as is the case for bilirubin; therefore they appear in the biliary system in few minutes and their concentration in liver paren-chyma is usually halved in 15–20 min after the maximum uptake, usually reached in 3–5 min.

Since endogenous bilirubin competes for the same membrane transporter, hyperbilirubinemia, as in jaundice, can impair the radiopharmaceuti-cal uptake. In this case, the standard dose (around 185 MBq in adults) can be increased proportion-ally, to guarantee an adequate visualization of the liver and the biliary system.

1.1.2 Patient Preparation

Patients should fast for 6–10 h (minimum 4 h, maximum 24 h). Of note, the fasting period must not exceed 24 h, to avoid excessive bile concen-tration and retention in the biliary tree, which can determine false-positive readings. The same con-sideration applies to total parenteral nutrition. Therefore, it is advisable to postpone the exami-nation or, alternatively, to pretreat the patient with cholecystokinetic drugs (e.g., sincalide), if allowed.

Smoking and alcohol consumption should be avoided during the 24 h preceding the examina-tion, because they can interfere with radiophar-maceutical absorption and/or excretion.

Some drugs may influence the sphincter of Oddi function (e.g., opiates) or gallbladder con-traction (atropine, somatostatin analogues, sin-calide). It is possible to exploit some pharmacological effects to test, for instance, the

gallbladder filling, administering morphine, or gallbladder contraction after sincalide.

Therefore, a detailed pharmacological history is mandatory during the examination, as in most scintigraphic studies.

When biliary atresia is suspected in neonates and infants, it is highly recommended to prevent abdominal skin contamination due to micturition. The positioning of a urine-collection bag will markedly simplify image interpretation.

1.1.3 Acquisition Protocol

Dynamic acquisition (matrix 128×128, 30–60 s/frame) in the anterior projection (patient lying supine) starts immediately after i.v. tracer injec-tion, using a large field-of-view (LFOV) gamma camera, fitted with a low-energy high-resolution (LEHR) parallel-hole collimator.

The field of view includes the whole liver, the upper abdomen, and at least a portion of the car-diac region.

The usual duration of the acquisition is between 45 and 60 min. Delayed images are acquired (most often after a lipid-rich meal) as the clinical situation requires (e.g., non-visualization of the bowel), up to 24 h after injection.

Tomographic images (single-photon emission tomography, SPET) can be useful when a biliary leakage is suspected, particularly if hybrid SPET/CT is available.

A double-head gamma camera is preferred, fitted with LEHR parallel-hole collimator, to keep the acquisition duration around 25–30 min (matrix 128×128, 360 degrees orbit, 120 frames, 25–30 s/frame).

1.1.4 Image Evaluation

Visual evaluation of all the images represents the first essential step. The parameters to consider are liver uptake, visualization of the intrahepatic tree and extrahepatic biliary ducts, gallbladder visualization (if any), and timing of radiotracer appearance in the small bowel.

Time-activity curves (region of interest drawn on heart, liver, main branches of the biliary tree and bile ducts, gallbladder, and small bowel) may help in image interpretation. The most used

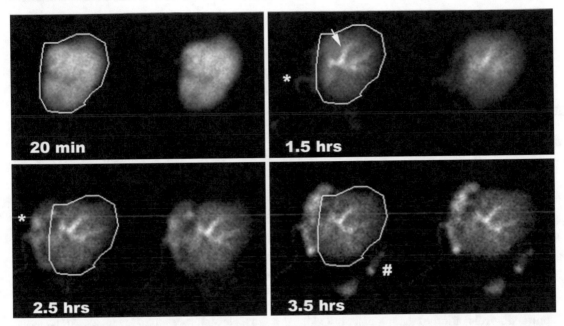

Fig. 1 ^{99m}Tc-IDA derivates in a child after S2–S3 left split liver transplantation. Upper left: two frames (5 min each) 20 min after the injection demonstrating good uptake of the graft. Upper right: two frames (5 min each) 1.5 h after injection showing dilatation of the intrahepatic biliary tree (white arrow) and initial visualization of the drainage (asterisk), clearly visible at 2.5 and 3.5 h. At 3.5 h the biliodigestive anastomosis (hash) can be seen

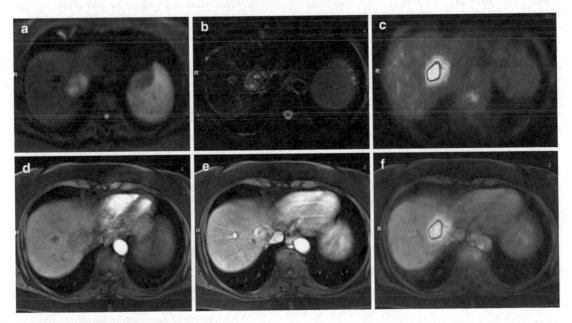

Fig. 2 18F-FDG PET/MR in a patient affected by hepatocellular carcinoma. In S8 an area of intense uptake (SUV Max 11) of the radiopharmaceutical corresponding to the lateral portion of an area (40 × 30 mm) previously treated. (**a**) DWI (b800); (**b**) T2 TSE fat saturated; (**c**) 18F-FDG PET; (**d**) T1 postcontrast (arterial phase); (**e**) T1 postcontrast (venous phase); (**f**): fused **c** + **e**

numerical parameters are liver-Tmax (time needed to reach the maximal activity in liver parenchyma), liver-T50 (time needed to reach 50% of maximum activity), and gallbladder ejection fraction (the percentage difference in background-corrected activity between maximum gallbladder filling and post-emptying image).

Circulating activity decreases fast in normal patients, reaching a nadir in around 5 min. The liver parenchymal uptake shows an early increase, with a maximum between 10 and 20 min postinjection, followed by a fast decrease, leaving very low activity at 60 min.

The intrahepatic biliary tree is usually visualized between 5 and 20 min postinjection, whereas the visualization of the gallbladder is highly variable, depending on its filling status and on the contraction/relaxation of the sphincter of Oddi.

The radiotracer usually reaches the small bowel in 20–40 min.

Bowel non-visualization, even after 24 h, is highly suggestive of biliary atresia in icteric neonates and infants, whereas biliary obstruction leads to variable delays in bile outflow and bowel visualization.

Acute cholecystitis is characterized by non-visualization of the gallbladder, even 60 min postinjection and after morphine administration. Sometimes, a thin rim of enhanced uptake is present in the gallbladder bed (rim sign).

The radiotracer appears in the abdominal cavity in case of biliary leakage.

Bilio-digestive anastomosis, using a bowel loop as biliary reservoir, is prone to acute and chronic cholangitis and the hepatic-biliary scintigraphy can identify the stasis in a malfunctioning bowel loop, which is a major risk factor.

1.1.5 Main Indications

Functional assessment of biliary function/post-surgical hyperplasia
  Biliary atresia
  Integrity of biliary tree/biliary extravasation
  Acute cholecystitis
  Patency of bilio-enteric surgical anastomosis
  Enterogastric reflux

1.2 Liver PET Studies

Positron-emission tomography (PET) uses positron-emitting radiopharmaceuticals and plays a crucial role in many diagnostic protocols, particularly in oncology, where the most widely used tracer is 18F-fluoro-deoxy-glucose (18F-FDG). PET scans are typical hybrid examinations, obtained on a combined PET and CT scanner (PET/CT). In recent years the first clinical hybrid PET/MR scanners have been introduced, opening exciting perspectives.

18F-FDG depicts the glucose metabolism and shows a physiologic uptake in the liver parenchyma. Therefore, it is useful to identify lesions with metabolic activity greater than the surrounding liver, as in the case of most metastatic lesions and in cholangiocarcinoma.

The glycolytic activity of hepatocellular carcinoma (HCC) does not differ, in many cases, from the normal liver metabolism, but increases significantly in high-grade lesions, when the tumor becomes more aggressive and is less differentiated. Therefore, the degree of 18F-FDG uptake corresponds roughly to the aggressiveness of HCC and can contribute to the grading of the disease.

Labelled choline, either with 11C or with 18F, detects low-grade HCC and has been proposed to stage at least the more complex cases of HCC, particularly aiming at extrahepatic disease.

18F-FDG and labelled choline are ideal candidates for the characterization of doubtful hepatic lesions, as is the case in multifocal disease after treatment, whether by TACE or by microwave ablation. The introduction of hybrid PET/MR scanners opens further perspectives in this evolving field.

Metastatic liver involvement at diagnosis is frequent in neuroendocrine tumors arising in the gastroenteric tract or in the pancreas (NET-GEP). NET-GEP metastasis shows a variable uptake of 18F-FDG, which is proportional to their aggressiveness. The same holds true for the primary tumor, which is often very small. Somatostatin receptors (SSR) are highly expressed in the vast majority of NET-GEP and radiolabelled compounds have been targeted both to their diagnosis and treatment. The most efficient PET radiopharmaceuticals are the DOTA compounds (DOTATOC, DOTANOC, and DOTANOE), labelled with 68Ga. They share a high affinity for the SSR-2, which is widely expressed in NET-GEP and represents an excellent opportunity for the evaluation of the primary tumor and of the metastatic disease, including the liver.

The treatment of metastatic NET-GEP is often difficult, even if they are often slow-growing tumors, because the disease can be already diffuse at the diagnosis. Radiometabolic therapy can control the disease with very limited side effects, using for instance DOTATE labeled with a beta-emitter (177 LU). The integrated approach of lesion characterization and radio-metabolic treatment represents a classical example of theranostics.

Further Reading

Barseghyan K, Ramanathan R, Chavez T, Harlan S, Lin CH, Mitsinikos T, McLean C (2018) Utility of hepatobiliary scintigraphy in diagnosing or excluding biliary atresia in premature neonates and full-term infants with conjugated hyperbilirubinemia who received parenteral nutrition. J Matern Fetal Neonatal Med 31(24):3249–3254

Bodei L, Weber WA (2018) Somatostatin receptor imaging of neuroendocrine tumors: from agonists to antagonists. J Nucl Med 59(6):907–908

Bodei L, Kwekkeboom DJ, Kidd M, Modlin IM, Krenning EP (2016) Radiolabeled somatostatin analogue therapy of gastroenteropancreatic cancer. Semin Nucl Med 46(3):225–238

Bodei L, Ambrosini V, Herrmann K, Modlin I (2017) Current concepts in(68)Ga-DOTATATE imaging of neuroendocrine neoplasms: interpretation, biodistribution, dosimetry, and molecular strategies. J Nucl Med 58(11):1718–1726

Christensen CT, Peacock JG, Vroman PJ, Banks KP (2018) Scintigraphic findings beyond ejection fraction on hepatobiliary scintigraphy: are they correlated with chronic gallbladder disease? Clin Nucl Med 43(10):721

Cremonesi M, Ferrari ME, Bodei L, Chiesa C, Sarnelli A, Garibaldi C, Pacilio M, Strigari L, Summers PE, Orecchia R, Grana CM, Botta F (2018) Correlation of dose with toxicity and tumour response to (90)Y- and (177)Lu-PRRT provides the basis for optimization through individualized treatment planning. Eur J Nucl Med Mol Imaging 45(13):2426–2441

Hepatobiliary (2019). http://snmmi.files.cms-plus.com/docs/Hepatobiliary_Scintigraphy_V4.0b.pdf. Accessed 15 June 2019

Kim JR, Hwang JY, Yoon HM, Jung AY, Lee JS, Kim JS, Namgoong JM, Kim DY, Oh SH, Kim KM, Cho YA (2018) Risk estimation for biliary atresia in patients with neonatal cholestasis: development and validation of a risk score. Radiology 288(1):262–269

Krishnamurthy GT, Krishnamurthy S (2009) Nuclear hepatology: a textbook of hepatobiliary diseases, 2nd edn. Springer, Berlin. ISBN: 978-3-642-00647-0

Liao X, Wei J, Li Y, Zhong J, Liu Z, Liao S, Li Q, Wei C (2018) 18F-FDG PET with or without CT in the diagnosis of extrahepatic metastases or local residual/recurrent hepatocellular carcinoma. Medicine (Baltimore) 97(34):e11970

Mallick B, Bhattacharya A, Gupta P, Rathod S, Dahiya D, Dutta U (2018) Cholecystocolic fistula diagnosis with hepatobiliary scintigraphy: a case report. JGH Open 3(1):91–93. https://doi.org/10.1002/jgh3.12104. eCollection 2019 Feb

Mandelia A, Lal R, Mutt N (2017) Role of hepatobiliary scintigraphy and preoperative liver biopsy for exclusion of biliary atresia in neonatal cholestasis syndrome. Indian J Pediatr 84(9):685–690

Matesan M, Bermo M, Cruite I, Shih CH, Elojeimy S, Behnia F, Lewis D, Vesselle H (2017) Biliary leak in the postsurgical abdomen: a primer to HIDA scan interpretation. Semin Nucl Med 47(6):618–629

Miner LT, Tulchinsky M (2018) Detecting intestinal malrotation on hepatobiliary scintigraphy: making a case for a better standardized reporting template. Clin Nucl Med 43(4):289–293

Oberg K, Krenning E, Sundin A, Bodei L, Kidd M et al (2016) A Delphic consensus assessment: imaging and biomarkers in gastroenteropancreatic neuroendocrine tumor disease management. Endocr Connect 5(5):174–187

Rassam F, Zhang T, Cieslak KP, Lavini C, Stoker J, Bennink RJ, van Gulik TM, van Vliet LJ, Runge JH, Vos FM (2019) Comparison between dynamic gadoxetate-enhanced MRI and (99m)Tc-mebrofenin hepatobiliary scintigraphy with SPECT for quantitative assessment of liver function. Eur Radiol 29:5063

Smit Duijzentkunst DA, Kwekkeboom DJ, Bodei L (2017) Somatostatin receptor 2-targeting compounds. J Nucl Med 58(Suppl 2):54S–60S

Snyder E, Lopez PP (2019) Hepatobiliary Iminodiacetic Acid (HIDA) scan. 2019 mar 25.StatPearls [internet]. StatPearls Publishing, Treasure Island, FL. http://www.ncbi.nlm.nih.gov/books/NBK539781/

Vélez-Gutierrez C, Gutierrez-Villamil C, Arevalo-Leal S, Mejía-Hernandez G, Marín-Oyaga V (2019) Hepatobiliary scintigraphy in the study of complications in adult patients after liver transplant. Description of the experience. Rev Esp Med Nucl Imagen Mol 38(4):207–211

Wang L, Yang Y, Chen Y, Zhan J (2018) Early differential diagnosis methods of biliary atresia: a meta-analysis. Pediatr Surg Int 34(4):363–380. Review

Watanabe A, Harimoto N, Araki K, Yoshizumi T, Arima K, Yamashita Y, Baba H, Tetsuya H, Kuwano H, Shirabe K (2018) A new strategy based on fluorodeoxyglucose-positron emission tomography for managing liver metastasis from colorectal cancer. J Surg Oncol 118(7):1088–1095

Yamamoto M, Tahara H, Hamaoka M, Shimizu S, Kuroda S, Ohira M, Ide K, Kobayashi T, Ohdan H (2018) Utility of hepatobiliary scintigraphy for recurrent reflux cholangitis following choledochojejunostomy: a case report. Int J Surg Case Rep 42:104–108

Zhang W, Fang C, Liu H, Chen Y (2019) FDG PET/CT imaging of hepatocellular carcinoma with bile duct tumor thrombus. Clin Nucl Med 44(2):130–132

Liver Biopsy

Valentina Bernardinello, Silvia Ceccato,
Antonio Giangregorio, Serena Magnaguagno,
Filippo Crimí, and Emilio Quaia

Contents

Liver biopsy is considered nowadays the most reliable tool to diagnose diffuse hepatic disease, despite improvements in serological and radiological techniques. The indications for this invasive technique must be weighed against the small, but not negligible, risk of complications (Tannapfel et al. 2012).

V. Bernardinello · S. Ceccato · A. Giangregorio
S. Magnaguagno · F. Crimí · E. Quaia (✉)
Radiology Unit, Department of Medicine - DIMED,
University of Padova, Padova, Italy
e-mail: emilio.quaia@unipd.it

© Springer Nature Switzerland AG 2021
E. Quaia (ed.), *Imaging of the Liver and Intra-hepatic Biliary Tract*,
Medical Radiology, Diagnostic Imaging, https://doi.org/10.1007/978-3-030-38983-3_7

The diagnostic accuracy of liver biopsy encloses several factors, e.g. patient cooperation, operator skills and experience, use of image guidance or assistance, biopsy technique, needle gauge, type of needle, number of biopsy passes, nature of the underlying histology and lesion size (Szymczak et al. 2012).

Nowadays liver biopsy might be taken percutaneously (via a needle through the skin or with an endoluminal biliary biopsy during percutaneous transhepatic biliary drainage) and transvenously (through the blood vessels).

1 Percutaneous Liver Biopsy

1.1 Historical Background

Paul Ehrlich is credited with the first liver aspiration in 1883 and subsequently the first percutaneous liver biopsy for diagnostic purposes was reported in 1923 (Bingel 1923). The technique has been modified since then, and over the past 50 years it has become a central investigation of hepatic disease. The low mortality (0.01–0.17%) and the relatively low morbidity of this procedure have meant that liver biopsy has become widely used (Sherlock and Dooley 1997).

1.2 Introduction

Correct diagnosis of hepatic lesions has a fundamental importance in oncology as it allows patients with malignant lesions to undergo the most appropriate treatment and those with benign lesions to avoid surgical interventions. Despite improvements in serological and radiological techniques, currently liver biopsy remains the most reliable method to obtain a suspicious lesion sample and a correct diagnosis (Bravo et al. 2001; Dezsofi and Knisely 2014; Myers et al. 2008; Rockey et al. 2009).

Percutaneous liver biopsy is a safe and effective invasive procedure, provided that the indications, contraindications, risk factors for complications and failure are considered carefully (El-Shabrawi et al. 2012; Holtz et al. 1993; Matos et al. 2012; Mogahed et al. 2016; Ozawa et al. 1994; Potter et al. 2011; Sparchez 2005; Westheim et al. 2012).

There are a number of variables within the literature that influence the diagnostic adequacy and accuracy of liver biopsy that include patient cooperation and body habitus, operator grade and experience (Szymczak et al. 2012), use of image guidance or assistance, biopsy technique, needle gauge, type of needle, number of biopsy samples, nature of the underlying histology and lesion size (Howlett et al. 2012).

US is the first choice for the guidance of percutaneous biopsy of hepatic lesions, to reduce the risk of complications (Kader et al. 2003).

US has a lot of advantages, including real-time capability, absence of radiation hazard, easy accessibility and low cost. But on the other hand, US cannot recognize all focal hepatic lesions.

1.3 Patient Selection

Not all patients with liver injury may undergo a percutaneous liver biopsy. Patients must be evaluated to recognize who can be submitted to the procedure (indications, alternative methods).

Radiologist should know the medical history of a patient and previous imaging studies (Lee et al. 2012; Veltri et al. 2017).

Then, it is necessary to check the patient's medications and suspend any anticoagulant/antiplatelet medications (Aspirin/Plavix discontinued 7–10 days prior and resumed 48–72 h post-procedure; warfarin discontinued 5–7 days prior and resumed the day following the procedure; heparin should be withheld 6–12 h prior to the procedure) (Gopal et al. 2011).

If the patient has any type of coagulation anomalies, these must be corrected (e.g. low platelet count, INR, PT, APTT, chronic renal failure, haemodialysis) (Douketis et al. 2012;

Hinojar et al. 2015; Patel et al. 2012; Rockey et al. 2009; Scheimann et al. 2000; Veltri et al. 2017).

Patients with cardiovascular issues (coronary stents, prosthetic valves) should be evaluated by a cardiologist, to be able to suspend therapy safely (Gopal et al. 2011).

1.4   Contraindications

Even though image-guided percutaneous liver biopsy is a relatively non-invasive procedure, there are defined absolute and relative contraindications (Bravo et al. 2001; Gopal et al. 2011; Rockey et al. 2009). The first ones prohibit the

procedure, and the second ones allow it to be performed (Figs. 1, 2, 3, 4, 5 and 6).

Identifying contraindications is important to avoid the major complications associated with the procedure (Mogahed et al. 2016).

The relative contraindications include all those conditions that increase the risk of complications. They should be promptly recognized and, when possible, corrected. They include the inability of the patient to cooperate (in this case general anaesthesia may be considered), coagulopathies, use of antiplatelet/anticoagulant drugs within 7–10 days (e.g. coumadin), presence of ascites (if difficult to reach the liver, the solution is to precede the biopsy with a paracentesis), obesity, known focal hepatic lesions (with histological

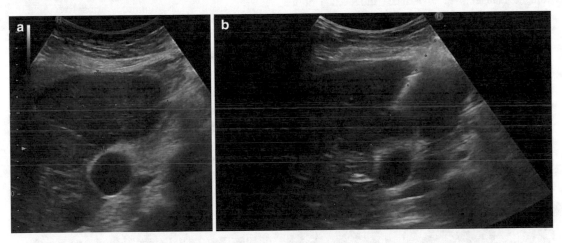

Fig. 1 Percutaneous biopsy of a lesion in the left lobe of the liver. (**a**) Pre-biopsy observation; (**b**) biopsy of the lesion with evidence of needle tracking

Fig. 2 Percutaneous liver biopsy materials: iodine solution, lidocaine hydrochloride 2%, formaldehyde solution, guide brackets, sterile probe cover and sterile ultrasound gel, 18G side-cutting biopsy needle

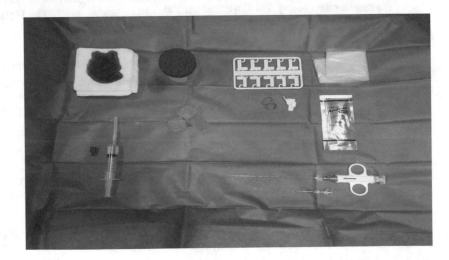

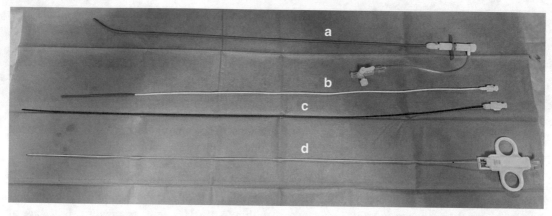

Fig. 3 Semi-automatic transjugular liver biopsy system: The four different parts from top to bottom are (**a**) the blue 7-French curved-ended sheathing catheter equipped with its antireflux valve, (**b**) the white 5-French end-hole straight catheter used to facilitate introduction of the sheathing catheter, (**c**) the black 5-French end-hole catheter which will be coaxially inserted into the sheathing catheter before descending on a stiff metal guide wire and (**d**) the biopsy needle in the "armed" position

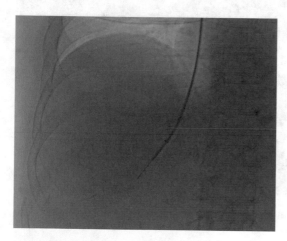

Fig. 4 Transjugular liver biopsy: Tru-Cut technique. The sheathing catheter is within the right hepatic vein and the needle moves forward in the hepatic parenchyma

diagnosis), vascular anomalies, bacterial cholangitis, unavailability of blood products for transfusion and premature infant.

Absolute contraindications are rare and include uncorrected severe coagulopathy (prothrombin time 3–5 s more than control, platelet count <50,000/mm, INR >1.5, prolonged bleeding time >10 min, factor VIII or IX deficiency, von Willebrand disease, hereditary bleeding disorders, sickle cell anaemia), intrahepatic abscess, history of unexplained bleeding (e.g. hyperfibrinolysis), hepatic infection, extrahepatic biliary obstruction, hydatid cyst (it causes anaphylaxis), lack of a safe access and refusal of consent.

1.5 Patient Preparation

The first step before performing a percutaneous liver biopsy is to obtain the informed consent by the patient (Scheimann et al. 2000; Veltri et al. 2017).

On the day of procedure, the patient must be fasting. Basal vital signs (blood pressure, heart rate, respiratory rate) and O_2 saturation are monitored (Davignon et al. 1979; Eachempati 2013; Fleming et al. 2011; Horan et al. 1987; Park 1996). An intravenous access is taken (Gopal et al. 2011).

Uncooperative patients (e.g. children) require sedation and the biopsy procedure is performed in an OR.

1.6 Procedure

A supine position is required with the right hand of the patient comfortably resting behind the head. In case of multiple hepatic lesions, it is necessary to recognize the target lesion (accessibility). A preliminary US exam is performed before the procedure to localize the lesion and a proper

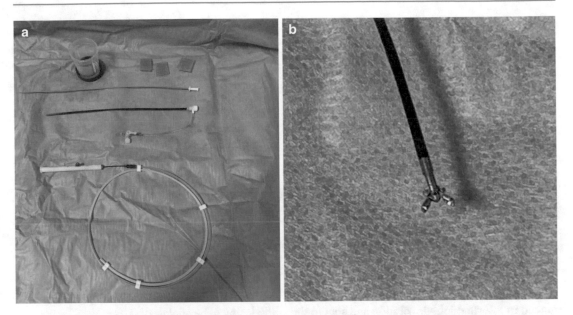

Fig. 5 Percutaneous Transhepatic Cholangio-Biopsy forceps device. (**a**) Materials; (**b**) detail of the forceps tail

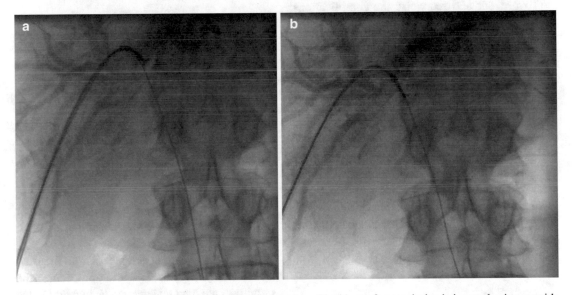

Fig. 6 Percutaneous Transhepatic Cholangio-Biopsy procedure. The biopsy forceps device is inserted using a guide wire, positioned over the biliary obstruction, (**a**) and then is pushed open within the tissue (**b**)

site for the biopsy (away from gallbladder, large vessels or bile ducts, lung, kidney—Fig 1a); a mark is made on the patient's skin (Mogahed et al. 2016; Veltri et al. 2017; Al Knawy and Shiffman 2007; McGrath and Sabharwal 2011).

The biopsy site is sterilized using iodine solution (for patients with iodine allergy, using Citroclorex 2%). Asepsis is required; the operator uses a sterile pack to cover the region of interest and a sterile probe cover with a sterile adapter.

Before biopsy, it is necessary to use a local anaesthetic with lidocaine hydrochloride 2%, injected between the skin and the hepatic capsule (for children, lidocaine 1%). It is important to ensure that anaesthetic is not injected into a vascular structure (Rockey et al. 2009; Mogahed et al. 2016; Veltri et al. 2017; McGrath and Sabharwal 2011; Lorentzen et al. 2015).

Patient must be collaborative; in particular he/she has to hold his breath during procedure. In patients who have difficulty complying with breath holding, they may be allowed to breathe once the needle tip is deep into the liver capsular surface (Gopal et al. 2011).

Biopsy is performed using an 18G side-cutting biopsy needle and by tracking needle penetration on US (Fig. 1b). US confirms the achievement of the tissue core and the absence of immediate complications. In case of failure or inadequate sample, biopsy can be repeated, but in the eventuality of repeated unsuccessful attempts, the biopsy can be reprogrammed another day (Howlett et al. 2012). The sample is quickly placed in a formaldehyde solution and sent to the histological analyses.

To prevent and recognize the complications, an US scan post-procedure is useful.

1.7 Post-procedure

Patient is kept in for rest and monitored for 6 h after the biopsy (basal vital signs and O_2 saturation). Only conscious patients can eat. A dosage of haemoglobin after the procedure can control and prevent the anaemia; in patients with haemoglobin level drop and hypotension, a transfusion is required. In case of pain, analgesics can be administered to the patient. Rest from lifting heavy weights and physical activity is recommended for 48 h post-procedure (Mogahed et al. 2016; Gopal et al. 2011).

1.8 Materials and Devices

The liver biopsy devices (Fig. 2) used most are the core-aspiration needles (Menghini, Jamshidi or Klatskin style) and sheathed cutting needles (either manual or spring loaded, often referred to as a "Tru-Cut style" in reference to one of the earliest cutting devices).

The cutting needle devices pass into the hepatic parenchyma using a troughed needle before an outer sheath or hood slides over this to secure a core of tissue. The calibre of (most) current cutting needles is about 18 gauge. Conversely, the traditional core-aspiration technique relies on suction generated via a syringe in conjunction with a flat or a bevelled (Menghini or Klatskin) needle tip. Newer automated core needle devices have recently emerged; these utilize a tiny inflection of the cannula at its tip, which serves to trap the specimen and obviates the need for suction (Howlett et al. 2012).

To avoid multiple steps through the liver parenchyma, increasing the risk of bleeding, it is very common to use a needle with Chiba tip, equipped with cannula with Chiba and internal chuck.

The radiologist can place the Chiba needle and through it, he/she can take several samples of the lesion to be analysed.

1.9 Complications

In only 13% of cases patients develop complications after the procedure (Bravo et al. 2001; Rockey et al. 2009; Veltri et al. 2017; Gopal et al. 2011; Howlett et al. 2013). Liver cirrhosis, malignancy, advanced age, impaired coagulation and number of passes are risk factors for serious complications in adults (McGill et al. 1990; Wawrzynowicz-Syczewska et al. 2002).

The biopsy complications are divided into major and minor (Cadranel et al. 2000; Neuberger et al. 2004; Pawa et al. 2007; Perrault et al. 1978; Stone and Mayberry 1996).

Major complications are bleeding in the peritoneal cavity (within 2 h after procedure, the symptoms are hypotension and tachycardia), due to a penetration in a branch of artery or portal vein (Atwell et al. 2010); biliary peritonitis or pleuritis (after a puncture of a bile duct or gallbladder perforation); haemobilia (GU bleeding, biliary pain and jaundice); intrahepatic hematoma; haemothorax; bacteraemia, septicaemia; shock; and death (1:10,000).

Minor complications are pain (84% patients); vasovagal reactions (mild transient hypotension); intrahepatic or subcapsular haematomas (often asymptomatic); pancreatitis after biopsy of an echinococcal cyst; puncture of adjacent abdominal organs; pneumothorax; pneumoperitoneum; pneumoscrotum; subcutaneous emphysema; subphrenic abscess; infection; and breaking of biopsy needle.

2 Transjugular Liver Biopsy

2.1 Introduction

In most patients, percutaneous biopsy is the preferred method to obtain hepatic tissue for its simplicity, ease and safety.

However, there are conditions, such as ascites and haemostatic defect, where percutaneous access is contraindicated because it is associated with a high risk of haemoperitoneum, which can be life threatening (Tobkes and Nord 1995).

In these cases, transjugular biopsy of the liver has become an accepted alternative method to obtain liver tissue specimens (Rosch et al. 1973) and it is generally considered effective, safe and well tolerated and major complications are extremely rare (Dohan et al. 2015).

2.2 Indications

Severe coagulation disorder and moderate or severe ascites resulting from advanced chronic liver disease or fulminant hepatic failure are the commonest indications for transjugular liver biopsy (McAfee et al. 1992).

In particular, transjugular liver biopsy can be performed in early acute liver failure for diagnostic, prognostic or therapeutic purpose, for example in acute alcoholic hepatitis, due to the need for specific corticosteroid treatment and the frequency of haemostatic disorders (Donaldson et al. 1993; Rockey et al. 2009).

In fact, liver biopsy via the venous system is performed without penetrating the liver capsule, and consequently it reduces the risk of bleeding (Rosch et al. 1973; Tobkes and Nord 1995).

Biopsy via the intravenous system is also chosen when additional procedures such as the measurement of the hepatic venous pressure gradient are required as part of the diagnostic evaluation, so that it is possible to perform both procedures through the same jugular access (McAfee et al. 1992).

Other less common reasons for using a transjugular approach to liver biopsy include previously failed percutaneous liver biopsy; a small, hard, cirrhotic liver; obesity with a difficult-to-identify flank site; and comorbidities that could lead to excessive bleeding during percutaneous biopsy (i.e. suspected vascular tumour, haemodialysis and chronic renal insufficiency or peliosis) (McAfee et al. 1992; Rockey et al. 2009).

Finally, transjugular liver biopsy can be an option in selected focal liver lesion, especially in case of previous failed percutaneous biopsy. In this circumstance, it is necessary to use ultrasound (US) or computed tomographic (CT) guidance for obtaining needle biopsy specimens (Ble et al. 2014).

2.3 Contraindications

There is no specific contraindication for transjugular liver biopsy, and for each patient risks and benefits should be considered (Ble et al. 2014).

The main limits are thrombosis of the right internal jugular vein or inability to access it.

Although, in this case, there are other possibilities to perform the venous access, such as via the right external jugular vein, the left internal jugular vein or the femoral vein, these should be the final chance, because they are riskier than the conventional route (Yavuz et al. 2007).

Another limit for transjugular liver biopsy is hepatic venous occlusion; in such cases some authors have described the transcaval biopsy technique as a proven, safe and viable option for obtaining liver samples (Mammen et al. 2008).

Other contraindications for transjugular liver biopsy described in literature are hydatid cysts, cholangitis and thrombosis of the hepatic veins (Dohan et al. 2014).

2.4 Patient Preparation

Patient should be informed about the technique and its risks; he/she must have fasted for at least 6 h and a written informed consent should be obtained. Moreover, clotting studies, serum creatinine and an adequate management of anti-coagulant therapy are required before the exam.

There is no consensus regarding the need for antibiotic prophylaxis and it should be managed on a case-by-case basis. The transjugular liver biopsy is performed in an interventional radiology room, under strictly aseptic conditions, and patient's vital signs (blood pressure, oxygen saturation, electrocardiographic parameters and heart rate) are monitored during the procedure. A peripheral venous access should be placed, and oxygen may be administered via a nasal cannula.

Light conscious sedation with benzodiazepines may be employed to relieve anxiety and minor discomfort (in particular, midazolam does not influence hepatic haemodynamics), while general anaesthesia is necessary for uncooperative and paediatric patients.

2.5   Procedure

The patient is positioned supine, with the head slightly turned in the opposite direction of the puncture site (preferentially right internal jugular vein).

Previous US evaluation gives precise information of topographic location of the right internal jugular vein and confirms its permeability; if this access is not feasible, left internal jugular, external jugular, subclavian or even femoral vein can be used (Ble et al. 2014; Dohan et al. 2014; Kalambokis et al. 2007).

After skin disinfection, positioning of a sterile drop and subcutaneous local anaesthetic infiltration, under ultrasonographic guidance, the right internal jugular vein is punctured using an 18-gauge needle connected to a saline-filled syringe.

Under fluoroscopic control, a 0.035-in. J-tipped guidewire is inserted into the vein and a 9–10 French (11 cm long) introducer is passed through according to Seldinger technique over the guide wire.

A 5-French end-hole catheter and a J-tipped 0.035-in. flexible hydrophilic guide are launched through the introducer via the superior vena cava,

right atrium, inferior vena cava and right hepatic vein or an appropriate alternative hepatic vein and a hepatic venogram is obtained to confirm the correct position of the catheter (3–4 cm from the inferior vena cava). Hepatic venous pressure gradient (HVPG) can be measured at this point. Once hepatic venous pressure gradient is measured, the catheter for the biopsy should be placed.

The specimens could be obtained by Menghini technique (aspiration system, using Colapinto needle) or Tru-Cut technique (cutting system) (Figs. 3 and 4).

Menghini technique: A 9-French tetrafluoroethylene (TFE) sheath catheter with curved tip is positioned into the hepatic vein and then the Colapinto needle is advanced into the sheath until it reaches the hepatic vein and successively is moved forward 1–2 cm into the liver parenchyma, with the patient holding his/her breath. To perform the puncture, a syringe is attached to the edge of the needle and aspiration force should be applied while puncturing.

Tru-Cut technique: A 7-French curved-end sheathing catheter is introduced into the hepatic vein and the sampling system is introduced coaxially to carry out the biopsy.

The direction of the needle tip is based on the hepatic vein selected: anteriorly if the right hepatic vein is catheterized or posteriorly if the median vein is catheterized. Biopsy through the left hepatic vein is used less because of a higher risk of extracapsular puncture due to lower left lobe dimensions. The starting point of the biopsy should be at 3–4 cm from the hepatic vein. It is important to remember that the semi-automatic sampling system moves forward for at least 24 mm and because of this the procedure should be checked regularly to ensure that the distal end of the biopsy needle is not too close to the liver capsule to reduce the risk of capsular rupture or bleeding. Moreover, after each pass, contrast medium should be injected to detect possible contrast leak.

If the liver specimen is absent or inadequate, other attempts may be made until success is achieved. It is recommended to take three biopsy samples, but two samples seem to be sufficient (depending on the size of the first two samples and their degrees of fragmentation).

There are no specific indications about postoperative care of these patients; however the authors recommend to monitor patient's vital signs for the next 2–4 h. Additionally if the capsule has been punctured the patient should be observed closely for at least 12 h.

In case of increased right upper quadrant pain, dyspnoea or vital sign change, it is mandatory to perform further exams and appropriate explorations to detect potential complications.

2.6 Complications

The total rate of complications in a systematic review of 62 series was 7.1%, divided into minor complications (6.5%), major complications (0.5%) and death (0.09%) (Kalambokis et al. 2007).

According to the Society of Interventional Radiology, minor complications are transitory abdominal pain, capsule perforation without haemodynamic effect, pyrexia, limited intrahepatic haematoma and other very exceptional complications such as a biliary fistula, or hepatic artery aneurysm. Other minor complications related to the puncture of the internal jugular vein such as neck pain, haematoma in the neck, accidental puncture of the carotid artery and even pneumothorax are much rarer when US guidance is used.

Major complications (Dohan et al. 2014, 2015) consist of haemoperitoneum, large hepatic haematoma, ventricular arrhythmia, pneumothorax, inferior vena cava or renal vein perforation and respiratory arrest. Death occurs almost exclusively due to hemoperitoneum and ventricular arrhythmia.

3 Percutaneous Transhepatic Cholangio-Biopsy (PTCB)

3.1 Introduction

Tumours affecting the biliary system, despite the recent advances in diagnostic imaging, are often too small to have specific imaging findings to allow the differentiation between the malignant structures from benign ones (Ierardi et al. 2014). In these cases, tissue sampling becomes essential to diagnose the real nature of the obstruction; according to the current European Society for Medical Oncology (ESMO) guidelines, histological confirmation is mandatory before any nonsurgical treatment such as chemotherapy, radiation therapy and biliary stenting (Valle et al. 2016). Percutaneous FNAB with US or CT guidance is often unsuccessful in biliary tumours (Jung et al. 2002).

Endoluminal techniques used for obtaining biliary samples can be shortly divided into those that require a percutaneous or an endoscopic access tract. Percutaneous-based methods include percutaneous transhepatic cholangiography (PTC), brush cytology, and cholangioscopy, while endoscopy-based methods include endoscopic retrograde cholangiopancreatography (ERCP) and endoscopic ultrasound (EUS). When accessing the biliary tree using ERCP- and PTC-based methods, either washings or brushings can be taken and sent for cytology (Patel et al. 2015).

Cytological sampling performed during percutaneous transhepatic biliary drainage (PTBD) or endoscopic retrograde cholangiopancreatography (ERCP) has been proven to be safe and popular (Ierardi et al. 2014) and represents the most commonly used technique since it is relatively simple and requires little time, but offers insufficient sensitivity of 30–60% (Kulaksiz et al. 2011; Selvaggi 2004; Rossi et al. 2004; Volmar et al. 2006).

PTBD is today considered a well-established, non-surgical method of relieving obstructive jaundice; collection of bile for cytologic examination is easy but often non-diagnostic (Jung et al. 2002). Endoluminal biliary biopsy during PTBD has been first reported almost 40 years ago (Elyaderani and Gabriele 1980) and several studies have described the safety and efficacy of the method using different forceps sets (Inchingolo et al. 2018; Andrade et al. 2017; Li et al. 2014, 2016; Park et al. 2017). The transluminal approach offers a direct and accurate route for the biopsy of biliary tumours, and a specimen can be obtained from a region that appears abnormal on a cholangiogram even when the tumour responsible for the stricture is not clearly visible at CT or at US. Forceps biopsy also enables the acquisition of deeper samples than does brush cytology. Forceps biopsy procedures were reported during PTBD to have greater accuracy and sensitivity (80–90%), with a specificity of 100% (Ierardi et al. 2014; Jung et al. 2002); this technique, however, has shown a poor negative predictive value.

PTCB is usually performed to diagnose the nature of a biliary obstruction. The lesions responsible for this obstruction, in most cases, are cholangiocarcinoma, HCC, fibrous tissue from chronic inflammation of the bile duct, metastatic lymph nodes or masses that compress the bile duct, and metastatic invasion of the biliary tree. Most of the studies on this technique show that the sensitivity of forceps biopsy with malignant tumours other than cholangiocarcinoma is lower that its sensitivity in patients with cholangiocarcinoma, so we can say that cancer originating in the biliary system is the best indication for PTBC (Jung et al. 2002; Li et al. 2016).

3.2   Contraindications

No absolute contraindications to the procedure are reported in literature.

Relative contraindications are, more or less, the same of the other interventional procedures on the liver and biliary tract that are sepsis, cholangitis, coagulopathy and allergy to iodinated contrast; in addition, large ascites can displace the liver from the abdominal wall, increasing the technical difficulty of percutaneous intervention.

3.3   Procedure

Usually the procedure is performed during conscious sedation (Jung et al. 2002) and under local anaesthesia at the puncture site (Inchingolo et al. 2018). Some authors (Ierardi et al. 2014; Andrade et al. 2017; Jung et al. 2002) recommend the administration of broad-spectrum antibiotics for both the drainage and the biopsy procedures. Heart rate, electrocardiographic trace, oxygen saturation, respiratory frequency and blood pressure are usually monitored throughout the procedure (Ierardi et al. 2014).

PTCB can be performed during the placement of the biliary drainage or some days after, for alleviation of cholangitis and haemobilia (Andrade et al. 2017; Jung et al. 2002).

Following percutaneous transhepatic access, a cholangiography has to be performed to identify the site of the obstruction. Then, under fluoroscopic guidance, the biliary obstruction is negotiated using a catheter and a hydrophilic guide wire. After lesion crossing, a sheath is positioned within the obstruction, over a super-stiff guide wire, positioned within the duodenum. The super-stiff guide wire is left for safety; then the biopsy forceps device is inserted by the wire, through the sheath, and is pushed and advanced open within the lesion under fluoroscopic guidance, using the sheath for support, trying to obtain specimens at the centre of the stricture (Figs. 5 and 6). Usually four hands are necessary for this procedure. Three to five biopsy specimens are taken from the lesion; they are fixed with formalin and sent to the pathology department for analysis. Then an internal–external biliary draining catheter is positioned; if the obstruction cannot be outdated, an external drainage has to be placed. Finally, a cholangiogram is performed to evaluate the potential extravasation of contrast material from the biopsy site (Ierardi et al. 2014; Inchingolo et al. 2018; Andrade et al. 2017; Jung et al. 2002).

3.4   Complications

Complications are rare (4–6%) (Jung et al. 2002; Park et al. 2017; Li et al. 2014), and are usually haemobilia or biloma. No major complications are reported in literature (Ierardi et al. 2014; Inchingolo et al. 2018).

Theoretically, PTCB could cause vascular or bile duct rupture leading to bile leakage and haemobilia, but this is rare in practice because, even if portal bile duct structures lie adjacent to the lumen, fat and fibrous connective tissue fill the spaces between them (Li et al. 2016). The complications reported are usually caused by the puncture of the liver or by the drainage process rather than by the biopsy procedure (Ierardi et al. 2014; Jung et al. 2002; Park et al. 2017; Perez-Johnsto et al. 2018) and can also be infection or tumour seeding along the course of the biliary catheter (Venkatanarasimha et al. 2017).

References

Al Knawy B, Shiffman M (2007) Percutaneous liver biopsy in clinical practice. Liver Int 27:1166–1173

Andrade GV, Santos MA, Meira MR, Meira MD (2017) Percutaneous trans biliary biopsy. Rev Col Bras Cir 44(1):107–108

Atwell TD, Smith RL, Hesley GK, Callstrom MR, Schleck CD, Harmsen WS et al (2010) Incidence of bleeding after 15,181 percutaneous biopsies and the role of aspirin. Am J Roentgenol 194(3):784–789

Beckmann M, Bahr M, Hadem J et al (2009) Clinical relevance of transjugular liver biopsy in comparison with percutaneous and laparoscopic liver biopsy. Gastroenterol Res Pract 9:1e7

Bingel A (1923) Ueber die parenchympunktion der leber. Verh Dtsch Ges Inn Med 35:210–212

Ble M, Procopet B, Miquel R, Hernandez-Gea V, Garcia-Pagan JC (2014) Transjugular liver biopsy. Clin Liver Dis 18(4):767–778

Bravo AA, Sheth SG, Chopra S (2001) Liver biopsy. N Engl J Med 344(7):15

Cadranel JF, Rufat P, Degos F (2000) Practices of liver biopsy in France: results of a prospective nationwide survey. For the Group of Epidemiology of the French Association for the Study of the Liver (AFEF). Hepatology 32(3):477–481

Cholongitas E, Quaglia A, Samonakis D et al (2006) Transjugular liver biopsy: how good is it for accurate histological interpretation? Gut 55:1789–1794

Davignon A, Rautaharju P, Boiselle E, Soumis F, Megelas M, Choquette A (1979) Normal ECG standards for infants and children. Pediatr Cardiol 1:123–131

Dezsofi A, Knisely SA (2014) Liver biopsy in children: who, whom, what, when, where, why? Clin Res Hepatol Gastroenterol 38(4):395–398

Dohan A, Guerrache Y, Boudiaf M, Gavini J-P, Kaci R, Soyer P (2014) Transjugular liver biopsy: indications, technique and results. Diagn Intervent Imaging 95(1):11–15

Dohan A, Guerrache Y, Dautry R, Boudiaf M, Ledref O, Sirol M et al (2015) Major complications due to transjugular liver biopsy: incidence, management and outcome. Diagn Interv Imaging 96(6):571–577

Donaldson BW, Gopinath R, Wanless IR, Phillips MJ, Cameron R, Roberts EA et al (1993) The role of transjugular liver biopsy in fulminant liver failure: relation to other prognostic indicators. Hepatology 18:1370–1374

Douketis JD, Spyropoulos AC, Spencer FA, Mayr M, Jaffer AK, Eckman MH et al (2012) Perioperative management of antithrombotic therapy: antithrombotic therapy and prevention of thrombosis, 9th ed. American College of Chest Physicians Evidence-Based Clinical Practice Guidelines. Chest 141(2 Suppl):e326S–50S

Eachempati SR (2013) Oxygen Desaturation (Hypoxia). In: Approach to Critically Ill Patient (Critical care medicine). The Merck Manual of Diagnosis and Therapy (19th ed.)

El-Shabrawi MH, El-Karaksy HM, Okahsa SH, Amal NM, El-Batran G, Badr KA (2012) Outpatient blind percutaneous liver biopsy in infants and children: is it safe? Saudi J Gastroenterol 18:26–33

Elyaderani MK, Gabriele OF (1980) Brush and forceps biopsy of biliary ducts via percutaneous transhepatic catheterization. Radiology 135:777–778

Fleming S, Thompson M, Stevens R, Heneghan C, Plüddemann A, Maconochie I et al (2011) Normal ranges of heart rate and respiratory rate in children from birth to 18 years of age: a systematic review of observational studies. Lancet 377:1011

Gopal RV, Sheehan D, Bermudez-Allende M, Hussain S (2011) Imaging-guided parenchymal liver biopsy: how we do it. J Clin Imaging Sci 1:30

Hinojar R, Jimenez-Natcher JJ, Fernandez-Golfin C, Zamorano JL (2015) New oral anticoagulants: a practical guide for physicians. Eur Heart J Cardiovasc Pharmacother 1(2):134–145

Holtz T, Moseley RH, Scheiman JM (1993) Liver biopsy in fever of unknown origin. A reappraisal. J Clin Gastroenterol 17:29–32

Horan MJ, Falkner B, Kimm SYS (1987) Report of the second task force on blood pressure control in children. Pediatrics 79:1–25

Howlett DC, Drinkwater KJ, Lawrence D, Barter S, Nicholson T (2012) Findings of the UK National audit evaluating image-guided or image-assisted liver biopsy. Part I. Procedural aspects, diagnostic adequacy, and accuracy. Radiology 265:819–831

Howlett DC, Drinkwater KJ, Lawrence D, Barter S, Nicholson T (2013) Findings of the UK National audit evaluating image-guided or image-assisted liver biopsy. Part II. Minor and major complications and procedure-related mortality. Radiology 266:226–235

Ierardi AM, Mangini M, Fontana F, Floridi F, De Marchi G, Petrillo M, Capasso R, Chini C, Cocozza E, Cuffari S, Segato S, Rotondo A, Carrafiello G (2014) Usefulness and safety of biliary percutaneous transluminal forceps biopsy (PTFB): our experience. Minimally Invasive Therapy 23:96–101

Inchingolo R, Spiliopoulos S, Nestola M, Nardella M (2018) Outcomes of percutaneous transluminal biopsy of biliary lesions using a dedicated forceps system. Acta Radiol 60(5):602–607

Jung GS, Huh JD, Lee SU, Han BH, Chang HK, Cho YD (2002) Bile duct: analysis of percutaneous transluminal forceps biopsy in 130 patients suspected of having malignant biliary obstruction. Radiology 224:725–730

Kader HA, Bellah R, Maller ES, Mamula P, Piccoli DA, Markowitz JE (2003) The utility of ultrasound site selection for pediatric percutaneous liver biopsy. J Pediatr Gastroenterol Nutr 36:364–367

Kalambokis G, Manousou P, Vibhakorn S et al (2007) Transjugular liver biopsy – indications, adequacy, quality of specimens, and complications – a systematic review. J Hepatol 47:284–294

Kulaksiz H, Strnad P, Rompp A, von Figura G, Barth T, Esposito I (2011) A novel method of forceps biopsy improves the diagnosis of proximal biliary malignancies. Dig Dis Sci 56:596–601

Lee MJ, Fanelli F, Haage P, Hausegger K, Van Lienden KP (2012) Patient safety in interventional radiology: a CIRSE IR checklist. Cardiovasc Intervent Radiol 35(2):244–246

Li TF, Ren KW, Han XW, Li WC, Ren JL, Jiao DC, Li Z, Ma J (2014) Percutaneous transhepatic cholangio biopsy to determine the pathological cause of anastomotic stenosis after cholangiojejunostomy for malignant obstructive jaundice. Clin Radiol 69:13e17

Li Z, Li TF, Ren JZ, Li WC, Ren JL, Shui SF, Han YW (2016) Value of percutaneous transhepatic cholangio biopsy for pathologic diagnosis of obstructive jaundice: analysis of 826 cases. Acta Radiol 58(1):3–9

Lorentzen T, Nolsøe CP, Ewertsen C, Nielsen MB, Leen E, Havre RF et al (2015) EFSUMB Guidelines on Interventional Ultrasound (INVUS), Part I. General aspects (long version). Ultraschall Med 36(5):E1–E14

Mammen T, Keshava SN, Eapen CE, Raghuram L, Moses V, Gopi K et al (2008) Transjugular liver biopsy: a retrospective analysis of 601 cases. J Vasc Interv Radiol 19:351–358

Matos H, Noruegas MJ, Goncalves I, Sanches C (2012) Effectiveness and safety of ultrasound-guided percutaneous liver biopsy in children. Pediatr Radiol 42:1322–1325

McAfee JH, Keeffe EB, Lee RG, Rösch J (1992) Transjugular liver biopsy. Hepatology 15:726–732

McGill DB, Rakela J, Zinsmeister AR, Ott BJ (1990) A 21-year experience with major hemorrhage after percutaneous liver biopsy. Gastroenterology 99:1396–1400

McGrath A, Sabharwal T (2011) General principles of biopsy and drainage. In: Gervais DA, Sabharwal T (eds) Interventional radiology procedures in biopsy and drainage. Springer-Verlag, London, pp 1–10

Mogahed EA, Mansy YA, Al Hawi Y, El-Sayed R, El-Raziky M, El-Karaksy H (2016) Blind percutaneous liver biopsy in infants and children: comparison of safety and efficacy of percussion technique and ultrasound assisted technique. Pan-Arab Association of Gastroenterology. Elsevier, Amsterdam

Myers RP, Fong A, Shaheen AA (2008) Utilization rates, complications and costs of percutaneous liver biopsy: a population-based study including 4275 biopsies. Liver Int 28:705–712

Neuberger J, Grant A, Day C, Saxseena S (2004) Guidelines for the use of liver biopsy in clinical practice. British Society of Gastroenterology, London, England

Ozawa K, Mori K, Morimoto T (1994) Evaluation of hepatic function. Curr Opin Gen Surg 17:23

Papatheodoridis GV, Patch D, Watkinson A, Tibballs J, Burroughs AK (1999) Transjugular liver biopsy in the 1990s: a 2-year audit. Aliment Pharmacol Ther 13:603–608

Park MK (1996) Pediatric cardiology for practitioners, 3rd edn. Mosby, St. Louis

Park JG, Jung GS, Yun JH, Yun BC, Lee SU, Han BH, Ko JH (2017) Percutaneous transluminal forceps biopsy in patients suspected of having malignant biliary obstruction: factors influencing the outcomes of 271 patients. Eur Radiol 27:4291–4297

Patel IJ, Davidson JC, Nikolic B, Salazar GM, Schwartzberg MS, Walker TG et al (2012) Consensus guidelines for periprocedural management of coagulation status and hemostasis risk in percutaneous image-guided interventions. J Vasc Interv Radiol 23(6):727–736

Patel P, Rangarajan B, Mangat K (2015) Improved accuracy of percutaneous biopsy using "cross and push" technique for patients suspected with malignant biliary strictures. Cardiovasc Intervent Radiol 38:1005–1010

Pawa S, Ehrinpreis M, Mutchnick M, Janisse J, Dhar R, Siddiqui FA (2007) Percutaneous liver biopsy is safe in chronic hepatitis C patients with end-stage renal disease. Clin Gastroenterol Hepatol 5(11):1316–1320

Perez-Johnsto R, Deipoly AR, Covey AM (2018) Percutaneous biliary interventions. Gastroenterol Clin N Am 47(3):621–641

Perrault J, McGill DB, Ott BJ, Taylor WF (1978) Liver biopsy: complications in 1000 inpatients and outpatients. Gastroenterology 74(1):103–106

Potter C, Hogan MJ, Henry-Kendjorsky K, Balint J, Barnard JA (2011) Safety of pediatric percutaneous liver biopsy performed by interventional radiologists. J Pediatr Gastroenterol Nutr 53:202–206

Rockey D, Caldwell S, Goodman Z, Nelson R, Smith A (2009) American Association for the Study of Liver Diseases. Liver biopsy. Hepatology 49:1017–1044

Rosch J, Lakin PC, Antonovic R, Dotter CT (1973) Transjugular approach to liver biopsy and transhepatic cholangiography. N Engl J Med 289:227–231

Rossi M, Cantisani V, Salvatori FM, Rebonato A, Greco L, Giglio L (2004) Histologic assessment of biliary obstruction with different percutaneous endoluminal techniques. BMC Med Imaging 4:3

Scheimann AO, Barrios JM, Al-Tawil YS, Gray KM, Gilger MA (2000) Percutaneous liver biopsy in children: impact of sonography and spring-loaded biopsy needles. J Pediatr Gastroenterol Nutr 31:536–539

Selvaggi SM (2004) Biliary brushing cytology. Cytopathology 15:74–79

Sherlock S, Dooley J (1997) Diseases of the liver and biliary system, 10th edn. Blackwell Scientific, London

Shin JL, Teitel J, Swain MG, Bain VG, Adams PC, Croitorou K et al (2005) A Canadian multicenter retrospective study evaluating transjugular liver biopsy in patients with congenital bleeding disorders and hepatitis C: is it safe and useful? Am J Hematol 78: 85–93

Sparchez Z (2005) Complications after percutaneous liver biopsy in diffuse hepatopathies. Rom J Gastroenterol 14:379–384

Stone MA, Mayberry JF (1996) An audit of ultrasound guided liver biopsies: a need for evidence-based practice. Hepato-Gastroenterology 43(8):432–434

Szymczak A, Simon K, Inglot M, Gladysz A (2012) Safety and effectiveness of blind percutaneous liver biopsy: analysis of 1412 procedures. Hepat Mon 12:32–37

Tannapfel A, Dienes H-P, Lohse AW (2012) The indications for liver biopsy. Dtsch Arztebl Int 109(27–28):477–483

Tobkes AI, Nord HJ (1995) Liver biopsy: review of methodology and complications. Dig Dis 13:267–274

Valle JW, Borbath I, Khan SA (2016) Biliary cancer: ESMO clinical practice guidelines. Ann Oncol 27:28–37

Veltri A, Bargellini I, Giorgi L, Matos Silva Almeida PA, Akhan O (2017) CIRSE Guidelines on Percutaneous Needle Biopsy (PNB). Springer Science+Business Media, New York. and the Cardiovascular and Interventional Radiological Society of Europe

Venkatanarasimha N, Damodharan K, Gogna A, Leong S, Too CW, Patel A, Tay KH, Tan BS, Lo R, Irani F (2017) Diagnosis and management of complications from percutaneous biliary tract interventions. Radiographics 37:665–680

Volmar KE, Vollmer RT, Routbort MJ, Creager AJ (2006) Pancreatic and bile duct brushing cytology in 1000 cases: review of findings and comparison of preparation methods. Cancer 108:231–238

Wawrzynowicz-Syczewska M, Kruszewski T, Boron-Kaczmarska A (2002) Complications of percutaneous liver biopsy. Rom J Gastroenterol 11:105–107

Westheim BH, Ostensen AB, Aagenaes I, Sanengen T, Almaas R (2012) Evaluation of risk factors for bleeding after liver biopsy in children. J Pediatr Gastroenterol Nutr 55:82–87

Yavuz K, Geyik S, Barton RE et al (2007) Transjugular liver biopsy via the left internal jugular vein. J Vasc Interv Radiol 18:237–241

Hepatic Angiography and Vascular Interventional Radiology

Alessandro Pauro, Amalia Lupi, Chiara Mattolin, Mirko Lazzarin, and Emilio Quaia

Contents

A. Pauro · A. Lupi · C. Mattolin · M. Lazzarin
E. Quaia (✉)
Radiology Unit, Department of Medicine - DIMED,
University of Padova, Padova, Italy
e-mail: emilio.quaia@unipd.it

© Springer Nature Switzerland AG 2021
E. Quaia (ed.), *Imaging of the Liver and Intra-hepatic Biliary Tract*,
Medical Radiology, Diagnostic Imaging, https://doi.org/10.1007/978-3-030-38983-3_8

1 Introduction

Interventional radiology plays a double role in the imaging of the vascular diseases of the liver: diagnostic and interventional, each with individual claims but often closely related.

Ultrasonography (US) and contrast-enhanced cross-sectional imaging (mainly CT angiography and less frequently MR angiography) represent important noninvasive diagnostic tools in the study of hepatic vascular diseases.

Nowadays US with color Doppler mode is a safe technology mostly used in the follow-up and early detection of abnormal hepatic vascular flow. Although in the literature there are many useful criteria in the diagnostic process, they are not properly easy to study in a substantial number of patients. In this context contrast-enhanced ultrasonography (CEUS) is spreading as an alternative tool in assessing hepatic vessel patency (for example in portal thrombosis study).

CT angiography is a high-performance noninvasive imaging that, despite its static nature, is often essential before any therapeutic approach because it provides a panoramic anatomy of hepatic vessels.

On the other hand, interventional radiology holds a central position in the diagnostic process of hepatic vascular disease, in particular through the opportunity to perform highly sensitive dynamic exams, by making angiography the diagnostic gold standard in many vascular abnormalities.

While the utility of diagnostic angiography could be questioned given the number of noninvasive imaging techniques, its interventional role continues to grow. Many vascular interventional procedures are increasingly gaining ground: percutaneous transluminal angioplasty, stent placement, arterial embolization, transjugular intrahepatic portosystemic shunt, and portal embolization.

It is important to underline that interventional radiology is not in opposition to traditional surgical approaches, but it is complementary to it. This is especially true with regard to vascular complications following liver transplantation, where critical patients have to be handled by a multidisciplinary team, in particular during the first 30 days after surgery characterized by a greater number of complications, usually with high mortality rate.

1.1 Hepatic Artery Angiography

Diagnostic hepatic artery angiography, even including celiac and superior mesenteric arteries, is performed under conscious sedation to determine liver arterial supply and patency of the portal vein in a later phase. Variant hepatic artery anatomy is present almost in half of the population. This evaluation is usually done using the femoral route; brachial or radial approaches are also feasible, especially in cases with bilateral femoro-iliac occlusion, extremely tortuous iliac axes, or femoral surgical grafts.

The technique includes the infiltration of the skin and subcutaneous tissue with a small amount of local anesthetic (lidocaine 1%) before puncturing the common femoral, brachial, or radial artery; single-wall puncture is preferable. Therefore a short 0.035″ guidewire is advanced to introduce a 4–5 French sheath. Especially in the presence of atheromatous or calcified iliac arteries, a 0.035″ hydrophilic coated guidewire is advanced in the abdominal aorta, in order to move a diagnostic catheter (with a Rosch Celiac, Cobra 1, or Sidewinder configuration) towards the celiac artery. After the catheterization of the celiac artery, which is approximately at the level of T12, a selective angiography is performed injecting 30 mL of iodinated nonionic contrast, preferably at high concentration (320/370 mgI/mL), at 5 mL/s. When the diagnostic problem is focused on the arterial supply, arterial and parenchymal phases are usually performed, with a frame rate of acquisition of at least 3 frames/s in the first phase and of 2 frames/s in the parenchymal one. Long acquisition is used to visualize the portal system.

1.2 Hepatic and Portal Vein Technique

Venous access is necessary to perform several diagnostic or therapeutic hepatic interventional radiology procedures, via jugular vein, like hepatic vein pressure gradient (HVPG) measurement or transjugular intrahepatic portosystemic shunt (TIPS), and percutaneously for the portal access, like portal embolization.

Local anesthesia (i.e., lidocaine) on the access site is performed; subsequently venous puncture is done under ultrasound guidance with the Seldinger technique.

An access system is then positioned, appropriately as per type, caliber, and length for the materials necessary for the procedure.

Further details are provided in the dedicated sections of this chapter.

2 Hepatic Vein Pressure Gradient (HVPG)

2.1 Introduction

Portal hypertension (PH) is a frequent clinical syndrome defined as a pathological increase in portal pressure gradient (PPG) which is the difference in pressure between the portal vein and the inferior vena cava and represents the perfusion pressure of the liver with portal blood.

The normal range of the PPG is 1–5 mmHg; values between 5 and 9 mmHg represent subclinical portal hypertension.

When the PPG increases to ≥10 mmHg, complications of portal hypertension can arise; these complications incorporate formation of portosystemic collaterals, varices (e.g., esophageal, gastric, and hemorrhoids), congestive gastropathy, hypersplenism, disturbance in the metabolism of drugs or endogenous substances that are normally eliminated by the liver, and severe ones, such as upper gastrointestinal bleeding resulting from ruptured gastroesophageal varices, ascites, spontaneous bacterial peritonitis, hepatorenal syndrome, porto-pulmonary hypertension, and hepatic encephalopathy.

The causes of portal hypertension can be classified according to their anatomical location as prehepatic (involving the splenic, mesenteric, or portal veins, e.g., portal vein thrombosis), intrahepatic (parenchymal liver disease), and posthe-

patic (diseases involving the hepatic venous outflow, e.g., Budd-Chiari syndrome).

Hepatic cirrhosis is the main cause of this syndrome in Western countries; it is the 14th most common cause of death worldwide but 4th in central Europe (Tsochatzis et al. 2014).

The measurement of the portal vein pressure was first attempted by Hallion and Francois-Frank but was invasive and impractical in terms of clinical practice (Hallion and Francois-Frank 1896).

Myers and Taylor first described the measurement of wedged hepatic venous pressure (WHVP), which reflected sinusoidal pressure, an indirect measure of PVP (Myers and Taylor 1951).

The currently preferred technique for determining portal venous pressure involves, through catheterization of the hepatic vein, measurement of the hepatic venous pressure gradient (HVPG) which is the difference between the WHVP and the free hepatic venous pressure (FHVP):

$$HVPG = WHVP\text{-}FHVP$$

This method has almost totally replaced direct measurement of portal pressure by more invasive techniques, such as splenic pulp puncture and percutaneous transhepatic or transvenous catheterization of the portal vein. These last direct techniques for determining the portal pressure gradient require the simultaneous puncture of a hepatic vein and are used only in specific cases, almost entirely to determine presinusoidal portal hypertension.

The WHVP is measured by occluding the hepatic vein; stopping the blood flow causes the static column of blood to equalize in pressure with the proximal vascular territory, in this case, the hepatic sinusoids. So WHVP is a measure of hepatic sinusoidal pressure, not of portal pressure. In the normal liver WHVP is slightly lower (approximately 1 mmHg) than portal pressure; this fact is due to the low-resistant sinusoidal system that dissipates most of the pressure (Groszmann and Wongcharatrawee 2004). In liver cirrhosis the connections between sinusoids are disrupted by the presence of fibrous septa and nodule formation and consequently the static column of blood created by occluding the hepatic vein cannot be dispersed (Bosch et al. 2006). So in this case WHVP gives an accurate estimate of portal pressure gradient (PPG) (Perello et al. 1999).

FHVP is a measure of the pressure of the unoccluded hepatic vein.

There are two techniques for measuring WHVP: catheter advancement technique and balloon occlusion technique. In the former, the catheter is pushed down in the hepatic vein until it cannot be advanced further; this results in a complete obstruction of the venous flow and the pressure recorded in this occluded position is the WHVP.

The second one, the balloon occlusion technique, was validated by Groszmann et al. (1979). It requires the use of a balloon-tipped catheter; inflation and deflation of the balloon within the hepatic vein allow measurement of wedged and free pressures without the need to advance and retract the catheter for each WHVP and FHVP determination.

Using the catheter advancement technique the WHVP is measured in a small hepatic venule. Keiding and Vilstrup showed different values of the WHVP when the catheter is advanced in different hepatic veins and the heterogeneity of sinusoidal involvement in diseases like liver cirrhosis is probably the cause of these differences (Keiding and Vilstrup 2002; Maharaj et al. 1986).

In contrast, the balloon occlusion technique is preferred because it allows measurement in the hepatic veins at the lobar and sublobar levels. The obtained pressure is an average of pressures in several segments of the liver and thus represents more accurately the true portal venous pressure (Groszmann and Wongcharatrawee 2004).

2.2   Technique

Patient should be informed about the technique and its risks; he/she must have fasted for at least 6 h and a written informed consent should be provided.

Clotting studies, serum creatinine, and an adequate management of anticoagulant therapy are required before the exam. A peripheral venous access should be placed.

The procedure is performed in an interventional radiology room, under strictly aseptic conditions, and patient's vital signs (blood pressure, digital oxygen saturation, electrocardiographic parameters, and heart rate) are monitored during the procedure.

Conscious sedation with low-dose midazolam (0.02 mg/kg intravenously) increases patient comfort and relieves anxiety without modifying hepatic pressures (Steinlauf et al. 1999).

Previous US evaluation gives precise information of topographic location of the right internal jugular vein and confirms its permeability; if this access is not feasible, left internal jugular, antecubital vein, or femoral vein can be used.

Doppler US should be used to facilitate venous localization and puncture and to avoid complications.

After skin's disinfection, positioning of a sterile drop, and subcutaneous local anesthetic infiltration, under US guidance, the right internal jugular vein is punctured using an 18-gauge needle connected to a saline-filled syringe.

Under fluoroscopic control, a 0.035 in. J-tipped guidewire is inserted into the vein and the introducer is passed through according to Seldinger technique over the guidewire.

A J-tipped 0.035 in. flexible hydrophilic guide and an end-hole catheter or a balloon-tipped catheter are inserted through the introducer via the superior vena cava, right atrium, inferior vena cava, and right hepatic vein or an appropriate alternative hepatic vein.

FHVP is measured by maintaining the tip of the catheter "free" in the hepatic vein, at 2–4 cm from its opening into the inferior vena cava (Fig. 1). The FHVP should be similar in value to the inferior vena cava (IVC) pressure; IVC pressure should be measured at the level of the hepatic vein ostium. A difference of >2 mmHg signifies that the catheter is probably inadequately placed or that a hepatic vein obstruction exists.

WHVP is measured by occluding the hepatic vein, either by "wedging" the catheter into a small branch of a hepatic vein or by inflating a balloon at the tip of the catheter.

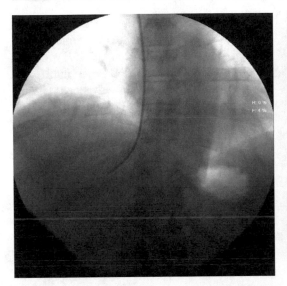

Fig. 1 The measurement of the free hepatic vein pressure

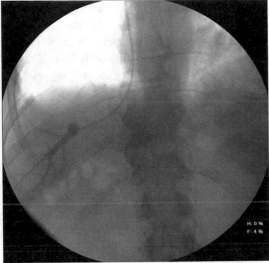

Fig. 3 The measurement of the WHVP with the balloon occlusion technique; note that with this technique a greater volume of hepatic parenchyma is examined compared to the catheter advancement technique

should not be considered and a new reading is taken and occlusion reconfirmed.

It is important that the WHVP readings should always be taken before injecting the contrast medium; otherwise the value would be falsely high and the catheter should be carefully washed with heparinized saline solutions before taking each set of readings.

As mentioned above the use of a balloon-tipped catheter, the preferred technique, reduces measurement variability.

FHVP and WHVP should be measured until the value remains stable and all measurements should be taken at least in duplicate (Groszmann and Wongcharatrawee 2004; Kumar et al. 2008).

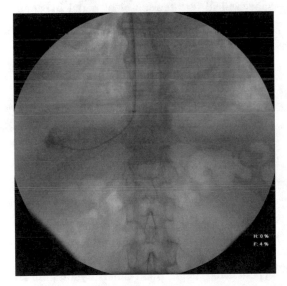

Fig. 2 The measurement of the WHVP with the catheter advancement technique

2.3 Complications

There are no absolute contraindications to HVPG measurement.

If the patient is allergic to iodine contrast medium it can be avoided and CO_2 can be used instead.

In the presence of known episodes of cardiac arrhythmia the catheter in the right cardiac atrium must be moved carefully.

The slow injection of 2–5 mL of contrast dye confirms the accurate occlusion of the hepatic vein; this method should be in a typical "wedged" pattern (sinusoidogram) without observing any reflux of the contrast or its washout through shunts with other hepatic veins (Figs. 2 and 3). If adequate occlusion is not achieved, the reading

Although coagulation disorders are common in patients with cirrhosis, only cases of severe thrombocytopenia (platelet levels <20,000/dL) or a low prothrombin ratio (below 30%) call for the replacement of platelets or transfusion of fresh frozen plasma.

The procedure of measuring the HVPG has proved to be extremely safe and usually carries only a modest discomfort (Bosch et al. 2009). Complications are infrequent (<1% of cases); most of them are related to local injury at the venous access site (e.g., leakage, hematoma, arteriovenous fistulae) and with the use of US guidance for performing the venous puncture this risk is greatly reduced.

Passage of the catheter through the right atrium might cause supraventricular arrhythmias (most commonly ectopic beats), but these are self-limited in most cases.

In the medical literature there are no reports of serious complications.

In Berzigotti et al. (2013) experience no fatalities have occurred in over 12,000 procedures in 30 years. In addition, hepatic vein catheterization offers the possibility to perform liver biopsies in patients with poor coagulation and contraindications for transcutaneous liver biopsies (Huet and Pomier-Layrargues 2004).

2.4 Indications

Normal portal pressure (determined by the HVPG) ranges from 1 to 5 mmHg. Pressure above this limit defines the presence of portal hypertension, regardless of clinical evidence (D'Amico and Garcia-Tsao 2001; Groszmann et al. 2003).

An HVPG value of 6–9 mmHg corresponds to preclinical sinusoidal portal hypertension, whereas clinically significant portal hypertension is diagnosed when HVPG is ≥10 mmHg, at which point clinical manifestations of portal hypertensive syndrome, such as varices, bleeding, gastropathy, and ascites, might appear (Garcia-Tsao et al. 1985; Groszmann et al. 1990, 2005; Ripoll et al. 2007).

HVPG measurement is the gold standard method to assess the presence of clinically significant portal hypertension (CSPH) CSPH, which is defined as HVPG ≥10 mmHg, in patients with compensated advanced chronic liver disease (cACLD) (De Franchis 2015).

In addition to diagnosing portal hypertension by pressure criteria, the patterns of the HVPG, WHVP, and FHVP obtained during portal pressure measurement can be used to delineate the types of portal hypertension and its possible causes.

Any condition that interferes with the blood flow from the spleno-mesenteric-portal axis to the inferior vena cava can cause portal hypertension so the latter is classified according to the site of obstruction as prehepatic, intrahepatic, and posthepatic.

Intrahepatic portal hypertension can be further subclassified into presinusoidal portal hypertension (e.g., schistosomiasis, sarcoidosis, tuberculosis), sinusoidal portal hypertension (e.g., cirrhosis), and postsinusoidal portal hypertension.

In patients with portal hypertension of unknown causes a normal HVPG with normal WHVP and FHVP is typical of prehepatic and presinusoidal intrahepatic portal hypertension. In these cases the catheter is not in continuity with the actual area of increased resistance, so the recorded pressure will be that of the normal sinusoids. The finding of an increased HVPG owing to an increase in WHVP indicates an intrahepatic sinusoidal hypertension, which is most frequently due to cirrhosis. In postsinusoidal intrahepatic portal hypertension and in posthepatic portal hypertension (e.g., Budd-Chiari syndrome) an increased FHVP and WHVP are found, while the HVPG remains normal.

The measurement of the HVPG moreover manages the clinical evolution of liver disease and the pharmacological therapy.

The main therapeutic goal for portal hypertension should be preventing its complications, such as varices hemorrhage, ascites, spontaneous bacterial peritonitis, and hepatorenal syndrome.

It has been demonstrated that there are threshold HVPGs necessary for the development of ascites and gastroesophageal varices, respectively, 8–10 mmHg for ascites and 10–12 mmHg for varices (Bosch et al. 1986; Rector 1986).

It was demonstrated that varices never bleed when the HVPG is less than 12 mmHg (Groszmann et al. 1990). A reduction in the HVPG to less than 12 mmHg is considered the single most useful prognostic indicator of portal hypertension complications and is the most important goal in pharmacologic therapy of portal hypertension.

In addition Feu and colleagues demonstrated that a 20% or greater reduction in HVPG from baseline after the initiation of beta-blocker therapy is associated with a significant reduction in the risk of variceal bleeding, even if the absolute HVPG of less than 12 mmHg is not reached (Feu et al. 1995).

It has been well demonstrated by many studies that the HVPG is a reliable parameter for predicting survival in cirrhotic patients (Vorobioff et al. 1996; Gluud et al. 1988; Merkel et al. 1992).

Transition from a compensated to a decompensated stage of cirrhosis is marked by the development of the complications of portal hypertension and the risk of developing these complications can be reduced by decreasing the portal pressure.

Albrades et al. (2014) showed that in cirrhotic patients treated pharmacologically for the prevention of variceal rebleeding, the long-term probability of survival was significantly higher for those who had an HVPG reduction of 20% or more from baseline or to less than 12 mmHg (defined as HVPG responders) than for nonresponders.

HVPG also is linked with the hepatocellular carcinoma (HCC).

Ripoll and colleagues showed that in patients with cirrhosis the risk of developing HCC is considerably higher in patients with clinically significant portal hypertension (HVPG ≥10 mmHg) than who have HVPG values <10 mmHg (Ripoll et al. 2009).

Moreover, in patients with well-compensated cirrhosis and resectable HCC, the presence of clinically significant portal hypertension markedly increases the risk of unresolved hepatic decompensation occurring within 3 months of hepatic resection (Llovet et al. 1999; Forner and Bruix 2009).

Thus according to Barcellona Clinic Liver Cancer (BCLC) staging surgical resection for HCC should be restricted to patients without clinically significant portal hypertension.

3 Transjugular Intrahepatic Portosystemic Shunt (TIPS)

3.1 Introduction

Transjugular intrahepatic portosystemic shunt (TIPS) is a direct communication between the portal system and the systemic venous circulation (Fig. 4) and allows the correction of portal hypertension in order to obtain a decrease of the hepatic vein pressure gradient (HVPG) at a value <12 mmHg or a reduction of at least 20% thanks to the portal decompression through a low-resistance vascular pathway (Reiberger et al. 2017).

3.1.1 TIPS History

TIPS discovery occurred in the 1960s, thanks to an accidental portal access during the first transjugular cholangiographic investigations; subsequently, in 1969, Rösch et al. advanced the hypotheses of a "radiologic portocaval shunt" (Rösch et al. 1969). Thirteen years later Colapinto et al. performed the first human balloon-dilated transjugular portosystemic shunt, but only the application of a metallic stent by Richter et al. guaranteed a longer term TIPS patency revealing TIPS as a valid alternative to the surgical portosystemic shunts (Colapinto et al. 1983; Richter et al. 1989).

With expanded polytetrafluoroethylene (e-PTFE)-covered stents TIPS procedure gained more and more acceptance as a treatment for the complications of portal hypertension until in 2004 Gore Viatorr® endoprostheses were designed for a longer TIPS patency and to date represents a well-accepted minimally invasive nonsurgical method for the establishment of a bypass in a congested hepatic vascular bed (Saad 2014).

Fig. 4 Scheme of an intrahepatic shunt between hepatic vein (HV) and right portal vein (RPV)

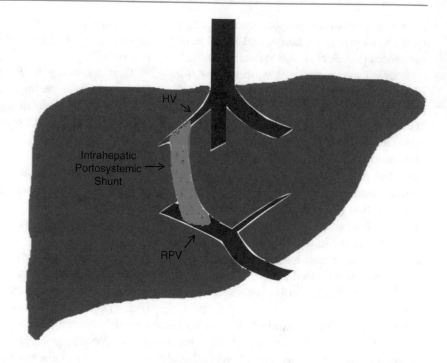

3.2 Indications

TIPS represents the treatment for some portal hypertension complications, mainly variceal hemorrhage and refractory ascites (Copelan et al. 2014; Fagiuoli et al. 2017).

3.2.1 Variceal Hemorrhage

In portal hypertension a hepatofugal portal circulation may be established, due to a diffuse parenchymal obstacle or a vascular obstruction, and the blood flow gathers its way back to the right heart reaching the vena cava system through anatomical venous shunts, the portosystemic anastomosis (Wachsberg et al. 2002).

When portal hypertension is such that HVPG >10 mmHg, the flow in the esophageal and para-esophageal varices gets prominent and the higher the gradient the higher the likelihood of variceal hemorrhage, with 12 mmHg considered as gradient threshold for bleeding (Garcia-Tsao et al. 1985). Risk factors for variceal bleeding are the stage of liver disease (i.e., Child-Pugh class A, B, or C) and the superficial aspect and dimensions of the varices (F1, F2, or F3 according to JRSPH classification) (Beppu et al. 1981). Gold standard

for esophageal varix diagnosis is esophago-gastro-duodenoscopy (EGDS), which must be performed at the moment of cirrhosis diagnosis and then repeated for periodical follow-up (Garcia-Tsao et al. 2007).

About 50% of cirrhotic patients develop esophageal varices and since variceal hemorrhage is a life-threatening complication associated with higher morbidity and mortality rate (10–20% of patients die within 6 weeks), its prevention is of primary interest to consent the improvement of survival rates (Garcia-Tsao et al. 2007; Triantos and Kalafateli 2014; Garcia-Tsao and Bosch 2010).

Nowadays preventive therapy of esophageal varices mainly employs endoscopic procedures (i.e., endoscopic variceal band ligation, EVL; endoscopic injection sclerotherapy, EIS) (Kim 2014). When the rupture of varices occurs, there is a severe gastrointestinal hemorrhage that manifests itself through hematemesis and, sometimes, melena or hematochezia; in these cases, once the hemodynamic stabilization is achieved, the therapeutic protocol (Baveno V) foresees the combination of pharmacologic, antibiotic, and endoscopic treatment, and the latter should be performed ideally between 6 and 12 h from admission, especially when cirrhosis is suspected (De Franchis 2010).

The insertion of the Sengstaken-Blakemore tube in the esophagus is effective in most cases (up to 80%) in which conventional medical and endoscopic treatments fail; however the bleeding relapses are constant after the decompression of the balloons (esophageal and gastric); therefore this procedure should be considered as a bridge therapy to a definitive therapeutic intervention (Kim 2014).

TIPS positioning is strongly advised as secondary prevention of esophageal variceal rebleeding, to treat uncontrollable variceal hemorrhage and portal hypertension gastropathy, or when ascites is concomitant to variceal hemorrhage (Copelan et al. 2014).

Furthermore, recent meta-analyses confirmed the superiority of TIPS over EVL in preventing rebleeding of esophageal varices and high-risk patients (i.e., Child-Pugh class C10-13 patients, Child-Pugh class B patients with active variceal bleeding, patients with HVPG >20 mmHg) treated with early TIPS intervention (<72 h) are more likely to survive or to not show significant bleeding than after an endoscopic treatment (Zheng et al. 2008; Deltenre et al. 2015).

3.2.2 Refractory Ascites

Ascites is associated with cirrhosis in 75% of cases and develops in 50% of cirrhotic patients, representing the most common manifestation of decompensation (Moore and Aithal 2006).

It is defined as an accumulation of fluid in the abdominal cavity in amounts above 250 mL and up to 10 L or more, due to two main pathogenetic mechanisms: portal hypertension that induces extravasation of fluids from the congested hepatic sinusoids and splanchnic capillaries, and renal sodium retention. This mechanism perpetuates in a vicious cycle, leading towards a progressive deterioration of the patient's conditions (Salerno et al. 2010).

At early stage of ascites-complicated cirrhosis, a therapeutic strategy that maintains a negative sodium balance, reducing its intake (that should be between 5 and 5.2 g NaCl/die, to avoid malnutrition) and increasing its renal excretion by diuretics administration, is sufficient (Runyon 2004; Wong 2012).

The evaluation of diuretic therapy effectiveness foresees patient's weight daily monitoring; up to 10% of patients do not obtain satisfactory results, due to the refractoriness of ascites at maximal doses of diuretics or due to their side effects (i.e., dysionemia, renal failure, encephalopathy), and therefore requires the execution of evacuative paracentesis (Moore and Aithal 2006).

Due to the poor prognosis of patients with refractory ascites, liver transplantation should be considered, but TIPS seems to improve the transplant-free survival of these patients and is preferable to repeated paracentesis of large volumes (Salerno et al. 2007; Garcia-Tsao 2005). Indeed natriuresis improves within a month after TIPS positioning; however, in order to obtain ascites clearance, patients should follow a sodium-restricted diet for a while, or continue diuretic therapy and within 12 months from TIPS procedure 80% of them achieve a complete resolution of ascites.

3.2.3 Other Portal Hypertension-Related Conditions

In changes of the gastric mucosa (i.e., *portal hypertensive gastropathy*, PHG) endoscopically described as "snakeskin" lesions, TIPS positioning may improve gastric perfusion (Copelan et al. 2014).

Hydrothorax can be found in cirrhotic patients (5%) with refractory ascites because of the migration of ascitic fluid through the diaphragm into the pleural cavity (Strauss and Boyer 1997). At its first diagnosis, an investigative thoracentesis for the differential diagnosis should be performed; evacuative thoracenteses may be necessary in addition to salt restriction and use of diuretic drugs. In this situation TIPS can help in relieving hydrothorax-related respiratory discomfort (Dhanasekaran et al. 2010).

Budd-Chiari syndrome is a rare condition caused by an occlusion of the hepatic veins (2 out of 3), due to thrombosis or ab extrinsic compression, in which TIPS represents the most common interventional measure, recommended in case of thrombolytic therapy failure (pharmacological and interventional), low functional liver reserve, or HVPG >10 mmHg, or is considered as a bridge therapy to liver transplantation (Ryu et al. 1999).

In case of advanced cirrhosis and clinically significant portal hypertension, systemic and splanchnic vasodilatation compromises renal perfusion causing acute kidney injury (AKI) and *hepatorenal syndrome* (HRS). Patients with HRS-AKI have more than one indication for TIPS placement, which may improve renal function (Rossle and Gerbes 2010).

Hepatopulmonary syndrome (HPS) occurs when a hepatopathic patient experiences dyspnea and hypoxemia due to an abnormal gas exchange, caused by vasodilatation of pulmonary capillaries. There is no evidence for TIPS effectiveness on this, but neither for TIPS to be unsafe if placed in these patients in order to treat other concomitant complications of portal hypertension (Martínez-Pallí et al. 2005).

Other particular conditions for TIPS positioning could be to maintain or achieve eligibility for liver transplantation with mild portal vein thrombosis, to reduce morbidity and mortality prior to extrahepatic major surgery, as access for portal or mesenteric endovascular intervention (i.e., thrombolysis, thromboaspiration) or as palliative measure in oncologic patients (Wallace et al. 2004).

On the contrary, TIPS should never be established in patients with no proven portal hypertension or in clinical conditions that may increase the risk of post-intervention complications (Krajina et al. 2012; Dariushnia et al. 2016), such as elevated right or left heart pressure, severe pulmonary hypertension, heart failure or sever cardiac valvular insufficiency, rapidly progressive liver failure, severe uncontrolled hepatic encephalopathy, uncontrolled systemic infections or sepsis, polycystic liver disease, extensive primary or metastatic hepatic malignancy, and severe uncorrectable coagulopathy.

Finally, TIPS should never be performed as primary prophylaxis of gastroesophageal variceal hemorrhage, with the exception of selected high-risk patients.

3.3 Preoperative Assessment

3.3.1 Anatomical References

For liver anatomy, refer to Chap. 2; here are some considerations related to the specific procedure.

Liver's vascularization is composed of two different types of afferents, the hepatic artery proper and the portal vein. The hepatic artery proper is the only liver arterial blood provider, and accounts only for the 25% of the hepatic blood needs; the remaining 75% of liver blood supply is granted by the portal vein that divides into two lobar veins, the right and left portal vein (RPV, LPV): this bifurcation may be extrahepatic (48%) and intrahepatic (26%), or in correspondence of the hepatic hilum (26%) (Schultz et al. 1994). The short but capacious RPV (see Chap. 2 for anatomical details) continues on the same direction of the portal trunk, with just a slight change of the axial angle and divide in the right anterior branch of portal vein (RAPV) and right posterior branch of portal vein (RPPV) which subdivide into superior and inferior segmental branches to supply the right lobe of the liver; the LPV is long twice as much as the RPV, but has half of its caliber and arises from the portal vein's trunk with an acute angle. The LPV turns medially toward the ligamentum teres, supplying the lateral segments (II and III) of the left lobe and describes a wide and anteriorly concave curve and ends in the superior and inferior segmental branches of segment IV. The cystic vein drains into the RPV or, sometimes, into the PV's trunk, while the ligamentum venosum (or umbilical vein, normally nonfunctional) drains into the LPV.

Despite the relative infrequency of portal vein anatomic variants (15%), four different variants of portal vein branching have been categorized according to Cheng et al. (1996):

- Type I represents the classical anatomy mentioned above (65–75%).
- Type II consists of the trifurcation of the portal trunk: RAPV, RPPV, and LPV (9–11%).
- Type III occurs when the RPPV is the first collateral of the portal trunk which ends with RAPV and LPV (5–13%).
- Type IV is characterized by the emergence on the RAPV from the distal tract of the LPV.

Even if the portal bifurcation absence is rare (1%), when unrecognized it can seriously compromise TIPS procedure's success.

The venous drainage of the liver occurs through three hepatic veins, which converge into the inferior vena cava (IVC): the right hepatic vein (RHV); the middle hepatic vein (MHV) which may drain into the IVC with a common trunk with the left hepatic vein (LHV) in 60% of population; and the LHV. These three venous trunks receive blood from smaller veins, the collector canals, which originate from the merging of the sublobular veins, the very first venous structure draining the hepatic functional unit. Anatomical variants of this district, such as accessory hepatic veins, are not infrequent, as the presence of supernumerary hepatic veins; the absence of one or more hepatic veins might be observed, too.

Normal and variant anatomy of the portal branching and hepatic veins should be accurately acknowledged and identified on preoperative computed tomography (CT) scan, considering that the vessels involved in a desired TIPS should be the right hepatic vein and the right portal vein (Saad et al. 2008).

Portal vein variants of interest when creating a TIPS are type II and III. Furthermore, since the portal vein puncture may cause bleeding when accomplished externally to the hepatic parenchyma, the location of the portal vein bifurcation should be considered prior to TIPS positioning.

Abdominal ultrasound and CT are employed also for the assessment of portal vein patency and the presence of primary or metastatic hepatic malignancy (Fig. 5).

3.3.2 Medical Evaluation

The evaluation of cardiac performance status, hepatic functional reserve, renal function and coagulation capacity are mandatory prior to a TIPS intervention (Chana et al. 2016).

An abnormal thrombocytic count and coagulopathy, not infrequent in cirrhotic patients, should be adjusted prior to the intervention; although there are controversies on the cutoffs to be obtained before the procedure, a platelet count >50,000/mm^3 and an INR <1.5 are advisable. Platelet infusion as well as fresh frozen plasma may be used for the correction of INR and thrombocytic count, respectively.

It should be considered also that TIPS intervention foresees the use of generous amounts of contrast agent that may furtherly deteriorate an already compromised renal function.

Since portosystemic hepatic encephalopathy (PHE) is a possible complication of TIPS creation, the presence of hepatic encephalopathy (HE) must be evaluated before the intervention.

Such a comprehensive medical workup may not be feasible in emergency scenarios; nevertheless a baseline hemato-chemical and bio-humoral screening should always be performed and a strict control for the maintenance of hemodynamic stability is required (Krajina et al. 2012).

MELD score allows the stratification of patients' survival prognosis in accordance to the

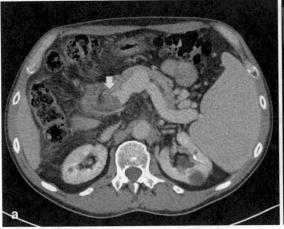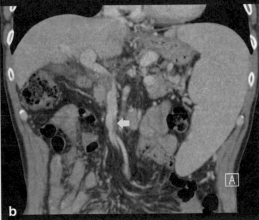

Fig. 5 Preoperative CT scan showing portal and mesenteric vein thrombus (arrows in A and B)

risk of post-TIPS hepatic decompensation (Farsad and Kolbeck 2014): when MELD score is >20 (or CTP score >C13) TIPS intervention is avoided, except for patients with hepatorenal syndrome who present a particularly high level of creatinine value.

Twenty-four hours prior to the intervention, prophylactic broad-spectrum antibiotic therapy (i.e., ceftriaxone intravenous administration) has begun and in case of known allergy to iodinated contrast medium, premedication with corticosteroids is recommended at least 12 h before the procedure.

A paracentesis (accompanied by volume replacement) can be performed the day before the procedure if needed: this allows the reduction of the angle between the hepatic veins and the inferior vena cava, and therefore an easier access to the hepatic venous system, in addition to better fluoroscopic images. If the presence of hydrothorax severely compromises the patient's respiratory performance, drainage should be considered.

Finally, fasting is required at least within 6 h before the procedure and informed consent must not be forgotten.

3.4 Procedure

For the TIPS positioning procedure, as well as for other interventional radiology procedures, a multidisciplinary team composed of interventional radiologist(s), anesthetist, radiology technician, and specialized nurse is required.

The patient, lying upon an angiographic table, is positioned with the head slightly turned to the left. Factors related to the patient's status will affect the choice between deep sedation and general anesthesia (Chana et al. 2016). Conscious sedation induced by sedative agents with a short action (e.g., midazolam, propofol, and fentanyl) may be employed together with supplemental oxygen supply. Many patients complain of great discomfort due to prolonged time in obliged supine position and balloon dilatation of the intrahepatic tracts; furthermore there is no guarantee of airway protection and ventilation may be compromised, so the feasibility of a prompt shift

to general anesthesia should always be ensured. General anesthesia on the other hand is the preferred choice of many operators, especially when procedural complications occur. To permit a quick post-procedural recovery, the most appropriate dosage of short-acting agents should be aimed. Tracheal intubation is the safest option as it prevents the occurrence of chemical pneumonia due to gastric reflux during the procedure. Furthermore, controlled ventilation permits breath holds whenever the radiologist needs the patient to be motionless, like during the most delicate phases of the shunt creation. In case of emergency TIPS positioning, general anesthesia and airway protection with tracheal intubation are mandatory.

Continuous cardiac activity monitoring with ECG is required and extreme caution should be paid while maneuvering the guidewire through the right atrium, because arrhythmic events may follow accidental cardiac inner wall stimulation.

At least two cross-matched blood units should be available during the procedure. It should be kept in mind that patients who experienced variceal bleeding are likely to have undergone multiple transfusions in the past: extended crossmatching is required by the possible presence of atypical antibodies in the blood.

3.4.1 Materials

3.4.1.1 TIPS Set and Stent

To date, five different sets to perform a transjugular venous hepatic access are available: the Ring, the Rösch-Uchida and the Haskal set provided by Cook Medical (Bloomington, IN, USA), the AngioDynamics set (Albany, NY, USA), and the Gore set (W. L. Gore & Associates, Inc., Newark, DE, USA).

The shunt can be created with bare metal stents (Wallstent™ Boston Scientific, Marlborough, MA, USA) or graft stents covered in expanded polytetrafluoroethylene (Gore Viatorr® ePTFE-coated stent grafts); the latter, nearly exclusively used for TIPS creation, is constituted by auto-expandable Nitinol covered in its last 4/5 by a thin layer of ePTFE and its employment results to be safe and effective (Vignali et al. 2005). Because of its low permeability to mucin and bile, the outer surface of this device inhibits the hyperplastic growth of the nearby liver parenchyma. While the ePTFE-covered portion (4–8 cm) is designed to be placed in the intrahepatic and hepatic venous tracts, the bare part (2 cm) of the stent is planned to be positioned in the portal vein.

The stent's diameter (8, 10, or 12 mm) is chosen taking into account the HVPG, the patient's age, his/her general clinical conditions, his/her hepatic encephalopathy grade, and his/her cardiac performance status (Fanelli et al. 2006; Schepis et al. 2018).

3.4.1.2 Balloons

Before and after TIPS placement, angiographic balloons are used for pre-dilatation of the intrahepatic tract and for dilatation of the stent after being completely released. The two types of balloon most used nowadays are Mustang balloon dilatation catheter (Boston Scientific, Marlborough, MA, USA) and ATB PTA dilatation catheter (Cook Medical, Bloomington, IN, USA).

3.4.2 Technique

TIPS creation can be considered a multistep procedure divided into four main phases (Keller et al. 2016) (Fig. 6).

3.4.2.1 Jugular Vein Puncture

The midportion of the right internal jugular vein is the preferred access point because the apex of the lung is usually lower and on this side it is possible to establish a more direct path for the achievement of the hepatic vein district. Since the common carotid artery is located next to this vein, the puncture should be performed under ultrasound guidance with an 18 G needle at the apex of the triangle drawn from the two ends of the sternocleidomastoid muscle. Successful access occurs in 75–99% of cases, depending on the experience of the operators. If the right jugular vein should not be available (e.g., agenesis, occlusion, or surgical ligation), the right external jugular vein, the left internal jugular vein, or the subclavian vein may be chosen.

For the technique of performing jugular venous access under ultrasound guidance, see the introductory part of the chapter.

3.4.2.2 Hepatic Vein Cannulation

Once in the jugular vein, a 0.035″ guidewire is driven down to the inferior vena cava. Passing through the atrial chamber caution is required for the avoidance of extrasystole. Then, a 12 F introducer sheath is advanced in the right atrium. Once the path to the inferior vena cava is gained, a curved catheter is used for the catheterization of the hepatic vein and the venous district's anatomy is eventually studied with a venogram (iodinated contrast or CO_2 may be used).

3.4.2.3 Portal Vein Access

Subsequently, the metal cannula of the TIPS set is used to direct the stylet, anteriorly when aiming the RPV or posteriorly when aiming the LPV, through the hepatic parenchyma for 4–5 cm. The stylet's access point to the portal vein should ideally be 1–2 cm from the portal bifurcation; this allows the Gore Viatorr® TIPS stent graft to assume a gentle curve that optimizes the shunt flow, reducing the risk of excessive turbulence and consequent obstruction.

After the removal of the stylet and a slow needle retraction together with a gentle syringe aspiration, once blood withdrawal is observed, contrast medium is injected to check whether the landing site is in the targeted portal vein or not.

Several attempts may be required for the attainment of a successful puncture, especially in cirrhotic patients who usually present a distorted intrahepatic vascular anatomy. Ultrasound guidance may be employed to facilitate the intrahepatic puncture and minimize the risk of hemorrhage. This is the most critical step of TIPS procedure, as it may be complicated by hepatic capsule perforation, hepatic artery puncture, biliary duct puncture, or extrahepatic portal tract puncture.

The degree of portal hypertension is then determined by measuring the HVPG, as discussed before in this chapter.

A portography is finally performed for an appropriate portal system anatomy study, the

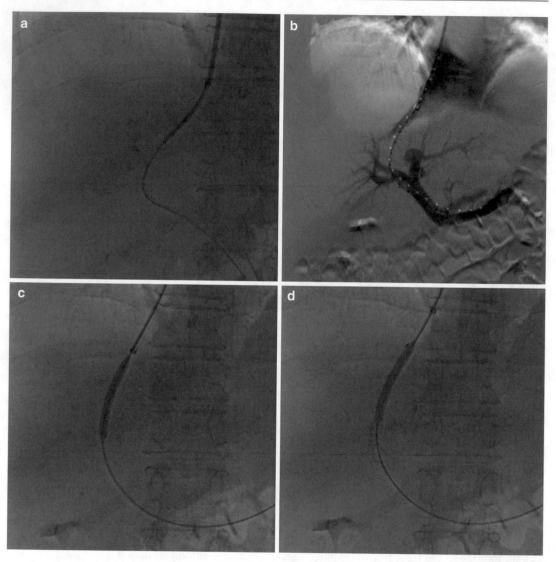

Fig. 6 After catheter-blocked transhepatic portography through a sheath placed in the right hepatic vein and transhepatic puncture (not shown), the portal system is achieved (**a**) and direct portography is performed using a marked pigtail catheter used for choosing the right length of stent (**b**); (**c**) dilatation of the transhepatic tract with angiographic balloon; (**d**) post-dilatation of the Gore Viatorr® stent

measurements of the shunt's length, and the definition of varices. Very curved shunt courses require to take into account a 1–2 cm longer stent graft compared to the measured shunt's length.

3.4.2.4 Stent Graft Deployment

Dilatation by an angiographic balloon of the intraparenchymal tract of the shunt precedes the placement of the stent that is subdivided into two steps: the release of the uncovered portion of the stent and then of the covered portion. A 12F introducer sheath is advanced in the portal system for at least 3 cm. Once the stent graft has been introduced in it, this can gently be unsheathed to permit the endoprosthesis' uncovered portion expansion in the portal vein. This is a delicate phase as a wrong positioning of this stent graft's portion cannot be corrected; moreover, in liver-transplant candidates, the positioning of both TIPS ends is particularly critical and has to be as precise as possible (Krajina et al. 2012). The introducer sheath is then retracted until a higher resistance, due to the transition from the portal vein tract to the intrahepatic tract, is felt; continuing in the retraction of the introducer into the inferior vena cava or the right atrium, the stent is allowed to be completely released with the proximal end at the junction of the chosen hepatic vein with the inferior vena cava. Keeping the system firmly still, the PTFE-covered portion is then deployed by pulling its constraining cord.

Stent dilatation by angiographic balloon is then performed; under-dilatation may be chosen to target a precise HVPG value or prevent excessive shunt.

To prevent thrombus formation inside the TIPS endoprosthesis 5000 IU of heparin could be administered immediately after its positioning.

Finally, a portogram is performed to check the shunt's functioning and another HVPG measurement is obtained to calculate the ΔHVPG: the procedure's hemodynamic success is achieved if HVPG is reduced to a value <12 mmHg or at least 20%.

3.4.3 Challenges

Compared to surgical shunts, TIPS procedure has lower mortality and morbidity rates: a fatal periprocedural complication occurs in 1.7% of patients (range 0.6–4.3%) (Krajina et al. 2012). Some procedural related events that may cause the patient's death, like extrahepatic portal vein puncture (2%), hepatic arterial vessel laceration (1%), or transcapsular puncture with transjugular needle (<1%) should be avoided. Other nonfatal periprocedural complications include neck hematoma due to accidental carotid puncture (1%), pneumothorax due to an overly low attempt of jugular puncture (<1%), and biliary duct lesion with consequent hemobilia (10%).

3.4.3.1 Portal Vein Thrombosis

In the case of cirrhosis complicated by PVT, the TIPS positioning requires, in addition to the venous transjugular access, portal access via transhepatic or trans-splenic track. Portal recanalization attempts can also be undertaken (Lombardo et al. 2018) (Fig. 7).

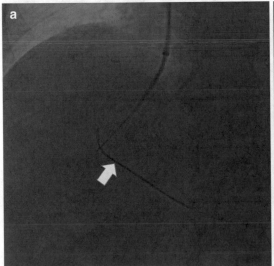
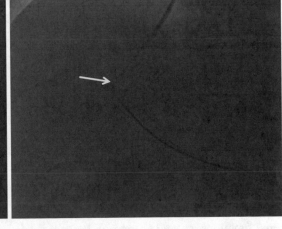

Fig. 7 Transhepatic puncture in a patient with portal thrombosis. Gooseneck catheter introduced via trans-splenic percutaneous access (yellow arrow in **a**) used to catch the guidewire introduced via transjugular access (thin yellow arrow in **b**), allowing to reach the portal system

3.5   Follow-Up

In patients that after the intervention present normal coagulative parameters, prophylactic anticoagulation therapy should be initiated (12,500 IU of heparin per 500 mL of physiological solution for the first 24 h, and subsequently 0.4 mg of low-molecular-weight heparin—LMWH—twice a day for at least 1 week). Further anticoagulation is not recommended, except for patients who underwent TIPS positioning with Budd-Chiari syndrome indication (i.e., massive hepatic vein thrombosis) or who experience PVT: in these cases INR target is >2 (Krajina et al. 2012).

The prophylactic antibiotic therapy initiated before the intervention has to be prolonged for at least 48 h after the procedure.

Post-procedure hospitalization foresees the evaluation of the liver's functional status. Whenever clinical abnormal findings should be encountered, the recovery is prolonged for further investigations and management.

TIPS patency should be evaluated with US examination within 1–5 days from the procedure.

After TIPS creation, the worsening or outbreak of HE may be detected by the evaluation of sleep pattern behaviors, working capacity, and changes of personality and of speech abilities. Psychometric tests are useful tools for the detection of subclinical HE (Campagna et al. 2017).

Impaired liver function may follow TIPS intervention: liver sufferance is presented with abnormal increase of serum bilirubin concentration.

Patients should be signed off only when their clinical status is sufficiently good and no laboratory examinations are out of range. At discharge, patients are provided with detailed dietary instructions as well as with prophylactic therapy for PHE.

Follow-up in patients with TIPS foresees a periodic evaluation of nutritional status, functional status, grade of encephalopathy, liver and renal functions, as well as status of the pathology for which TIPS was indicated. This allows to understand if the clinical endpoints of each patient have been reached or not and to perform further examinations or modify the therapy appropriately.

3.5.1   Ultrasonographic Examination

Due to its noninvasive nature, US is the first-line examination method for patients with TIPS. In patients who received a Wallstent™ (bare metal stent), the first investigation should be performed 24 h after the procedure, aiming the ruling out of the immediate onset of complications such as stent occlusion or insufficient shunt flow (if these are encountered, a prompt TIPS angiographic revision is required) (ŽiŽka et al. 2000). On the contrary, patients who underwent the positioning of a Gore Viatorr® TIPS endoprosthesis have no recommendation for such early examination. This is due to the fact that a thin air layer may be trapped between the stent's ePTFE sheets, impeding a proper TIPS insonation and resulting in a false-positive evaluation for occlusion (Ferral et al. 2016). Therefore, the first radiological evaluation of these patients should be carried out 5–10 days after the intervention. From then on, follow-up should be performed every 6 months even if shorter intervals (i.e., 3 months) between one and another examination may be required in case of critical patients (Darcy 2012). Furthermore, the success of radiological follow-up also depends on the patients' compliance to attend such clinical investigations. US is employed for the assessment of the liver's anatomy as well as for the ruling out of nodular lesions, but it is a valid method for the detection of shunt malfunctioning and occlusion too (85–100% sensitivity; 96–100% specificity) (Kanterman et al. 1997).

The caliber of the portal vein and of the stent graft should be measured for the evaluation, respectively, of possible excessive ectasia or stenoses. Ultimately, the TIPS diameter, measured on its proximal, middle, and distal tracts, is compared to the nominal caliber of the endoprosthesis' design. Color Doppler US could give information about the intra-TIPS blood flow and the assessment of TIPS patency, in addition to portal blood flow direction (Feldstein et al. 1996).

The baseline portal vein blood flow speed (V_{max} 10–20 cm/s) rises two- to fourfold after the insertion of TIPS in the hepatic parenchyma. Therefore, in patients with TIPS, a portal vein blood flow slower than 30 cm/s is suspicious of TIPS malfunctioning, and a blood flow speed lower than 20 cm/s is most likely indicative of endoprosthesis stenosis (ŽiŽka et al. 2000).

For ePTFE-covered stents, mean intra-TIPS flow rates <90 cm/s or >250 cm/s have to be considered suggestive of TIPS malfunctioning and hence worthy of further investigation (i.e., angiographic revision), even if there are no cutoff values in literature.

Contrast-enhanced ultrasound (CEUS) allows a direct evaluation of the TIPS patency and may serve as a complementary tool to the otherwise insufficient ultrasonographic investigation by showing enhancement defects or even a total absence of enhancement (Micol et al. 2012). Thus, in the follow-up of patients with TIPS, CEUS could play a bridge role between Doppler ultrasound examination and angiographic TIPS revision (Figs. 8 and 9).

The contrast agent used for CEUS consists of sulfur hexafluoride microbubbles stabilized by a shell of phospholipids that allows a notable increase of the ultrasound backscatter with or without contrast medium flowing movement and has the capability to entirely remain in the bloodstream and not permeate into the extravascular space.

The use of CEUS contrast agents has been demonstrated to be safe with a very rare incidence of side effects (Piscaglia and Bolondi 2006). There is no need for a laboratory workup prior to the examination and it is enough to keep the patient monitored for at least 15 min after the contrast agent injection. Ultrasound contrast agent administration is forbidden in patients affected by allergy to sulfur hexafluoride or any other component, cardiac right-to-left shunt, severe pulmonary hypertension, uncontrollable

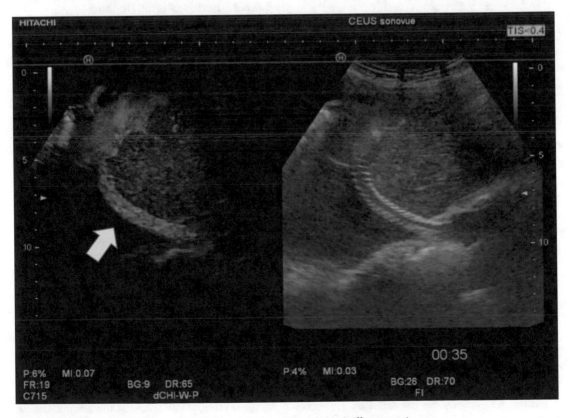

Fig. 8 Contrast-enhanced ultrasound well demonstrating stent patency (yellow arrow)

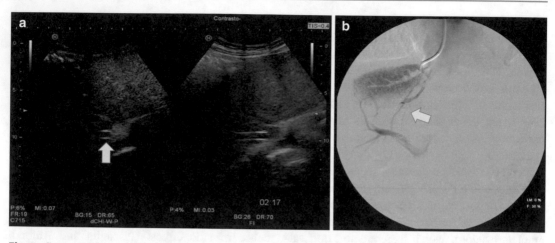

Fig. 9 Contrast-enhanced ultrasound showing stent occlusion (yellow arrow in **a**) then confirmed at TIPS revision (yellow arrow in **b**, DSA image)

Table 1 Main complications related to TIPS procedure

Complications	Frequency (%)
Arterial injuries	2
Nontarget TIPS insertion	Rare
Liver capsule transgression	33
Acute hepatic encephalopathy	5–35
Acute hepatic failure	Rare
Early acute occlusion	<5
Hernia incarceration	25
Infection	1

hypertension, acute respiratory distress syndrome, and severe cardiac disease that contraindicates the use of dobutamine.

Informed consent should always be obtained before the use of ultrasound contrast agent as well.

3.5.2 Complications

The complications can be technical (i.e., related to the procedure), or resulting from the successful realization of the shunt, or directly related to the TIPS; the main conditions are listed in Table 1 (Gaba et al. 2011).

3.5.2.1 Arterial Injury

The accidental puncture of an arterial branch during the procedure may lead to the development of a fistula, which must be corrected by embolization or covered stents to treat hemorrhage (Fig. 10).

3.5.2.2 Acute Hepatic Failure

Hepatic parenchymal ischemia can occur due to reduced sinusoidal flow and can be treated by reducing the caliber of the stent (Fig. 11).

3.5.2.3 Portosystemic Hepatic Encephalopathy (PHE)

The most common medical complication of TIPS positioning is a higher incidence of PHE, a medical condition caused by an excess of toxins in the central nervous system because of bypass of bloodstream hepatic filter and characterized by confusion, disorientation, obtundation, anomalous sleep patterns, and a general compromised quality of life (Riggio et al. 2008; Madoff et al. 2004).

Clinical classification of PHE, that may be classified as episodic, recurrent, or persistent according to its periodicity, is based on the West-Haven criteria or Glasgow coma scale (GCS). The main risk factors for the reoccurrence or new outbreak of PHE are history of PHE, older age, bigger shunt caliber, creatinine blood levels, hyponatremia, and liver dysfunction. Such TIPS complication may be prevented by aiming a lower HVPG reduction, reaching a compromise between portal hypertension decrease and control of excessive blood shunting. Furthermore, treatment of precipitating factors prior to TIPS positioning assures a lower risk of PHE outbreak. Medical prophylaxis foresees the administration of lactulose, which causes ammonia to transform into ammonium, excreted in stool.

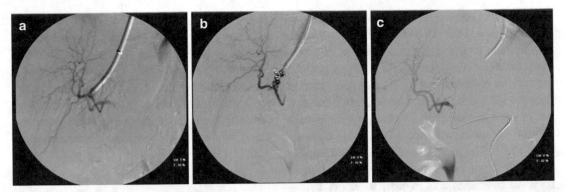

Fig. 10 Accidental puncture of an arterial branch during TIPS creation (**a**), treated by embolization with spirals (**b**, **c**)

Fig. 11 Ischemia of the VI hepatic segment and part of the VII segment after creation of TIPS

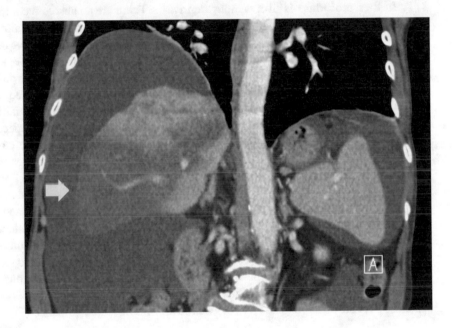

PHE has been encountered in up to 35% of patients who underwent TIPS intervention, but among these only 8% are refractory to medical management; in this case a re-intervention to reduce the flow of shunting blood could be necessary and liver transplantation should be considered.

4 Portal Venous Embolization (PVE)

4.1 Introduction

Surgery is nowadays the gold standard for radical treatment in patients with primitive neoplastic or metastatic liver disease. The available options are liver transplant or resection. Because of the limited number of organs available, liver resection is the most common procedure in the treatment of neoplastic liver disease. In more than 45% of patients extended liver surgery is needed to achieve clear margins and liver ability to regenerate has allowed larger and larger resection. However, the wider the resections the higher the risk for the patient of liver insufficiency. This is more pronounced in the early postoperative period, with a mortality rate ranging from 3.2% to 7% after major liver resections that reaches 32% in patients with cirrhosis (Broering et al. 2002).

In order to support a rapid growth of the future liver remnant (FLR) in 1965 portal vein ligation was initially reported in humans as part of a two-stage extended hepatectomy. In 1982 preoperative portal vein embolization (PVE) was performed in patients with cholangiocarcinoma, while the first use of preoperative PVE for patients with hepatocellular carcinoma was reported in 1986 (Makuuchi et al. 1990). The main aim of PVE is the complete occlusion of the portal branches feeding the future resected liver segments in order to induce hypertrophy of the FLR and atrophy of the embolized liver parenchyma (Denys et al. 2010).

A further procedure is liver venous deprivation (LVD). It consists in the simultaneous embolization of right portal vein (RPV) and the right and/or intermediate hepatic veins, in order to increase the damage to the embolized liver leading to increased hypertrophy of the contralateral parenchyma (Panaro et al. 2019).

Since its original description indications for PVE have been expanded and now include any primary or metastatic liver cancer requiring better FLR prior to hepatectomy.

4.2 PVE and Surgical Portal Ligature

The effectiveness of right portal vein occlusion in large hepatic resections is well known but it is still unsure whether surgical portal ligation has to be preferred over the interventional PVE, or vice versa.

In literature there are studies that proved that PVE can reach a FLR growth between 10% and 46% after 2–8 weeks (Liu and Zhu 2009). Similarly other studies found a growth of 38% in 8 weeks after surgical portal ligation (Aussilhou et al. 2008). In conclusion there is still no evidence that can help choose between interventional and surgical treatment (Pandanaboyana et al. 2015).

4.3 Technical Considerations

There are no absolute contraindications to PVE.

Relative contraindications are uncorrectable coagulopathy, tumor invasion of the portal vein, tumor precluding transhepatic access, biliary dilatation (pre-procedural positioning of a biliary drainage is recommended in these cases), portal hypertension, and renal failure.

Intravenous broad-spectrum antibiotic prophylaxis is given on the day of the procedure to minimize the possibilities of biliary sepsis.

Local anesthetic (1% lidocaine hydrochloride) and intravenous sedatives are administered.

Ultrasonography is used to find the best route to the portal venous system; it is recommended not to pass through the tumor during the access in order to avoid neoplastic seeding.

Under sterile conditions a 21-gauge needle is used to enter the portal system by ultrasonic or fluoroscopic guidance (Fig. 12).

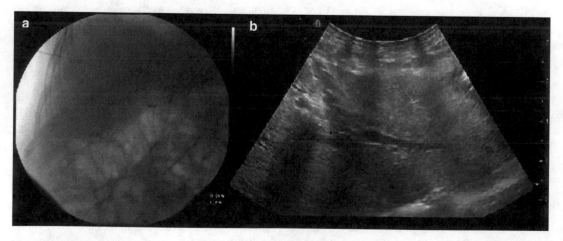

Fig. 12 (a) Fluoroscopic guided access to portal system with a 21-gauge needle. (b) US-guided access to portal system with a 21 Gauge needle

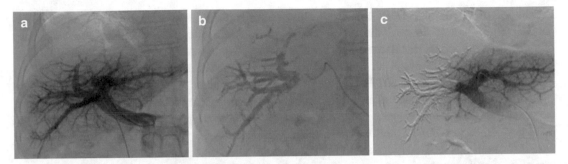

Fig. 13 (**a**) Portography realized with a 5F catheter and a contralateral access. (**b**) Following portal embolization. (**c**) Post-procedure portography confirming the effectiveness of the treatment

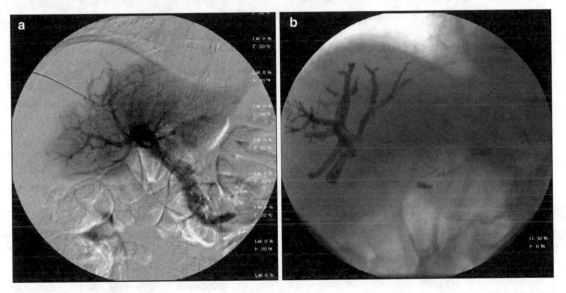

Fig. 14 (**a**) Portography performed with a 5 French catheter inserted with an ipsilateral access. (**b**) Mix of NBCA and Lipiodol in the right lobe following PVE

The percutaneous procedure can be performed using an ipsilateral or contralateral percutaneous access.

The ipsilateral approach has the advantage that it does not damage the FLR, but it is more technically difficult because of the sharp angulation encountered in cannulating portal branches. It consists of the puncture of a peripheral right portal vein and a 180° reverse-curved catheter to embolize ipsilateral portal branches (Fig. 13).

The contralateral approach has the advantage of cannulation without pronounced angulation and allows a prograde delivering of embolic agents and contrast; nonetheless it may injure the FLR. In the contralateral approach the portal vein of segment three is usually punctured as it is the most anterior branch (Fig. 14).

In both cases at least 1 cm proximal to the main portal vein should be left untouched, in order to allow surgical control during the resection. Five-French materials are usually recommended.

It has also been described a trans-ileocolic approach that is now rarely used. It requires general anesthesia and a surgical incision to extract a portion of the ileum in order to cannulate an ileocolic vein.

A final portography must be performed to verify the correctness of the procedure, the complete occlusion of targeted liver segments, and redistribution of flow to the FLR branches only. Embolization has to involve the entire portal branch with its distal ramification to prevent porto-portal shunts (Denys et al. 2010; Liu and Zhu 2009; Narula and Aloia 2017).

There are various embolic agents that can be used but any large randomized study has ever been performed to compare their efficacy; up-to-date information is derived from small retrospective studies and expert opinion.

Two products are not recommended in PVE: gelfoam because of the high rate of recanalization and alcohol because of a significant post-procedural morbidity (parenchymal necrosis and venous thrombosis).

Recommended embolic agents are cyanoacrylate and microspheres. N-butyl-cyanoacrylate (NBCA) has been used mixed to lipiodol showing good results and low morbidity. Spherical microparticles are mostly used in North America and are associated with coil embolization at the end of the procedure; most teams start with 300–500 µm particles followed by 700–900 µm spheres (Denys et al. 2010).

4.4   Complications

CIRSE guidelines indicate a minor and major post-procedural complication rate of less than 20–25% and 5%, respectively (Denys et al. 2010).

Puncture-related complications include mechanical injuries to vessel, biliary structure, and pleura (Narula and Aloia 2017). They are the majority of complications, so that many authors advice for the ipsilateral approach.

The most common complication of percutaneous transhepatic procedures is hemorrhage; after PVE it occurs in 2–4% of patients. Bleeding can present as subcapsular hematoma or hemoperitoneum and it can be immediate or delayed. Bleeding sources include intercostal artery, portal vein, hepatic vein, and hepatic artery. Transarterial embolization can be an effective treatment.

Biliary injuries are usually less common because biliary puncture is rarer and it becomes symptomatic less frequently. The main manifestations are bile leak, which necessitate biliary drainage, and hemobilia treated with embolization of the underlying artero-biliary fistula.

Pneumothorax and hemothorax can also happen but they are rare.

Embolization-related injuries are non-targeted embolization, portal vein thrombosis, liver infarction, portal hypertension, post-embolization syndrome, and recanalization (Narula and Aloia 2017).

Non-targeted embolization strongly depends on the embolic materials. Especially for inexperienced operators, liquid embolic materials can flow distally and inadvertently embolize areas of the FLR, forcing the surgeon to enlarge the resection (Fig. 15).

PVT is one of the most dangerous complications because it can cause acute liver failure and jeopardize post-PVE surgery; immediate treatment is mandatory (Yeom and Shin 2015).

Post-embolization syndrome includes minor symptoms such as abdominal pain, fever, nausea, and vomiting. It happens rarer than in arterial embolization probably because PVE mainly activates apoptosis mechanism rather than ischemic necrosis so inflammatory mediator release is limited.

Half of the patients after PVE show little liver enzyme alteration 3 days after the embolization which returns to baseline after 7–10 days (Liu and Zhu 2009).

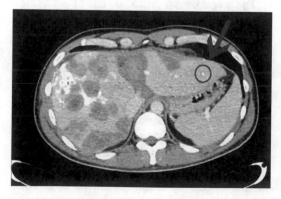

Fig. 15 Radiopaque material in the left hepatic lobe in a non-targeted PVE

Complications are more frequent in patients with chronic liver disease overall.

4.5 Outcome

The degree of hypertrophy and the time interval through which it manifests after PVE have a great variability among patients. In patients with a normal functioning liver the regeneration time is about 2 weeks and it grows 12–21 cm³/day. Otherwise in patients with cirrhosis the growth is limited to 9 cm³/day (Madoff et al. 2002).

There are several factors that inhibit FLR growth, such as pre-procedural chemotherapy, high bilirubin levels, and diabetes mellitus.

The risk of neoplastic progression after PVE is still under debate. Several studies report a risk of neoplastic progression of 25% during the period the FLR growth is expected (Hoekstra et al. 2012). Some patients with liver metastasis from colon-rectal cancer had a pre-procedural chemotherapy, because literature reports that the risk of disease progression is low if the time between the end of chemotherapy and PVE is short (Simoneau et al. 2015).

Regarding the two-stage hepatectomy (resection of the lesions in the FLR followed by PVE and subsequently by the resection of the contralateral neoplastic lobe) the survival rate at 5 years is between 51% and 32% with a median survival time of 39.6 months (Brouquet et al. 2011; Narita et al. 2011).

5 Posttransplant Vascular Complications

5.1 Introduction

Vascular complications (VCs) following orthotopic liver transplantation (OLTx) are linked to a high incidence of both graft loss and mortality.

After the transplant the hepatic artery becomes the primary blood supply to the graft and the only one to the biliary tree; although liver parenchyma is partially supplied by the portal vein, the absence of hepatic arterial flow (possible native collaterals are lost) can lead to acute graft ischemia and biliary tree complications.

For this reason it is really important to have a good timing of diagnosis and to perform the best therapeutic management in order to improve the outcomes of liver allograft recipients.

In a recent review the overall incidence of VCs in adult patients was quite different among different centers (Piardi et al. 2016). However, it is around 7% in deceased donor liver transplantation and around 13% in case of living donor liver transplant.

In order to detect complications correlated with OLTx, physicians should perform careful surveillance with US and, in particular to detect VCs, using color and Doppler mode.

Once a suspected VC is recognized, it must be evaluated with second-level imaging examinations, as CT angiography or angiography. In case of confirmation of VCs it has to be managed promptly.

While in the past the surgical treatment was considered the first approach towards these complications, nowadays the advances in endovascular intervention have increased and made it a viable therapeutic option.

With regard to the type and entity of VCs, we can perform surgical revascularization, retransplantation, percutaneous transluminal angioplasty with or without stenting, intra-arterial thrombolysis, embolization, or conservative approach (Chen et al. 2014).

In this text, for the sake of simplicity, we will distinguish the VCs that regard the blood inflow from the ones that regard the blood outflow. Kinking or sudden bleeding, stenosis, and thrombosis can arise at any of the vascular anastomoses, although with a different rate: arterial complications are the most common (overall incidence 5–10%), accounting for more than 50%, VCs after OLTx, while both portal and caval venous complications are less frequent (in both cases overall incidence about 2%) (Piardi et al. 2016).

The knowledge of postoperative anatomy is the key to assess the best management.

OLTx involves four anastomotic sites, each with specific VCs:

- Hepatic artery anastomosis: conduits or jump grafts or end-to-end anastomosis, typically end-to-end hepatic artery anastomosis
- Portal vein anastomosis: commonly end-to-end recipient portal vein to donor portal vein anastomosis
- Hepatic veins/inferior vena cava anastomosis: piggyback reconstruction, interposition; caval anastomosis for whole grafts; end-to-end anastomosis between the graft hepatic venous outflow and the recipient hepatic veins (split graft)
- Common bile duct anastomosis

5.2   Arterial Complications

A transplanted liver maintains a dual-inflow blood supply as a native one, portal and arterial, but after OLTx, the arterial blood gives a major contribution to the irroration of the hepatic graft, perfusing both liver parenchyma and biliary tree.

It is important to remember that in an OLTx recipient there are no arterial collateral vessels (which could prevent liver parenchymal ischemia during a hepatic artery occlusion) due to total hepatectomy, and if arterial inflow is reduced, the allograft may survive only if new arterial collaterals have developed due to insufficient portal inflow (Panaro et al. 2011). Arterial collaterals can develop as early as within 2 weeks.

The hepatic artery complications following OLTx are:

- Thrombosis
- Stenosis
- Pseudoaneurysm and rupture
- Splenic steal syndrome

Furthermore, although the definition of early and late complications is a problem, in this text complications will be classified in this way: early, with maximum onset within 1 month of transplant, and late, with onset more than 1 month after transplant.

We would like to underline the importance of early complications, because they are associated with higher graft loss and mortality rates.

5.2.1   Hepatic Artery Thrombosis (HAT)

HAT is defined as a complete thrombotic occlusion of the hepatic artery and it represents the most frequent and severe VCs following OLTx.

HAT is the second leading cause of graft loss after primary nonfunction (Meek et al. 2018).

In a systematic review a HAT overall incidence of 4.4% was reported after OLTx. In adults, the incidence of HAT was 2.9% (Bekker et al. 2009). Late HAT is less prevalent, counting for less than 2% of cases.

HAT can be classified in early HAT and late HAT, each one characterized by different clinical expressions, depending on the timing of the onset and on the existence of arterial collateral vessels.

While early HAT has an acute presentation with variable but severe clinical course (from an elevation in liver enzyme to ischemic biliary necrosis, primary dysfunction, and graft loss), late HAT, due to existence of collaterals, is usually less serious with 15–23% mortality rate and the majority of patients are asymptomatic or can present biliary complications (Nikeghbalian et al. 2007; Stange et al. 2003; Gunsar et al. 2003).

Most patients with early HAT presented acute fulminant hepatic failure (30%). In most cases, they undergo a retransplant (81%) (Pareja et al. 2010).

Up to 20% of HAT cases are probably due to surgical technical problems in the arterial anastomosis (such as technical imperfections, kinking, stenotic anastomosis). There are many other causes, often unacknowledged, as the median arcuate ligament celiac artery compression, which discussion is beyond the purpose of this chapter.

5.2.1.1   Diagnosis

Early diagnosis is pivotal to treat the complication and to try to prevent graft loss.

During allograft recipient follow-up it is mandatory to recognize patients with abnormal biological findings and/or morphological (ultrasonography) exams suggestive of HAT.

Doppler US is the gold standard for screening protocols (Vaidya et al. 2007).

Abdominal contrast-enhanced computed tomography (CT) angiography or DSA usually allows to confirm the diagnosis: in particular, DSA may detect predisposing anatomical anomalies and allow therapeutic management at the same time.

US diagnosis of hepatic artery thrombosis is based on the absence of Doppler arterial signal at the hilus as well as in the intrahepatic arterial branches.

In 2010 Pareja et al. established a screening protocol for early HAT: Doppler US within 48 h after OLTx and 7 days later. If this was not conclusive, they performed CEUS or CT. There are many other ultrasound protocols suggested in the literature (Murata et al. 2016).

Once diagnosis of HAT has been confirmed, arteriography or a retransplantation, depending on the degree of liver graft damage, must be performed.

In HAT follow-up, collaterals can be identified during angiography examination as early as 2 weeks after OLTx.

After the first month, considering that intimal hyperplasia can induce progressive hepatic artery stenosis and secondary late HAT, a yearly Doppler US assessment should be performed.

5.2.1.2 Therapeutic Management and Prognosis

In general, the therapeutic options for management of HAT are revascularization (surgical or endovascular), retransplantation, and observation (20% of cases).

Traditional percutaneous endovascular revascularization includes intra-arterial thrombolysis (IAT), percutaneous transluminal angioplasty (PTA), and stent placement.

Endoluminal success is defined as the complete resolution of the thrombus without residual thrombus or arterial anatomic defects that reduce the arterial diameter lumen more than 50% (Saad et al. 2007) (Fig. 16).

Murata et al. reported an overall technical success with endovascular treatment of 77.8% (Murata et al. 2016).

Even if efficacy (around 50% in literature) and safety of thrombolytic treatment are proven, also with different drugs (urokinase, streptokinase, alteplase) and doses, there are no currently specific guidelines for thrombolytic therapy. Furthermore, considering that anatomic defects can lead to rethrombosis, IAT should be associated with underlying anatomic defect treatment if

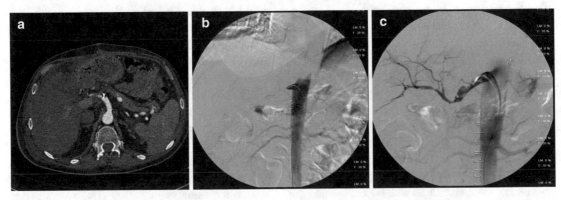

Fig. 16 Direct anastomosis of the donor hepatic artery to the supraceliac aorta with extension graft. Supraceliac arterial graft occlusion. (**a**) Contrast-enhanced CT, axial scan, arterial phase. Extensive peri-anastomotic stenosis of arterial inflow; intraparenchymal arterial branches were patent. (**b**) DSA confirmed graft occlusion; hepatic artery and its intraparenchymal branches are not displayed. (**c**) Intra-arterial thrombolysis was performed and partial patency of arterial graft was restored (not complete endoluminal success). There is a residual discrepancy between donor and recipient hepatic arteries with persistent filling defects

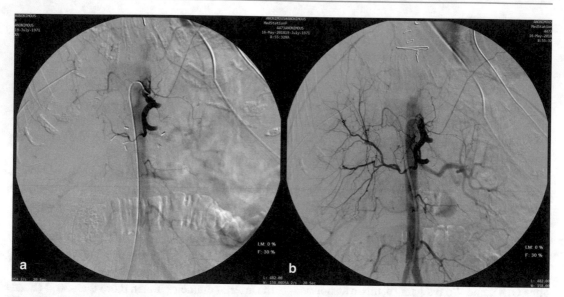

Fig. 17 (**a**) Digital subtraction angiography (DSA) shows celiac trunk stenosis and complete occlusion of left hepatic artery; right hepatic artery is patent but of narrow caliber. (**b**) After balloon angioplasty (PTA) and stent placement in celiac trunk and intra-arterial thrombolysis and PTA in hepatic artery main branches, DSA shows optimal results (good caliber of celiac trunk, left hepatic artery patent, and minimal residual stenosis of right hepatic artery) with improved hepatic arterial inflow

present: association of IAT with PTA and/or stenting showed better efficacy and survival rates when compared to IAT alone (Zhang et al. 2017) (Fig. 17).

In Zhou et al.'s experience, early diagnosis and treatment of HAT are very important for successful revascularization by thrombolysis because urokinase therapy is more effective when the clots are fresh. In the same study the quantity of urokinase used in patients with HAT was as much as 950,000 units to nine million units (Zhou et al. 2005).

Dose and timing of IAT may vary; Zhou et al. recommend the administration of a 100,000–250,000 IU bolus, followed by a second infusion of 250,000–750,000 IU 30 min later in case of unsatisfactory result. After this, a continuous perfusion of 50,000–100,000 UI/h is administered for 12–24 h. During the treatment, at least every 12 h, a DSA imaging is performed.

The catheter sheath should be maintained for 2–3 days after initial recanalization of the hepatic artery so that thrombus recurrence can be detected and rethrombolysis can be performed immediately.

Thrombolysis is stopped if no significant differences during monitoring or if bleeding complications occur.

Finally, some patients could survive without revascularization or retransplantation. Fouzas et al. (2012) described how these patients with hepatic artery thrombosis can develop arterial collaterals, which maintain adequate blood inflow and allow conservative treatment (Fig. 18).

Based on the relative lack of utility of revascularization of late HAT and the contraindication to early postoperative thrombolysis, Saad et al. proposed that the clinical utility window of IAT should be from 1–3 weeks to 1–3 months post-transplantation, unless there are contraindications (Saad et al. 2007).

Despite encouraging results of endovascular interventions, the efficacy and risk of complications (mainly represented by hemorrhage risk) make this therapeutic option still controversial. Moreover, in some cases, endovascular approach is not conclusive and anastomotic revision and retransplantation are necessary.

In a meta-analysis of 2009 HAT was a major cause of graft loss (53.1%) and mortality (33.3%) in the early postoperative period (Bekker et al. 2009).

The main complication of thrombolysis is anastomotic and intra-abdominal bleeding (about 20% of cases in literature). More safer and effec-

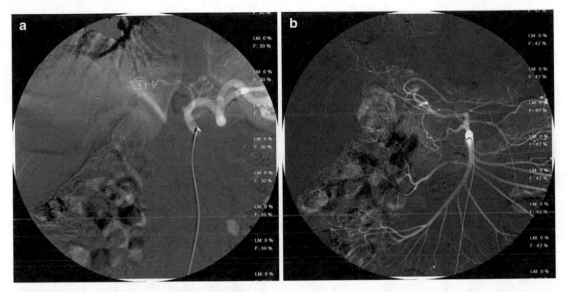

Fig. 18 (**a**) Celiac axis DSA shows complete occlusion of the proper hepatic artery; left gastric artery is patent and hypertrophic, with hepatic collaterals. (**b**) Same patient, superior mesenteric artery (SMA) angiogram: hypertrophic peripancreatic arcades provide collaterals from the SMA to the intraparenchymal hepatic artery

tive therapy can be obtained if the infusion catheter is placed inside the thrombus (Figueras et al. 1995). Furthermore selective thrombolysis has several advantages, such as a smaller thrombolytic dose and a highly localized concentration with a little influence on systemic coagulation.

The complications of PTA include thrombosis, vascular dissection, pseudoaneurysm, and arterial rupture with arterial bleeding (up to 5% of cases).

In recent years the use of Penumbra System (PS; Penumbra, Alameda, Calif) has been described to perform thromboaspiration of thrombi in the hepatic artery of patients with high risk of thrombus fragmentation-distal embolization and bleeding (Gandini et al. 2016).

Meek et al. tried to treat HAT using a mechanical endovascular approach, a stent retriever device for revascularization (Meek et al. 2018).

5.2.2 Hepatic Artery Stenosis (HAS)

HAS following OLTx can be defined as a narrowing of the hepatic artery diameter, more or less extended along the vessel; significant HAS is defined on angiography as a narrowing of the hepatic artery diameter greater than 50% (Saad et al. 2005).

HAS occurs from 2% to 13% of transplants (Piardi et al. 2016). It was assumed that HAS can progress to HAT considering that HAS and HAT are part of the same contiguous ischemic spectrum.

Similar to HAT, HAS may be divided into two groups: early HAS and late HAS. Chen et al. reported an overall HAS incidence of 2.8%, with an early HAS incidence of 40% vs. a late HAS incidence of 60% (Chen et al. 2009).

In several studies, up to 60% of the cases HAS occur at the level of the hepatic artery anastomosis (Fig. 19).

Patients with HAT can show a variable symptomatology, ranging from normal liver function to transplant failure secondary to ischemia or necrosis; most commonly, they only present with abnormal liver function tests; for this reason, most HAS are detected during routine Doppler US screening.

5.2.2.1 Diagnosis

Doppler US efficiency in the early diagnosis of HAS has been reported in several studies.

Dodd III et al. criteria for HAS diagnosis consist of a tardus parvus waveform: resistive index (RI) less than 0.5, systolic acceleration time (SAT) greater than 0.08 s, and peak systolic velocity (PSV)

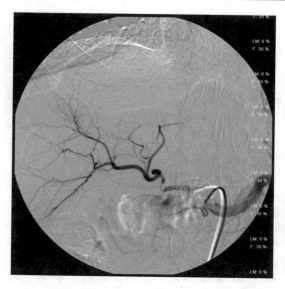

Fig. 19 DSA shows a focal >70% narrowing and kinking of the hepatic artery. Surgical arterial anastomotic revision was performed

greater than 200 cm/s (Dodd III et al. 1994). Intrahepatic arterial branches have to be visualized.

To exclude HAT with the development of collateral vessels, that shows a dampening of the systolic peak with normal RI, similar to tardus parvus waveform, it is necessary to detect a focal poststenotic systolic peak velocity greater than 200 cm/s, diagnostic for hepatic artery stenosis (Zheng et al. 2017; Hom et al. 2006).

With regard to the many questionable cases and considering that measuring the acceleration time is hard and imprecise, arterial RI should be used solely as a screening method for detecting abnormality of arterial flow and further imaging methods such as contrast-enhancement CT angiography and standard angiography are used to confirm the diagnosis. Conventional angiography is the gold standard for HAS diagnosis (Frongillo et al. 2013).

5.2.2.2 Therapeutic Management and Prognosis

The therapeutic management of HAS includes surgical revision, retransplant, or percutaneous endovascular interventions (PTA with or without stent placement).

Endovascular treatment success has been defined by luminal restoration with 30% residual stenosis and without consequences such as dissection (rate limiting or not) or arterial leaks/rupture (Saad et al. 2005).

It is demonstrated that early HAS management with PTA has 6-month HAT rate of 19%, compared to HAT rate of 65% in untreated patients with HAS.

Similar to Abbasoglu et al. (1997), Saad et al. (2005) reported 81% successful PTA treatment of significant HAS, with incidence of immediate complications (dissection and arterial rupture) around 7% and of delayed complications (HAT) within 30 days of PTA occurring in 5% of cases.

Different rates of restenosis have been reported in literature, from no restenosis to rates as high as 75%. It is been proved that repeated endovascular treatment of recurring HAS improves the rate of success (Sommacale et al. 2013).

Ueno et al. (2006) documented that hepatic artery stent placement is feasible and shows low complication rate.

Stent placement has been employed when there was >30% residual stenosis or when a flow-limiting dissection was present.

Saad et al. (2005 and 2007) reported that restenosis after a stent placement occurred later than after angioplasty alone (Fig. 20).

Prompt early diagnosis of HAS and percutaneous endovascular revascularization are usually successful with long-term graft and patient survival, in particular if stenosis is not associated with biliary complications.

The reported risk of procedural complications after endovascular treatment of HAS is quite variable, ranging from 0% to 23% in the literature.

In pediatric patients stent placement is recommended only if angioplasty fails or if other procedure-related VCs occur (hepatic artery dissection or rupture) because its long-term patency is not known and a possible retransplantation has to be taken into account considering the patient's age (Miraglia et al. 2009).

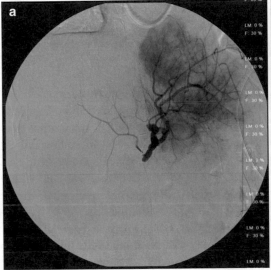

Fig. 20 (a) Celiac axis DSA shows patent arterial anastomosis between the recipient's celiac trunk and donor's superior mesenteric artery (SMA); the right hepatic artery arises from SMA in donor and after OLTx, in recipient, its caliber is narrow in the origin site. (b) Post-balloon angioplasty (PTA) and stent placement DSA shows suboptimal results with residual <30% stenosis and improved arterial hepatic inflow

5.2.3 Hepatic Artery Pseudoaneurysm (HAP)

HAP is defined as a pulsating, encapsulated hematoma in communication with the lumen of a ruptured vessel (Sueyoshi et al. 2005): blood leaks through the artery wall and it pools outside of it.

There is a persistent communication between the hepatic artery, patent, and resultant perfused sac; it is contained by the media or adventitia or simply by soft-tissue structures surrounding the injured vessel (Saad et al. 2005).

Post-OLTx HAPs are classified as intra- or extrahepatic; while intrahepatic ones are uncommon and secondary to percutaneous transhepatic interventions, extrahepatic HAPs are more common (69–100% of post-OLTx HAP) and usually due to local infection, from both bacterial and fungal organisms, in anastomotic site.

Additionally, HAPs have been described secondary to salvage procedures related to thrombolysis and angioplasty for hepatic artery (Fistouris et al. 2006).

The clinical presentation is not specific: from asymptomatic state to abdominal pain with fever, and from self-limiting hemobilia to hemorrhagic shock.

5.2.3.1 Diagnosis

The diagnosis of HAP is made by Doppler US, contrast-enhanced CT angiography, or DSA, but almost 50% of HAP is not recognized before rupture (Volpin et al. 2014).

5.2.3.2 Therapeutic Management and Prognosis

The management of HAP can be carried out by a surgical team (mainly hepatic artery ligation) or an interventional radiologist.

Hepatic artery ligation mortality rate is quite variable: from high mortality rate of 60% to 35%.

There are only few case reports of patients treated with endovascular approach because of the low incidence of this VC. Different techniques are available: intentional occlusive embolization (in order to produce an intentional thrombosis of the hepatic artery to stop bleeding without preserving arterial inflow) and bare stents and covered stents. Selective embolization (in order to perform an intentional thrombosis of the pseudoaneurysm with preservation of the arterial inflow) is usually reserved for intrahepatic HAP.

The use of coil has been reported to embolize the hepatic artery and the HAP exclusion with a covered stent inserted into the hepatic artery.

Embolization can lead to subsequent graft ischemia. Furthermore, a large percentage of these pseudoaneurysms are mycotic, and a stent graft may become an infectious nidus, reducing the survival of the graft.

Detecting HAP before rupture should improve outcome, with 100% successful therapy; from this perspective, it seems legit in the early management of HAP to perform prompt percutaneous endovascular approach, to take time and stabilize patients. Surgical intervention is an option if endovascular management has failed or once patients are stabilized (Piardi et al. 2016).

5.2.4 Hepatic Artery Rupture (HAR)

HAR is defined as a severe hemorrhage from the trunk or from a main branch of the hepatic artery, resulting in the absence of the arterial blood supply of the graft.

Clinical presentation is always sudden hemorrhage: hemoperitoneum, gastrointestinal bleeding, hematoma, and hemobilia.

5.2.4.1 Therapeutic Management and Prognosis

It is usually a complication of HAP or of its treatment; it requires an aggressive treatment, usually emergency major surgery: anastomotic revision, aorto-hepatic grafting, hepatic artery ligation, or emergency/elective retransplantation.

However, some endovascular possibilities are available. Goldsmith et al. (2017) placed a bare-metal self-expanding stent and did a prolonged balloon tamponade; if this treatment was not successful they used a covered balloon-expandable coronary stents (2.5–3.5 mm) off-label.

Other options for treating active extravasation include embolization of the hepatic artery when low-profile covered stents are not available or cannot be delivered to the site of vessel injury.

Anyway, the reported mortality rate for endovascular management is high.

Kim et al. (2004) underlined that endovascular treatment of hepatic artery rupture is not always feasible, listing some critical points in this kind of approach, in particular the difficulty of superselective catheterization of bleeding arteries.

5.2.5 Arterial Steal Syndromes

The arterial steal syndromes, currently diagnosed on DSA, are characterized by low arterial flow towards the graft caused by a shift of flow into an enlarged splenic artery (splenic artery steal syndrome, the most frequent) or into the gastroduodenal artery (gastroduodenal artery steal syndrome). Overall incidence is 4.7%.

On Doppler US, there is a high RI of the hepatic artery with absent diastolic flow.

DSA is required for the diagnosis: slow hepatic artery flow as opposed to splenic artery flow in the absence of significant hepatic artery anatomical defects, often associated with large caliber of the splenic artery with earlier preferential splenic parenchymal perfusion compared to the liver (Nüssler et al. 2003).

Endovascular proximal splenic artery embolization is currently considered the best approach towards this syndrome; it can reverse flow abnormalities and improve liver function tests in most cases. Coil embolization of the splenic artery has been reported to be safe and effective.

Common complications of splenic artery embolization include splenic infarction, abscess formation, and sepsis (Zhu et al. 2011).

5.2.6 Non-hepatic Arterial Bleeding

OLTx is often associated with abdominal bleeding, especially during early postoperative period. A study reported a 9% overall incidence of postoperative abdominal bleeding within 1 month (Jung et al. 2012).

The most frequent non-hepatic arterial bleeding sites are the inferior phrenic arteries (the right ones are especially important because they can act as extrahepatic collateral vessels), the right and left epigastric arteries, and the intercostal arteries.

The treatment of the rupture of these vessels is performed mainly by transarterial embolization with microcoils.

5.3 Venous Complications

Venous VC linked to OLTx overall incidence is less than 3%, quite lower than arterial VCs (Pawlak et al. 2003; Pérez-Saborido et al. 2011).

Like arterial VCs, they represent an important cause of morbidity and mortality after OLTx, especially if they occur in the early postoperative period (Woo et al. 2007).

Furthermore, the dramatic nature of these complications lies in its higher incidence in pediatric transplants than in adult transplants (Orlandini et al. 2014).

Venous VCs after OLTx shall include portal (thrombosis and stenosis) and caval (thrombosis, stenosis, and kinking) problems.

As arterial VCs, they can be distinguished in early or late complications.

Currently, a vast majority of authors agree on endovascular intervention management of venous complications considering the good outcomes.

5.4 Portal Vein Complications

The incidence of portal vein complications after liver transplantation is low, ranging from 1% to 3% of patients. These complications are more common with split liver and also in pediatric transplantation.

5.4.1 Portal Vein Thrombosis (PVT)

The incidence of PVT following OLTx is between 0.3% and 2.6% (Piardi et al. 2016), occurring more frequently within 3 months after transplant (Kyoden et al. 2008).

Similar to HAT, the clinical presentation depends on the timing of thrombosis and portal hypertension development: when it occurs early, there is a severe acute liver insufficiency with graft failure; meanwhile if it occurs later, portocaval collateral circulation could exist and the clinical course will be mild (abdominal pain and/or elevated liver enzymes).

The most common causes of PVT are technical surgical errors related to venous redundancy and kinking and/or stenosis of the anastomosis. Other reported risk factors exist, such as early

PVT caused by coronary vein steal after OLTx, but their discussion is beyond the aims of this chapter (Koo et al. 2008).

PVT has been associated with technical surgical problems, discrepancy between donor and recipient calibers, and hypercoagulability state; furthermore it can occur also in the case of elevated downstream flow resistance, such as in inferior vena cava stricture, or low portal inflow, related to arterial steal syndromes (see below) (Girometti et al. 2014).

5.4.1.1 Diagnosis

Portal VCs are usually detected by Doppler US or CEUS.

Doppler US is the most used examination: it should document the absence of flow in the main extrahepatic trunk, with or without definite delineation of an intraluminal echogenic thrombus on B-mode. There is not a specific protocol, but it is recommended to perform a daily evaluation of the main liver vessels.

Recently the use of CEUS has been proposed to avoid frequent false-positive results after preliminary Doppler US (Lee et al. 2013).

Furthermore, contrast-enhanced CT or contrast-enhanced MR should be used in patients who have been diagnosed with PVT by US to achieve a detailed characterization (collateral mapping, detection of local factors, and complications) (Rodrigues et al. 2017).

The invasive angiographic approach is reserved for the cases with uncertain diagnosis on noninvasive imaging and it is used when an endovascular treatment could be performed. On portography, stenosis is considered hemodynamically significant when the prestenotic/poststenotic pressure gradient is >5 mmHg.

5.4.1.2 Therapeutic Management and Prognosis

The Yerdel classification system of PVT is based on partial or complete obstruction of the lumen and extension into the splenic vein or superior mesenteric vein (SMV) (Yerdel et al. 2000). The approach to surgical management and portal vein reconstruction is dictated by the grade of PVT.

Conservative management with anticoagulation (vitamin K antagonists or heparins) is the current mainstay of treatment of PVT, getting thrombosis and secondary complications under control.

Kaneko et al. (2003) described a case of an OLTx recipient treated conservatively with anticoagulation after an early diagnosis of PVT.

However PVT remains a life-threatening event associated with a high rate of graft loss or death and in patients not responding to anticoagulation (with thrombus extension or worsening symptoms) an alternative approach should be considered.

If in the past the first choice of treatment of PVT was the surgical approach, through thrombectomy, anastomosis revision, or retransplantation, currently, except early PVT, percutaneous endovascular procedures are the first-line treatment for PVT following OLTx, and the portal VCs in general.

These include percutaneous thrombolytic therapy, transhepatic portal vein angioplasty with or without stent placement, and thrombectomy (Chamarthy et al. 2016).

Percutaneous thrombolysis involves administration of low-dose thrombolytic agents close to the clot; it can be direct using transhepatic, transsplenic, and transjugular intrahepatic portal venous accesses or indirect when thrombolytic drugs are administered into the superior mesenteric artery.

Transjugular intrahepatic puncture is the most used approach in PVT and it is usually followed by TIPS to enhance venous outflow (Saad 2012).

Another advantage of the TIPS approach is that it may reduce the risk of intraperitoneal bleeding.

The main complications of endovascular thrombolytic therapy are risk of vessel injury, re-thrombosis, and pulmonary embolism and bradycardia if performed after creation of TIPS.

While the disadvantages of TIPS approach are that it takes longer, has more complications, and may need anesthesia, the percutaneous direct approach may have an increased bleeding risk.

Endovascular thrombectomy requires mechanical thrombus fragmentation by means of pigtail catheter, balloons, or dedicated devices (balloon thrombectomy, rheolytic thrombectomy, and suction thrombectomy) (Seedial et al. 2018).

The fragmented thrombus should be aspired using an aspiration catheter or a thrombectomy device (Uflacker 2003).

This method is mainly used in patients with contraindications to thrombolytic agents, but it may be associated with thrombolysis: the main reason of thrombolysis failure is the size of the thrombus and fragmentation facilitates the action of thrombolytic agents. In addition, thrombolysis dissolves the smaller thrombi not targetable by mechanical actions.

Percutaneous thrombectomy can also be performed through the TIPS by pulling a Fogarty catheter from the portal vein and into the IVC (Saad 2012).

Balloon angioplasty with or without stenting is meaningful in case of residual or refractory thrombosis of previous thrombolysis/thrombectomy because it can treat the underlying causes of PVT; it increases luminal gain, helps to decrease the risk of recurrent thrombosis, and removes any residual thrombus (Baccarani et al. 2001).

Moreover, initial angioplasty and/or stenting can help to restore the patency of the portal vein without prolonged thrombolysis and it reduces the risk of intrahepatic embolism that might occur during a thrombectomy or thrombolytic procedure (Adani et al. 2007).

The risks of this management are the suture dehiscence during angioplasty, the long-term patency rate being not excellent, and the interference of the stent with future surgical treatment.

To summarize, according to the time of onset of thrombosis, the management is different:

- Complete PVT within the first 48 h post-OLTx: surgical approach is mandatory (revision of the anastomosis or retransplantation).
- PVT at 48 h and within 30 days post-OLTx (early PVT): primarily endovascular approach, regardless of complete or partial PVT.
- Later than 30 days (late PVT): management depends on clinical course; if liver function

tests are normal, observation may be justified (there is the development of hepatoportal collaterals), while if PVT is symptomatic it should be treated with percutaneous or surgical approach. In particular, if liver function exams are stable and the intrahepatic portal vein is patent due to cavernous transformation, a conservative management is to be considered (Shibata et al. 2005).

PVT is associated with poor survival without treatment, whereas the success rate with different endovascular methods ranges from 68% to 100% with mortality and morbidity rates of 0% and 11%, respectively (Cavallari et al. 2001).

Durham et al. (1994) reported that technical success is probably around 55–70% and the mid- to long-term patency is probably as high as 50–60%.

5.4.2 Portal Vein Stenosis (PVS)

PVS is a rare vascular complication, with incidence rate reported to be less than 3% (Woo et al. 2007).

If treated late, it could lead to portal hypertension and its corollary signs, up to graft dysfunction.

In the past, surgical treatments have been considered the standard for PVS; recently percutaneous endovascular management has become established due to its minimal invasiveness and low complication and high success rates (Vignali et al. 2004).

Early PVS evolves into an early thrombosis if not treated promptly.

Most patients with PVS are asymptomatic; when symptomatic they may show signs of portal hypertension (gastroesophageal varices, ascites, and splenomegaly). Abnormal liver function tests are not constant.

Similar to PVT, the main risk factors of PVS are surgical technical complications: in children with split OLTx and living-donor liver graft there are a relatively short donor portal vein segment and usually a mismatched diameter between native portal vein segment and donors' one.

Other predisposing factors for portal complications are preexisting thrombosis and large portocaval collaterals.

Late PVS may have different etiologies and be secondary to fibrosis or intimal hyperplasia.

5.4.2.1 Diagnosis

Doppler US is the first examination to screen for VCs, but definite and objective criteria for PVS do not exist (Piardi et al. 2016).

The PVS criteria for diagnosis include narrowing portal caliber, abnormal velocities at the anastomotic site (PSV greater than 125 cm/s; anastomotic to preanastomotic segment PSV rate greater than 3:1), and scarcity of flow of the intrahepatic portal vein. If findings are suggestive of PVS, contrast-enhanced CT should be performed to confirm the diagnosis (more than 50% narrowing of the main portal venous diameter with or without poststenotic dilatation).

Contrast-enhanced CT or MRI angiography could also be used to detect a focal stenosis because it is hard to investigate by Doppler US.

When a patient is asymptomatic, indirect portography is an option to detect a PVS; percutaneous transhepatic portography is performed when the measurement of portal pressure gradients is required. Criteria for diagnosing PVS are stenosis more than 50% of the main portal venous diameter and a pressure gradient across the stenosis >5 mmHg.

Although a pre-post-anastomotic pressure gradient >5 mmHg has been considered diagnostic of PVS, there are no standard criteria to define a pressure gradient as significant. Park et al. showed that trans-stenotic pressure gradient does not appear to be directly related to the clinical and therapeutic results (Park et al. 2005).

If PVS is suspected, operative therapeutic management is necessary to prevent PVT and other complications. Some authors recommend the use of anticoagulant therapy for the prevention of recurrent PVT (Sanada et al. 2010).

5.4.2.2 Therapeutic Management and Prognosis

As in arterial VCs, classically and especially in very early portal VCs, surgical treatment (anastomotic revision or retransplantation) was usually performed, while nowadays interventional radiology is the first-line treatment for PVS following OLTx.

The approach can be transhepatic or transjugular, and unlike in PVT the most used is the first one (Glanemann et al. 2001).

In case of asymptomatic patients with PVS diagnosis and normal hepatic function test, management may be conservative and an appropriate follow-up is normally sufficient (Kaneko et al. 2003).

Percutaneous treatment includes balloon angioplasty with or without stent placement, or primary stent placement (Ko et al. 2007).

Technical success of the procedure was defined as <30% residual stenosis at portography with the absence of varices or collateral circulation (Park et al. 2005).

Shibata et al. (2005) reported that a single-balloon dilatation was sufficient to maintain portal vein patency with relative low recurrence rate (28.6%); similar results have been experienced by Park and colleagues.

Stents have usually been used to treat recurrent and elastic portal venous stenosis following balloon angioplasty. Majority early PVS is secondary to technical factors (tight suture line, discrepancy of the PV size) that does not benefit from balloon angioplasty alone.

Ko et al. (2007) performed primary stent placement rather than balloon angioplasty with positive technical and clinical outcome in almost 78% of patients.

Wei et al. (2009) performed first balloon angioplasty and then placed a balloon-expandable metallic stent in order to reduce the incidence "jump forward" of the stent (the most common displacement during stent deployment), achieving promising results although PVT or stent-edge stenosis may occur.

It seems reasonable that angioplasty with stenting can restore the normal portal flow once and for all, reducing the number of procedure-related complications, especially in PVS with fibrosis or intimal hyperplasia etiology (most late PVS).

5.5 Caval Complications

Hepatic blood outflow obstruction following OLTx is mainly related to VCs in caval anastomosis site, i.e., kinking, stenosis, or thrombosis of inferior vena cava or hepatic veins.

These VCs are relatively uncommon, with a reported incidence of less than 2% (Zhang et al. 2017).

Hepatic vein stenosis is more likely to occur after living-related transplants because the preservation of the recipient IVC with the piggyback technique has been associated with an increased risk of thrombosis or stenosis.

Clinical course of hepatic vein occlusion may vary from mildly abnormal liver function tests to an acute Budd-Chiari syndrome with abdominal pain, ascites, and hepatomegaly, or from lower limb edema and pericardial and pleural effusion to hypotension leading to allograft loss and multiorgan failure.

Almost 20% of patients are asymptomatic because chronic hepatic venous obstruction is associated with intrahepatic and portosystemic collateral vessels.

Usually, technical factors lead to venous obstruction in the early postoperative period, whereas the delayed presentation may be related to intimal hyperplasia, perivascular fibrosis, or extrinsic caval compression (Darcy 2007).

5.5.1 Diagnosis

Diagnosis should be achieved by Doppler US, contrast-enhanced CT, and RM, and finally, if findings are suggestive of venous outflow impairment, by cavography.

Although Doppler US is useful, venography and pressure measurements are still considered to be the gold standard.

Usually the gradient across the hepatic venous anastomosis is assessed to prove the diagnosis: a gradient higher than 10 mmHg is one commonly used threshold, but a gradient ranging from 3 to 20 mmHg has been considered to be the threshold of abnormality in different studies.

For this reason, stenoses have to be validated considering symptoms and response to treatments.

5.5.2 Therapeutic Management and Prognosis

Modified piggyback consists of a complete resection of the recipient inferior caval vein and interposition of the donor intrahepatic part of the vena cava with two end-to-end anastomoses; it is reported a three-vein technique for anastomosis with a low rate of these VCs.

Except for severe allograft dysfunction and multiorgan failure requiring retransplantation, percutaneous radiological intervention is the first-line treatment for liver blood outflow VCs in order to attempt to rescue the outflow patency, reserving surgery for a lower number of cases.

Endovascular management can be performed by transjugular approach or percutaneous transhepatic access.

Technical success is defined as morphologic improvement or as elimination or significant reduction of the trans-stenotic pressure gradient; venous outflow VCs are often treated with 100% success rate (Wang et al. 2005).

Thrombolysis has been described to treat anastomotic stenosis with superimposed thrombosis (Borsa et al. 1999). Mechanical thrombolytic devices may also be used to avoid bleeding.

Balloon angioplasty can restore anastomotic patency in almost 100% of cases, but the recurrence rate is high; however it is possible to repeat balloon dilatations (Cheng et al. 2005).

PTA associated with stent placement seems to have a higher rate of success than PTA alone, ranging from 73% to 100% in the literature (Ko et al. 2002).

While thrombolysis and angioplasty may cause anastomotic bleeding, stent migration is an infrequent but reported complication, not only during the procedure but also later, related to changes in the size of the IVC.

During PTA, a close monitoring is required since prolonged balloon inflation reduces blood return to the heart.

Considering the high incidence of restenosis, stenting may be preferable in adults, while in pediatric patients stenting may not be the best option: considering the potential growth of children repeated PTA is probably a better strategy.

References

Abbasoglu O, Levy MF, Vodapally MS, Goldstein RM, Husberg BS, Gonwa TA, Klintmalm GB (1997) Hepatic artery stenosis after liver transplantation—incidence, presentation, treatment, and long-term outcome. Transplantation 63:250–255

Abraldes JG, Tarantino I, Turnes J et al (2003) Hemodynamic response to pharmacological treatment of portal hypertension and long-term prognosis of cirrhosis. Hepatology 37:902–908

Abraldes JG, Tandon P, Yap J (2014) The adult survivor with variceal bleeding. Clin Liver Dis 4(4):89–92

Adani GL, Baccarani U, Risaliti A (2007) Percutaneous transhepatic portography for the treatment of early portal vein thrombosis after surgery. Cardiovasc Intervent Radiol 30:1222–1226

Aussilhou B, Lesurtel M, Sauvanet A, Farges O, Dokmak S, Goasguen N, Silbert A, Vilgrain V, Belghiti J (2008) Right portal vein ligation is as efficient as portal vein embolization to induce hypertrophy of the left liver remnant. J Gastrointest Surg 12:297–303

Baccarani U, Gasparini D, Risaliti A, Vianello V, Adani GL, Sainz M, Sponza M, Bresadola F (2001) Percutaneous mechanical fragmentation and stent placement for the treatment of early posttransplantation portal vein thrombosis. Transplantation 72:1572–1582

Bekker J, Ploem S, de Jong KP (2009) Early hepatic artery thrombosis after liver transplantation: a systematic review of the incidence, outcome and risk factors. Am J Transplant 9:746–757

Beppu K, Inokuchi K, Koyanagi N, Nakayama S, Sakata H, Kitano S, Kobayashi M (1981) Prediction of variceal hemorrhage by esophageal endoscopy. Gastrointest Endosc 27(4):213–218

Berzigotti A, Seijo S, Reverter E et al (2013) Assessing portal hypertension in liver diseases. Expert Rev Gastroenterol Hepatol 7(2):141–155

Borsa JJ, Daly CP, Fontaine AB et al (1999) Treatment of inferior vena cava anastomotic stenoses with the Wallstent endoprosthesis after orthotopic liver transplantation. J Vasc Interv Radiol 10(1):17–22

Bosch J, Mastai R, Kravetz D et al (1986) Hemodynamic evaluation of patients with portal hypertension. Semin Liver Dis 6(4):309–317

Bosch J, Garcia-Pagan JC, Berzigotti A et al (2006) Measurement of portal pressure and its role in the management of chronic liver disease. Semin Liver Dis 26:348–362

Bosch J, Abraldes JG, Berzigotti A (2009) The clinical use of HVPG measurements in chronic liver disease. Nat Rev Gastroenterol Hepatol 6(10):573–582

Broering DC, Hillert C, Krupski G et al (2002) Portal vein embolization vs. portal vein ligation for induction of hypertrophy of the future liver remnant. J Gastrointest Surg 6:905–913

Brouquet A, Abdalla E, Kopetz S, Garrett C, Overman M, Eng C et al (2011) High survival rate after two-stage resection of advanced colorectal liver metastases: response-based selection and complete resection define outcome. J Clin Oncol 29(8):1083–1090

Campagna F, Montagnese S, Ridola L, Senzolo M, Schiff S, De Rui M et al (2017) The animal naming test: an easy tool for the assessment of hepatic encephalopathy: Campagna et al. Hepatology 66:198–208

Cavallari A, Vivarelli M, Bellusci R, Jovine E, Mazziotti A, Rossi C (2001) Treatment of vascular complications following liver transplantation: multidisciplinary approach. Hepato-Gastroenterology 48:179–183

Chamarthy MR, Anderson ME, Pillai AK, Kalva SP (2016) Thrombolysis and transjugular intrahepatic portosystemic shunt creation for acute and subacute portal vein thrombosis. Tech Vasc Interv Radiol 19:42–51

Chana A, James M, Veale P (2016) Anaesthesia for transjugular intrahepatic portosystemic shunt insertion. BJA Educ 16:405–409

Chen GH, Wang GY, Yang Y, Li H, Lu MQ, Cai CJ, Wang GS, Xu C, Yi SH, Zhang JF, Fu BS (2009) Single-center experience of therapeutic management of hepatic artery stenosis after orthotopic liver transplantation. Report of 20 cases. Eur Surg Res 42:21–27

Chen J, Weinstein J, Black S, Spain J, Brady PS, Dowell JD (2014) Surgical and endovascular treatment of hepatic arterial complications following liver transplant. Clin Transpl 28:1305–1312

Cheng YF, Huang TL, Lee TY, Chen TY, Chen CL (1996) Variation of the intrahepatic portal vein; angiographic demonstration and application in living-related hepatic transplantation. Transplant Proc 28:1667–1668

Cheng YF, Chen CL, Huang TL et al (2005) Angioplasty treatment of hepatic vein stenosis in pediatric liver transplants: long-term results. Transpl Int 18:556–561

Colapinto RF, Stronell RD, Gildiner M, Ritchie AC, Langer B, Taylor BR, Blendis LM (1983) Formation of intrahepatic portosystemic shunts using a balloon dilatation catheter: preliminary clinical experience. AJR Am J Roentgenol 140:709–714

Copelan A, Kapoor B, Sands M (2014) Transjugular intrahepatic portosystemic shunt: indications, contraindications, and patient work-up. Semin Interv Radiol 31:235–242

D'Amico G, Garcia-Tsao G (2001) Diagnosis of portal hypertension. How and when? In: de Franchis R (ed) Portal hypertension. In: Proceedings of the third Baveno international consensus workshop on definitions, methodology and therapeutic strategies. Blackwell Science, Oxford, UK, pp 36–64

Darcy M (2007) Management of venous outflow complications after liver transplantation. Tech Vas Intervent Radiol 10(3):240–245

Darcy M (2012) Evaluation and management of transjugular intrahepatic portosystemic shunts. Am J Roentgenol 199:730–736

Dariushnia SR, Haskal ZJ, Midia M, Martin LG, Walker TG, Kalva SP et al (2016) Quality improvement guidelines for transjugular intrahepatic portosystemic shunts. J Vasc Interv Radiol 27:1–7

De Franchis R (2010) Baveno V faculty: revising consensus in portal hypertension: report of the Baveno V consensus workshop on methodology of diagnosis and therapy in portal hypertension. J Hepatol 53:762–768

De Franchis R (2015) Expanding consensus in portal hypertension Report of the Baveno VI Consensus Workshop: stratifying risk and individualizing care for portal hypertension. J Hepatol 63:743–752

Deltenre P, Trépo E, Rudler M, Monescillo A, Fraga M, Denys A et al (2015) Early transjugular intrahepatic portosystemic shunt in cirrhotic patients with acute variceal bleeding: a systematic review and meta-analysis of controlled trials. Eur J Gastroenterol Hepatol 27:e1–e9

Denys A, Bize P, Demartines N, Deschamps F, De Baere T (2010) Quality improvement for portal vein embolization. Cardiovasc Intervent Radiol 33(3):452–456

Dhanasekaran R, West JK, Gonzales PC, Subramanian R, Parekh S, Spivey JR et al (2010) Transjugular intrahepatic portosystemic shunt for symptomatic refractory hepatic hydrothorax in patients with cirrhosis. Am J Gastroenterol 105:635–641

Dodd GD III, Memel DS, Zajko AB, Baron RL, Santaguida LA (1994) Hepatic artery stenosis and thrombosis in transplant recipients: Doppler diagnosis with resistive index and systolic acceleration time. Radiology 192(3):657–661

Durham JD, LaBerge JM, Altman S, Kam I, Everson GT, Gordon RL, Kumpe DA (1994) Portal vein thrombolysis and closure of competitive shunts following liver transplantation. J Vasc Interv Radiol 5:611–615; discussion 616–618

Fagiuoli S, Bruno R, Debernardi Venon W, Schepis F, Vizzutti F et al (2017) Consensus conference on TIPS management: techniques, indications, contraindications. Dig Liver Dis 49:121–137

Fanelli F, Salvatori FM, Corona M, Bruni A, Pucci A, Boatta E et al (2006) Stent graft in TIPS: technical and procedural aspects. Radiol Med (Torino) 111:709–723

Farsad K, Kolbeck KJ (2014) Clinical and radiologic evaluation of patients before TIPS creation. Am J Roentgenol 203:739–745

Feldstein VA, Patel MD, LaBerge JM (1996) Transjugular intrahepatic portosystemic shunts: accuracy of Doppler US in determination of patency and detection of stenoses. Radiology 201:141–147

Ferral H, Gomez-Reyes E, Fimmel CJ (2016) Post-transjugular intrahepatic portosystemic shunt follow-up and management in the VIATORR era. Tech Vasc Interv Radiol 19:82–88

Feu F, Garcia-Pagan JC, Bosch J et al (1995) Relation between portal pressure response to pharmacotherapy and risk of recurrent variceal hemorrhage in patients with cirrhosis. Lancet 346:1056–1059

Figueras J, Busquets J, Diminguez J et al (1995) Intra-arterial thrombosis in the treatment of acute hepatic artery thrombosis after liver transplantation. Transplantation 59:1356

Fistouris J, Herlenius G, Beackman L et al (2006) Pseudoaneurysm of the hepatic artery following liver transplantation. Transplant Proc 38:2679

Forner A, Bruix J (2009) East meets the west: portal pressure predicts outcome of surgical resection for hepatocellular carcinoma. Nat Clin Pract Gastroenterol Hepatol 6:14–15

Fouzas I, Sklavos A, Bismpa K, Paxiadakis I, Antoniadis N, Giakoustidis D, Katsiki E, Tatsou N, Mouloudi E, Karapanagiotou A, Tsitlakidis A, Karakatsanis A, Patsiaoura K, Petridis A, Gakis D, Imvrios D, Papanikolaou V (2012) Hepatic artery thrombosis after orthotopic liver transplantation: 3 patients with collateral formation and conservative treatment. Transplant Proc 44:2741–2744

Frongillo F, Grossi U, Lirosi MC, Nure E, Sganga G, Avolio AW, Inchingolo R, Di Stasi C, Rinaldi P, Agnes S (2013) Incidence, management, and results of hepatic artery stenosis after liver transplantation in the era of donor to recipient match. Transplant Proc 45:2722–2725

Gaba RC, Khiatani VL, Knuttinen MG, Omene BO, Carrillo TC, Bui JT, Owens CA (2011) Comprehensive review of TIPS technical complications and how to avoid them. Am J Roentgenol 196:675–685

Gandini R, Konda D, Toti L, Abrignani S, Merolla S, Tisone G, Floris R (2016) Endovascular mechanical thromboaspiration of right hepatic arterial thrombosis after liver transplantation. Cardio Vascular Intervent Radiol 40(4):621–624

Garcia-Tsao G (2005) Transjugular intrahepatic portosystemic shunt in the management of refractory ascites. Semin Interv Radiol 22:278–286

Garcia Tsao G, Bosch J (2010) Management of varices and variceal hemorrhage in cirrhosis. New Engl J Med 362(9):823–832

Garcia-Tsao G, Groszmann RJ, Fisher RL et al (1985) Portal pressure, presence of gastroesophageal varices and variceal bleeding. Hepatology 5:419–424

Garcia Tsao G, Sanyal AJ, Grace ND, Carey W (2007) Prevention and management of gastroesophageal varices and variceal hemorrhage in cirrhosis. Hepatology 46:922–938

Girometti R, Como G, Bazzocchi M, Zuiani C (2014) Post-operative imaging in liver transplantation: state-of-the-art and future perspectives. World J Gastroenterol 20(20):6180–6200

Glanemann M, Settmacher U, Langrehr JM, Kling N, Hidajat N, Stange B, Staffa G, Bechstein WO, Neuhaus P (2001) Portal vein angioplasty using a transjugular, intrahepatic approach for treatment of extrahepatic portal vein stenosis after liver transplantation. Transpl Int 14:48–51

Gluud C, Henriksen JH, Nielsen G (1988) Prognostic indicators in alcoholic cirrhotic men. Hepatology 8:222–227

Goldsmith LE, Wiebke K, Seal J, Brinster C, Smith TA, Bazan HA, Sternbergh WC (2017) Complications after endovascular treatment of hepatic artery stenosis after liver transplantation. J Vasc Surg 66(5):1488–1496

Groszmann RJ, Wongcharatrawee S (2004) The hepatic venous pressure gradient: anything worth doing should be done right. Hepatology 39:280–282

Groszmann RJ, Glickman M, Blei AT et al (1979) Wedged and free hepatic venous pressure measured with a balloon catheter. Gastroenterology 76:253–258

Groszmann RJ, Bosch J, Grace ND et al (1990) Hemodynamic events in a prospective randomized trial of propranolol versus placebo in the prevention of a first variceal hemorrhage. Gastroenterology 99:1401–1407

Groszmann RJ, Garcia-Tsao G, Makuch R et al (2003) Multicenter randomized placebo-controlled trial of non-selective b-blockers in the prevention of the complications of portal hypertension: final results and identification of a predictive factor. Hepatology 38:206

Groszmann RJ, Garcia-Tsao G, Bosch J et al (2005) Beta-blockers to prevent gastroesophageal varices in patients with cirrhosis. N Engl J Med 353:2254–2261

Gunsar F, Rolando N, Pastacaldi S, Patch D, Raimondo ML, Davidson B, Rolles K, Burroughs AK (2003) Late hepatic artery thrombosis after orthotopic liver transplantation. Liver Transpl 9(6):605–611

Hallion L, Francois-Frank CA (1896) Recherches experimentales executees a l'aide d'um novel appareil volumetrique sur l'innervation vaso-motrice de l'intestin. Arch Physiol Norm Pathol 8:493–508

Hoekstra LT, Van Lienden KP et al (2012) Tumor progression after preoperative portal vein embolization. Ann Surg 256(5):812–817

Hom BK, Shrestha R, Palmer SL, Katz MD, Selby RR, Asatryan Z, Wells JK, Grant EG (2006) Prospective evaluation of vascular complications after liver transplantation: comparison of conventional and microbubble contrast-enhanced US. Radiology 241:267–274

Huct PM, Pomier-Layrargues G (2004) The hepatic venous pressure gradient: "remixed and revisited". Hepatology 39(2):295–298

Jung JW, Hwang S, Namgoong JM, Yoon SY, Park CS, Park YH, Lee HJ, Park HW, Park GC, Jung DH, Song GW, Ha TY, Ahn CS, Kim KH, Moon DB, Ko GY, Sung KB, Lee SG (2012) Incidence and management of postoperative abdominal bleeding after liver transplantation. Transplant Proc 44:765–768

Kaneko J, Sugawara Y, Ohkubo T, Matsui Y, Kokudo N, Makuuchi M (2003) Successful conservative therapy for portal vein thrombosis after living donor liver transplantation. Abdom Imaging 28:58–59

Kanterman RY, Darcy MD, Middleton WD, Sterling KM, Teefey SA, Pilgram TK (1997) Doppler sonography findings associated with transjugular intrahepatic portosystemic shunt malfunction. Am J Roentgenol 168:467–472

Keiding S, Vilstrup H (2002) Intrahepatic heterogeneity of hepatic venous pressure gradient in human cirrhosis. Scand J Gastroenterol 37:960–964

Keller FS, Farsad K, Rösch J (2016) The transjugular intrahepatic portosystemic shunt: technique and instruments. Tech Vasc Interv Radiol 19:2–9

Kim YD (2014) Management of acute variceal bleeding. Clin Endosc 47:308–314

Kim JH, Ko GY, Yoon HK et al (2004) Causes of arterial bleeding after living donor liver transplantation and the results of transcatheter arterial embolization. Korean J Radiol 5:164

Ko GY, Sung KB, Yoon HK et al (2002) Endovascular treatment of hepatic venous outflow obstruction after living-donor liver transplantation. J Vasc Interv Radiol 13:591–599

Ko GY, Sung KB, Yoon HK, Lee S (2007) Early posttransplantation portal vein stenosis following living donor liver transplantation: percutaneous transhepatic primary stent placement. Liver Transpl 13:530–536

Koo BY, Yu HC, So MC, Jin GY, Kwak HS, Cho BH (2008) Endovascular management of early portal vein thrombosis caused by coronary vein steal after liver transplantation and its outcome. Clin Transpl 22:668–671

Krajina A, Hulek P, Fejfar T, Valek V (2012) Quality improvement guidelines for transjugular intrahepatic portosystemic shunt (TIPS). Cardiovasc Intervent Radiol 35:1295–1300

Kumar A, Sharma P, Sarin SK (2008) Hepatic venous pressure gradient measurement: time to learn! Indian J Gastroenterol 27:74–80

Kyoden Y, Tamura S, Sugawara Y, Matsui Y, Togashi J, Kaneko J, Kokudo N, Makuuchi M (2008) Portal vein complications after adult-to-adult living donor liver transplantation. Transpl Int 21:1136–1144

Lee SJ, Kim KW, Kim SY, Park YS, Lee J, Kim HJ, Lee JS, Song GW, Hwang S, Lee SG (2013) Contrast-enhanced sonography for screening of vascular complication in recipients following living donor liver transplantation. J Clin Ultrasound 41:305–312

Liu H, Zhu S (2009) Present status and future perspectives of preoperative portal vein embolization. Am J Surg 197:686–690

Llovet JM, Fuster J, Bruix J (1999) Intention-to-treat analysis of surgical treatment for early hepatocellular carcinoma: resection versus transplantation. Hepatology 30:1434–1440

Lombardo S, Espejo JJ, Pérez-Montilla ME, Zurera LJ, Gonzalez-Galilea A (2018) The keys for successful TIPS in patients with portal vein thrombosis and cavernous transformation. Australas Radiol 60:94–104

Madoff DC, Marshall EH et al (2002) Transhepatic portal vein embolization: anatomy, indications, and technical considerations. Radiographics 22(5):1063–1076

Madoff DC, Wallace MJ, Ahrar K, Saxon RR (2004) TIPS-related hepatic encephalopathy: management options with novel endovascular techniques. Radiographics 24:21–36

Maharaj B, Maharaj RJ, Leary WP et al (1986) Sampling variability and its influence on the diagnostic yield of percutaneous needle biopsy of the liver. Lancet 1:523–525

Makuuchi M, Thai BL et al (1990) Preoperative portal embolization to increase safety of major hepatectomy for hilar bile duct carcinoma: a preliminary report. Surgery 107(5):521–527

Martínez-Pallí G, Drake BB, García-Pagán J-C, Barberà J-A, Arguedas MR, Rodriguez-Roisin R et al (2005) Effect of transjugular intrahepatic portosystemic shunt on pulmonary gas exchange in patients with portal hypertension and hepatopulmonary syndrome. World J Gastroenterol 11:6858–6862

Meek JC, McDougal Jonathan S, Borja-Cacho D, Meek ME (2018) Use of a mechanical thrombectomy device to treat early hepatic artery thrombosis after orthotopic liver transplant. Radiol Case Rep 13(2):522–526

Merkel C, Bolognesi M, Bellon S et al (1992) Prognostic usefulness of hepatic vein catheterization in patients with cirrhosis and esophageal varices. Gastroenterology 102:973–979

Micol C, Marsot J, Boublay N, Pilleul F, Berthezene Y, Rode A (2012) Contrast-enhanced ultrasound: a new method for TIPS follow-up. Abdom Imaging 37:252–260

Miraglia R, Maruzzelli L, Caruso S, Milazzo M, Marrone G, Mamone G, Carollo V, Gruttadauria S, Luca A, Gridelli B (2009) Interventional radiology procedures in adult patients who underwent liver transplantation. World J Gastroenterol 15:684–693

Moore KP, Aithal GP (2006) Guidelines on the management of ascites in cirrhosis. Gut 55:vi1–vi12

Murata S, Mizuno S, Kato H, Tanemura A, Kuriyama N, Azumi Y, Kishiwada M, Usui M, Sakurai H, Fujimori M, Yamanaka T, Nakatsuka A, Yamakado K, Isaji S (2016) Technical feasibility and clinical outcomes of interventional endovascular treatment for hepatic artery thrombosis after living-donor liver transplantation. Transplant Proc 48:1142–1148

Myers JD, Taylor WJ (1951) An estimation of portal venous pressure by occlusive catheterization of a hepatic venule. J Clin Invest 30:662–663

Narita M, Oussoultzoglou E et al (2011) Two-stage hepatectomy for multiple bilobar colorectal liver metastases. Br J Surg 98(10):1463–1475

Narula N, Aloia TA (2017) Portal vein embolization in extended liver resection. Langenbeck's Arch Surg 402(5):727–735

Nikeghbalian S, Kazemi K, Davari HR, Salahi H, Bahador A, Jalaeian H, Khosravi MB, Ghaffari S, Lahsaee M, Alizadeh M, Rasekhi AR, Nejatollahi SM, Malek-Hosseini SA (2007) Early hepatic artery thrombosis after liver transplantation: diagnosis and treatment. Transplant Proc 39(4):1195–1196

Nüssler N, Settmacher U, Haase R, Stange B, Heise M, Neuhaus P (2003) Diagnosis and treatment of arterial steal syndromes in liver transplant recipients. Liver Transpl 9:596–602

Orlandini M, Feier FH, Jaeger B, Kieling C, Vieira SG, Zanotelli ML (2014) Frequency of and factors associated with vascular complications after pediatric liver transplantation. J Pediatr 90:169–175

Panaro F, Gallix B, Bouyabrine H, Ramos J, Addeo P, Testa G, Carabalona JP, Pageaux G, Domergue J,

Navarro F (2011) Liver transplantation and spontaneous neovascularization after arterial thrombosis: "the neovascularized liver". Transpl Int 24:949–957

Panaro F, Giannone F, Riviere B, Sgarbura O, Cusumano C, Deshayes E, Navarro F, Guiu B, Quenet F (2019) Perioperative impact of liver venous deprivation compared with portal venous embolization in patients undergoing right hepatectomy: preliminary results from the pioneer center. Hepatobiliary Surg Nutr 8(4):329–337

Pandanaboyana S, Bell R et al (2015) A systematic review and meta-analysis of portal vein ligation versus portal vein embolization for elective liver resection. Surgery 157(4):690–698

Pareja E, Cortes M, Navarro R et al (2010) Vascular complications after orthotopic liver transplantation: hepatic artery thrombosis. Transplant Proc 42:2970–2972

Park KB, Choo SW, Do YS, Shin SW, Cho SG, Choo IW (2005) Percutaneous angioplasty of portal vein stenosis that complicates liver transplantation: the mid-term therapeutic results. Korean J Radiol 6: 161–166

Pawlak J, Grodzicki M, Leowska E, Małkowski P, Michałowicz B, Nyckowski P, Rowiński O, Pacho R, Zieniewicz K, Andrzejewska M, Ołdakowska U, Grzelak I, Patkowski W, Alsharabi A, Remiszewski P, Dudek K, Krawczyk M (2003) Vascular complications after liver transplantation. Transplant Proc 35:2313–2315

Perello A, Escorsell A, Bru C et al (1999) Wedged hepatic venous pressure adequately reflects portal pressure in hepatitis C virus-related cirrhosis. Hepatology 30:1393–1397

Pérez-Saborido B, Pacheco-Sánchez D, Barrera-Rebollo A, Asensio-Díaz E, Pinto-Fuentes P, Sarmentero-Prieto JC, Rodríguez-Vielba P, Martínez-Díaz R, Gonzalo-Martín M, Rodríguez M, Calero Aguilar H, Pintado-Garrido R, García-Pajares F, Anta-Román A (2011) Incidence, management, and results of vascular complications after liver transplantation. Transplant Proc 43:749–750

Piardi T, Lhuaire M, Bruno O, Memeo R, Pessaux P, Kianmanesh R, Sommacale D (2016) Vascular complications following liver transplantation: a literature review of advances in 2015. World J Hepatol 8(1):36–57

Piscaglia F, Bolondi L (2006) The safety of Sonovue® in abdominal applications: retrospective analysis of 23188 investigations. Ultrasound Med Biol 32:1369–1375

Rector WG (1986) Portal hypertension: a permissive factor only in the development of ascites and variceal bleeding. Liver 6:221–226

Reiberger T, Püspök A, Schoder M, Baumann-Durchschein F, Bucsics T, Datz C et al (2017) Austrian consensus guidelines on the management and treatment of portal hypertension (Billroth III). Wien Klin Wochenschr 129:135–158. https://doi.org/10.1007/s00508-017-1262

Richter GM, Palmaz JC, Noldge G, Rossle M, Siegerstetter V, Franke M, Wenz W (1989) The transjugular intrahepatic portosystemic stent-shunt. A new nonsurgical percutaneous method. Radiologe 29:406–411

Riggio O, Angeloni S, Salvatori FM, De Santis A, Cerini F, Farcomeni A et al (2008) Incidence, natural history, and risk factors of hepatic encephalopathy after transjugular intrahepatic portosystemic shunt with polytetrafluoroethylene-covered stent grafts. Am J Gastroenterol 103:2738–2746

Ripoll C, Groszmann RJ, Garcia-Tsao G et al (2007) Hepatic venous pressure gradient predicts clinical decompensation in patients with compensated cirrhosis. Gastroenterology 133:481–488

Ripoll C, Groszmann RJ, Garcia-Tsao G et al (2009) Hepatic venous pressure gradient predicts development of hepatocellular carcinoma independently of severity of cirrhosis. J Hepatol 50:923–928

Rodrigues SG, Maurer Martin H, Baumgartner I, De Gottardi A, Berzigotti A. (2017) Imaging and minimally invasive endovascular therapy in the management of portal vein thrombosis. Abdom Radiol.

Rösch J, Hanafee WN, Snow H (1969) Transjugular portal venography and radiologic portacaval shunt: an experimental study. Radiology 92:1112–1114

Rossle M, Gerbes AL (2010) TIPS for the treatment of refractory ascites, hepatorenal syndrome and hepatic hydrothorax: a critical update. Gut 59:988–1000

Runyon BA (2004) Management of adult patients with ascites due to cirrhosis. Hepatology 39:841–856

Ryu RK, Durham JD, Krysl J, Shrestha R, Shrestha R, Everson GT et al (1999) Role of TIPS as a bridge to hepatic transplantation in Budd-Chiari syndrome. J Vasc Interv Radiol 10:799–805

Saad WEA (2012) Liver transplant-related vascular disease. In: Dake M, Geshwind J-F, eds. Abrams angiography: interventional radiology 3rd ed.

Saad WEA (2014) The history and future of transjugular intrahepatic portosystemic shunt: food for thought. Semin Interv Radiol 31:258–261

Saad NEA, Saad WEA, Davies MG, Waldman DL, Fultz PJ, Rubens DJ (2005) Pseudoaneurysms and the role of minimally invasive techniques in their management. Radiographics 25:S173–S189

Saad WEA, Davies MG, Saad NEA, Westesson KE, Patel NC, Sahler LG, Lee DE, Kitanosono T, Sasson T, Waldman DL (2007) Catheter thrombolysis of thrombosed hepatic arteries in liver transplant recipients: predictors of success and role of thrombolysis. Vasc Endovasc Surg 41:19–26

Saad NEA, Darcy M, Saad WEA (2008) Portal anatomic variants relevant to transjugular intrahepatic portosystemic shunt. Tech Vasc Interv Radiol 11:203–207

Salerno F, Cammà C, Enea M, Rössle M, Wong F (2007) Transjugular intrahepatic portosystemic shunt for refractory ascites: a meta-analysis of individual patient data. Gastroenterology 133:825–834

Salerno F, Guevara M, Bernardi M, Moreau R, Wong F, Angeli P et al (2010) Refractory ascites: pathogenesis, definition and therapy of a severe complication in patients with cirrhosis. Liver Int 30:937–947

Sanada Y, Kawano Y, Mizuta K, Egami S, Hayashida M, Wakiya T, Fujiwara T, Sakuma Y, Hydo M, Nakata M, Yasuda Y, Kawarasaki H (2010) Strategy to prevent recurrent portal vein stenosis following interventional radiology in pediatric liver transplantation. Liver Transpl 16:332–339

Schepis F, Vizzutti F, Garcia-Tsao G, Marzocchi G, Rega L, De Maria N et al (2018) Under-dilated TIPS associate with efficacy and reduced encephalopathy in a prospective, non-randomized study of patients with cirrhosis. Clin Gastroenterol Hepatol 16(7):1153. e7–1162.e7

Schultz SR, LaBerge JM, Gordon RL, Warren RS (1994) Anatomy of the portal vein bifurcation: intra- versus extrahepatic location—implications for transjugular intrahepatic portosystemic shunts. J Vasc Interv Radiol 5:457–459

Seedial S, Mouli S, Desai K (2018) Acute portal vein thrombosis: current trends in medical and endovascular management. Semin Interv Radiol 35(3): 198–202

Shibata T, Itoh K, Kubo T, Maetani Y, Shibata T, Togashi K, Tanaka K (2005) Percutaneous transhepatic balloon dilation of portal venous stenosis in patients with living donor liver transplantation. Radiology 235:1078–1083

Simoneau E, Hassanain M et al (2015) Portal vein embolization and its effect on tumour progression for colorectal cancer liver metastases. Br J Surg 102(10):1240–1249

Sommacale D, Aoyagi T, Dondero F, Sibert A, Bruno O, Fteriche S, Francoz C, Durand F, Belghiti J (2013) Repeat endovascular treatment of recurring hepatic artery stenoses in orthotopic liver transplantation. Transpl Int 26:608–615

Stange BJ, Glanemann M, Nuessler NC, Settmacher U, Steinmuller T, Neuhaus P (2003) Hepatic artery thrombosis after adult liver transplantation. Liver Transpl 9:612–620

Steinlauf AF, Garcia-Tsao G, Zakko MF et al (1999) Low-dose midazolam sedation: an option for patients undergoing serial hepatic venous pressure measurements. Hepatology 29:1070–1073

Strauss RM, Boyer TD (1997) Hepatic hydrothorax. Semin Liver Dis 17:227–232

Sueyoshi E, Sakamoto I, Nakashima K, Minami K, Hayashi K (2005) Visceral and peripheral arterial pseudoaneurysms. AJR 185:741–749

Triantos C, Kalafateli M (2014) Endoscopic treatment of esophageal varices in patients with liver cirrhosis. World J Gastroenterol 20:13015–13026

Tsochatzis EA, Bosch J, Burroughs AK (2014) Liver cirrhosis. Lancet 383:1749–1761

Ueno T, Jones G, Martin A, Ikegami T, Sanchez EQ, Chinnakotla S, Randall HB, Levy MF, Goldstein RM, Klintmalm GB (2006) Clinical outcomes from hepatic

artery stenting in liver transplantation. Liver Transpl 12:422–427

Uflacker R (2003) Applications of percutaneous mechanical thrombectomy in transjugular intrahepatic portosystemic shunt and portal vein thrombosis. Tech Vasc Interv Radiol 6:59–69

Vaidya S, Dighe M, Kolokythas O et al (2007) Liver transplantation: vascular complications. Ultrasound Q 23:239

Vignali C, Cioni R, Petruzzi P, Cicorelli A, Bargellini I, Perri M, Urbani L, Filipponi F, Bartolozzi C (2004) Role of interventional radiology in the management of vascular complications after liver transplantation. Transplant Proc 36:552–554

Vignali C, Bargellini I, Grosso M, Passalacqua G, Maglione F, Pedrazzini F et al (2005) TIPS with expanded polytetrafluoroethylene-covered stent: results of an Italian multicenter study. Am J Roentgenol 185:472–480

Volpin E, Pessaux P, Sauvanet A, Sibert A, Kianmanesh R, Durand F, Belghiti J, Sommacale D (2014) Preservation of the arterial vascularisation after hepatic artery pseudoaneurysm following orthotopic liver transplantation: long-term results. Ann Transplant 19:346–352

Vorobioff J, Groszmann RJ, Picabea E et al (1996) Prognostic value of hepatic venous pressure measurement in alcoholic cirrhosis: a 10-year prospective study. Gastroenterology 111:701–709

Wachsberg RH, Bahramipour P, Sophocleous CT et al (2002) Hepatofugal flow in the portal venous system: pathophysiology, imaging findings, and diagnostic pitfalls. Radiographics 22:123–140

Wallace MJ, Madoff DC, Ahrar K, Warneke CL (2004) Transjugular intrahepatic portosystemic shunts: experience in the oncology setting. Cancer 101: 337–345

Wang SL, Sze DY, Busque S et al (2005) Treatment of hepatic venous outflow obstruction after piggyback liver transplantation. Radiology 236:352–359

Wei BJ, Zhai RY, Wang JF, Dai DK, Yu P (2009) Percutaneous portal venoplasty and stenting for anastomotic stenosis after liver transplantation. World J Gastroenterol 15:1880–1885

Wong F (2012) Management of ascites in cirrhosis. J Gastroenterol Hepatol 27:11–20

Woo DH, Laberge JM, Gordon RL, Wilson MW, Kerlan RK (2007) Management of portal venous complications after liver transplantation. Tech Vasc Interv Radiol 10:233–239

Yeom YK, Shin JH (2015) Complications of portal vein embolization: evaluation on cross sectional imaging. Korean J Radiol 16(5):1079–1085

Yerdel MA, Gunson B, Mirza D et al (2000) Portal vein thrombosis in adults undergoing liver transplantation: risk factors, screening, management, and outcome. Transplantation 69(9):1873–1881

Zhang ZY, Jin L, Chen G, Su TH, Zhu ZJ, Sun LY, Wang ZC, Xiao GW (2017) Balloon dilatation for treatment of hepatic venous outflow obstruction following pediatric liver transplantation. World J Gastroenterol 23(46):8227–8234

Zheng M, Chen Y, Bai J, Zeng Q, You J, Jin R et al (2008) Transjugular intrahepatic portosystemic shunt versus endoscopic therapy in the secondary prophylaxis of variceal rebleeding in cirrhotic patients: meta-analysis update. J Clin Gastroenterol 42:507–516

Zheng BW, Tan YY, Fu BS, Tong G, Wu T, Wu LL, Meng XC, Zheng RQ, Yi SH, Ren J (2017) Tardus parvus waveforms in Doppler ultrasonography for hepatic artery stenosis after liver transplantation: can a new cut-off value guide the next step? Abdom Radiol 43(7):1634–1641

Zhou J, Fan J, Wang JH, Wu ZQ, Qiu SJ, Shen YH, Shi YH, Huang XW, Wang Z, Tang ZY, Wang YQ (2005) Continuous transcatheter arterial thrombolysis for early hepatic artery thrombosis after liver transplantation. Transplant Proc 37:4426–4429

Zhu X, Tam MD, Pierce G et al (2011) Utility of the Amplatzer vascular plug in splenic artery embolization: a comparison study with conventional coil technique. Cardiovasc Intervent Radiol 34: 522–531

Žižka J, Eliáš P, Krajina A, Michl A, Lojík M, Ryška P et al (2000) Value of doppler sonography in revealing transjugular intrahepatic portosystemic shunt malfunction: a 5-year experience in 216 patients. Am J Roentgenol 175:141–148

Intrahepatic Biliary Tract Interventional Radiology

Alessandro Rago, Francesca Zavan, Sofia Moschi,
Paolo De Vincentis, Filippo Crimí,
and Emilio Quaia

Contents

A. Rago · F. Zavan · S. Moschi · P. De Vincentis
F. Crimí · E. Quaia (✉)
Radiology Unit, Department of Medicine - DIMED,
University of Padova, Padova, Italy
e-mail: emilio.quaia@unipd.it

© Springer Nature Switzerland AG 2021
E. Quaia (ed.), *Imaging of the Liver and Intra-hepatic Biliary Tract*,
Medical Radiology, Diagnostic Imaging, https://doi.org/10.1007/978-3-030-38983-3_9

Abstract

This chapter focuses on the technical aspects of diagnostic cholangiography and nonvascular interventional procedures on the liver, such as percutaneous transhepatic biliary drainage, biliary stenting, percutaneous transhepatic biliary stone removal, and percutaneous cholecystostomy.

Technique, indications, contraindications, and complications are discussed for each procedure.

1   Introduction

Interventional radiology of the biliary tract includes procedures well established since 1970s, when the first percutaneous transhepatic cholangiography was performed (Pomerantz 2009).

This technique became widespread over the years, thanks to technical advances, because it showed to be helpful, next to traditional surgery, in diagnosis and in treatment of biliary obstructions or leaks. Even with the subsequent spread of endoscopic techniques, percutaneous biliary interventions still have an important role, particularly in case of technical failure of endoscopy or in case of its impossibility for example due to patient's postsurgical altered anatomy.

These procedures include diagnostic cholangiography, biliary drainage and stent placement, cholecystostomy placement, and percutaneous management of biliary calculi.

To perform all these procedures fluoroscopy, ultrasound (US), computed tomography (CT), and magnetic resonance imaging (MRI) have to be used together both to study biliary tract and its pathologies and to guide interventional maneuvers.

Chiba needles, guidewires, drainages, catheters, balloon catheters, and different types of stents are currently used for biliary interventional radiology, but there are continuous improvements in design and materials of these tools that will hopefully lead to further developments in this field.

2   Percutaneous Transhepatic Cholangiography (PTC)

PTC is a diagnostic procedure that involves the placement of a needle into the peripheral biliary ducts under US and fluoroscopy guidance followed by contrast injection to delineate biliary anatomy and potential biliary disease (Saad et al. 2010).

2.1   Indications

Indications of PTC are listed in Table 1. Coagulopathy is a relative contraindication

Table 1 Percutaneous transhepatic cholangiography (Saad et al. 2010)

Percutaneous transhepatic cholangiography: indications
– Define the level of obstruction in patients with dilated bile ducts
– Evaluate for the presence of suspected bile duct stones
– Determine the etiology of cholangitis
– Evaluate the suspected bile duct inflammatory disorders
– Demonstrate the site of bile duct leak
– Determinate the etiology of transplanted hepatic graft dysfunction

to PTC; coagulation values should be corrected as necessary.

2.2 Technique

PTC is usually performed with sterile technique under US and fluoroscopy guidance. Lidocaine 2% is used for local anesthesia at the puncture site. Two approaches have been described: right-sided approach is intercostal and the needle is inserted the intercostal space anterior to the midaxillary line, in a 25-degree cranial direction. The left-sided approach is subxiphoid.

The correct needle position can be confirmed by contrast injection; if the position is correct the contrast material will slowly move away from the needle and fills the tubular structure.

If the contrast material does not move away from the needle, parenchymal extravasation must be suspected.

2.3 Success Rate

The overall success rate is 97.8% for dilated bile ducts and 70% for non-dilated ducts (Harbin et al. 1980).

2.4 Complications

Complications of PTC should be low. They include sepsis, cholangitis, bile leak, hemobilia, and pneumothorax (Ginat and Saad 2008).

3 Percutaneous Transhepatic Biliary Drainage (PTDB)

PTBD is an image-guided procedure used to access and study the biliary tree. It is performed with fluoroscopic assistance and the aid of US. This technique allows an external or internal drainage of the bile when the biliary route is obstructed or damaged, not permitting a correct flow of the fluid into the duodenum.

In this situation the main biochemical finding is hyperbilirubinemia (>3 g/dL) that clinically presents with jaundice and pruritus; it can be present as dilatation of the biliary system (Covey and Brown 2008).

Evaluation of the biliary system with US prior to percutaneous intervention is recommended (Fig. 1). When possible the positioning of an internal/external biliary drainage is always preferred that allows the physiological passage of the bile into the duodenum and at the same time

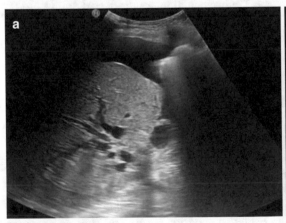 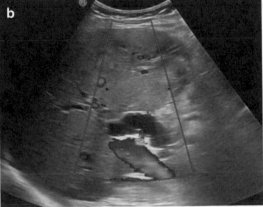

Fig. 1 (**a, b**) Ultrasound (US) in pre-procedural workup before percutaneous transhepatic biliary drainage (PTDB). (**a**) US longitudinal scan of the abdomen of a patient with dilatation of intrahepatic biliary ducts and ascites which represents a relative contraindication to PTDB. (**b**) US longitudinal scan of the abdomen shows a dilatation of the common bile duct. Color Doppler US exam may help in differentiating the biliary tree from the hepatic vessels

drains part of the fluid outward. Occasionally an external drainage catheter is required at the first attempt in the presence of significant biliary sepsis or when the site of obstruction cannot be crossed (Shawyer et al. 2013).

3.1 Indications

The indications include treatment of cholangitis, bile duct damage, and obstructive jaundice with dilatation of the biliary tree as a result of malignant or benign biliary stenosis (Garcarek et al. 2012). Endoscopic retrograde cholangiopancreatography (ERCP) is the preferred access route to the biliary tree. PTBD is considered when ERCP is unsuccessful or contraindicated (e.g., anatomic variation) or when it cannot offer a good palliation in terms of durability (Chandrashekhara et al. 2016) or even when biliary tract obstruction involves the intra-hepatic or proximal extra-hepatic biliary tract. Indications of PTBD are listed in Table 2.

Table 2 PTBD indications (from Chandrashekhara et al. 2016 modified)

Altered anatomy that prevents ERCP
Benign biliary obstruction
Cholelithiasis/choledocholithiasis
Bacterial cholangitis
Ischemic cholangitis
Sclerosing cholangitis
Postsurgical stricture of the common bile duct
Postsurgical stricture of the biliodigestive anastomosis
Malignant biliary obstruction
Palliative drainage of unresectable biliary tumor
Pancreatic neoplasm extrinsically compressing the distal bile duct (Asadi et al. 2016)
Metastases from nonbiliary cancers (Iwasaki et al. 1996)
Liver hilar lymphadenopathy
Hyperbilirubinemia that contraindicates initiation of chemotherapy
Access biliary system for further intraductal interventions (biopsy, stent placement, and transhepatic brachytherapy)
Bile leak
Iatrogenic (Jabłońska and Lampe 2009)
Post-traumatic

Table 3 PTBD contraindications (from Pomerantz 2009 modified)

Absolute
In case of emergency there are no absolute contraindications
Uncorrectable coagulopathy
Relative
INR >1.5
History of allergy to iodinated contrast agents
Platelet counts <50,000
Ascites (drainage prior to procedure is recommended)
Multiple hepatic cysts (Morgan and Adam 1998)

3.2 Contraindications

Contraindications of PTDB are classified in Table 3.

3.3 Materials

- Local anesthetic (5–10 mL of 1% lidocaine) and syringe
- Puncture fine needle 18–21 G
- Coaxial percutaneous access kit
- Guidewires: curved stiff hydrophilic wire (0.035 in.), super-stiff wire (long floppy tip)
- Catheters: dilators (at least 4–9 F), biliary manipulation catheter (Kessel and Robertson 2017 modified)
- Drains: pigtail internal/external drain 8–14 F
- Sutures or catheter-retention device

3.4 Procedure Preparations

The patient should be preferably fasting for at least 6 h prior to the procedure. It is important to explain the procedure and its possible complications to the patient, obtaining informed consent. Collect patient history and previous clinical data, including blood tests (especially INR, platelet counts, AST/ALT, bilirubin, and creatinine). Establish good i.v. access and start an adequate antibiotic coverage. For pain alleviation, i.v. analgesics can be administered. The review of the previous imaging studies of the liver and the biliary system allows the operator to determine

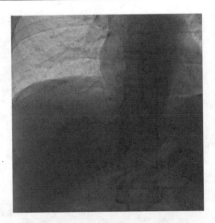

Fig. 2 A biliary brunch of the left hepatic lobe is cannulated through percutaneous ultrasound-guided access

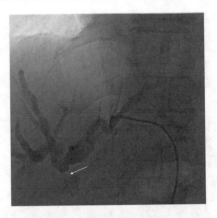

Fig. 3 Dilated and tortuous intrahepatic bile ducts that have narrow stenosis (arrow) downstream from the confluence of the main bile ducts

which main hepatic duct is primarily involved and to select the best target to access (Fig. 2).

Preprocedural abdominal US is fundamental to assess the state of the liver and of the biliary tree (evaluation of intrahepatic biliary tract diameter, site of obstruction and localization of primary or metastatic masses). Deep sedation might be required to place a biliary drainage "ex novo" (Tae-Hoon Kim 2006).

3.5 Techniques

The operator can choose to use the right (subcostal) or left ductal (subxiphoid) approach, although each technique has its strength and limitations.

The left approach is relatively easier and safer to perform, but performer's hand is more exposed to radiation.

The right approach allows the drainage of a greater number of hepatic segments and performer is less exposed to X-ray, but it is more painful for the patient and is more affected by respiration movements.

In case of cholangiocarcinoma involving the hilum, a bilateral access may be required to allow a correct drainage of both right and left biliary hemi-systems (Nimura et al. 2000).

When the suitable bile duct is targeted under US guidance, local anesthesia of the puncture site with 1% lidocaine is administered. An 18–21 G puncture fine needle is then introduced to access the targeted biliary duct.

It is recommended to guide the needle to a peripheral portion of the liver, avoiding central and hilar regions, due to lower risk of major vascular injury involving a branch of the portal vein or hepatic artery.

When the outflow of bile starts, a 0.035 in. hydrophilic guidewire is passed through the puncture needle with fluoroscopy assistance and subsequent dilatations of the entry point are performed for an eventual placement of a catheter sheath introducer. Deep sedation might be required since dilatation of the cutaneous entry point and adjacent Glisson's capsule can be very painful.

After demonstrating the site of obstruction/damage of the biliary tract with an intraprocedural cholangiography, a guidewire is used to cross the pathological duct and then to place a drainage pigtail catheter with its curled tip in the duodenum, beyond the ampulla.

A final cholangiography with contrast injection is necessary to verify the correct functioning of the PTBD (Figs. 3, 4, and 5).

3.6 Postprocedural Care

Postprocedural care includes daily saline irrigation of the tube, monitoring of bile volume drained, and determination of bilirubin and alkaline phosphatase blood levels. All patients should be closely monitored for any evidence of sepsis and/or hemorrhage (Pomerantz 2009).

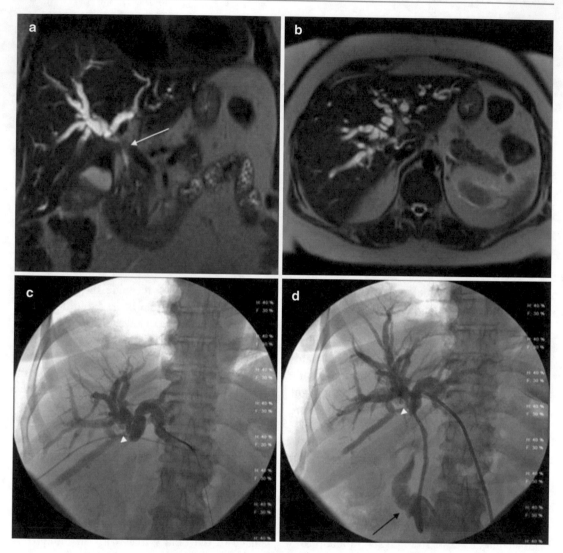

Fig. 4 (**a–d**) Magnetic resonance cholangiopancreatography (MRCP). Coronal (**a**) and axial (**b**) MRCP T2-HASTE MRI sequences of a patient with diffuse intrahepatic biliary dilatation due to a mass stenosing primary biliary confluence (white arrow). Cholangiography of the same patient before (**c**) and after (**d**) the insertion of a percutaneous transhepatic biliary drainage with its distal tip in the duodenum (black arrow). White arrowheads indicate the stenosis of the biliary ducts at the confluence

The external drainage is usually allowed to outflow in the drainage bag for about 24–48 h, and then the catheter is capped to direct the flow of the bile into the bowel.

3.7 Success Rate

Thanks to increased expertise and better instrumentation, observed technical success rate of PTBD is ~90–95%, with very few complications observed nowadays (Chandrashekhara et al. 2016).

3.8 Complications

Patients should be monitored carefully for 24 h after drainage for signs of bleeding or sepsis (Ferrucci et al. 1980). With proper technique, especially with peripheral bile duct puncture, serious bleeding complications can be avoided (Covey and Brown 2008). Because hepatic artery and portal vein branches run along the biliary tree in the liver (portal triad), it is possible that some blood could pass into the bile duct during the procedure, resulting in transient hemobilia.

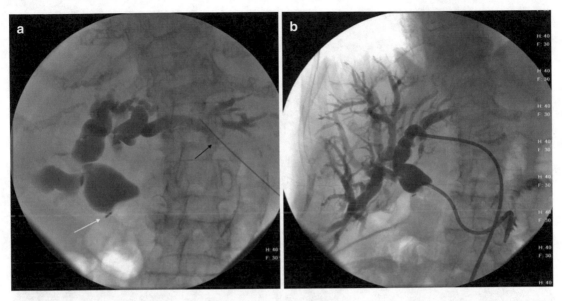

Fig. 5 (**a**, **b**) Cholangiography before (**a**) and after (**b**) the positioning of PTBD with left ductal (subxiphoid) approach (black arrow). The cholangiography demonstrates the obstruction of the common bile duct in biliodi-gestive anastomosis (white arrow). A final cholangiography with contrast injection is necessary to verify the correct functioning of the PTBD

These complications can be reduced with adequate antibiotic coverage and by keeping the biliary manipulation to minimum (Burke et al. 2003).

One of the most dangerous complications is hemorrhage caused by intraprocedural lesion of a main branch of the hepatic artery (Figs. 6 and 7) (Mueller et al. 1982). Complications can occur immediately after the procedure or in the following 24–48 h (Table 4).

4 Biliary Stenting

Biliary stenting is a well-known and established procedure since decades. Endoscopic and percutaneous approaches are both validated techniques that are chosen mostly based on the location of the pathology in the biliary tract and on postsurgical anatomy of upper gastrointestinal tract (Shawyer et al. 2013). Nevertheless, the percutaneous approach allows to reach precisely the biliary duct that needs to be treated (Li et al. 2016).

4.1 Indications and Stent Types

The main indications for biliary stent placement are the following:

- Treatment of benign biliary strictures, particularly the recurrent ones that are not responsive to bilioplasty, a procedure that consists of sequential (usually 1–3 sessions with interval of 2–3 weeks) prolonged balloon dilatations of the stenosis using balloon catheters (Ng et al. 2015; Shawyer et al. 2013). Benign biliary strictures can be consequent to inflammatory events, infective or autoimmune cholangitis, radiant therapy, ischemic events, or iatrogenic causes (such as postsurgery biliary duct injury or liver transplantation) (Fidelman 2015).
- Palliative treatment of malignant biliary strictures that generally have as its main causes cholangiocarcinomas, pancreatic tumors, liver carcinomas or metastasis, gallbladder tumors, lymphomas, and lymph node metastasis (Leng et al. 2014).

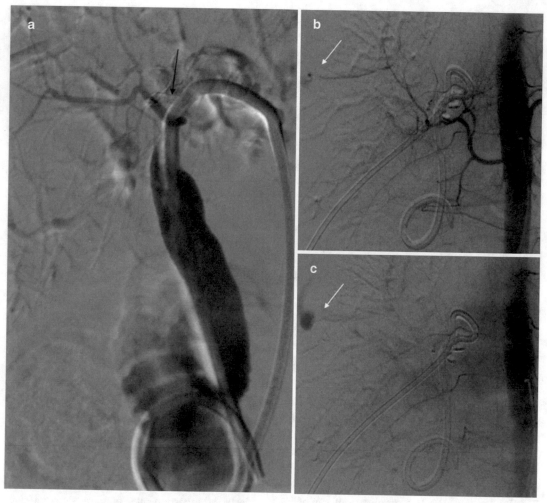

Fig. 6 (a–c) Postprocedural bleeding. (a) Cholangiogram shows a hepatic artery branch in communication with the biliary tree after positioning PTDB (black arrow). Celiac axis angiogram of another patient shows contrast extrava- sation of a distal branch of the hepatic artery (white arrows) in different phases (b), (c) as a complication of the insertion of a PTDB

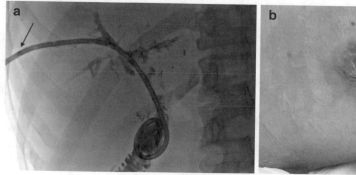
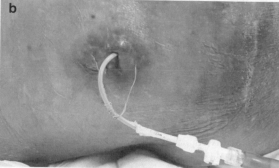

Fig. 7 (a, b) Catheter dislodgement. (a) Cholangiogram shows distal marker and some side holes of drainage cath- eter outside the biliary tree (black arrow). (b) Photograph of the same patience: the imbibition of the skin around the percutaneous access can lead to rupture of the sutures and dislodgement of the catheter

Table 4 Classification of PTBD complications (from Saad et al. 2010 modified)

	Immediate/periprocedural complications	Delayed complications
Minor	– Pain	– Pericatheter leak
Major	– Hemobilia – Pneumothorax – Sepsis/cholangitis – Subcapsular hematoma	– Hemorrhage – Hemobilia/pseudoaneurysm – Bile peritonitis – Dislodged catheter (Fig. 7) – Catheter occlusion by tumor ingrowth – Pancreatitis – Pleural effusion/empyema – Electrolyte depletion due to high-output external drainage

In fact a prolonged obstruction of biliary tract causes cholestasis that can lead to pruritus, jaundice, cholangitis, and hepatic dysfunction, greatly reducing the quality of life of patients (Li et al. 2016).

Moreover re-establishing a good liver function through an effective drainage of the biliary tract is fundamental for chemotherapy administration in oncologic patients (Furuse et al. 2008).

For all these reasons, percutaneous or endoscopic biliary stenting is considered fundamental for treatment of both benign and malignant biliary strictures.

A more recent indication for biliary stenting, thanks to the development of retrievable stents, is represented by the treatment of biliary leaks. Usage of retrievable stents to treat bile leakage has shown to be effective (Páramo et al. 2017), because stent placement into the damaged biliary duct, giving a least resistance way for bile flow, consents biliary duct healing (Ng et al. 2015).

For all these indications, different kinds of biliary stents are available:

– Plastic stents
– Metal stents, uncovered and covered
– Biodegradable stents

4.1.1 Plastic Stents

Plastic stents are devices made of radiopaque polyethylene and can be placed both endoscopically and percutaneously (Mauro et al. 2008) (Fig. 8). In the former case the size of the stent can be up to 12 Fr, according to the size of the endoscope's channel; in the latter case the stent size reaches 14 Fr, which however results in a large intrahepatic tract that can cause discomfort for the patient and more complications (Tsetis et al. 2016).

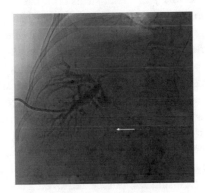

Fig. 8 Plastic stent (arrow) in the common bile duct seen at fluoroscopy. It is possible to see that it is occluded as, performing the cholangiography, it is not opacified by contrast material

Anyhow, despite the large percutaneous hepatic tract they need, their lumen is relatively small and thus they are more subject to an early occlusion. Moreover they showed to be more prone to migration (15% of incidence).

Nevertheless these stents have the advantage of being less expensive than other types and can be retrieved endoscopically when occluded or no longer useful (Mauro et al. 2008).

Considering all these features, plastic stents are mainly used to treat recurrent benign biliary strictures (Mauro et al. 2008) and to consent a temporary drainage of biliary tract as a bridge to surgery or to a medical resolution of malignant stenosis (for example caused by lymphoma or metastatic lymph nodes) (Di Sena et al. 2005).

Sometimes plastic stents are even used for palliation in malignant biliary strictures, especially in cases with an expected survival of less than 3 months (because of their low-term patency rates) (Soderlund and Linder 2006).

4.1.2 Metallic Stents

Self-expanding uncovered metal stents are widely used for palliative treatment of malignant biliary strictures, particularly in patients with an expected survival of at least 4.5 months (Soderlund and Linder 2006). These stents in fact have long-term patency rates due to their large diameter: they can reach a lumen up to 30 Fr when placed into biliary tract, even if they are generally mounted over 6–7 Fr carrying catheters (Tsetis et al. 2016).

Superiority of metal stents compared to plastic stents concerning patency rates has widely been proved by several studies over the years (Soderlund and Linder 2006; Mukai et al. 2013).

Moreover these devices, once made of stainless steel, are actually made of nitinol (an alloy of nickel and titanium), an MR-compatible material that has good flexibility, radial force, and thermal shape memory (Shawyer et al. 2013) (Fig. 9).

Nevertheless uncovered metal stents, once placed into the biliary tract, can be subject to loss of patency and cannot be removed because of epithelization of metal struts and tumor ingrowth.

For these reasons uncovered permanent metal stents are not recommended for the treatment of benign biliary strictures but only for confirmed malignant biliary strictures (Kapoor et al. 2018).

Considering all this, during the years retrievable-covered metal stents have been developed that can be placed and removed both percutaneously and endoscopically.

These stents are made of a tubular metal mesh covered by a polytetrafluoroethylene, polyure-

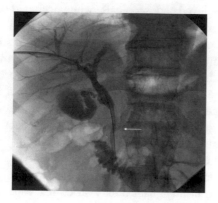

Fig. 9 Metal stent (arrow) in the common bile duct seen at fluoroscopy

thane, or silicone layer. This membrane allows to prevent tumor ingrowth and to avoid integration of the stent within the biliary wall, making it removable if needed (Tsetis et al. 2016).

For these reasons usage of covered retrievable stents has been proposed not only to treat malignant biliary strictures, but also to treat benign biliary strictures (Gwon et al. 2008) and biliary leaks (Gwon et al. 2011).

Removal of these stents is usually realized approximately after 6–8 weeks when used to treat benign biliary strictures and after 3 months when used to treat biliary leaks; anyway clinic always influences this timing of removal (Shawyer et al. 2013).

At the same time the layer of covered metal stent makes them more prone to migration and to occlusion of cystic duct and main pancreatic duct causing cholecystitis and pancreatitis (Tsetis et al. 2016).

To treat malignant hilar biliary strictures, when often more than one stent is needed for a satisfactory result, metal stents with larger gaps between their struts have been designed too. The less dense mesh in the central portion of the stent in fact consents the insertion of a second stent into the first one (Tsetis et al. 2016).

4.1.3 Biodegradable Stents

Biodegradable stents are recently introduced devices made of polydioxanone (PDX), a radiolucent biodegradable polymer that degrades by hydrolysis in 3–6 months, and with radiopaque platinum markers at the extremities to allow interventional radiologists to understand where to place them (Kapoor et al. 2018) (Fig. 10).

These devices are mainly used to treat benign biliary strictures, particularly the refractory ones (Mauri et al. 2013).

Use of these stents is not yet widespread as they are available only as custom-made devices (Kapoor et al. 2018); anyway they showed to have a good radial force, flexibility, and remodeling effect of strictures. Moreover, being degradable, they do not need to be removed with a further endoscopic procedure and stent migration does not represent a problem (Siiki et al. 2018).

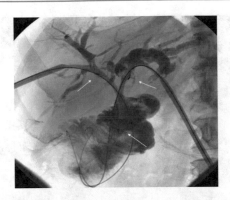

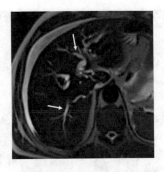

Fig. 11 T2w MRI axial image of dilated intrahepatic bile ducts (arrows)

Fig. 10 Double-biodegradable stents placed in the common bile duct and in left and right main hepatic ducts. It is possible to see the radiopaque markers at their extremities (arrows)

4.2 Procedure Preparation

Patient's preparation to biliary stent placement should include:

- Performing a biopsy of biliary duct, to confirm the underlying etiology of the stricture (benign or malignant) (Mauro et al. 2008).
- Performing imaging studies, particularly MRI (Fig. 11), to determine the location and length of the stenosis or of the bile duct injury, in order to choose the better approach for the procedure and the correct size of the stent.
- Imaging can also be useful to preventively identify the eventual presence of anatomic variants of biliary tree and ascites, both things that can make the procedure more difficult (Shawyer et al. 2013; Thompson et al. 2013).
- Eventual positioning of an internal-external drainage for 1–2 weeks before stent release, to consent decompression of biliary tree, cleaning from eventual clots and debris, and treatment of cholangitis if present.
- Review of coagulation parameters and them correction if found abnormal (normal values include INR <1.5 and platelet count >50,000/mm³) (Kapoor et al. 2018; Gwon et al. 2013).
- Review of renal function parameters to exclude a kidney failure.
- Exclusion of allergy to iodinated contrast agents.
- Exclusion of intercurrent presence of infection or sepsis.
- Eventual antibiotic prophylaxis (Mauro et al. 2008).

4.3 Techniques

CT or MRI is fundamental to choose the best approach to biliary tree to place correctly the stent; the target should be draining more than 50% of the liver (Vienne et al. 2010).

In most cases a right lobe approach is preferred, because it has a lower rate of complication and because right biliary ducts drain the majority of the liver (Kapoor et al. 2018).

After a fluoroscopic or US-guided puncture of the biliary tree with a 21-gauge Chiba needle, a sheath with a side arm (large enough to leave the stent go through it) has to be placed in the intrahepatic bile duct chosen. The tip of the sheath should be placed proximally to the stricture, in order to leave enough space for the interventional radiologist's maneuvers (Fidelman 2015).

Injecting the side arm of the sheath is then possible to obtain a cholangiogram that consents to estimate the site and extension of the stenosis and to select proper caliber and length of the stent (Sutter and Ryu 2015).

Performing the cholangiogram in a right anterior oblique projection can consent a better visualization of the confluence of the principal right and left bile ducts.

A 0.035″ guidewire has then to be used to cross the obstruction; a 5 French angled-tip catheter can be used to give more support to the guidewire, thus making this maneuver easier. The catheter, after being pushed in the duodenum through the stenosis, is also fundamental to consent the exchange of the first guidewire with a stiffer one.

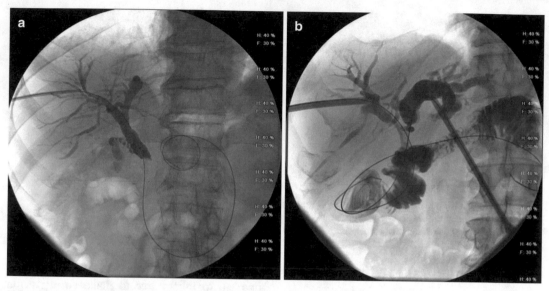

Fig. 12 (**a**) Cholangiogram from a sheath placed in right bile ducts and 0.035″ guidewire passed through the stenosis into the duodenum; (**b**) cholangiogram through sheaths placed in both hepatic lobes and 0.035″ guidewires passed through the biliary tract into the duodenum

Sometimes a microwire and a microcatheter are needed to cross particularly tight stenosis: the microcatheter is then used to pass a stiff microwire across the obstruction that can be used as a platform for balloon dilatation and for the passage of the 5 F catheter across the stenosis (Fidelman 2015) (Fig. 12).

Anyway pre-stent deployment balloon dilation of malignant stricture is not recommended routinely because this maneuver can cause bleeding and subsequent overgrowth of the tumor with possible early stent occlusion.

Using the stiff guidewire as support, the stent is then deployed; in order to reduce the risk of overgrowth of the tumor at the stent margins, the device is usually placed across the stricture with a safety margin of 2 cm at both proximal and distal ends of the stricture itself (Das et al. 2017).

A post-deployment cholangiogram injecting the sheath has always to be done, to assess the correct placement of the stent and if a good passage of the contrast medium in the duodenum has been obtained without residual stenosis (Maillard et al. 2012).

If the control cholangiogram shows a persistent narrow tract within the stent, post-deployment balloon dilation can be performed (Das et al. 2017); however the expansion of self-expandable

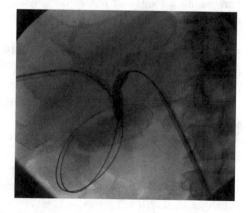

Fig. 13 Pre-stent deployment balloon dilatation using balloon catheters mounted over 0.035″ stiff guidewires

stents continues even after their release in biliary tract, so post-deployment balloon dilation should not be routinely made (Sutter and Ryu 2015).

In particular cases, especially with hilar bile duct stenosis, a bilateral stent insertion can be considered, even if the benefit to drain both hepatic lobes is still debated (Li et al. 2016) (Fig. 13).

There are two bilateral stent placement techniques:

- Side by side that consists of the placement at the same time of two parallel metallic stents:

These stents drain the bile ducts of both hepatic lobes and then become parallel and close when reaching the common hepatic duct, where they cannot expand completely and can possibly collapse instead.

- Stent in stent that consists first of the placement of a metallic stent across the biliary hilar stricture to drain a hepatic lobe, and subsequently the deployment of a second metallic stent into the first one to drain the contralateral hepatic lobe. The second stent is placed through the mesh of the first one, thus creating an overlap of part of the stents that helps in increasing their radial force and preventing stent migration or collapse (Corvino et al. 2016).

The stent-in-stent technique provides a T-shaped stent configuration (that requests a unilateral percutaneous access and is preferred when there is an obtuse angle between right and left hepatic ducts) or a Y-shaped stent configuration (that requests a bilateral percutaneous access and is preferred when there is an acute angle between right and left hepatic ducts) (Das et al. 2017).

4.4 Postprocedural Care

As postprocedural care after stent placement, it is a good rule to leave an internal-external drainage or a 5 French catheter through the stent to the duodenum for protection (Fig. 14); this drainage or catheter can then be removed in a few days after checking the good functioning of the stent (Maillard et al. 2012).

4.5 Success Rate

Technical success is considered as the correct positioning of the stent in the desired place in biliary ducts with a good passage of contrast material through the stricture to the duodenum. This condition is reached almost always in 100% of cases (Gwon et al. 2013; Li et al. 2016; Corvino et al. 2016).

Clinical success is defined as a successful removal of the temporary protection drainage catheter and the reduction in serum total bilirubin

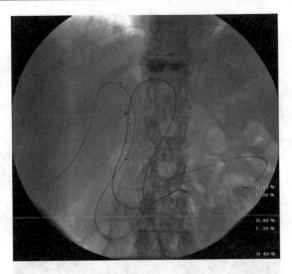

Fig. 14 5-French internal and external catheters left for protection through two biodegradable stents to the small bowel

level of 30% after 1 week or 50% after 2 weeks or 75% after 1 month, compared with pretreatment bilirubin level. Clinical success rates are comprised between 84.7% and 91.6% (Li et al. 2016; Gwon et al. 2013; Corvino et al. 2016; Zhang et al. 2018; Yi et al. 2012).

For benign biliary strictures, treated with retrievable covered metal stents or biodegradable stents, a residual stenosis of less than 20–30% should be considered a success (Saad 2008). In different studies rates from 75% to 90% of stenosis resolution have been reported (Kapoor et al. 2018).

4.6 Complications

Biliary stent placement is a procedure affected by the same general complications as all other percutaneous biliary interventions. These complications include hemorrhage or bleeding, pneumothorax, hemothorax, biliary tract and gallbladder damages, and sepsis (Thompson et al. 2013). However major complications are rare, with a rate between 0.5% and 2.5% (Kapoor et al. 2018).

Particular complications of biliary stents are as follows:

- Stent occlusion that can be acute for obstructive formation of clots, or chronic for tumor ingrowth (between stent mesh), tumor overgrowth (at proximal or distal end of the stent),

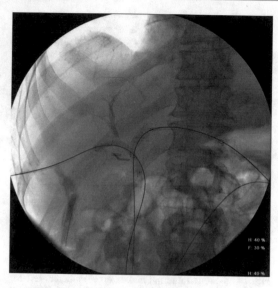

Fig. 15 Bilateral metal stents placed at hepatic hilum with a Y-shaped configuration seen at fluoroscopy

sludge incrustation, or stone formation (Venkatanarasimha et al. 2017). Time between stent placement and stent occlusion is defined as stent patency time (Gwon et al. 2013). A study reported patency rates of metal stents of 73.5% at 3 months, 53.1% at 6 months, and 36.1% at 12 months (Li et al. 2016). Another study reported patency rates of 95–97% at 1 month, 83–87% at 3 months, 74–78% at 6 months, and 50–56% at 12 months (Kullman et al. 2010). Moreover patency time rates have been reported to be often longer for covered metallic stents than for uncovered metallic stents (Kapoor et al. 2018; Saleem et al. 2011). In general tumor ingrowth and overgrowth are more frequent in uncovered metallic stents; sludge incrustation instead is more frequent in plastic and covered metallic stents. Anyway, in case of occlusion, it is possible to repeat an intervention on biliary tree and place an additional stent to resolve the obstruction (Tsetis et al. 2016) (Figs. 15 and 16).

- Stent migration that is more frequent with plastic stents and covered metallic stents: With these stents in fact it can reach a rate up to 20% (Kapoor et al. 2018).
- Stent fracture that occurs in 7–11% of metallic stents (Venkatanarasimha et al. 2017).

- Stent-related infections or inflammation: In particular cholecystitis and pancreatitis can be consequent to a covered metal stent placed above cystic duct and pancreatic main duct outlet in common bile duct (Tsetis et al. 2016; Shawyer et al. 2013). Cholangitis instead has shown to be more frequent with biodegradable stent placement, maybe consequent to irritation of bile ducts by products of stent degradation (Siiki et al. 2018).

5 Percutaneous Transhepatic Biliary Stone Removal

Symptomatic gallstones affect 260,000 Americans each year (Mauro et al. 2008); 7–20% of patients with cholecystolithiasis also have stones in the bile duct (Garcia-Vila et al. 2004; Bin et al. 2018) and 2–5% of patients present with residual biliary stones after biliary tract surgery (Garcia-Garcia and Lanciego 2004).

Biliary stones can be asymptomatic for years or can cause symptoms (nausea, vomiting, abdominal pain, postprandial fullness) and/or severe complications such as cholangitis, jaundice, or pancreatitis.

The majority of patients are treated definitively with surgery and, with the advent of laparoscopic cholecystectomy, surgeons can treat patients less invasively with a quicker recovery.

Even in the setting of laparoscopic cholecystectomy, some patients will not be suitable for surgery because of significant comorbidities: this group of patients can greatly benefit from percutaneous drainage and stone extraction.

Patients with symptomatic gallstones often simultaneously have calculi in the intrahepatic or extrahepatic bile ducts as well. Endoscopic retrograde cholangiopancreatography (ERCP) has been available since the 1970s and is nowadays considered the main technique to remove such stones in the majority of patients (Mauro et al. 2008; Garcia-Vila et al. 2004).

The procedure though can be difficult in patients with challenging or surgically altered anatomy (duodenal diverticulum, impacted stones larger than 15 mm, patients who have pre-

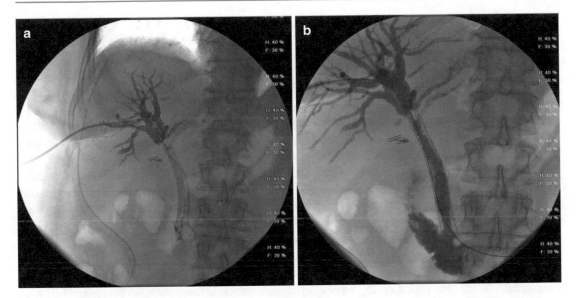

Fig. 16 (a) Occluded metallic stent seen at cholangiography, with dilated intrahepatic bile ducts. (b) After the placement of a second stent into the first one, stent patency is re-established

viously undergone biliary reconstruction as in Billroth II or Roux-en-Y surgery) in which endoscopic techniques are more prone to failure or the bile ducts may be inaccessible (Mauro et al. 2008; Copelan and Kapoor 2015).

In these patients, the radiological percutaneous treatment is a fundamental option: the technique has been developed and made popular by Burhenne in the 1980s (Burhenne 1980).

5.1 Indications

The principal indication for percutaneous transhepatic biliary stone removal is the treatment of symptomatic calculi in patients who are not eligible for surgery, e.g., patients with intrahepatic duct stones virtually out of endoscopic reach: these patients usually have recently undergone gallstone or biliary surgery and still have a T-tube in place, so the surgeon would refer these patients for interventional radiological management as first-line treatment (Mauro et al. 2008).

The percutaneous treatment of biliary stones is recommended also for patients in which ERCP has failed or is impracticable (as in case of surgically altered anatomy) (Mauro et al. 2008).

5.2 Contraindications

The main absolute contraindication is the presence of an incorrigible bleeding diathesis since hemorrhagic complications are a significant source of morbidity and mortality, especially in case of large-bore percutaneous transhepatic tracts.

Among relative contraindications we find stone-related active infection and excessively dilated biliary ducts: in these cases, preliminary placement of an appropriate drainage catheter is indicated to "cool off" the infectious process or reduce duct dilatation (Mauro et al. 2008).

5.3 Procedure

5.3.1 Patient Preparation

Patient should be preferably fasting or on liquid diet for at least 4–6 h prior to the procedure.

Usually, pre-procedure antibiotic prophylaxis and sedation are required (Mauro et al. 2008).

Before and during the procedure the patient vital signs have to be monitored and 0.25 mg of somatostatin or 0.1 mg of octreotide can be administered to protect the pancreas; additionally, 1 mg of glucagon can be useful to relax the sphincter of Oddi (Garcia-Vila et al. 2004; Clouse and Falchuk 1985).

5.3.2 Pre-intervention

The way of access to the biliary tree is variable and time dependent and noninvasive imaging acquired before the procedure can help plan the route of access and the intervention.

Patients who have recently had a cholecystectomy with retained calculi might have a T-tube in place that can be used as an access. In the other patients, the access is the same as in percutaneous biliary drainage (see below).

Approximately half of the patients with biliary stones will have multiple calculi: a careful search has to be made during preliminary cholangiography. If all the intrahepatic stones are located in one hepatic lobe, most of the operators prefer to access the opposite lobe to have a wider angle when entering the ducts containing the stones.

5.3.3 Access

• T-tube access:

A preliminary cholangiogram is performed through the T-tube which is then removed and replaced with a vascular sheath using a guidewire.

• De novo access:

US- and fluoroscopy-guided liver puncture under local anesthesia is performed with sterile technique, usually to the right lobe, even if a left lobe or bilateral access can be carried out depending on the specific patient conditions and location of calculi (Mauro et al. 2008; Hwang et al. 1993).

Using a guidewire through the needle, a vascular sheath is placed within the hepatic duct.

In some cases, the procedure can be two staged: firstly an internal/external biliary drainage catheter is positioned to reduce biliary tree dilatation or to "cool off" a cholangitis. Subsequently the drainage is replaced with a vascular sheath of the appropriate caliber using a guidewire (Mauro et al. 2008; Hwang et al. 1993).

5.3.4 Stone Extraction

Independently on the access, a safety guidewire is then pushed into the small bowel.

A cholangiography is performed through the vascular sheath to show and confirm the stone or stone location.

A 10 or 12 mm angioplasty or a valvuloplasty balloon is then placed across the ampulla of Vater and inflated for up to 3 min: the sphincteroplasty can be repeated twice, if necessary, also with an occlusion balloon. Many authors suggest 12 mm as maximum balloon size, but in some cases a dilatation up to 22–23 mm has been performed (Mauro et al. 2008; Park et al. 1987; Bin et al. 2018; Garcia-Vila et al. 2004).

Two kinds of balloon can be used to fragment the stones: angioplasty or occlusion balloons, depending on the calculi morphological characteristics. The balloon diameter is chosen on the size of the largest stone (Mauro et al. 2008; Garcia-Garcia and Lanciego 2004; Garcia-Vila et al. 2004; Gil et al. 2000).

When stones exceed 12–15 mm, other devices and techniques are necessary, such as the use of fragmentation basket (e.g., Dormia basket) (Mauro et al. 2008; Hwang et al. 1993).

The stones and their fragments are then carefully flushed (high-frequency pulsed flushing) and/or pushed into the small bowel with an angioplasty balloon through the dilated papilla (Shin et al. 2014).

After cholangiography has confirmed complete clearance of the stones, an internal/external drainage catheter is placed across the sphincter of Oddi in the small bowel (Figs. 17 and 18).

5.4 Postprocedural Care

In our institute, an internal-external biliary drainage catheter is left in place after the procedure and replaced with one of the progressively smaller calibers to facilitate the healing process of the intrahepatic and percutaneous tracts. A cholangiography is usually performed before removal of the drainage to ensure complete clearance of the calculi.

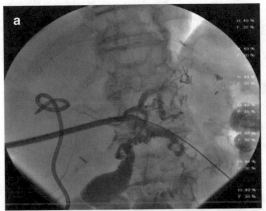

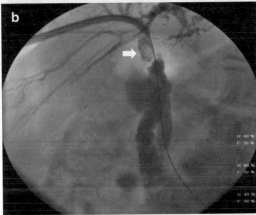

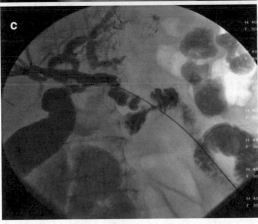

Fig. 17 (**a–c**) Stone impacted in the pre-papillary region (white arrow). (**b**) During the attempt to push it down, the stone migrates cranially (white arrow: stone). (**c**) Postprocedural cholangiography control with the guidewire in place: the contrast medium drainage appears satisfactory, but the stone was not removed

The short-term complications are assessed and managed before discharge.

Long-term complications such as refluxing cholangitis and calculi recurrence are monitored over time.

Patients with more complex clinical situation are managed conjointly with the referring hepatobiliary surgeon and/or gastroenterologist (Mauro et al. 2008).

5.5 Success Rate

Success is achieved in more than 90–99.5% of cases (Mauro et al. 2008; Garcia-Vila et al. 2004; Shin et al. 2017). Most patients are completely cleared of calculi in one treatment session.

Success is more probable in patients with ductal stones related to cholecystitis than in the ones with disease involving the intrahepatic ducts (Mauro et al. 2008).

5.6 Complications

According to literature, the overall morbidity rate of percutaneous transhepatic biliary stone removal varies between 2% and 13.5% and the overall mortality rate varies between 0% and 1.7% (Garcia-Vila et al. 2004); in case of major complications the mortality rate within 30 days is approximately 4% (Stokes et al. 1989).

The most reported and common complications according to literature are the following (Mauro et al. 2008; Garcia-Vila et al. 2004; Bin et al. 2018):

- Related to bile leakage, ranging from simple loculated biloma to severe bile peritonitis.
- Pancreatitis, which can occur in 8–12% of patients and has a mortality rate of 0.5–1% (Bergman et al. 1997; Freeman et al. 1996).
- Bleeding complications such as hemobilia, which can be severe in 12% of cases (Bonnel et al. 1991) and needs to be treated with arterial embolization; when not clinically relevant, cold saline irrigation can be sufficient (Garcia-Garcia and Lanciego 2004).

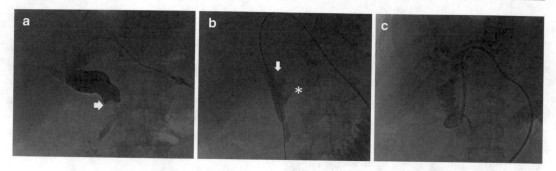

Fig. 18 (**a–c**) Stone impacted in the pre-papillary region (white arrow) with thin contrast medium passage to the duodenum and important dilatation of the common bile duct upstream. (**b**) During the attempt to push it down, the stone migrates cranially and gets stuck between the balloon and the bile duct wall (white arrow: stone; white asterisk: angioplasty balloon). (**c**) An internal-external biliary drainage catheter is then placed in order to reduce the biliary duct dilatation before attempting to remove the stone again

Bowel perforation is another fearsome complication and, with pancreatitis and hemorrhage, represents the most serious complication (Garcia-Vila et al. 2004).

Infective complications are less common and include symptomatic bacteremia, biliary duct infection and cholangitis, and liver or subcutaneous abscess (Mauro et al. 2008; Bin et al. 2018; Garcia-Garcia and Lanciego 2004).

Partial success of the procedure, with residual stones in the biliary tree, occurs in 3–4% of cases (Gandini et al. 1990).

6 Percutaneous Cholecystostomy (PC)

6.1 Introduction

PC is a therapeutic procedure that involves the sterile placement of a needle into the gallbladder with the use of imaging guidance to aspirated bile. This is commonly followed by sterile placement of a tube for external drainage of gallbladder contents, which completes the procedure (Saad et al. 2010).

PC was first described in 1979 as a cholangitis treatment in a patient with obstructive jaundice and it was first performed in 1980 in a patient with empyema of the gallbladder (Radder et al. 1980).

Since then, there was an increasing acceptance and awareness towards PC and many studies reported on its employment in different subsets of patients (Li et al. 2018).

6.2 Indications

PC tube placement is performed to manage acute cholecystitis (Tokyo 2018 stage III) or remove gallstones.

It is also used to decompress the biliary tract and dilate biliary benign or malignant strictures. Indications of PC are listed in Table 5.

The Tokyo Guidelines 2018 define the severity grading for acute cholecystitis and can help the clinician with the management of this pathology (Yokoe et al. 2018) (Table 6).

6.3 Contraindications

Coagulopathy is the most common contraindication. Other contraindications of PC include many conditions such as gallbladder cancer, perforated and decompressed gallbladder, and bowel interposition between the gallbladder and the point of puncture.

6.4 Preparation

Preprocedural preparation requires reviewing of any previous US or CT images to evaluate the type of gallbladder access.

Table 5 Cholecystostomy indications (from Saad et al. 2010)

Cholecystostomy indications
Gallbladder access (>95%)
– Management of cholecystitis
– Portal for dissolution/removal of stones
Biliary tract access (<5%)
– Decompress obstructed biliary tract
– Divert bile from bile duct defect
– Provide a portal of access to the biliary tract for therapeutic purpose

Table 6 Tokyo Guidelines 2018, severity grading for acute cholecystitis (from Okamoto, et al. 2018)

Grade III (severe) acute cholecystitis
"Grade III" acute cholecystitis is associated with dysfunction of any one of the following organs/systems:
1. Cardiovascular dysfunction: hypotension requiring treatment with dopamine ≥ 5 µg/kg per min, or any dose of norepinephrine
2. Neurological dysfunction: decreased level of consciousness
3. Respiratory dysfunction: PaO_2/FiO_2 ratio <300
4. Renal dysfunction: oliguria, creatinine >2.0 mg/dL
5. Hepatic dysfunction: PT-INR >1.5
6. Hematological dysfunction: platelet count <100,000/mm³
Grade II (moderate) acute cholecystitis
"Grade II" acute cholecystitis is associated with any one of the following conditions:
1. Elevated WBC count (>18,000/mm³)
2. Palpable tender mass in the right abdominal quadrant
3. Duration of complaints >72 h
4. Marked local inflammation (gangrenous cholecystitis, pericholecystic abscess, hepatic abscess, biliary peritonitis, emphysematous cholecystitis)
Grade I (mild) acute cholecystitis
"Grade I" acute cholecystitis does not meet the criteria of "Grade II" or "Grade II" acute cholecystitis. It can also be defined as acute cholecystitis in healthy patients with no organ dysfunction and mild inflammatory changes in the gallbladder, making cholecystectomy a safe low-risk operative procedure

Prophylactic antibiotics are given 12 h prior to the procedure and coagulation values should be checked and corrected as necessary. The optimal coagulation values are INR <1.5 and platelets >50,000.

6.5 Technique

PC is usually performed under US (rarely CT) and fluoroscopy guidance (Little et al. 2013).

Two approaches have been described: transhepatic and transperitoneal (Gulaya et al. 2016).

Transhepatic access has the advantages of lower risk of bile leak and catheter dislodgement and provides quicker maturation of catheter tract. Transperitoneal approach is considered more suitable in patients with liver disease and coagulopathy.

Two techniques have been described including Seldinger and trocar technique (Akhan et al. 2002).

The Seldinger technique consists of inserting a needle (18 G) into the gallbladder under local anesthesia (lidocaine 1%) and US guidance. The correct needle position can be confirmed by bile aspiration and contrast injection. A guidewire is then advanced into the gallbladder and the needle is removed.

Pigtail catheter (8–12 F) can be advanced over the guidewire within the gallbladder lumen (Figs. 19 and 20).

6.6 Success Rate

Technical success rates for percutaneous cholecystostomy are around 95%. The causes of technical failure include small gallbladder, porcelain gallbladder, and thin gallbladder wall.

6.7 Complications

The complication rate is low (around 8%). They include bile leaks, catheter dislodgement, haemobilia, and more rarely pneumothorax and bowel perforation (Park et al. 2018).

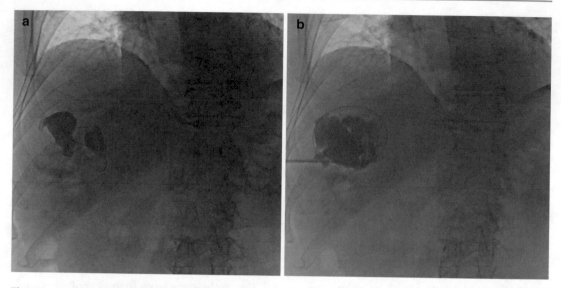

Fig. 19 (**a, b**) The hepatic collection adjacent the gallbladder is opacified through percutaneous ultrasound-guided access

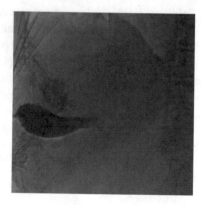

Fig. 20 The drainage (10 F) is positioned over the wire inside the gallbladder

References

Akhan O, Akıncı D, Özmen MN (2002) Percutaneous cholecystostomy. Eur J Radiol 43(3):229–236

Asadi H et al (2016) A review of percutaneous transhepatic biliary drainage at a tertiary referral centre. Clin Radiol 71(12):1312–13e7

Bergman JJ, Rauws EA, Fockens P et al (1997) Randomised trial of endoscopic balloon dilatation versus endoscopic sphincterotomy for removal of bile duct stones. Lancet 349:1124–1129

Bin L, De-Shun W, Pi-Kun C, Yong-Zheng W, Wu-Jie W, Wei W, Hai-Yang C, Dong L, Xiao L, Yancu H, Yu-Liang L (2018) Percutaneous transhepatic extraction and balloon dilation for simultaneous gallbladder stones and common bile duct stones: a novel technique. World J Gastroenterol 24(33):3799–3805

Bonnel D, Liguory CE, Cornud FE, Lefebvre JF (1991) Common bile duct and intrahepatic stones: results of transhepatic electrohydraulic lithotripsy in 50 patients. Radiology 180:345–348

Burhenne HJ (1980) Garland lecture. Percutaneous extraction of retained biliary tract stones: 661 patients. Am J Roentgenol 134(5):889–898

Burke DR et al (2003) Quality improvement guidelines for percutaneous transhepatic cholangiography and biliary drainage. J Vas Intervent Radiol 9(Pt 2):S243

Chandrashekhara SH et al (2016) Current status of percutaneous transhepatic biliary drainage in palliation of malignant obstructive jaundice: a review. Indian J Palliat Care 22(4):378

Clouse ME, Falchuk KR (1985) Percutaneous transhepatic removal of common duct stones: report of ten patients. Gastroenterology 85:815–819

Copelan A, Kapoor BS (2015) Choledocholithiasis: diagnosis and management. Tech Vasc Interv Radiol 18(4):244–255. https://doi.org/10.1053/j.tvir.2015.07.008

Corvino F, Centore L, Soreca E, Corvino A, Farbo V, Bencivenga A (2016) Percutaneous "Y" biliary stent placement in palliative treatment of type 4 malignant hilar stricture. J Gastrointest Oncol 7(2):255–261. https://doi.org/10.3978/j.issn.2078-6891.2015.069

Covey AM, Brown KT (2008) Percutaneous transhepatic biliary drainage. Tech Vasc Interv Radiol 11(1):14–20

Das A, Baliyan V, Gamanagatti S, Gupta AK (2017) Percutaneous biliary intervention: tips and tricks. Trop Gastroenterol 38(2):71–89

Di Sena V, Thuler FP, Macedo EP, Paulo GA, Della Libera E, Ferrari AP (2005) Obstructive jaundice secondary to bile duct involvement with Hodgkin's disease: a case report. Sao Paulo Med J 123(1):30–32

Ferrucci JT, Mueller PR, Harbin WP (1980) Percutaneous transhepatic biliary drainage: technique, results, and applications. Radiology 135(1):1–13

Fidelman N (2015) Benign biliary strictures: diagnostic evaluation and approaches to percutaneous treatment. Tech Vasc Interv Radiol 18(4):210–217

Freeman ML, Nelson DB, Sherman S et al (1996) Complications after endoscopic biliary sphincterotomy. N Engl J Med 335:909–918

Furuse J, Takada T, Miyazaki M, Miyakawa S, Tsukada K, Nagino M, Kondo S, Saito H, Tsuyuguchi T, Hirata K, Kimura F, Yoshitomi H, Nozawa S, Yoshida M, Wada K, Amano H, Miura F, Japanese Association of Biliary Surgery; Japanese Society of Hepato-Biliary-Pancreatic Surgery; Japan Society of Clinical Oncology (2008) Guidelines for chemotherapy of biliary tract and ampullary carcinomas. J Hepato-Biliary-Pancreat Surg 15(1):55–62. https://doi.org/10.1007/s00534-007-1280-z

Gandini G, Righi D, Regge D, Recchia S, Ferraris A, Fronda GR (1990) Percutaneous removal of biliary stones. Cardiovasc Intervent Radiol 13:245–251

Garcarek J et al (2012) Ten years single center experience in percutaneous transhepatic decompression of biliary tree in patients with malignant obstructive jaundice. Adv Clin Exp Med 21(5):621–632

Garcia-Garcia L, Lanciego L (2004) Percutaneous treatment of biliary stones: sphincteroplasty and occlusion balloon for the clearance of bile duct calculi. Am J Roentgenol 182:663–670

Garcia-Vila JH, Redondo-Ibanez M, Diaz-Ramon C (2004) Balloon sphincteroplasty and transpapillary elimination of bile duct stones: 10 years' experience. Am J Roentgenol 182:1451–1458

Gil S, De La Inglesia P, Verdù JF, De Espana F, Arenas J, Irurzun J (2000) Effectiveness and safety of balloon dilation of the papilla and the use of an occlusion balloon for clearance of the bile duct calculi. Am J Roentgenol 174:1455–1460

Ginat D, Saad WEA (2008) Cholecystostomy and transcholecystic biliary access. Tech Vasc Interv Radiol 11(1):2–13

Gulaya K, Desai SS, Sato K (2016) Percutaneous cholecystostomy: evidence-based current clinical practice. Seminars in interventional radiology, vol 33. Thieme Medical Publishers, New York

Gwon DI, Shim HJ, Kwak BK (2008) Retrievable biliary stent-graft in the treatment of benign biliary strictures. J Vasc Interv Radiol 19(9):1328–1335. https://doi.org/10.1016/j.jvir.2008.05.017

Gwon DI, Ko GY, Sung KB, Kim JH, Yoon HK (2011) Percutaneous transhepatic treatment of postoperative bile leaks: prospective evaluation of retrievable covered stent. J Vasc Interv Radiol 22(1):75–83. https://doi.org/10.1016/j.jvir.2010.10.004

Gwon DI, Ko GY, Kim JH, Shin JH, Kim KA, Yoon HK, Sung KB (2013) Percutaneous bilateral metallic stent placement using a stent-in-stent deployment technique in patients with malignant hilar biliary obstruction. Am J Roentgenol 200(4):909–914. https://doi.org/10.2214/AJR.12.8780

Harbin WP, Mueller PR, Ferrucci JT (1980) Transhepatic cholangiography: complications and use patterns of the fine-needle technique: a multi-institutional survey. Radiology 135(1):15–22. https://doi.org/10.1148/radiology.135.1.6987704

Hwang MH, Tsai CC, Mo LR, Yang CT, Yeh YH, Yau MP, Yueh SK (1993) Percutaneous choledochoscopic biliary tract stone removal: experience in 645 consecutive patients. Eur J Radiol 17:184–190

Iwasaki M et al (1996) Percutaneous transhepatic biliary drainage for the treatment of obstructive jaundice caused by metastases from nonbiliary and nonpancreatic cancers. Jpn J Clin Oncol 26(6):465–468

Jabłońska B, Lampe P (2009) Iatrogenic bile duct injuries: etiology, diagnosis and management. World J Gastroenterol 15(33):4097

Kapoor BS, Mauri G, Lorenz JM (2018) Management of biliary strictures: state-of-the-art review. Radiology 289(3):590–603. https://doi.org/10.1148/radiol.2018172424

Kessel D, Robertson I (2017) Biliary intervention. Interventional radiology survival guide, 3rd edn. Churchill Livingstone, London, UK

Kim T-H (2006) Safety and effectiveness of moderate sedation for radiologic non-vascular intervention. Korean J Radiol 7(2):125–130

Kullman E, Frozanpor F, Söderlund C, Linder S, Sandström P, Lindhoff-Larsson A, Toth E, Lindell G, Jonas E, Freedman J, Ljungman M, Rudberg C, Ohlin B, Zacharias R, Leijonmarck CE, Teder K, Ringman A, Persson G, Gözen M, Eriksson O (2010) Covered versus uncovered self-expandable nitinol stents in the palliative treatment of malignant distal biliary obstruction: results from a randomized, multicenter study. Gastrointest Endosc 72(5):915–923, https://doi.org/10.1016/j.gie.2010.07.036

Leng JJ, Zhang N, Dong JH (2014) Percutaneous transhepatic and endoscopic biliary drainage for malignant biliary tract obstruction: a meta-analysis. World J Surg Oncol 12(1):272

Li M, Li K, Qi X, Wu W, Zheng L, He C, Yin Z, Fan D, Zhang Z, Han G (2016) Percutaneous transhepatic biliary stent implantation for obstructive jaundice of perihilar cholangiocarcinoma: a prospective study on predictors of stent patency and survival in 92 patients. J Vasc Interv Radiol 27(7):1047.e2–1055.e2. https://doi.org/10.1016/j.jvir.2016.02.035

Li YL, Wong KH, Chiu KW et al (2018) Percutaneous cholecystostomy for high-risk patients with acute cholangitis. Medicine (Baltimore) 97(19):e0735

Little MW et al (2013) Percutaneous cholecystostomy: the radiologist's role in treating acute cholecystitis. Clin Radiol 68(7):654–660

Maillard M, Novellas S, Baudin G, Evesque L, Bellmann L, Gugenheim J, Chevallier P (2012) Placement of metallic biliary endoprostheses in complex hilar tumours. Diagn Interv Imaging 93(10):767–774. https://doi.org/10.1016/j.diii.2012.05.014

Mauri G, Michelozzi C, Melchiorre F, Poretti D, Tramarin M, Pedicini V, Solbiati L, Cornalba G, Sconfienza LM (2013) Biodegradable biliary stent implantation in the treatment of benign bilioplastic-refractory biliary strictures: preliminary experience. Eur Radiol 23(12):3304–3310. https://doi.org/10.1007/s00330-013-2947-2

Mauro MA, Murphy KPJ, Thomson KR, Venbrux AC, Zollikofer CL (2008) Image-guided interventions, vol 2. Saunders Elsevier, Amsterdam, pp 1423–1457

Morgan RA, Adam A (1998) "Percutaneous management of biliary obstruction." Hepatobiliary and Pancreatic Radiology Imaging and Intervention. Thieme, New York, pp 677–709

Mueller PR, Van Sonnenberg E, Ferrucci JT Jr (1982) Percutaneous biliary drainage: technical and catheter-related problems in 200 procedures. Am J Roentgenol 138(1):17–23

Mukai T, Yasuda I, Nakashima M, Doi S, Iwashita T, Iwata K, Kato T, Tomita E, Moriwaki H (2013) Metallic stents are more efficacious than plastic stents in unresectable malignant hilar biliary strictures: a randomized controlled trial. J Hepatobiliary Pancreat Sci 20(2):214–222. https://doi.org/10.1007/s00534-012-0508-8

Ng S, Tan KA, Anil G (2015) The role of interventional radiology in complications associated with liver transplantation. Clin Radiol 70(12):1323–1335. https://doi.org/10.1016/j.crad.2015.07.005

Nimura Y et al (2000) Aggressive preoperative management and extended surgery for hilar cholangiocarcinoma: Nagoya experience. J Hepato-Biliary-Pancreat Surg 7(2):155–162

Páramo M, García-Barquín P, Carrillo M, Millor Muruzábal M, Vivas I, Bilbao JI (2017) Treatment of benign biliary leaks with transhepatic placement of coated self-expanding metallic stents. Australas Radiol 59(1):47–55. https://doi.org/10.1016/j.rx.2016.09.004

Park JH, Choi BI, Han MC, Sung KB, Choo IW, Kim CW (1987) Percutaneous removal of residual intrahepatic stones. Radiology 163:619–623

Park JM et al (2018) Percutaneous cholecystostomy for biliary decompression in patients with cholangitis and pancreatitis. J Int Med Res 46(10):4120–4128

Pomerantz BJ (2009) Biliary tract interventions. Tech Vasc Interv Radiol 12(2):162–170

Radder RW (1980) Ultrasonically guided percutaneous catheter drainage for gallbladder empyema. Diagn Imaging 49(6):330–333

Saad WE (2008) Percutaneous management of postoperative anastomotic biliary strictures. Tech Vasc Interv Radiol 11(2):143–153. https://doi.org/10.1053/j.tvir.2008.07.008

Saad WEA et al (2010) Quality improvement guidelines for percutaneous transhepatic cholangiography, biliary drainage, and percutaneous cholecystostomy. J Vasc Interv Radiol 21(6):789–795

Saleem A, Leggett CL, Murad MH, Baron TH (2011) Meta-analysis of randomized trials comparing the patency of covered and uncovered self-expandable metal stents for palliation of distal malignant bile duct obstruction. Gastrointest Endosc 74(2):321.e1-3–327.e1-3. https://doi.org/10.1016/j.gie.2011.03.1249

Shawyer A, Goodwin MD, Gibson RN (2013) Interventional biliary radiology: current state-of-the-art and future directions. Imaging Med 5(6):525–538

Shin J, Shim H, Yoon H (2014) A single center study of biliary stone removal through the percutaneous transhepatic biliary drainage route: results of 695 patients. J Vasc Interv Radiol 25(3):S50

Shin JS, Shim HJ, Kwak BK, Yoon HK (2017) Biliary stone removal through the percutaneous transhepatic biliary drainage route, focusing on the balloon sphincteroplasty flushing technique: a single center study with 916 patients. Jpn J Radiol 35(8):440–447

Siiki A, Sand J, Laukkarinen J (2018) A systematic review of biodegradable biliary stents: promising biocompatibility without stent removal. Eur J Gastroenterol Hepatol 30(8):813–818. https://doi.org/10.1097/MEG.0000000000001167

Soderlund C, Linder S (2006) Covered metal versus plastic stents for malignant common bile duct stenosis: a prospective, randomized, controlled trial. Gastrointest Endosc 63(7):986–995

Stokes KR, Falchuk KR, Clouse ME (1989) Biliary duct stones: update on 54 cases after percutaneous transhepatic removal. Radiology 170:999–1001

Sutter CM, Ryu RK (2015) Percutaneous management of malignant biliary obstruction. Tech Vasc Interv Radiol 18(4):218–226. https://doi.org/10.1053/j.tvir.2015.07.005

Thompson CM, Saad NE, Quazi RR, Darcy MD, Picus DD, Menias CO (2013) Management of iatrogenic bile duct injuries: role of the interventional radiologist. Radiographics 33(1):117–134. https://doi.org/10.1148/rg.331125044

Tsetis D, Krokidis M, Negru D, Prassopoulos P (2016) Malignant biliary obstruction: the current role of interventional radiology. Ann Gastroenterol 29(1):33–36

Venkatanarasimha N, Damodharan K, Gogna A, Leong S, Too CW, Patel A, Tay KH, Tan BS, Lo R, Irani F (2017) Diagnosis and management of complications from percutaneous biliary tract interventions. Radiographics 37(2):665–680. https://doi.org/10.1148/rg.2017160159

Vienne A, Hobeika E, Gouya H, Lapidus N, Fritsch J, Choury AD, Chryssostalis A, Gaudric M, Pelletier G, Buffet C, Chaussade S, Prat F (2010) Prediction of drainage effectiveness during endoscopic stenting of malignant hilar strictures: the role of liver volume assessment. Gastrointest Endosc 72(4):728–735. https://doi.org/10.1016/j.gie.2010.06.040

Yi R, Gwon DI, Ko GY, Yoon HK, Kim JH, Shin JH, Sung KB (2012) Percutaneous unilateral placement of biliary covered metallic stent in patients with malignant hilar biliary obstruction and contralateral portal vein occlusion. Acta Radiol 53(7):742–749. https://doi.org/10.1258/ar.2012.120185

Yokoe M et al (2018) Tokyo Guidelines 2018: diagnostic criteria and severity grading of acute cholecystitis (with videos). J Hepatobiliary Pancreat Sci 25(1):41–54

Zhang JX, Wang B, Liu S, Zu QQ, Shi HB (2018) Predictors of recurrent biliary obstruction following percutaneous uncovered metal stent insertion in patients with distal malignant biliary obstruction: an analysis using a competing risk model. Cardiovasc Intervent Radiol 42:276. https://doi.org/10.1007/s00270-018-2107-9

Part III

Hepatic and Biliary Tract Non-Tumoral Pathology

Congenital and Development Disorders of the Liver

Anna Florio, Lorenzo Ugo, Filippo Crimí,
and Emilio Quaia

Contents

Abstract

In this chapter we present the congenital anomalies of the hepatic vasculature system and biliary tract. The alterations are determined during the complex development that occurs between the fourth and the tenth weeks of embryonic life together with the ductal plate malformation; they constitute the basis for the study and understanding of the following paragraphs.

A. Florio · L. Ugo · F. Crimí · E. Quaia (✉)
Radiology Unit, Department of Medicine - DIMED,
University of Padova, Padova, Italy
e-mail: emilio.quaia@unipd.it

1 Congenital Portosystemic Venous Shunt: Abernethy Malformation

1.1 Clinical Features

Congenital absence of the portal vein is an important finding as the complete loss of portal perfusion predisposes the liver to focal or diffuse hyperplastic or dysplastic changes, involving neurological, pulmonary, metabolic, and other systems. In 1793 John Abernethy, a surgeon, for the first time, described an autopsy of a 10-month-old female and showed termination of the portal vein (PV) in the inferior vena cava at

© Springer Nature Switzerland AG 2021

E. Quaia (ed.), *Imaging of the Liver and Intra-hepatic Biliary Tract*,
Medical Radiology, Diagnostic Imaging, https://doi.org/10.1007/978-3-030-38983-3_10

the level of the renal veins (complete portosystemic shunt) (Abernethy 1793). An aberrant development of the portal vein or vena cava in early embryonic life explains the genesis of congenital portosystemic shunts (CPSS) (Ghuman et al. 2016). Congenital portosystemic venous shunt (PSVS) has been explained by alterations in the embryological development of the portal system and inferior vena cava (IVC) with abnormal involution of the vitelline veins that occur between the fourth and tenth weeks of embryonic life (Bhargava et al. 2011) and maybe depends on the anatomical site (right or left) and level (proximal or distal) at which the vitelline veins fail to differentiate. Instead a patent ductus venosus (Kamimatsuse et al. 2010) acts as an intrahepatic shunt and may result in hypoplasia of the portal vein due to an alteration in hemodynamics from congenital heart defects. For further details see the section on embryology of the liver (chapter "Embryology and Development of the Liver").

Portosystemic shunts can be congenital or acquired due to portal hypertension. PSVS is a rare condition and is classified into two major categories, intrahepatic and extrahepatic variants according to the site of the shunt. Congenital extrahepatic portosystemic venous shunt (EPSVS) is a rare condition in which the porto-mesenteric blood drains into a systemic vein, bypassing the liver through a complete or partial shunt; in this condition the anastomoses are established between a systemic vein and the porto-mesenteric vasculature before division of the portal vein (PV). Morgan and Superina (1994) classified EPSVS into two types; in type 1 there is a complete diversion of portal blood into the systemic circulation (*end-to-side shunt*), with absent intrahepatic portal branches (Fig. 1). Moreover type 1 shunt is subdivided into two classes in which splenic vein (SV) and superior mesenteric vein (SMV) drain separately into a systemic vein—inferior vena cava (type 1a)—those in which drain together after joining to form a common trunk (type 1b) (Howard and Davenport 1997). In type 1 EPSVS liver is not perfused with portal blood because of complete shunt of portal blood flow into systemic circulation and liver transplantation is the only effective

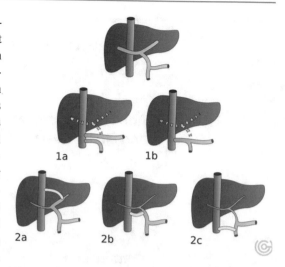

Fig. 1 Classification of congenital extrahepatic portosystemic shunts (blue line: inferior vena cava (IVC); red line: splenic vein (SV) and superior mesenteric vein (SMV) and portal vein branches; yellow line: shunt). Normal anatomy of hepatic vasculature in the first figure above. Shunts before main portal vein division with "congenital absence of portal vein." Type 1: end-to-side shunt; type 1a: splenic vein (SV) and superior mesenteric vein (SMV) drain separately into inferior vena cava (IVC); type 1b: the SV and SMV drain together after joining to form a common trunk without supplying the liver. Type 2: the portal vein (PV) is normal or hypoplastic. Type 2a shunts arise from portal vein branches and include the patent ductus venous. In type 2b the shunts arise from the main portal vein, its bifurcation, or porto-mesenteric confluence. Type 2c porto-hepatic shunt is peripheral and arises from gastric, mesenteric, or splenic veins

treatment in critical cases. In type 2 EPSVS (Lautz et al. 2011) the intrahepatic portal vein (PV) is intact, but some of the portal flow is switched into a systemic vein through a *side-to-side shunt* (Fig. 1). Patients with type 1a EPSVS shunt are usually girls with cardiac or other congenital anomalies, including biliary atresia, oculo-auriculo-vertebral dysplasia (Goldenhar syndrome), situs inversus and polysplenia (Marois et al. 1979), and hepatic masses (Motoori et al. 1997). Type 1b EPSVS shunt usually occurs in boys without other associated anomalies or hepatic masses (Kohda et al. 1999). Patients with type 2 EPSVS shunts do not present gender preference and have fewer associated malformations (Murray et al. 2003).

Type 2 exhibits partial shunting and a hypoplastic portal vein with preserved hepatic flow and is subdivided into three forms: shunt type 2a arising from left or right portal vein (includes patent ductus venosus) (Uchino et al. 1999); shunt type 2b arising from a position between the bifurcation of the portal vein and the spleno-mesenteric confluence (Mboyo et al. 1995); and shunt type 2c arising from the mesenteric (or its superior rectal tributaries), gastric, or splenic veins and flowing into the renal vein, azygos vein, iliac veins, or their branches (Mizoguchi et al. 2001). In this case persistent portal circulation allows shunt surgical closure or embolization (Hu et al. 2008; Stringer 2008).

Intrahepatic portosystemic venous shunt (IPSVS) is an abnormal intrahepatic communication >1 mm in diameter between the intrahepatic portal vein and the hepatic veins or IVC. Park et al. (1990) subdivided them into type 1 (a single large vessel runs from the right branch of portal vein to the posterior surface of the livers and enters inferior vena cava); type 2 (a localized peripheral shunt in one hepatic segment that has one or more communications between peripheral branches of portal and hepatic veins); type 3 (an aneurysmal communication between peripheral portal vein and hepatic veins); type 4 (multiple communications between peripheral portal and hepatic veins are present in both lobes); and type 5 (persistent ductus venosus). The first two types are the most common. Embolization or surgery is performed if the shunt is symptomatic.

Congenital portosystemic venous shunts (PSVS) are rare (1/30,000 births) (Bernard et al. 2012) and their clinical manifestations are various and can be divided into three types:

– *Conditions due to the abnormal liver development*: adenoma, focal nodular hyperplasia (Grazioli et al. 2000), hemangioma due to the alteration in local hemodynamics, hepatic ischemia with the compensatory increase in arterial flow, and associated elevated circulating levels of hepatic growth factors (e.g., insulin, glucagon, hepatocyte growth factor). Possible evolution into hepatoblastoma and hepatocellular carcinoma has been reported (Pupulim et al. 2013).

– *Shunt-related symptoms* such as hepatic encephalopathy for the increase of serum levels of ammonia, galactose, and other toxic metabolites that cannot be absorbed by the failing liver (Murray et al. 2003); hepato-pulmonary syndrome and pulmonary hypertension due to the deviation of vasoactive mediators in the systemic circulation, with consequent dilation of intrapulmonary vessels, are the most prominent manifestations caused by long-term portosystemic shunting (Sokollik et al. 2013).

– *Symptoms secondary to the congenital anomalies associated* (Badea et al. 2012) with abnormalities such as polysplenia (Newman et al. 2010), congenital heart disease (septal defects, patent ductus arteriosus, tetralogy of Fallot), biliary system (congenital biliary atresia, choledochal cyst), malrotation, duodenal atresia, annular pancreas, situs inversus, anomalies of the renal tract (cystic dysplasia of kidneys), skeletal anomalies (radial hypoplasia), Down syndrome (Figs. 2 and 3), and Turner syndrome (Kim et al. 2012) (Table 1).

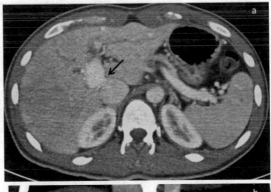

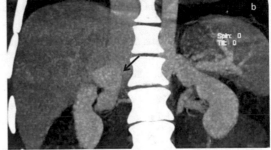

Fig. 2 Type 2. Contrast-enhanced CT, transverse (**a**) and coronal (**b**) planes. Portal vein is patent. Shunt (black arrow) between the intrahepatic portal vein and the inferior vena cava (**a**) placed cranially to the right renal vein (**b**) and caudally to the hepatic veins

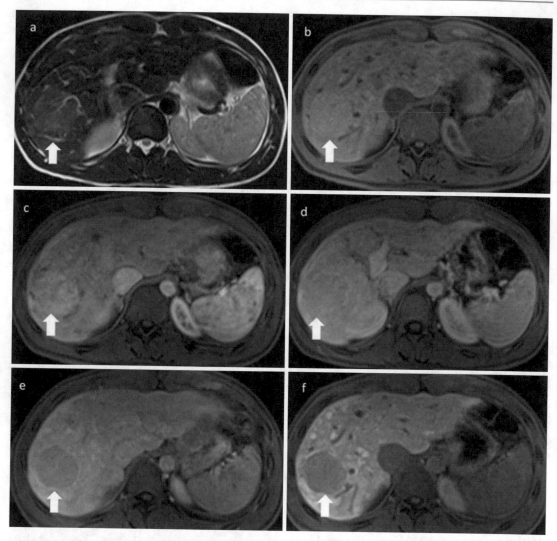

Fig. 3 Hepatic adenoma proven histologically in a 26-year-old boy with Down syndrome and Abernethy syndrome. On MR mass of 4 cm in the right hepatic lobe tenuously hyperintense on T2-w (**a**) and iso-hyperintense on T1-w fat sat pre-contrast (**b**) and post-contrast enhancement: tenuously hyperintense on arterial phase (**c**), isointense on portal phase (**d**), hypointense on late phase (**e**) and hepatobiliary phase (**f**)

Table 1 Congenital anomalies associated with congenital portosystemic shunt

Cardiovascular	*Gastrointestinal*
Atrial ventricular septal defect	Polysplenia
Patent ductus arteriosus	Biliary atresia
Ventricular septal defect	Choledochal cyst
Tetralogy of Fallot	Annular pancreas
Dextrocardia[*]	Duodenal atresia
Mesocardia[*]	*Genitourinary anomalies*
Congenital stenosis of aortic valve[*]	Multicystic dysplastic kidney
Vascular anomalies	Bilateral ureteropelvic stenosis
Double inferior vena cava	Vesicoureteral reflux
Interruption of the inferior vena cava	Crossed fused renal ectopia
Genetic syndromes	Hypospadias
Down, Bannayan-Riley-Ruvalcaba, Turner, Holt-Oram, Grazioli and Goldenhar, LEOPARD, Rendu-Osler-Weber, Noonan	*Cutaneous vascular malformations and tumors*
	Skeletal anomalies
	[*]Rarely observed

1.2 Imaging Findings

Most often, the diagnosis is made primarily with US and Doppler US when patients undergo an US scan for other reasons. CT angiography (Prokop 2000) and MR angiography (MRA) are used for further classification of the shunt and assessment of accompanying anomalies. DSA is necessary when results of the other tests disagree or are inconclusive for hepatic and portal vein pressure measurement or when TIPS positioning and portal vein embolization are necessary. About imaging CT or MR (Gallego et al. 2004) combined with Doppler US permits a comprehensive evaluation of morphologic and functional abnormalities of the portal system.

According to the diagnostic criteria proposed by Ohwada et al. (1994), it is possible to diagnose congenital portosystemic shunts in the absence of hypersplenism and portal hypertension; in the absence of remarkable microscopic change in liver samples, and not like those that occur in the course of idiopathic portal hypertension, hepatitis, or cirrhosis, the portal vein must be hypoplastic without arterio-portal fistula; there are no previous stories of abdominal surgery or inflammation.

US is the first-choice test because it is noninvasive and does not expose to ionizing radiation and it is neither necessary to seduce young patients. The experience and a good operator, associated with a careful knowledge of the anatomy of the hepatic and abdominal vessels and related venous abnormalities, contribute to accurate diagnosis of EPSVS (Hu et al. 2008). A decrease in the size of the liver or an increase in echogenicity of the periportal spaces can be observed; however these findings are nonspecific. The US findings include abnormal cystic or tubular, anechoic, serpiginous vascular structures which seem to communicate the portal with the systemic circulation (Tsitouridis et al. 2009). Moreover, this method is also widely used for prenatal screening or as an intraoperative investigation technique (Achiron et al. 2009). US may fail to accurately demonstrate the associated extrahepatic shunts (Massin et al. 1999; Nakasaki et al. 1989). Therefore, once the anomaly has been identified, it is passed to Doppler US which

is useful for determining the flow direction of the identified vessels (Konno et al. 1997). Doppler US study can confirm the vascular nature of the structures and calculate the shunt ratio (total blood flow volume in the shunt divided by the blood flow in the portal vein). It has been recommended that a shunt ratio greater than 60% should be corrected to prevent complications (Ohwada et al. 1994).

These patients usually do not present portal hypertension imaging characteristics such as ascites, varices, or splenomegaly (Murray et al. 2003). CT and MRI are useful to confirm the diagnosis of congenital portosystemic shunt and to identify the absent vessels and the type of vascular malformation (Gallego et al. 2004; Kornprat et al. 2005). Post-processing techniques, such as maximum intensity projection, multiplanar reformation, and volume rendering, provide additional information. MRA can also confirm congenital absence of portal vein and visualize the portosystemic shunt (Kornprat et al. 2005). Multidetector CT has also been shown to show small vascular branches and has a spatial resolution higher than the MRI (Prokop 2000). However, the use of CT in evaluating these patients is not regularly recommended because it involves exposure to ionizing radiation, as these are very often paediatric patients. MRI is also a reliable and noninvasive diagnostic modality for the portal venous system (Usuki and Miyamoto 1998). MR imaging can be used in the diagnosis of congenital portosystemic shunt but the definitive diagnosis can only be made with catheter DSA (Matsuoka et al. 1992) and with additional histological analysis of the hepatic parenchyma that demonstrates the absence of hepatic portal venules within the portal triad (Collard et al. 2006). However, DSA has the disadvantage of exposure to radiation and requires anesthesia and a vascular puncture with its complications. DSA is not the gold standard for children, even if it is safe enough (Usuki and Miyamoto 1998). For these reasons DSA is reserved only in cases in which treatment is considered necessary. Indirect mesenteric porto-venography is usually the angiographic technique used to clarify the anatomy of the portal system and depict the characteristics of an extrahepatic shunt. This technique is performed during the visceral phase of mesenteric arteriography. When it cannot provide a distinct image of the shunt, transhepatic percutaneous portography may be required. With this technique, selective embolization can be performed in type 2 shunt as a possible therapy. Transvenous liver biopsy and measurement of pressure gradients can also be performed at the same time (Hu et al. 2008). Finally the portal scintigraphy performed with rectal administration of iodine 123-iodoamphetamine may be for the evaluation of type 2 shunts and for calculating the shunt ratio. The portosystemic shunt index is calculated dividing the lung accounts for the liver and lung counts (Kashiwagi et al. 1988). Shunt reports of more than 5% are considered abnormal (Uchino et al. 1996). If a portosystemic shunt is present, the isotope is detected in liver and lungs simultaneously.

Imaging is useful also for the evaluation of focal hepatic lesions (regenerative nodular hyperplasia, focal nodular hyperplasia, or hepatocellular adenoma) (Goo 2007) that very often occur in patients with this malformation and that present a histological variety in the nature of the nodules but their growth and development seem to depend on the degree of arterial supply. In particular regenerative nodular hyperplasia and focal nodular hyperplasia are more often atypical than in patients with normal livers and may enlarge over time; for complete and chronic portal deprivation often there are atypias (Kim et al. 2004).

Nodular regenerative lesions on MRI are homogeneous, well defined, and frequently multiple; on T1-w images are hyperintense, on T2-w images are more variable, and on T2-w images are isointense to slightly hyperintense. The lesions show arterial hyperenhancement and remain isointense to slightly hyperintense on portal venous, equilibrium, and delayed-phase images. This tendency for these lesions to remain hyperintense on portal venous and delayed phases is different from other benign lesions that become isointense as well as from HCC that shows venous phase washout and appears hypointense to the liver parenchyma (Alonso-Gamarra et al. 2011). The contrastographic behavior is the same also on CT and CEUS (Bartolozzi and Lencioni 2001). Another aspect that distinguishes them is the absence of fat (present instead in the adenoma), calcification, and hemorrhage. Some may be surrounded by a peripheral hypointense border on MRI, hypodense border on the CT images, and a hypoechoic border on US, due to sinusoidal dilation and marked congestion in the surrounding liver (the "sign of the halo") (Wanless 1990). A "coral atoll-like appearance" has also been reported on US for nodular regenerative hyperplasia. This refers to a peripheral hyperechoic rim surrounding a focal liver lesion (Caturelli et al. 2011).

MRI of the brain (Córdoba 2011) may reveal deposition of paramagnetic substances in the basal ganglia related to chronic portosystemic shunting and white matter atrophy or a hyperintense basal ganglia (globus pallidus) on T1-w images.

For this rare condition it is important to focalize the presence or absence of hepatic portal vein supply and the course of the shunt to decide the appropriate therapeutic option; imaging plays a crucial role in the diagnosis and follow-up of patients.

2 Simple Cysts

The detection of hepatic cysts in subjects who undergo an imaging examination for other reasons is not infrequent. The finding of hepatic cysts is more common in women (Farges and Aussilhou 2012). Based on margins and content, hepatic cysts can be divided into simple and complex cysts. This distinction is important because it may be necessary to make further diagnoses and treatments. Simple hepatic cysts are generally round or ovoid structures that have a subtle wall. Microscopically, the liver cysts contain serous liquid, bile-like fluid, and are covered with a single layer of cuboidal epithelial cells, and a thin rim of fibrous stroma around. Their origin derives from aberrant bile ducts that have lost communication with the biliary tree and continue to secrete intraluminal fluid (Benhamou and

Menu 1994). Probably they originate from hamartomatous tissue (Van Sonnenberg et al. 1994). Hepatic cysts are common and are presumed to be present in almost 2.5% of the population. They are almost always asymptomatic. They can also reach considerable sizes of up to 30 cm (Mathieu et al. 1997). Complex cysts (Table 2) have internal septa, wall thickening, or nodularity, which may present contrast enhancement to radiological investigations; the fluid contains debris, or proteinaceous or hemorrhagic material. Complex cysts may be of neoplastic, inflammatory, infectious, or post-traumatic origin or even present other etiologies (Vachha et al. 2011). Intracystic hemorrhage is a rare complication of simple cysts and usually presents with severe abdominal pain (Salemis et al. 2007), although in some cases it may be completely asymptomatic (Kitajima et al. 2003). Hepatic cysts are generally asymptomatic and treatment with aspiration sclerotherapy or with laparoscopic or open surgical fenestration techniques (Moorthy et al. 2001) of the cyst may be necessary when they reach large dimensions to avoid complications such as biliary obstruction, rupture with hemorrhage, and hemoperitoneum.

The feedback of the following characteristics allows an highly likely diagnosis of cyst: spherical or oval in shape, with smooth and sharp edges and strong echoes of the rear walls (which indicate an interface fluid/well-defined tissue) in an anechoic content (i.e., cavity filled with liquid), without septa (Spiegel et al. 1978). After CEUS, simple cysts (or those complicated by hemorrhage or infection) show no vascularization of contents and walls in all the vascular phases (Vidili et al. 2018). On CT a simple hepatic cyst appears round or ovoid, well defined, homogeneous, with hypo-attenuation (0–10 UH) which does not improve after intravenous contrast medium administration. The uncomplicated cysts are almost never septate (Murphy et al. 1989). MRI also shows a well-defined lesion content liquid that does not show contrast enhancement. On the basis of these features, imaging alone is sufficient to establish an accurate diagnosis (Figs. 4 and 5) and follow-up of a simple hepatic cyst (Mathieu et al. 1997).

3 Ductal Plate Malformation

Ductal plate malformations represent a complex continuum of pathological abnormalities encountered depending on the level of the biliary tree affected (intrahepatic and/or extrahepatic biliary ducts; large, medium, or smaller intrahepatic biliary ducts) during embryogenesis. Jorgensen

Table 2 US findings of hepatic cyst

Simple cyst	Complex cyst
Thin, smooth walls	Mural irregularity or nodularity
Zero to two septa	Septated
Anechoic content	Debris, calcification, fluid levels

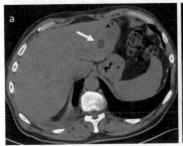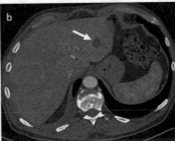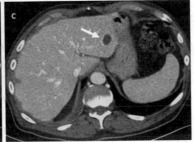

Fig. 4 Simple hepatic cyst (arrow) on (**a**) unenhanced and contrast-enhanced CT on (**b**) hepatic arterial and (**c**) portal venous phase

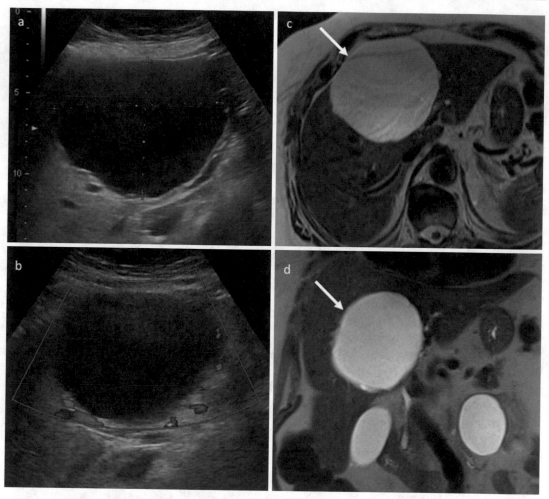

Fig. 5 Large hepatic cyst (calipers) with diffuse posterior acoustic enhancement on grayscale US (**a**) and on color Doppler US (**b**); T2-w turbo spin-echo MRI sequence on transverse (**c**) and coronal planes (**d**). The cystic lesion (arrow) appears hyperintense without evidence of peripheral capsule or septa

(1977) was the first to describe ductal plate malformations in 1977. The ductal plate is a transient structure along the branches of the portal vein, in the embryonic life, and corresponding to the most immature state of the bile duct. During the first 8 weeks after fertilization, the developing liver is composed only of hepatoblasts, along portal vein; no bile ducts have yet formed (Desmet 1992). These hepatoblasts are bipotential cells and are capable of differentiating into hepatocytes or cholangiocytes (bile duct cells)

(Dcsmct 1992; Krause et al. 2002). The hepatoblast cell layer in contact with mesenchyme surrounding the portal vein produces cytokeratins 8 and 18 present in the hepatoblasts, to which is added the cytokeratin 7 marker of the biliary cells. This layer of cells joins with a second layer to create a double-epithelial cylinder of biliary cell type, called the ductal plate (Lonergan et al. 2000). A narrow lumen is present between these ductal plate layers. During the next several weeks, ductal plate remodeling occurs in three phases. First, several focal dilatations, called peripheral tubules, form between the two ductal plate layers and become the intrahepatic bile ducts (Hassan and Ellethy 2014). Second, with continued remodeling of the ductal plate, the hepatic artery branch appears in the periportal mesenchyme. Finally, the peripheral tubules become incorporated into the periportal mesenchyme, and residual non-tubular segments of the ductal plate disappear by apoptosis. Thus, within each portal triad, a tubular bile duct is surrounded by portal connective tissue. Any interruption in the remodeling of the ductal plate may result in persistence of the excess embryonic epithelial duct structures, called exactly ductal plate malformation (Jorgensen 1977) which can affect the intra- or extrahepatic biliary ductal system further delineating the spectrum of clinic-pathological appearances; for example, malformations of the larger extrahepatic biliary ducts result in choledochal cysts; involvement of large- and medium-sized intrahepatic ducts results in Caroli disease and autosomal dominant polycystic liver disease—ADPLD—(for the latter see chapter "Fibropohlycystic Liver Diseases"), respectively; small-sized intrahepatic duct involvement results in biliary hamartomas and congenital hepatic fibrosis (Fig. 6).

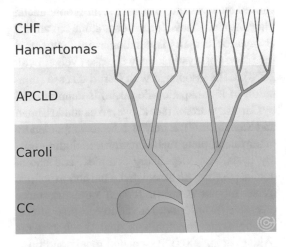

Fig. 6 Schematic illustration showing the types of ductal plate malformations depending on the duct size affected. *CHF* congenital hepatic fibrosis, *APLD* adult polycystic liver disease, *CC* choledochal cysts

3.1   Biliary Hamartomas

Biliary hamartomas (BH), also known as micro-hamartomas or von Meyenburg complex, because initially described by the Swiss pathologist Hanns von Meyenburg in 1918, are considered as malformation of small intralobular bile ducts (Yonem et al. 2006) embedded in abundant fibrous stroma; they are benign hepatic lesions resulting from developmental malformation of the ductal plate (Desmet 2005). According to Raynaud et al. (2011) there are three main mechanisms that can explain the malformations of the ductal plate, in particular when the apicobasal polarity is systematically interrupted. These mechanisms consist of abnormal differentiation of hepatoblasts in bile cells, abnormal maturation of the primitive biliary structure in bile ducts, and abnormal expansion of the duct. BH are a rare and usually isolated asymptomatic entity, and are usually discovered incidentally (Karahan et al. 2007). They are seen in 5.6% of adults and 0.9% of children at autopsy, and often are associated with polycystic kidney and liver disease (Redston and Wanless 1996). Patients with BH have relatively small cystic lesions, ranging in size from less than 5–10 mm in diameter (Luo et al. 1998), but some may reach up to 3 cm and BH are multiple, up to about 10, scattered throughout both liver lobes, predominantly in the subcapsular and periportal areas. Microscopically, they consist of irregularly shaped, dilated, branching bile ducts surrounded by abundant fibrous stroma. The ducts have a cuboidal epithelial lining and can contain bile or amorphous materials (Duran-Vega et al. 2000). Typically, BH appear well circumscribed but not encapsulated and might be exchanged with hepatic metastases, lymphoma, and simple liver cysts. In addition, BH are associated with increased risk of hepatobiliary carcinomas (Brancatelli et al. 2005). It is asymptomatic and does not compromise liver function. Definitive diagnosis requires liver biopsy (Zheng et al. 2005).

Imaging findings are usually not specific. On US BH present as innumerable tiny hypoechoic or hyperechoic lesion and are distributed uniformly throughout the liver that often appears exactly heterogeneous and coarse (Pech et al. 2016). These tiny micronodules may demonstrate "comet-tail artifacts" (Lev-Toaff et al. 1995) which explains why they are difficult to differentiate from aerobilia and from intrahepatic stones. Bright echogenic foci without mass effect can be seen and are attributed to periductal fibrosis crowding the interface between dilated bile ducts (Tan et al. 1989). Differences in echogenicity may be due to the size of the dilated bile duct component, which, at a certain size, would behave like other microcystic structures and demonstrate echogenicity. The lesions that affect all segments of the liver give a "honeycomb" (Ryu et al. 2012) pattern with heterogeneous echo texture (Zheng et al. 2005). On CT the lesions are depicted as multiple, round, hypoattenuated lesions without enhancement after contrast medium administration and with dimension of less than 15 mm distributed throughout the liver (Brancatelli et al. 2005) in the subcapsular and periportal areas. They are difficult to characterize due to their small size and in some cases it is impossible to exclude the possibility that the lesions are small metastases, in particular in patients with known primary neoplasm. On precontrast T1- and T2-weighted MRI, lesions appear hypointense and hyperintense, respectively, and are generally well defined. On DWI MRI, they mimic cystic lesions. At MRCP (Fig. 7) the multiple tiny cystic lesions demonstrate no communication with the biliary tree. And also the nodules do not show enhancement after administration of hepatospecific contrast agents, because the lesions are independent and do not communicate with the biliary system (Mortele et al. 2002). The lesions may demonstrate thin rim enhancement with gadolinium, because the liver parenchyma that surrounds is compressed (Semelka et al. 1999). MRCP and, more generally, heavily T2-w MRI sequences are essential for differential diagnosis with Caroli disease (see below) (Krause et al. 2002). Differential diagnosis includes metastases, intrahepatic stones, peribiliary cysts, other ductal plate malformations such as Caroli disease and polycystic liver disease, and intrahepatic cholangiocarcinoma (Jain et al. 2010).

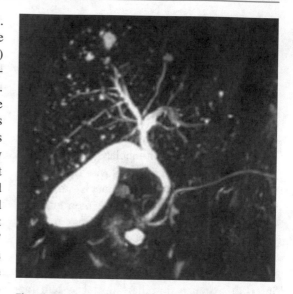

Fig. 7 Multiple biliary hamartomas in asymptomatic 55-year-old man. Three-dimensional T2-w MRCP with maximum intensity projection 3D reconstruction shows innumerable cysts that are nearly uniform in size and are distributed throughout the liver. The biliary tree has a normal appearance; MRI findings suggest biliary hamartomas

3.2 Congenital Hepatic Fibrosis (CHF)

CHF is a developmental malformation of ductal plate and is characterized by aberrant interlobular bile duct proliferation and periductal fibrosis. It is caused by a premature arrest in embryonic ductal plate into bile ducts. It can occur alone but almost always occurs in association with autosomal recessive polycystic kidney disease (Veigel et al. 2008). CHF associated with Caroli disease (dilatation of intrahepatic bile ducts) is denominated by Caroli syndrome (see above) (Ananthakrishnan and Saeian 2007); it may also be accompanied by other ductal plate malformations, including biliary cysts, von Meyenburg complex, and choledochal cyst or with associated renal abnormalities (renal tubular ectasia). It is a rare autosomal recessive disorder with a variable course affecting both the hepatobiliary and renal systems (Akhan et al. 2007). Associated renal conditions include renal dysplasia, autosomal recessive polycystic kidney disease (ARPKD) (Cobben et al. 1990), and nephronophthisis (medullary cystic disease). CHF appears both sporadically and in a familial form. The age of onset ranges from early childhood to the fifth and sixth decades of life (Veigel et al. 2008). CHF has been described in four clinical forms: portal hypertensive, cholangitic, mixed portal hypertensive-cholangitic, and latent forms (D'agata et al. 1994). Symptoms may manifest early in life, in childhood, or in adult life, and include portal hypertension and upper gastrointestinal hemorrhage from ruptured esophageal varices (Kerr et al. 1978). Major complications of CHF consist of ascending cholangitis, hepatic failure, cirrhosis, and an increased risk of HCC. CHF consists histologically of broad, densely collagenous fibrous bands surrounding otherwise normal hepatic lobules. The fibrous band contains numerous small, uniform bile ducts, some of which can be dilated and irregularly shaped and can contain bile and traces of mucin. The ductal lining consists of cuboidal or low columnar epithelial cells. The hepatic parenchyma is subdivided by the overgrowth of portal fibrous tissue, while the regenerative activities of subdivided parenchyma are not evident, thus differing from cirrhotic regenerative nodules. In addition, portal vein branches are hypoplastic or unidentifiable in the fibrous portal tracts. Arterial branches are normal or hypoplastic, while the veins appear reduced in size. Inflammatory changes are not seen (Desmet 1998). In typical CHF, cysts are not visible due to their very small size. Liver biopsy is essential for diagnosis, but because of the firm consistency of the liver it may be difficult.

Imaging with US, CT, and MRI has roles in the evaluation of CHF. On US, CHF demonstrates increased or heterogeneous echogenicity, hyperechoic portal triads, and poorly defined portal vessels, secondary to fibrosis and ductular proliferation (Lowe and Schlesinger 2007). US can also evaluate biliary duct and liver parenchymal abnormalities, such as bile duct dilatation, regenerative nodules, hepatosplenomegaly, and periportal thickening (Akhan et al. 2007). Doppler US studies can be utilized to evaluate the patency of the portal vein and the flow direction in the portal and hepatic veins and detect portal

hypertension in patients with suspected vascular complications related to liver cirrhosis. Zeitoun et al. (2004) retrospectively analyzed 18 patients with CHF. Suggestive morphological findings highly characteristic for CHF are hypertrophy of the left lateral segment and caudate, and normal or hypertrophic left medial segment and atrophic right lobe. Other hepatic elements related to CHF are varices, splenomegaly, portal hypertension, and periportal cuffing indicative of fibrotic process. CT may also demonstrate associated ductal plate abnormalities (biliary hamartoma, Caroli disease), and non-hepatic features such as renal abnormalities. On MRI periportal hepatic fibrosis is seen as high signal intensity among portal vessels on T2-w images and especially T2-w half-Fourier acquisition single-shot turbo spin-echo (HASTE) images beautifully depict these tiny proliferating ductules distributed along portal ramifications. MRCP (Ernst et al. 1998) can be utilized to detail the biliary tree, when associated with Caroli disease, and illustrates dilated biliary ducts. Presence of cholangitis may be assessed with post-gadolinium T1-weighted images or regenerative nodules may also be easily characterized.

Differential diagnosis includes cirrhosis due to other causes (alcohol, viral). Features that help discern the differential diagnosis are that the medial segment is normal in size or enlarged in CHF, but is usually small in patients with cirrhosis due to other causes. About complications of this disease, portal hypertension, esophageal varices, HCC (Ghadir et al. 2011), cholangiocarcinoma, amyloidosis, and adenomatous hyperplasia of the liver (Vilgrain et al. 2016) are reported in patients with CHF. Recurrent uncontrolled cholangitis is an indication for liver transplantation.

3.3 Caroli Disease and Caroli Syndrome

Caroli disease was first described by Caroli et al. (1958) as a congenital condition in which the larger (segmental) intrahepatic bile ducts are dilated. It is a rare complex autosomal recessive congenital disorder characterized by nonobstructive communicating saccular or fusiform dilatations of the large intrahepatic bile ducts. Important associations with Caroli disease include CHF ARPKD (Hussman et al. 1991; Jordon et al. 1989), choledochal cyst (Henry et al. 1987), medullary sponge kidney, and nephronophthisis (medullary cystic kidney disease) (Torra et al. 1997). If the defective remodeling involves the entire intrahepatic biliary tree, Caroli syndrome - CS - (a combination of Caroli disease and CHF) develops. CS is characterized by varying degrees of persistent embryonic bile duct structures, fibrosis, and ductal dilatation. In addition, Caroli disease and CS have also been associated with other hepatorenal fibrocystic diseases including Meckel–Gruber syndrome, cerebellar vermis hypo/aplasia, oligophrenia, ataxia congenital, coloboma, and hepatic fibrosis syndrome (COACH) syndrome, Joubert syndrome and related disorders, Bardet–Biedl syndrome, and oral–facial–digital syndrome. Caroli disease is very rare, with 1 case per 1,000,000 people (Freidman et al. 2007). The liver may be diffusely affected, or the ductal abnormalities more frequently may be localized to one segment or lobe, most commonly the left lobe (Boyle et al. 1989), and in any case less than 50% of the hepatic surface. The pathogenesis of Caroli disease is related to a partial or complete arrest of remodeling of the ductal plate of the large intrahepatic bile ducts (Desmet 1992). The molecular pathogenesis of Caroli disease and syndrome is incompletely understood. The dilated ducts are lined by biliary epithelium that may be hyperplastic and ulcerated. The age of presentation ranges from infants to young adults. About symptoms of Caroli disease the saccular or fusiform dilatation of bile ducts predisposes to stagnation of bile leading to the formation of biliary sludge, intraductal lithiasis, and bacterial cholangitis that may be complicated by septicemia and hepatic abscess formation. Other symptoms include abdominal pain from bile stasis or passage of stones, fever, and right upper quadrant pain when cholangitis is present (Murray-Lyon et al. 1972), which can present with fever and right upper quadrant pain. Jaundice is rarely present in these patients. Secondary biliary cirrhosis can occur due to biliary obstruction. Patients with CS can present with portal hypertension and its sequelae, ascites, and esophageal variceal hemorrhage. Pruritus and hepatomegaly are common. Children with CS usually have an earlier onset of symptoms and a more rapidly progressive disease because of the combined effects of cholangitis and portal hypertension. Caroli disease is a risk factor for malignancy, as neoplastic changes occur in 7% of patients (Arcement et al. 2000).

On US, Caroli's disease appears as well-defined intrahepatic cystic anechoic lesions and calculi or sludge within these cystic areas may increase the echogenicity and may also appear heterogeneous (Marchal et al. 1986). Similarly, contrast-enhanced CT and MRI demonstrate intrahepatic saccular or fusiform cystic areas with sizes measuring up to 5 cm, which often contains calculi and sludge. Peculiar sign is "the central dot sign" fibrovascular bundle lying centrally within the dilated duct that contains a portal vein radically that enhances with contrast (seen as hyper-enhancing or hyperintense focus), (Choi et al. 1990). On MRCP (Figs. 8 and 9) these cystic areas are seen communicating with the bile ducts and it is useful for demonstrating the characteristic features of saccular dilated, non-obstructed, intrahepatic bile ducts that communicate with the biliary tree (Brancatelli et al. 2005). The main differential consideration includes primary sclerosing cholangitis, polycystic liver disease (Fig. 10), and recurrent pyogenic cholangitis. Complications (Miller et al. 1995) are usually a consequence of bile stasis predisposing to recurrent cholangitis, abscess formation, biliary cirrhosis, and occasionally cholangiocarcinoma.

3.4 Choledochal Cyst

Choledochal cysts (Fig. 11) are a congenital dilatation of the extrahepatic and/or intrahepatic bile ducts. Choledochal cysts are classified into five

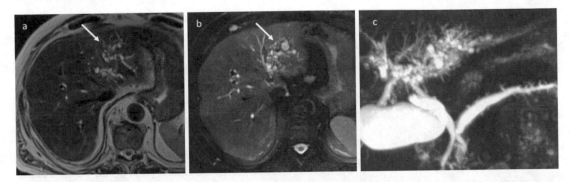

Fig. 8 Caroli disease. (**a**) TSE T2-weighted MRI sequence; (**b**) fat-saturated TSE T2-weighted MRI sequence; (**c**) MR cholangiography. Left liver lobe cystic lesions (arrows) connected with the intrahepatic biliary tree

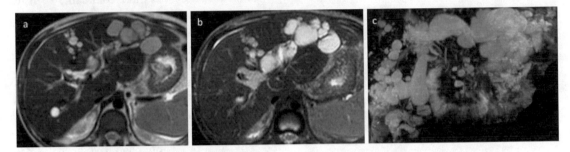

Fig. 9 Caroli disease. (**a**) TSE T2-weighted MRI sequence; (**b**) fat-saturated TSE T2-weighted MRI sequence; (**c**) MR cholangiography. Right and left liver lobe cystic lesions (arrows) connected with the intrahepatic biliary tree

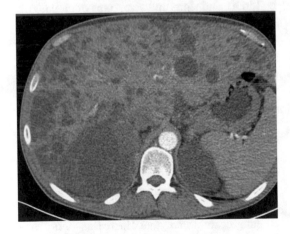

Fig. 10 Polycystic liver disease. Contrast-enhanced CT. Multiple cystic lesions with variable sizes on both liver segments

types based on the Todani modification of the Alonso-Lej classification (Lenriot et al. 1998).

Type I cystic (Ia), segmental (Ib), or fusiform (Ic) dilation of the common bile duct, as well as part or all of the common hepatic duct

and extrahepatic portions of the left and right hepatic ducts: A further group (Id, not represented) has been suggested with multiple extrahepatic cysts. Differentiation between the fusiform type and dilation of the bile duct secondary to obstruction is based on the absence of a previous history of gallstones or biliary surgery, a common bile duct diameter >30 mm, and presence of an anomalous bile duct junction shown on cholangiography (Lipsett et al. 1994). Type Ia cysts are associated with abnormal pancreaticobiliary junction and the cystic duct and gallbladder arise from the dilated common bile duct. Type Ib is segmental dilation of an extrahepatic bile duct, often the distal common bile duct. Type Ic is dilation of all the extrahepatic bile ducts and dilation extends from the pancreatobiliary junction, that is anomalous, to the extrahepatic portions of the left and right hepatic ducts. Type Id is cystic dilation of the common duct and cystic duct. This group accounts for 50–85% of all bile duct cysts.

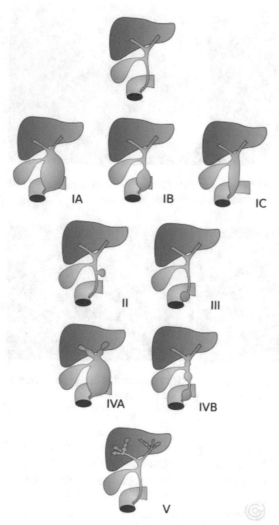

Fig. 11 Classification of choledochal cysts according to Todani modification of the Alonso-Lej classification

intrahepatic bile duct involvement: Type IVa shows intrahepatic and extrahepatic cystic dilations with a distinct change in duct caliber and/or a stricture at the hilum, features that help differentiate it from a type Ic cyst. Type IVb presents multiple extrahepatic cysts but no intrahepatic cysts. It is the second most common type of bile duct cyst (10%).

Type V is characterized by one or more cystic dilations of the intrahepatic ducts, without extrahepatic duct disease known as Caroli disease. It accounts for 1–5% of a bile duct cyst.

Choledochal cyst is more commonly seen in East Asian populations, with a female-to-male ratio of approximately 3.5:1 (Lipsett and Pitt 2003). The majority of patients (60%) are diagnosed before the age of 10 years but the disease can be diagnosed at any age (Sela-Herman and Scharschmidt 1996). Choledochal cysts may be an acquired condition thought to arise from an abnormal pancreaticobiliary junction. Cysts may be congenital or acquired and have been associated with a variety of anatomic abnormalities.

The clinical features include right upper quadrant mass, jaundice (more commonly seen in children), and signs and symptoms of cholangitis (more commonly seen in adults). Choledochal cysts vary in size and may contain as much as 10 L of bile. Microscopically, the cyst wall is fibrotic, thickened (in contrast to simple hepatic cyst which has a thin wall), and chronically inflamed. Bile can be seen within the wall. The epithelial lining of the cyst is usually denuded. When preserved, the lining consists of columnar epithelial cells. Intestinal metaplasia with abundant mucinous glands is a feature which is seen in almost all patients older than 15 years. Affected individuals have an increased risk of developing cholangiocarcinoma that increases with age (Nonomura et al. 1994).

About imaging at US, they appear as anechoic or hypoechoic fusiform or cystic lesions in the porta hepatis, which demonstrate communication with the biliary tree. The dilatated system may demonstrate echogenic sludge or stones. Transabdominal US has a sensitivity of 71–97% for diagnosing biliary cysts (Fulcher et al. 2001). Factors that may limit the usefulness of an

Type II cyst forms a diverticulum from the extrahepatic bile duct. It accounts for 2–3% of a bile duct cyst. It represents a true diverticulum. Saccular outpouching arises from the supraduodenal extrahepatic bile duct or the intrahepatic bile ducts.

Type III is cystic dilation (choledochocele) of the distal common bile duct lying mostly within the duodenal wall; it may arise embryologically as duodenal duplications involving the ampulla. It accounts for 1–5% of a bile duct cyst.

Type IV cysts are defined by the presence of multiple cysts and are subdivided based on their

US include the patient's body habitus and the presence of bowel gas that may limit visualization. CT and MRCP offer a noninvasive and accurate diagnosis. CT can detect all types of biliary cysts. It can demonstrate continuity of the cyst with the biliary tree and examine the relationship of the cyst to surrounding structures; it is useful for evaluating the presence of malignancy or for determining the extent of intrahepatic disease in patients with type IVA or V cysts. CT cholangiography with the usage of hepatobiliary excreted iodinated contrast (e.g. Meglumine iodoxamic acid) has been used in the past to delineate the anatomy of the biliary tree with high sensitivity (93%), but its sensitivity (64%) for imaging the pancreatic duct and for pancreatobiliary junction is poor (Lam et al. 1999). MRCP is considered the current gold standard for initial evaluation and diagnosis of choledochal cysts. MRCP techniques are able to accurately assess intra- and extrahepatic biliary anatomy and the pancreaticobiliary junction, and look for associated complications (Guo et al. 2012). On heavily T2-w sequences they are characterized by a hyperintense tubular, fusiform, or cystic structure. However, the detection of intraductal stones may be difficult on this sequence as the protein plugs commonly seen in the cysts are isointense to calculi and differentiation between the two is difficult. Hepatobiliary MR contrast agents allow for better visualization of the bile ducts (Figs. 12, 13, 14, and 15). Alternatively ERCP (Irie et al. 1998) can be used for diagnosis, but it is invasive and is associated with the risk of introducing infection into the dilated biliary system. It has a sensitivity of up to 100% for diagnosing biliary cysts (Keil et al. 2010).

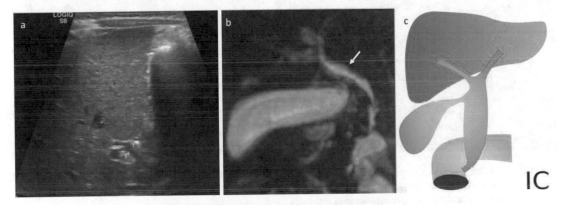

Fig. 12 Type IC choledochal cyst in a boy. (**a**) Transverse US and (**b**) MRCP image shows fusiform dilatation of the common bile duct (arrow) as shown in the scheme (**c**)

Fig. 13 Type IVa choledochal cyst MRCP image shows fusiform dilatation of the common bile duct and the intrahepatic bile duct

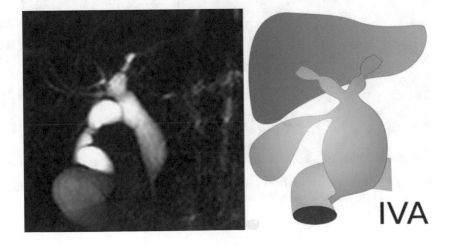

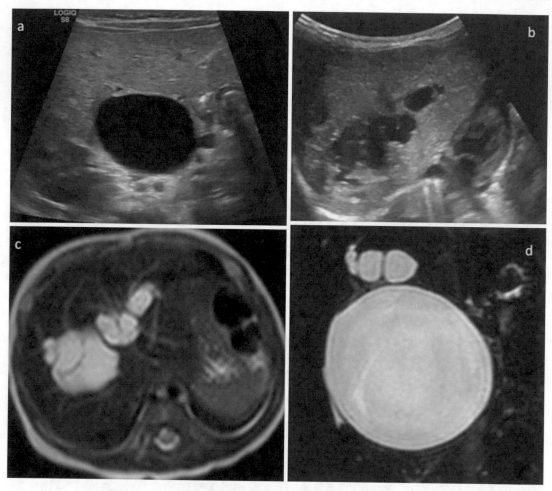

Fig. 14 Type IVa choledochal cyst: massive choledochal cyst on grayscale US (**a**) and (**b**), and on TSE T2-w MRI sequence axial (**c**) and coronal (**d**) planes, in a newborn with evidence of dilation of the common bile duct and intrahepatic bile duct

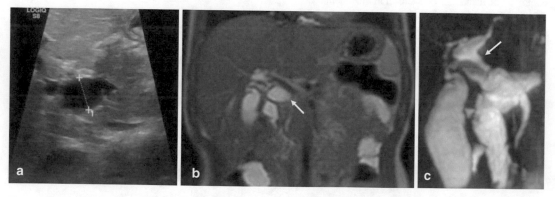

Fig. 15 Type IVa choledochal cyst US (**a**) and MRCP cholangiography images show dilatation of the common bile duct (arrow) (**b**) with evidence of the left intrahepatic bile duct (arrow) (**c**)

Biliary cysts should be differentiated from cysts that do not communicate with the biliary tree including pancreatic, mesenteric, and hepatic cysts and if doubt remains after cross-sectional imaging, hepatobiliary scintigraphy or endoscopic retrograde cholangiopancreatography (ERCP) can be performed to confirm that the cyst communicates with the biliary tree.

Choledochal cysts can be complicated by recurrent cholangitis, pancreatitis, cystolithiasis, and gallstones (70%) (Söreide et al. 2004).

4   Biliary Atresia

Also for this last paragraph, it is good to remember some notions of embryology of the liver (chap. 1 "Embryology and Development of the Liver") before reviewing the characteristics of diseases, biliary atresia (BA), and Alagille' syndrome (AGS).

Biliary atresia (BA) is a progressive, idiopathic, and severe neonatal disease caused by an inflammatory and fibrotic obliteration of the extrahepatic biliary tree. It results in cholestasis and progressive hepatic failure. BA occurs in 1 in 8000–18,000 live births and appears to be more frequent in Asians (Lin et al. 2011) and Africans than Europeans; it occurs in 1 in 15,000 live births in the United States (Hopkins et al. 2017) and it is more common in female than male children. Although the overall incidence is low, BA is the most common cause of neonatal jaundice for which surgery is indicated and the most common indication for liver transplantation in children because BA remains the most common cause of end-stage cirrhosis in children.

The possibility of BA is suggested by the clinical presentation of neonatal jaundice (Makin et al. 2009) and/or acholic stools. After the first 2 weeks of life, acholic stools and conjugated hyperbilirubinemia (cholestasis) must suggest BA as it represents 30–40% of the causes of biliary jaundice. BA is divided into three distinct clinical forms (Hartley et al. 2009) with different etiologic subgroups:

– BA without any other anomalies or malformations (isolated form 80% of patients): This pattern is sometimes referred to as "perinatal" BA, and (Schwarz et al. 2013) typically, these children are born without jaundice, but within the first 2 months of life, jaundice develops and stools become progressively acholic.
– BA in association with other congenital malformations (non-laterality defect, 5–10% of patients) is associated with major cardiovascular, gastrointestinal, and genitourinary malformations that include intestinal atresia, imperforate anus, kidney anomalies, and/or heart malformations (Schwarz et al. 2013) or chromosomal abnormalities such as trisomy 18, trisomy 21, or Turner syndrome.
– BA in association with laterality malformations (1–10% of patients): This pattern is also known as biliary atresia splenic malformation (BASM) or "embryonal" BA (Davenport et al. 1993). The laterality malformations include situs inversus, asplenia or polysplenia, intestinal malrotation, interrupted inferior vena cava, preduodenal portal vein, and cardiac anomalies.

In addition, cystic dilatation of biliary remnants may be seen in a small minority of cases of embryonal type biliary atresia (approximately 8% of cases); another variant is BA associated with cytomegalovirus (CMV) (Zani et al. 2015).

Several surgical classifications of BA have been proposed, for example Kasai classification (Kasai et al. 1976) that distinguishes type I (the common bile duct is obliterated while the proximal bile ducts are patent); type IIa (atresia of the hepatic duct, the cystic and common bile ducts are patent); type IIb (the cystic, common bile, and hepatic ducts are obliterated); and type III (atresia refers to discontinuity of the right and left hepatic ducts to the level of the porta hepatis, more than 90% of cases) (Fig. 16).

The pathogenesis of BA is incompletely understood but appears to be multifactorial; the genetic factors driving this inflammatory process and the molecular basis of phenotypic heteroge-

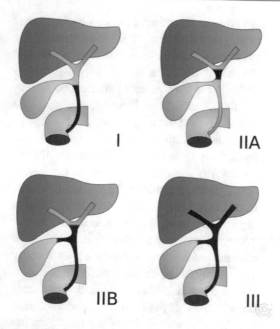

Fig. 16 Schematic illustration of biliary atresia

neity in affected infants remain undefined and many factors have been incriminated. Some of them may be related to a defect in early bile duct development (mainly observed in patients with several abnormalities) and some may arise during perinatal period, due to external factors, such as cytomegalovirus (Zani et al. 2015), reovirus (Szavay et al. 2002), rotavirus, environmental toxins and neonatal immune dysregulation. A possible association of congenital malformation with deletion of the gene GPC1, which is located on the longarm of chromosome 2 (2q37) (Al-Salem 2014)* and is usually responsible for identification of active and progressive inflammation, have been implicated in the pathogenesis of BA and early destruction of the biliary system. Finally, a definitive pathogenesis of BA remains uncertain.

After birth, most infants with BA are born at full term; the clinical triad of BA is jaundice (conjugated hyperbilirubinemia lasting beyond 2 weeks of life) (Wang 2015), acholic (white) stools, and dark urine, hepatosplenomegaly.

The first imaging examination to which the newborn is subjected is the US with the aim of evaluating the biliary tract and in the first instance to exclude other anatomical causes of cholestasis.

US evaluates the presence of liver masses, biliary ductal dilatation, choledochal cysts, vascular anomalies, signs of portal hypertension, and polysplenia. On US, furthermore, reduced gallbladder size (<15 mm) (Aziz et al. 2011) and shape (shrunk despite fasting), "triangular cord" sign (liver hilum, in the vicinity of the portal vein, appearing hyperechoic with thickness >4 mm) (So Mi Lee et al. 2015), gallbladder reduced contractility, and absence of the common bile duct can be suggestive of BA (Zhou et al. 2016). For evaluation of gallbladder contraction, the examination is repeated 60–90 min after the infant was fed. The volume of gallbladder is calculated using $V = 0.52 \times$ width $\times$ width $\times$ length. A diameter of the hepatic artery larger than 1.5 mm is considered as hepatic artery enlargement and it shows a sensitivity of 92%, a specificity of 87%, and an accuracy of 89% in the diagnosis of BA (Kim et al. 2007). In syndromic BA infants, US may show other features such as multiple spleens, preduodenal portal vein, absence of retrohepatic IVC, or abdominal situs inversus (Schwarz et al. 2013).

MRCP may be useful for the evaluation of the patency of intra- and extrahepatic biliary tree with reported diagnostic accuracy of 71–82% (Yang et al. 2009).

If no diagnosis emerges from the initial laboratory or imaging studies, hepatobiliary scintigraphy with a variety of 99mTc labelled iminodiacetic acid (IDA) agents is diagnostic imaging study that can be used to assess hepatocellular function and patency of the biliary system by tracing bile flow from the liver through the biliary system into the bowel. A lack of excretion of bile into the bowel is suggestive of extrahepatic occlusive disorders including BA (Kianifar et al. 2013). In case of failure to diagnose or when the gallbladder seems normal on US, cholangiography is needed to assess the morphology and patency of the biliary tree. Direct imaging of the biliary tree by cholangiography is performed either percutaneously (puncture of the gallbladder) (Lee et al. 2011) or endoscopically (ERCP) (Shanmugam et al. 2009). These procedures are invasive; however demonstration of a patent extrahepatic biliary tree effectively

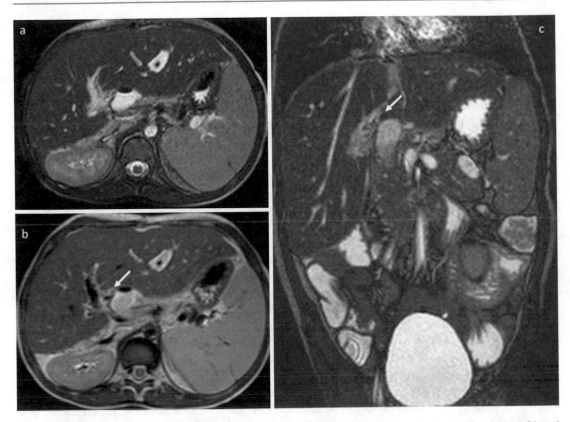

Fig. 17 Kasai portoenterostomy in a female with biliary atresia. TSE T2-w MRI sequences on transverse (**a**, **b**) and coronal planes (**c**)

excludes biliary atresia. At liver biopsy the main histopathologic features of BA are portal tracts with bile duct proliferation, portal tract edema, fibrosis and inflammation, and canalicular and bile duct bile plugs; the portal tracts are expanded by edema, neutrophilic infiltrate, and a prominent periportal ductular reaction (Kahn 2004). Portal fibrosis is progressive and the severity depends on the age at diagnosis and the duration of ductal obstruction. About 15% of cases show giant cell transformation of hepatocytes (Hussein et al. 2005). If BA is confirmed, Kasai hepatic portoenterostomy (HPE) is performed in the first months of life, in which the extrahepatic biliary system is surgically removed and replaced with a loop of intestine (Roux-en-Y anastomosis) that is connected directly to the portal area of the liver (Kasai and Suzuki 1959); it allows the restoration of bile flow and relief of obstruction (Fig. 17). The alternative is liver transplantation, when the

patients develop ascending cholangitis, progressive biliary cirrhosis, portal hypertension, esophageal varices, and ascites (Shneider et al. 2012). With the combination of HPE and liver transplantation, most children with BA now survive into adulthood (Hartley et al. 2009). About differential diagnosis, causes of neonatal cholestasis, such as Alagille syndrome, alpha-1-antitrypsin deficiency, sclerosing cholangitis with neonatal onset, and cystic fibrosis, must be excluded.

4.1 Alagille Syndrome

Alagille syndrome (AGS), also known as arteriohepatic dysplasia, is a complex, multisystemic, and an autosomal dominant disorder characterized by ductopenia (paucity of intrahepatic bile ducts) that causes cholestasis, in association with a wide range of extrahepatic subdivided into four main clinical abnormalities (Spinner et al. 2013): cardiac disease, skeletal abnormalities, ocular abnormalities, and characteristic facial features. This multisystem condition has an estimated frequency of 1 in 30,000 (Piccoli and Spinner 2001) and this disorder is localized to defects in the Notch signaling pathways: up to 98% are caused by mutations in JAG1, gene on chromosome 20p12, and 2% are caused by mutations in Notch-2 receptor, gene variant of unknown significance (Brennan and Kesavan 2017). JAG1 is a ligand of the Notch receptors; in turn the Notch activated by Jag1 plays a vital role in the regulation of cell differentiation, thereby controlling neurogenesis, hematopoiesis, myogenesis, somitogenesis, endocrinogenesis, and adipogenesis (Turnpenny and Ellard 2012). Disruption of the JAG1/Notch sequence leads to embryonic developmental abnormalities of many organs. Notch signaling has been shown to be essential in the development of the biliary tree during ductal plate remodeling because *JAG1* gene leads to overexpression of the hepatocyte growth factor (HGF) and that is thought to result in increased differentiation of the hepatic stem cells to hepatocytes and less to biliary cells, thus causing bile duct paucity. Of note, alteration in the expression of *JAG1* and Notch has also been reported in the course of chronic liver diseases (Fabris et al. 2007).

The hepatic phenotype is recognized by variable degrees of cholestasis, jaundice, and pruritus. Fibrosis is not a main feature of AGS and evolution to cirrhosis is rare; however in approximately 15% of cases it leads to liver transplantation (Emerick et al. 1999). In newborns with AGS, bile duct paucity is not always present and liver biopsy may demonstrate ductal proliferation portal inflammation, which may lead to a misdiagnosis of biliary atresia, and this is important because BA patients may undergo the Kasai procedure, which is not beneficial in AGS (Kaye et al. 2010); in late infancy and early childhood bile duct paucity appears to be progressive. Xanthomas, fatty deposits on the extensor surfaces, and failure to thrive due to fat malabsorption may also be there (Mouzaki et al. 2015). A small proportion of patients have no manifestations of liver disease.

About cardiac disease pulmonary vasculature is the most commonly involved. Peripheral pulmonary stenosis is the most common cardiac finding and the most common complex cardiac defect is tetralogy of Fallot; other cardiac malformations include ventricular septal defect, atrial septal defect, aortic stenosis, and coarctation of the aorta (Emerick et al. 1999).

The most common skeletal abnormalities are butterfly-shaped thoracic vertebrae, secondary to clefting abnormality of the vertebral bodies, narrowing of the interpedicular distance in the lumbar spine, pointed anterior process of C1, spina bifida occulta, and fusion of adjacent vertebrae and hemivertebrae, and absence of the 12th rib, a square shape of the proximal part of the fingers with tapering distal phalanges and extra digital flexion creases (Turnpenny et al. 2007). There may be an increase in pathological long-bone fractures in AGS, which may be due to cholestasis and/or an intrinsic defect of the bones.

Ocular abnormalities in individuals with AGS are posterior embryotoxon (a prominent Schwalbe's ring), a defect in the anterior chamber of the eye (Hingorani et al. 1999), and Axenfeld-Rieger anomaly, which is characterized by an abnormal pupil that is off-center (corectopia) or by extra holes in the iris that look like multiple pupils (polycoria). Other manifestations are microcornea, keratoconus, congenital macular dystrophy, shallow anterior chamber, exotropia, band keratopathy, and cataracts; diffuse hypopigmentation of the retinal fundus may occur.

Characteristic facial features are dysmorphic facies, broad forehead, deep-set eyes sometimes with upslanting palpebral fissures, prominent ears, straight nose with bulbous tip, and pointed chin giving the face a somewhat inverted triangular appearance (McDaniell et al. 2006).

Generally major criteria for diagnosis are considered as butterfly vertebrae, characteristic facies, and ocular abnormalities. Minor criteria include vascular accidents, intracranial bleeding, renal anomalies, xanthomas, supernumerary digital flexion creases, hypothyroidism, growth hormone insensitivity, pancreatic insufficiency, failure to thrive, growth retardation, and intellectual disability. Genetic test is mandatory for diagnosis.

As AGS is a multisystem disorder with a wide spectrum of clinical variability ranging from life-threatening liver or cardiac disease to only sub-clinical manifestations, such as mildly abnormal liver enzymes, a heart murmur, butterfly vertebrae, posterior embryotoxon, or characteristic facial features or neurovascular malformation, the diagnosis may be difficult because of the variable expressivity of the clinical manifestations. X-ray is useful for evaluation vertebrae. US, scintigraphy, and MRCP may be useful for evaluation of the patency of intra- and extrahepatic biliary tree (Yang et al. 2009). Definitive diagnosis of AGS about liver requires biopsy-proven paucity of interlobular bile ducts. US is useful for evaluation of hepatic masses (Fig. 18) and for evaluation of kidneys for structural problems such as small kidney, unilateral and bilateral multicystic kidney, dysplastic kidneys, horseshoe kidneys,

and ureteropelvic obstruction (McDaniell et al. 2006). Cerebral vasculopathy is an important feature of AGS and includes dolichoectasia, cerebral aneurysms, and moyamoya arteriopathy (progressive intracranial arterial occlusive showed "puff-of-smoke" appearance in DSA) (Connor et al. 2002). In the event of a serious head injury or neurological symptom, it is mandatory to aggressively and rapidly evaluate these children clinically and with appropriate imaging CT, MRI, and angiography (Doberentz et al. 2015). MRI screening in these patients is not validated yet. In addition to cerebral arterial abnormalities, alterations of venous development may be a feature of AGS in adults.

As for therapy, the severity and presentation of AGS determine the level of treatment, ranging from supportive care to standard medical management for cardiac and hepatic complications, including transplantation and cardiac surgeries in severe cases (Spinner et al. 2013). Prognosis of

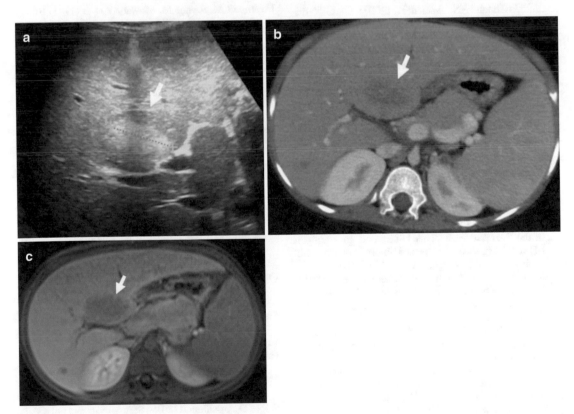

Fig. 18 Regenerative hepatic nodule (arrow) in the fourth hepatic segment on US (**a**), contrast-enhanced CT (**b**), and MRI (**c**) in a female 12-year-old with Alagille syndrome

AGS is also related to severity of organ involvement, with congenital heart disease, progressive liver disease, intracranial bleeding, and infection being the main contributors to increased mortality.

References

Abernethy J (1793) Account of two instances of uncommon formation in the viscera of the human body. Philos Trans R Soc Lond 17:292–299

Achiron R, Gindes L, Kivilevitch Z et al (2009) Prenatal diagnosis of congenital agenesis of the fetal portal venous system. Ultrasound Obstet Gynecol 34(6):643–646

Akhan O, Karaosmanoglu AD, Ergen B (2007) Imaging findings in congenital hepatic fibrosis. Eur J Radiol 61:18–24

Al-Salem A (ed) (2014) Biliary Atresia. An illustrated guide to pediatric surgery. Springer, New York

Alonso-Gamarra E, Parrón M, Pérez A et al (2011) Clinical and radiologic manifestations of congenital extrahepatic portosystemic shunts: a comprehensive review. Radiographics 31(3):707–722. https://doi.org/10.1148/rg.313105070

Ananthakrishnan AN, Saeian K (2007) Caroli's disease: identification and treatment strategy. Curr Gastroenterol Rep 9:151–155

Arcement CM, Towbin RB, Meza MP et al (2000) Intrahepatic chemoembolization in unresectable pediatric liver malignancies. Pediatr Radiol 30:779–785

Aziz S, Wild Y, Rosenthal P et al (2011) Pseudo gallbladder sign in biliary atresia—an imaging pitfall. Pediatr Radiol 41:620–626

Badea R, Serban A, Procopet B et al (2012) Education and imaging: hepatobiliary and pancreatic: Abernethy malformation congenital portocaval shunt. J Gastroenterol Hepatol 27:1875

Bartolozzi C, Lencioni R (2001) Contrast-specific ultrasound imaging of focal liver lesions. Prologue to a promising future. Eur Radiol 11(Supplement 3):13–14

Benhamou J, Menu Y (1994) Nonparasitic cystic disease of the liver and intrahepatic biliary tree. In: Blumgart LH (ed) Surgery of the liver and biliary tract. Churchill Livingstone, Edinburgh, UK, pp 1197–1210

Bernard O, Franchi-Abella S, Branchereau S et al (2012) Congenital portosystemic shunts in children: recognition, evaluation, and management. Semin Liver Dis 32(4):273–287

Bhargava P, Vaidya S, Kolokythas O et al (2011) Hepatic vascular shunts: embryology and imaging appearances. Br J Radiol 84:1142–1152

Boyle MJ, Doyle GD, McNulty JG (1989) Monolobar Caroli's disease. Am J Gastroenterol 84:1437–1444

Brancatelli G, Federle MP, Vilgrain V et al (2005) Fibropolycystic liver disease: CT and MR imaging findings. Radiographics 25:659–670

Brennan A, Kesavan A (2017) Novel heterozygous mutations in JAG1 and NOTCH2 genes in a neona-tal patient with Alagille syndrome. Case Rep Pediatr 2017:1368189. https://doi.org/10.1155/2017/1368189

Caroli J, Couinaud C, Soupault R et al (1958) New disease, undoubtedly congenital, of the bile ducts: unilobar cystic dilation of the hepatic ducts. Sem Hop 34:496–502

Caturelli E, Ghittoni G, Ranalli TV et al (2011) Nodular regenerative hyperplasia of the liver: coral atoll-like lesions on ultrasound are characteristic in predisposed patients. Br J Radiol 84(1003):129–134

Choi BI, Yeon KM, Kim SH et al (1990) Caroli disease: central dot sign in CT. Radiology 174:161–163

Cobben JM, Breuning H, Schoots C et al (1990) Congenital hepatic fibrosis in autosomal-dominant polycystic kidney disease. Kidney Int 38:880–885

Collard B, Maleux G, Heye S et al (2006) Value of carbon dioxide wedged venography and transvenous liver biopsy in the definitive diagnosis of Abernethy malformation. Abdom Imaging 31:315–319

Connor SE, Hewes D, Ball C et al (2002) Alagille syndrome associated with angiographic moyamoya. Childs Nerv Syst 18:186–190

Córdoba J (2011) New assessment of hepatic encephalopathy. J Hepatol 54:1030–1040

D'Agata ID, Jonas MM, Perez-Atayde AR et al (1994) Combined cystic disease of the liver and kidney. Semin Liver Dis 14:215–228

Davenport M, Savage M, Mowat AP et al (1993) Biliary atresia splenic malformation syndrome: an etiologic and prognostic subgroup. Surgery 113:662–668

Desmet VJ (1992) Congenital diseases of intrahepatic bile ducts: variations on the theme "ductal plate malformation". Hepatology 16:1069–1083

Desmet VJ (1998) Ludwig symposium on biliary disorders–part 1 pathogenesis of ductal plate abnormalities. Mayo Clin Proc 73:80–89

Desmet VJ (2005) Cystic diseases of the liver. From embryology to malformations. Gastroenterol Clin Biol 29:858–860

Doberentz E, Kuchelmeister K, Madea B (2015) Subarachnoid hemorrhage due to aneurysm rupture in a young woman with Alagille syndrome—a rare cause of sudden death. Leg Med (Tokyo) 17(5):309–312

Duran-Vega HC, Luna-Martinez J, Gonzalez-Guzman R et al (2000) Hamartoma of the bile ducts. Report of a case and review of the literature. Rev Gastroenterol Mex 65:124–128

Emerick KM, Rand EB, Goldmuntz E et al (1999) Features of Alagille syndrome in 92 patients: frequency and relation to prognosis. Hepatology 29:822–829

Ernst O, Gottrand F, Calvo M et al (1998) Congenital hepatic fibrosis: findings at MR cholangiopancreatography. Am J Roentgenol 170:409–412

Fabris L, Cadamuro M, Guido M et al (2007) Analysis of liver repair mechanisms in Alagille syndrome and biliary atresia reveals a role for notch signaling. Am J Pathol 171:641–653

Farges O, Aussilhou B (2012) Simple cysts and polycystic liver disease: surgical and non-surgical management. In: Jarnagin WR, Blumgart LH, editors. Blumgart's surgery of the liver, biliary tract and pancreas, 5th ed.

Philadelphia, PA: Saunders, 1066-1079 doi: https://doi.org/10.1016/B978-1-4377-1454-8.00118-1

Freidman JR, Piccoli D, Baldassano R (2007) Caroli disease. eMedicine. Available via DIALOG http://www.emedicine.com/ped/topic325.htm

Fulcher AS, Turner MA, Sanyal AJ (2001) Case 38: Caroli disease and renal tubular ectasia. Radiology 220:720–723

Gallego C, Miralles M, Marin C et al (2004) Congenital hepatic shunts. Radiographics 24:755–772

Ghadir MR, Bagheri M, Ghanooni AH (2011) Congenital hepatic fibrosis leading to cirrhosis and hepatocellular carcinoma: a case report. J Med Case Rep 5:160

Ghuman SS, Gupta S, Buxi TB et al (2016) The Abernethy malformation-myriad imaging manifestations of a single entity. Indian J Radiol Imaging 26:364–372

Goo HW (2007) Extrahepatic portosystemic shunt in congenital absence of the portal vein depicted by time-resolved contrast-enhanced MR angiography. Pediatr Radiol 37:706–709

Grazioli L, Alberti D, Olivetti L et al (2000) Congenital absence of portal vein with nodular regenerative hyperplasia of the liver. Eur Radiol 10(5):820–825

Guo WL, Huang SG, Wang J et al (2012) Imaging findings in 75 pediatric patients with pancreaticobiliary maljunction: a retrospective case study. Pediatr Surg Int 28(10):983–988

Hartley JL, Davenport M, Kelly DA (2009) Biliary atresia. Lancet 374:1704–1713

Hassan GMA, Ellethy AT (2014) Hepatic embryonic development and anomalies of the liver. J Gastroenterol Hepatol Res 38:407–414

Henry X, Marrasse E, Stoppa R et al (1987) The combination of Caroli's disease, cyst of the choledochus, congenital hepatic fibrosis and renal polykystosis. Proposal of a new classification of ectatic biliary dysembryoplasia of the common bile duct Apropos of a case. Chirurgie 113:834–843

Hingorani M, Nischal KK, Davies A et al (1999) Ocular abnormalities in Alagille syndrome. Ophthalmology 106:330–337

Hopkins PC, Yazigi N, Nylund CM (2017) Incidence of biliary atresia and timing of hepatoportoenterostomy in the United States. J Pediatr 187:253–257

Howard ER, Davenport M (1997) Congenital extrahepatic portocaval shunts - the Abernethy malformation. J Pediatr Surg 32:494–497

Hu GH, Shen LG, Yang J et al (2008) Insight into congenital absence of the portal vein: is it rare? World J Gastroenterol 14(39):5969–5979

Hussein A, Wyatt J, Guthrie A et al (2005) Kasai portoenterostomy – new insights from hepatic morphology. J Pediatr Surg 40:322–326

Hussman KL, Friedwald JP, Gollub MJ et al (1991) Caroli's disease associated with infantile polycystic kidney disease. Prenatal sonographic appearance. J Ultrasound Med 10:235–237

Irie H, Honda H, Jimi M et al (1998) Value of MR cholangiopancreatography in evaluating choledochal cysts. Am J Roentgenol 171:1381–1385

Jain D, Ahrens W, Finkelstein S (2010) Molecular evidence for the neo-plastic potential of hepatic von Meyenburg complexes. Appl Immunohistochem Mol Morphol 18:166–171

Jordon D, Harpaz N, Thung SN (1989) Caroli's disease and adult polycystic kidney disease: a rarely recognized association. Liver 9:30–35

Jorgensen MJ (1977) The ductal plate malformation. Acta Pathol Microbiol Scand Suppl 257:1–87

Kahn E (2004) Biliary atresia revisited. Pediatr Dev Pathol 7:109–124

Kamimatsuse A, Onitake Y, Kamei N et al (2010) Surgical intervention for patent ductus venosus. Pediatr Surg Int 26:1025–1030

Karahan OI, Kahriman G, Soyuer I et al (2007) Hepatic von Meyenburg complex simulating biliary cystadenocarcinoma. Clin Imaging 31:50–53

Kasai M, Suzuki S (1959) A new operation for "non-correctable" biliary atresia and portoenterostomy. Shijitsu 13:733–739

Kasai M, Sawaguchi M, Akiyama T et al (1976) A proposal of new classification of biliary atresia. J Jpn Soc Pediatr Surg 12:327–331

Kashiwagi T, Azuma M, Ikawa T et al (1988) Portosystemic shunting in portal hypertension: evaluation with portal scintigraphy with transrectally administered I-123 IMP. Radiology 169(1):137–140

Kaye AJ, Rand EB, Munoz PS et al (2010) Effect of Kasai procedure on hepatic outcome in Alagille syndrome. J Pediatr Gastroenterol Nutr 51:319–321

Keil R, Snajdauf J, Rygl M et al (2010) Diagnostic efficacy of ERCP in cholestatic infants and neonates a retrospective study on a large series. Endoscopy 42:121–112

Kerr D, Okonkwo S, Choa R (1978) Congenital hepatic fibrosis: the long-term prognosis. Gut 19:514–520

Kianifar HR, Tehranian S, Shojaei P et al (2013) Accuracy of hepatobiliary scintigraphy for differentiation of neonatal hepatitis from biliary atresia: systematic review and meta-analysis of the literature. Pediatr Radiol 43:905–919

Kim T, Murakami T, Sugihara E et al (2004) Hepatic nodular lesions associated with abnormal development of the portal vein. Am J Roentgenol 183:1333–1338

Kim WS, Cheon J-E, Youn BJ et al (2007) Hepatic arterial diameter measured with US: adjunct for US diagnosis of biliary atresia 1. Radiology 245:549–555

Kim MJ, Ko JS, Seo JK et al (2012) Clinical features of congenital portosystemic shunt in children. Eur J Pediatr 171:395–400

Kitajima Y, Okayama Y, Hirai M et al (2003) Intracystic hemorrhage of a simple liver cyst mimicking a biliary cystadenocarcinoma. J Gastroenterol 38:190–193

Kohda E, Saeki M, Nakano M et al (1999) Congenital absence of the portal vein in a boy. Pediatr Radiol 29:235–237

Konno K, Ishida H, Uno A et al (1997) Large extrahepatic portosystemic shunt without portal hypertension. Abdom Imaging 22:79–81

Kornprat P, Langner C, Fritz K et al (2005) Congenital absence of the portal vein in an adult woman: a case report. Wien Klin Wochenschr 117:58–62

Krause D, Cercueil JP, Dranssart M et al (2002) MRI for evaluating congenital bile duct abnormalities. J Comput Assist Tomogr 26:541–552

Lam WW, Lam TP, Saing H et al (1999) MR cholangiography and CT cholangiography of pediatric patients with choledochal cysts. Am J Roentgenol 173:401–405

Lautz TB, Tantemsapya N, Rowell E et al (2011) Management and classification of type II congenital portosystemic shunts. J Pediatr Surg 46(2):308–314

Lee SY, Kim GC, Choe BH et al (2011) Efficacy of US-guided percutaneous cholecysto-cholangiography for the early exclusion and type determination of biliary atresia. Radiology 261:916–922

Lenriot JP, Gigot JF, Segol P et al (1998) Bile duct cysts in adults: a multi-institutional retrospective study. Ann Surg 228:159–166

Lev-Toaff AS, Bach AM, Wechsler RJ et al (1995) The radiologic and pathologic spectrum of biliary hamartomas. Am J Roentgenol 165:309–313

Lin YC, Chang MH, Liao SF et al (2011) Decreasing rate of biliary atresia in Taiwan: a survey, 2004–2009. Pediatrics 128:530–536

Lipsett PA, Pitt HA (2003) Surgical treatment of choledochal cysts. J Hepato-Biliary-Pancreat Surg 10:352–359

Lipsett PA, Pitt HA, Colombani PM et al (1994) Choledochal cyst disease: a changing pattern of presentation. Ann Surg 220:644–652

Lonergan GJ, Rice RR, Suarez ES (2000) Autosomal recessive polycystic kidney disease: radiologic-pathologic correlation. Radiographics 20:837–855

Lowe LH, Schlesinger AE (2007) Hepatobiliary system, congenital abnormalities. In: Slovis TL (ed) Caffey's pediatric diagnostic imaging, 11th edn. Mosby, Elsevier, Philadelphia, pp 1861–1869

Luo TY, Itai Y, Eguchi N et al (1998) Von Meyenburg complexes of the liver: imaging findings. J Comput Assist Tomogr 22:372–378

Makin E, Quaglia A, Kvist N et al (2009) Congenital biliary atresia: liver injury begins at birth. J Pediatr Surg 44:630–633

Marchal GJ, Desmet VJ, Proesmans WC et al (1986) Caroli disease: high-frequency US and pathologic findings. Radiology 158:507–511

Marois D, van Haerden JA, Carpenter HA et al (1979) Congenital absence of the portal vein. Mayo Clin Proc 54:55–59

Massin M, Verloes A, Jamblin P (1999) Cardiac anomalies associated with congenital absence of the portal vein. Cardiol Young 9:522–525

Mathieu D, Vilgrain V, Mahfouz A et al (1997) Benign liver tumors. Magn Reson Imaging Clin N Am 5:255–288

Matsuoka Y, Ohtomo K, Okubo T et al (1992) Congenital absence of the portal vein. Gastrointest Radiol 17:31–33

Mboyo A, Lemouel A, Sohm O et al (1995) Congenital extra-hepatic portocaval shunt. Concerning a case of antenatal diagnosis. Eur J Pediatr Surg 5:243–245

McDaniell R, Warthen DM, Sanchez-Lara PA et al (2006) NOTCH2 mutations cause Alagille syndrome, a heterogeneous disorder of the NOTCH signaling pathway. Am J Hum Genet 79:169–173

Miller WJ, Sechtin AG, Campbell WL et al (1995) Imaging findings in Caroli's disease. Am J Roentgenol 165:333–337

Mizoguchi N, Sakura N, Ono H et al (2001) Congenital porto-left renal venous shunt as a cause of galactosaemia. J Inherit Metab Dis 24:72–78

Moorthy K, Mihssin N, Houghton PW (2001) The management of simple hepatic cysts: sclerotherapy or laparoscopic fenestration. Ann R Coll Surg Engl 83:409–414

Morgan G, Superina R (1994) Congenital absence of the portal vein: two cases and a proposed classification system for portosystemic vascular anomalies. J Pediatr Surg 29(9):1239–1241

Mortele B, Mortele K, Seynaeve P et al (2002) Hepatic bile duct hamartomas (von Meyenburg complexes): MR and MR cholangiography findings. J Comput Assist Tomogr 26(3):438–443

Motoori S, Shinozaki M, Goto N et al (1997) Case report: congenital absence of the portal vein associated with nodular hyperplasia in the liver. J Gastroenterol Hepatol 12:639–643

Mouzaki M, Bass LM, Sokol RJ (2015) Early life predictive markers of liver disease outcome in an international multicentre cohort of children with Alagille syndrome. Liver Int 36(5):755–760

Murphy BJ, Casillas J, Ros PR et al (1989) The CT appearance of cystic masses of the liver. Radiographics 9:307–322

Murray CP, Yoo SJ, Babyn PS (2003) Congenital extrahepatic portosystemic shunts. Pediatr Radiol 33(9):614–620

Murray-Lyon IM, Shilkin KB, Laws JW et al (1972) Non-obstructive dilatation of the intrahepatic biliary tree with cholangitis. Q J Med 41:477

Nakasaki H, Tanaka Y, Ohta M et al (1989) Congenital absence of the portal vein. Ann Surg 210(2):190–193

Newman B, Feinstein JA, Cohen RA et al (2010) (2010) Congenital extrahepatic portosystemic shunt associated with heterotaxy and polysplenia. Pediatr Radiol 40:1222–1230

Nonomura A, Mizukami Y, Matsubara F, Ueda H (1994) A case of choledochal cyst associated with adenocarcinoma exhibiting sarcomatous features. J Gastroenterol 29:669–675

Ohwada S, Hamada Y, Morishita Y et al (1994) Hepatic encephalopathy due to congenital splenorenal shunts: report of a case. Surg Today 24:145–149. https://doi.org/10.1007/BF0247339

Park JH, Cha SH, Han JK et al (1990) Intrahepatic portosystemic venous shunt. Am J Roentgenol 55(3):527–528

Pech L, Favelier S, Falcoz MT et al (2016) Imaging of von Meyenburg complexes. Diagn Interv Imaging 97(4):401–409. https://doi.org/10.1016/j.diii.2015.05.012

Piccoli DA, Spinner NB (2001) Alagille syndrome and the Jagged1 gene. Semin Liver Dis 21:525–534

Prokop M (2000) Multislice CT angiography. Eur J Radiol 36(2):86–96

Pupulim LF, Vullierme MP, Paradis V et al (2013) Congenital portosystemic shunts associated with liver tumours. Clin Radiol 68:362–369

Raynaud P, Tate J, Callens C et al (2011) A classification of ductal plate malformations based on distinct pathogenic mechanisms of biliary dysmorphogenesis. Hepatology 53:1959–1966

Redston MS, Wanless IR (1996) The hepatic von Meyenburg complex: prevalence and association with hepatic and renal cysts among 2843 autopsies. Mod Pathol 9:233–237

Ryu Y, Matsui O, Zen Y et al (2012) Multicystic biliary hamartoma: imaging findings in four cases. Abdom Imaging 35:543–554

Salemis NS, Georgoulis E, Gourgiotis S et al (2007) Spontaneous rupture of a giant non-parasitic hepatic cyst presenting as an acute surgical abdomen. Ann Hepatol 6:190–193

Schwarz KB, Haber BH, Rosenthal P et al (2013) Extrahepatic anomalies in infants with biliary atresia: results of a large prospective North American multicenter study. Hepatology 58:1724–1731

Sela-Herman S, Scharschmidt BF (1996) Choledochal cyst, a disease for all ages. Lancet 347:779–782

Semelka RC, Hussain SM, Marcos HB et al (1999) Biliary hamartomas: solitary and multiple lesions shown on current MR techniques including gadolinium enhancement. J Magn Reson Imaging 10:196–201

Shanmugam NP, Harrison PM, Devlin J et al (2009) (2009) Selective use of endoscopic retrograde chol angiopancreatography in the diagnosis of biliary atresia in infants younger than 100 days. J Pediatr Gastroenterol Nutr 49:435–441

Shneider BL, Abel B, Haber B et al (2012) Portal hypertension in children and young adults with biliary atresia. J Pediatr Gastroenterol Nutr 55:567–573

So Mi Lee MD, Jung-Eun Cheon MD, Choi YH et al (2015) Ultrasonographic diagnosis of biliary atresia based on a decision-making tree model. Korean J Radiol 16(6):1364–1372

Sokollik C, Bandsma RH, Gana JC et al (2013) Congenital portosystemic shunt: characterization of a multisystem disease. J Pediatr Gastroenterol Nutr 56:675–681

Söreide K, Körner H, Havnen J et al (2004) Bile duct cysts in adults. Br J Surg 12:1538–1548

Spiegel RM, King DL, Green WM (1978) Ultrasonography of primary cysts of the liver. Am J Roentgenol 131:235

Spinner N, Leonard L, Krantz I (2013) Alagille syndrome. In: Pagon RA, Adam MP, Ardinger HH et al (eds) Gene reviews. University of Washington, Seattle, WA

Stringer MD (2008) The clinical anatomy of congenital portosystemic venous shunts. Clin Anat 21:147–157

Szavay P, Leonhardt J, Czech-Schmidt G et al (2002) The role of reovirus type 3 infection in an established murine model for biliary atresia. Eur J Pediatr Surg 12:248–250

Tan A, Shen J, Hecht A (1989) Sonogram of multiple bile duct hamartomas. J Clin Ultrasound 17:667–669

Torra R, Badenas C, Darnell A et al (1997) Autosomal dominant polycystic kidney disease with anticipation and Caroli's disease associated with a PKD1 mutation. Rapid communication. Kidney Int 52:33–38

Tsitouridis I, Sotiriadis C, Michaelides M et al (2009) Intrahepatic portosystemic venous shunts: radiological evaluation. Diagn Interv Radiol 15:182–187

Turnpenny PD, Ellard S (2012) Alagille syndrome: pathogenesis, diagnosis and management. Eur J Hum Genet 20(3):251–257

Turnpenny PD, Alman B, Cornier AS et al (2007) Abnormal vertebral segmentation and the Notch signaling pathway in man. (Review). Dev Dyn 236:1456–1474

Uchino T, Endo F, Ikeda S et al (1996) Three brothers with progressive hepatic dysfunction and severe hepatic steatosis due to a patent ductus venosus. Gastroenterology 110(6):1964–1968

Uchino T, Matsuda I, Endo F (1999) The long-term prognosis of congenital portosystemic venous shunt. J Pediatr 135:254–256

Usuki N, Miyamoto T (1998) A case of congenital absence of the intrahepatic portal vein diagnosed by MR angiography. J Comput Assist Tomogr 22:728–729

Vachha B, Sun MR, Siewert B et al (2011) Cystic lesions of the liver. Am J Roentgenol 196:W355–W366. https://doi.org/10.2214/AJR.10.5292

Van Sonnenberg E, Wroblicka JT, D'Agostino HB et al (1994) Symptomatic hepatic cysts: percutaneous drainage and sclerosis. Radiology 190:387–392

Veigel MC, Prescott-Focht J, Rodriguez MG et al (2008) Fibropolycystic liver disease in children. Pediatr Radiol 30:779–785

Vidili G, De Sio I, D'Onofrio M (2018) SIUMB guidelines and recommendations for the correct use of ultrasound in the management of patients with focal liver disease. J Ultrasound 22:1–11. https://doi.org/10.1007/s40477-018-0343-0

Vilgrain V, Lagadec M, Ronot M (2016) Pitfalls in liver imaging. Radiology 278:34–51

Wang KS (2015) Section on surgery, committee on fetus and newborn, childhood liver disease research network newborn screening for biliary atresia. Pediatrics 136:1663–1669

Wanless IR (1990) Micronodular transformation (nodular regenerative hyperplasia) of the liver: a report of 64 cases among 2,500 autopsies and a new classification of benign hepatocellular nodules. Hepatology 11(5):787–797

Yang J-G, Ma D-Q, Peng Y et al (2009) Comparison of different diagnostic methods for differentiating biliary atresia from idiopathic neonatal hepatitis. Clin Imaging 33(6):439–446

Yonem O, Ozkayar N, Balkanci F et al (2006) Is congenital hepatic fibrosis a pure liver disease? Am J Gastroenterol 101:1253–1259

Zani A, Quaglia A, Hadzic N et al (2015) Cytomegalovirus-associated biliary atresia: an aetiological and prognostic subgroup. J Pediatr Surg 50:1739–1745. https://doi.org/10.1016/j.jpedsurg.2015.03.001

Zeitoun D, Brancatelli G, Colombat M et al (2004) Congenital hepatic fibrosis: CT findings in 18 adults. Radiology 231:109–116

Zheng RQ, Zhang B, Kudo M et al (2005) Imaging findings of biliary hamartomas. World J Gastroenterol 11:6354–6359

Zhou L, Shan Q, Tian W et al (2016) Ultrasound for the diagnosis of biliary atresia: a meta-analysis. Am J Roentgenol 206:73–82

Fibropolycystic Liver Diseases

Carlos Bilreiro and Inês Santiago

Contents

C. Bilreiro
PreClinical MRI Lab, Champalimaud Foundation,
Lisbon, Portugal

I. Santiago (✉)
PreClinical MRI Lab, Champalimaud Foundation,
Lisbon, Portugal

Radiology Department, Champalimaud Foundation,
Aveiro, Portugal

Nova Medical School, Lisbon, Portugal

Abstract

Fibropolycystic liver diseases are a group of congenital disorders with a common origin in ductal plate developmental abnormalities and varied fenotypes. They include the simple hepatic cysts, Caroli disease and syndrome, polycystic liver diseases, congenital hepatic fibrosis and biliary hamartomas. In this chapter, we first discuss the embryologic develo-

© Springer Nature Switzerland AG 2021
E. Quaia (ed.), *Imaging of the Liver and Intra-hepatic Biliary Tract*,
Medical Radiology, Diagnostic Imaging, https://doi.org/10.1007/978-3-030-38983-3_11

pent of the normal ductal plate and of the multiple ductal plate abnormalities. Then, we individually address the various fibropolycystic liver diseases with respect to their epidemiology, clinical features and therapeutic management, with a special emphasis on the description and illustration of their imaging findings.

1 Clinical Background

Fibropolycystic liver diseases represent a heterogeneous group of disorders, with a common origin in ductal plate development anomalies. These include the simple hepatic cysts, Caroli disease and syndrome, polycystic liver diseases, congenital hepatic fibrosis (CHF) and biliary hamartomas (von Meyenburg complexes).

1.1 Embryology: The Ductal Plate

During the fourth gestational week, the hepatic diverticulum arises from the ventral wall of the primitive midgut (Fig. 1a) (Ando 2010). This diverticulum then develops a cranially located pars hepatica, which originates in the liver primordium and the common hepatic duct. Caudally, a superior and an inferior bud also develops (Fig. 1b). The superior bud originates in the gallbladder and cystic and choledochal ducts, while the inferior bud originates in the ventral portion of the pancreas (Fig. 1c–e). The choledochal duct and ventral portion of the pancreas then rotate 180° and, by the sixth gestational week, reach their definitive location (Fig. 1f).

The ductal plate is formed in the eighth gestational week, originating from hepatoblasts in the liver primordium (Crawford 2002). These become

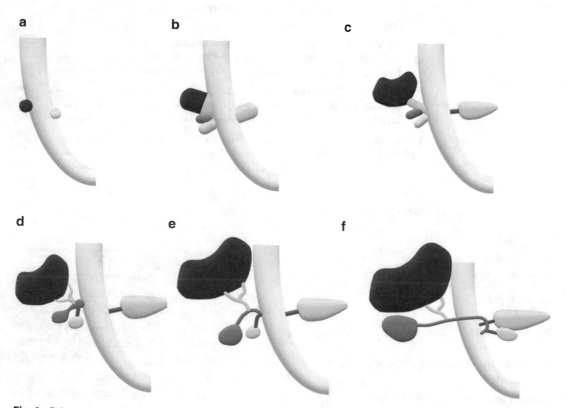

Fig. 1 Schematic representation of liver, pancreas, gallbladder, and biliary tree embryologic development from weeks 4 to 6, in chronological order from (**a–f**)

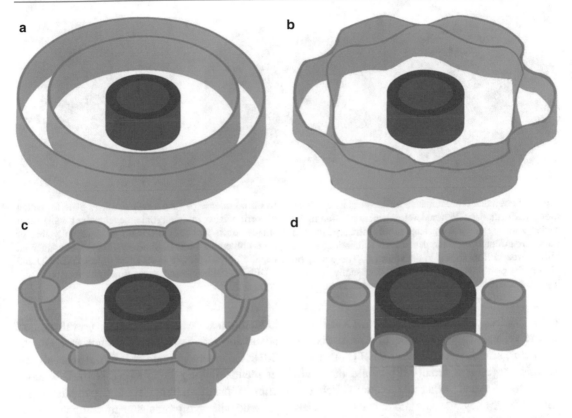

Fig. 2 Schematic representation of the ductal plate development, in chronological order from (**a–d**)

epithelial cells arranged in double-layer cylindrical structures, adjacent to the mesenchyme of portal vein branches (Fig. 2a). This process begins in the hepatic hilum and progresses in a centrifugal fashion to the liver periphery. Between the 11th and 13th weeks of gestation, the ductal plate begins a remodeling process, in which the ductal plates separate by apoptotic deletion of intervening cells and create progressively cylindrical structures (Fig. 2b, c). These structures then mature into a network of longitudinally arranged bile ducts, up until the postnatal period (Fig. 2d) (Crawford 2002; Lazaridis et al. 2004).

1.2 Development of Fibropolycystic Liver Diseases

Developmental disorders of the ductal plate are responsible for fibropolycystic liver diseases, as represented in Fig. 3. Depending on the anatomic site and caliber of branching duct disorder, different pathological entities may occur (Brancatelli et al. 2005; Santiago et al. 2012). Malformations of the larger extrahepatic bile ducts may create choledochal cysts (not reviewed in this chapter). Caroli disease is caused by large intrahepatic duct developmental abnormalities. Biliary atresia, not reviewed in this chapter, refers to underdevelopment of large intrahepatic and extrahepatic bile ducts. When medium-sized intrahepatic ducts are affected, polycystic liver disease may ensue. The malformation of smaller caliber intrahepatic ducts may cause CHF and biliary hamartomas (von Meyenburg complexes).

The pathological entities in this spectrum may occur simultaneously and in association with a common genetic background. Most frequently, ADPKD and ARPKD, with genetic defects in PKD1, PKD2, and PKHD1, respectively, may associate with polycystic liver disease, CHF, Caroli disease, and biliary hamartomas (Dell

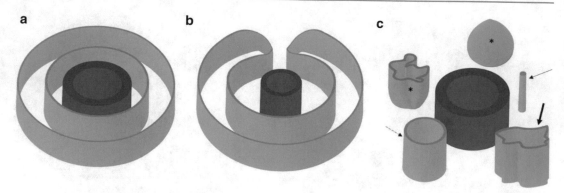

Fig. 3 Schematic representation of ductal plate development malformations. When development is arrested in the early gestational period, large-sized intrahepatic bile ducts are affected and saccular/fusiform dilatations of the biliary tree will be found in the adult (**a**). These may be pierced by portal mesenchyma, the latter usually containing an abnormally small portal venous branch, as observed in Caroli disease (**b**). An arrest in ductal plate formation occurring later in embryonic development will affect smaller ducts and may originate in abnormally thin or even obliterated ducts (thin arrows in **c**) as in congenital hepatic fibrosis, simple cysts (* in **c**) as in ADPKD and ADPLD, or biliary hamartomas (thick arrows in **c**)

2011; Mehta and Jim 2017). Also, Caroli syndrome refers to the presence of Caroli disease occurring simultaneously with CHF (both intrahepatic large- and small-caliber bile ducts are affected). Several other associations between congenital kidney diseases and ductal plate developmental anomalies have been described, mainly with CHF, including nephronophthisis type 3, Jeune syndrome, Joubert syndrome, Meckel syndrome, Bardet–Biedl syndrome, oral-facial-digital syndrome type 1, and Ivemark syndrome (Gunay-Aygun et al. 2008). Also, an isolated form of polycystic liver disease may occur (autosomal dominant polycystic liver disease—ADPLD), without kidney abnormalities, due to genetic defects in PRKCSH, SEC36, LRP5, and recently identified SEC61B and ALG8 (Drenth et al. 2004; Cnossen et al. 2014; Besse et al. 2017; van de Laarschot and Drenth 2018).

2 Simple Hepatic Cyst

2.1 Epidemiology, Clinical Features, and Management

The simple hepatic cyst is a benign cyst, lined by simple cuboidal or columnar biliary-type epithelium. It is a very common lesion, the second most common benign liver lesion in adults after hepatic hemangioma, with increasing prevalence in advancing age (van de Laarschot and Drenth 2018; Gaines and Sampson 1989). It is usually an incidental finding in imaging studies, without clinical manifestations. Rarely, patients might present with symptoms due to compression of adjacent structures, infection (Fig. 4e–h), hemorrhage, or rupture (Sayma et al. 2019; Yoshida et al. 2003). Simple hepatic cysts follow an invariably benign course and intervention is only needed in rare symptomatic cases or when the diagnosis is uncertain (Rogers et al. 2007).

2.2 Imaging Findings

In imaging studies, the diagnosis of simple hepatic cyst is usually straightforward (Fig. 4). In ultrasound imaging, it most frequently presents as a well-defined anechoic lesion, sometimes with lobulated contours (Gaines and Sampson 1989). Posterior acoustic enhancement might be seen, if the lesion is large enough. Fine septa in its interior might be observed, but without solid components or vascularization when using Doppler ultrasound. Simple hepatic cysts present as well-defined water density lesions in CT scans (Horton et al. 1999). In MRI, these appear as well-defined lesions, with homogeneous high signal intensity on T2- and low signal intensity

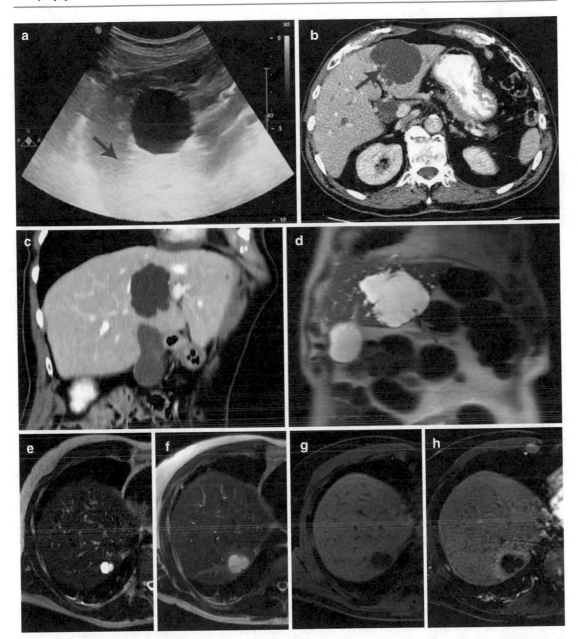

Fig. 4 Simple hepatic cysts are typically homogeneous and well-defined anechoic (**a**), hypoattenuating (**b** and **c**), and strongly T2 hyperintense lesions (**d** and **e**) on ultrasound, CT, and MR imaging, respectively. They typically exhibit posterior acoustic enhancement on ultrasound (arrow in **a**). Although more frequently round (**a**), they may also be lobulated (**b**, **e**) and sometimes present with thin regular septa (arrows in **b** and **d**), which should not enhance after IV contrast administration. An unusual complication of simple hepatic cysts is infection, which may present with an increase in cyst size (**f** vs. **e**), heterogeneous content sometimes with air-fluid or fluid-fluid levels (arrow in **f**), and contour blurring (**f**) with peripheral arterial hyperenhancement (**h** vs. **g**)

on T1-weighted images. There should be no enhancement of internal components after intravenous contrast administration in both CT and MRI (Horton et al. 1999; Elsayes et al. 2005). If enhancing internal components are seen, cystadenoma or cystadenocarcinoma should be the main diagnostic possibilities, when considering a primary liver lesion.

3 Caroli Disease and Syndrome

3.1 Epidemiology, Clinical Features, and Management

Caroli first described two forms of disease in the spectrum of the ductal plate malformations (Caroli et al. 1958). These became known as Caroli syndrome and Caroli disease. Both diseases affect the large-caliber intrahepatic bile ducts and Caroli syndrome also affects the small-caliber intrahepatic bile ducts, occurring with simultaneous CHF. Both are inherited in an autosomal recessive fashion and can be associated with ARPKD or ADPKD (Jordon et al. 1989). Abnormal ductal plate remodeling with persistence of dilated ductal plate remnants is thought to be the cause for Caroli disease (Fig. 3b) (Desmet 2005).

Patients with Caroli disease and syndrome might present with abdominal pain, enlarged liver, and recurrent episodes of cholangitis. Because Caroli syndrome is associated with CHF, these patients might present with signs of portal hypertension. As both diseases occur with cholestasis, intrahepatic sludge and stone formation are common. This also puts patients at a higher risk for developing cholangiocarcinoma (Bloustein 1977). The prognosis for both conditions is relatively poor, with frequent secondary biliary cirrhosis. Therapy mainly consists of antibiotics when acute cholangitis occurs; drainage procedures might be performed when there are liver abscesses. Liver transplantation is an important therapeutic option and, if the disease affects predominantly one liver lobe, partial hepatectomy might be performed with success (Ramond et al. 1984; Lendoire et al. 2011; Lendoire et al. 2007; Kassahun et al. 2005).

3.2 Imaging Findings

Typical imaging findings in Caroli disease include saccular and/or fusiform dilatation of intrahepatic bile ducts (Fig. 5a, b), often containing biliary sludge and stones (Brancatelli et al. 2005; Santiago et al. 2012; Mamone et al. 2019).

A classical finding is the "central dot sign" in CT and MRI studies (Fig. 6), which represents the central vascular bundle surrounded by the dilated biliary duct. The main differential diagnosis is with polycystic liver disease, which can be difficult. MRCP may help in this regard, when it shows communication of the intrahepatic bile ducts with the liver cysts (Fig. 5b). Another finding used to demonstrate communication with the biliary tree and perform this differential diagnosis is the presence of intracystic gadolinium, when performing MRI with intracellular hepato-specific contrast agents that undergo uptake by hepatocytes and are later secreted into the bile ducts, during the hepatobiliary phase (Fig. 5c–e) (Brancatelli et al. 2005; Santiago et al. 2012; Mamone et al. 2019; Lewis et al. 2016). The most used contrast agents in this regard are gadoxetic acid (Gd-EOB-DTPA) and gadobenate dimeglumine (Gd-BOPTA) (Lewis et al. 2016).

4 Polycystic Liver Disease

4.1 Epidemiology, Clinical Features, and Management

Polycystic liver diseases are characterized by the growth of multiple cysts in the liver, without communication to the biliary tree. These cysts are lined by functional biliary epithelium and usually grow progressively in size, ultimately replacing a significant portion of the liver parenchyma. These may occur in association with ADPKD and ARPKD, or in isolation as an autosomal dominant polycystic liver disease (ADPLD) (Cnossen and Drenth 2014). The most common of these disorders is ADPKD, with estimated prevalence ranging from 1:400 to 1:4033 births; a more recent review reports a prevalence of near 4:10,000 (or 1:2500) (Perugorria et al. 2014; Torres et al. 2007; Willey et al. 2017). ARPKD is significantly less common, with an estimated prevalence of 1:20,000 births and a high mortality rate shortly after birth; approximately half of newborns die of pulmonary complications (Perugorria et al. 2014; Torres et al. 2007; Zerres et al. 1998; Paul and VandenHeuvel 2014).

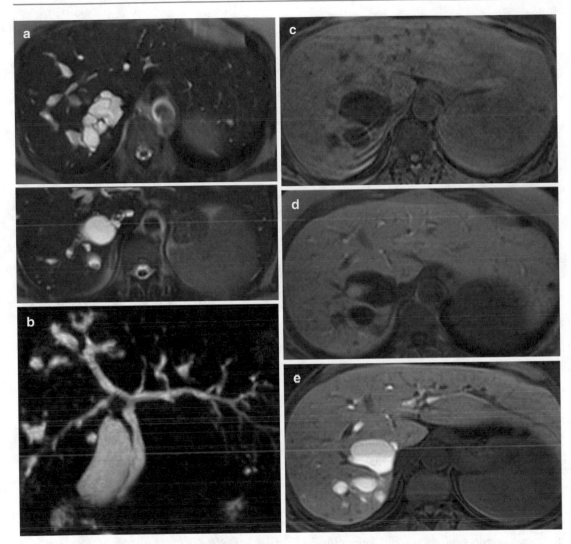

Fig. 5 Caroli disease presenting with lobulated cystic lesions predominantly located in the posterior sector of the right liver lobe (**a**) corresponding to saccular focal dilatations of the biliary tree (**b**). After Gd-EOB-DTPA administration, a progressive but slow filling of the cystic lesions on the hepatobiliary phase is observed, proving communication with the biliary tree (**c**: pre-contrast; **d**: post-contrast at 10 min; **e**: post-contrast at 3 h)

ADPLD is the rarest form of these diseases, with an estimated prevalence of 1:100,000 (Perugorria et al. 2014).

Several germline mutations have been identified in the development of these diseases. ADPKD and ARPKD are associated with germline mutations in PKD1, PKD2 and PKHD1, respectively, while ADPLD has been associated with mutations in PRKCSH, SEC63, LRP5, ALG8, and SEC61 (Drenth et al. 2004; Cnossen et al. 2014; Besse et al. 2017; van de Laarschot and Drenth 2018).

ADPKD usually manifests clinically in adulthood. Hypertension, hematuria, proteinuria, and recurrent pyelonephritis may dominate the initial presentation. A progression to end-stage chronic kidney disease occurs in approximately 45% of patients by the age of 60 years (Gabow 1993). The hallmark of this condition is the presence of renal cysts, affecting virtually all patients as age advances. The presence of liver cysts affects 30–70% of patients, more frequently women, possibly due to hormonal influences (Mamone et al. 2019). Treatment directed to liver cysts may

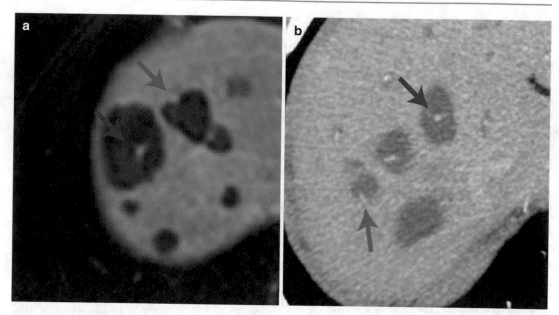

Fig. 6 Central dot sign. Two cases of Caroli disease exhibiting the characteristic central dot sign on post-contrast portal venous phase imaging are depicted, on MR (**a**) and CT (**b**). The central dot sign (red arrows) results from the piercing of the ectatic abnormal bile duct by the portal sheet. When it contains a portal venous branch, it is usually reduced in caliber, but the portal venous branch(es) may also be located at the periphery of the abnormal bile duct (blue arrows)

be necessary when there are complications: hemorrhage, infection, or compression of adjacent structures. Cyst drainage and antibiotics are the main therapeutic options when recurrent cyst infection occurs (Torres et al. 2007). New therapeutic options have emerged, and somatostatin analogue administration, namely lanreotide and octreotide, has shown efficacy in decreasing liver and kidney volume (van Keimpema et al. 2009; Hogan et al. 2010; Gevers et al. 2015). However, a recent trial concluded that lanreotide administration in late stages does not improve renal function and cannot be recommended for this specific purpose (Meijer et al. 2018).

ARPKD, on the other hand, manifests early in infancy and childhood, with strikingly enlarged kidneys with innumerable tiny cysts (Drenth et al. 2010). These abnormalities are nowadays frequently found during gestational ultrasound, sometimes with Potter syndrome (oligohydramnios with enlarged kidneys, pulmonary hypoplasia, characteristic facies, and contracted limbs with clubfeet). This condition has approximately

50% mortality rate in the neonatal period, and the children that survive early infancy present later with hypertension, frequently requiring multi-drug therapy (Bergmann et al. 2005). Also in later stages, children may present with dominant hepatobiliary clinical findings. The liver involvement is similar to CHF, with hepatic fibrosis and hyperplastic biliary ducts (Turkbey et al. 2009). Although liver function is frequently preserved until late stages, progressive hepatic fibrosis and portal hypertension ultimately lead to the development of esophageal varices with upper gastrointestinal bleeding and hypersplenism with pancytopenia (Drenth et al. 2010; Guay-Woodford and Desmond 2003). A combined liver-kidney transplant is usually considered early in the course of the disease. Caroli disease may be associated with ARPKD; therapeutic options due to hepatic cyst complications or liver function decline are similar as explained previously, namely cyst drainage, antibiotics, partial hepatectomy, and liver transplant.

ADPLD has a milder clinical course, unassociated with significant kidney disease. Renal cysts may occur, but as a mild sporadic finding when compared with ADPKD or ARPKD and without decrease in renal function (Mamone et al. 2019). Arbitrarily, the diagnosis can be made when there are more than 20 liver cysts, or more than 4 when there is a family history of ADPLD (van Keimpema et al. 2009). Patients are frequently asymptomatic until late adulthood. Symptoms may arise from compression of abdominal structures due to large cysts, cyst infection, hemorrhage, or rupture. Therapeutic intervention might be necessary in symptomatic patients; cyst aspiration, sclerotherapy, partial hepatectomy, or even liver transplantation can be considered (van Keimpema et al. 2008; Russell and Pinson 2007; Neijenhuis et al. 2019). Similar to ADPKD, the administration of somatostatin analogues has shown promise in reducing liver volume in ADPLD (van Keimpema et al. 2009; Hogan et al. 2010; Gevers et al. 2015).

4.2 Imaging Findings

Regarding imaging findings of each of these polycystic liver diseases, ADPKD and ADPLD may have similar hepatic features with liver enlargement and multiple cysts; however the major involvement of kidneys in ADPKD will help in the differential diagnosis (Fig. 7a, b). The size of cysts can vary from 1 mm to 12 cm (Brancatelli et al. 2005; Morgan et al. 2006). The hepatic cysts have similar imaging characteristics as simple cysts, presenting in ultrasound as well-defined anechoic lesions and in CT as well-defined water density lesions. In MRI, the multiple cysts are also seen with high signal intensity in T2-weighted images and low signal intensity in T1-weighted images. Complicated cysts appear with heterogeneous content in ultrasound, higher density in CT scans, and heterogeneous signal in MRI (high T1 signal intensity if hemorrhage is present) (Fig. 7c). A previously complicated cyst can develop peripheral calcifications (Santiago et al. 2012; Mamone et al.

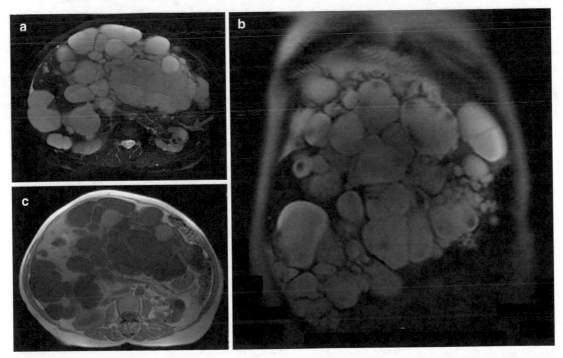

Fig. 7 Autosomal dominant polycystic liver disease. Numerous T2-hyperintense liver cysts of various sizes are depicted (**a**), causing massive hepatomegaly (**b**). Notice how the left kidney is relatively spared (arrow in **a**). Some cysts exhibit T1 hyperintensity (arrows in **c**) likely due to previous hemorrhage

2019). To perform the differential diagnosis with Caroli disease, MRCP and hepatospecific contrast-enhanced MRI have specific findings in this regard, as previously mentioned, with both modalities showing absence of communication of hepatic cysts with the biliary tree in ADPLD and ADPKD (Brancatelli et al. 2005; Santiago et al. 2012; Mamone et al. 2019). Also, peribiliary cysts have been associated with ADPLD and ADPKD (Mamone et al. 2019; Lewis et al. 2016). These are usually smaller than 10 mm and may present as a discrete string of cysts or tubular structures, developing within the periductal connective tissue. These also do not communicate with the biliary tree; however, they may cause biliary obstruction.

Imaging findings of ARPKD differ, however, as these are similar with CHF. Periportal fibrosis, irregular dilatation of the biliary tree, regenerative nodules, and a coarse liver texture may be observed (Lonergan et al. 2000). Portal hypertension eventually develops and imaging findings reflect this, with splenomegaly and venous collateral development with esophageal varices. Ultrasound may show the coarse liver texture, with echogenic portal tracts thought to represent periportal fibrosis. CT and MRI also depict these same findings, with better identification of regenerative nodules and findings related to portal hypertension. MRCP may accurately depict the intrahepatic bile ducts' irregular caliber (Jung et al. 1999).

5 Congenital Hepatic Fibrosis

5.1 Epidemiology, Clinical Features, and Management

In contrast to the majority of previously discussed disorders, where hepatic or renal cysts were a dominant finding, CHF is mainly characterized by the presence of periportal fibrosis and irregular-caliber bile ducts (Desmet 1992; Venkatanarasimha et al. 2011). Typically, CHF has been associated with ARPKD, representing different manifestations of a spectrum of diseases (Desmet 1992). However, CHF can also present as an isolated condition or in the context of Caroli syndrome. A

literature review reported 64% of CHF to appear associated with ARPKD, 25.6% associated with Caroli syndrome, and 9.5% in isolation (Srinath and Shneider 2012). Reports of association with ADPKD are rare (O'Brien et al. 2012).

Affected patients frequently maintain hepatocellular function until late stages of the disease (Mamone et al. 2019; Bergmann et al. 2005; Turkbey et al. 2009). Different forms of disease have been described: portal hypertensive, cholangitic, mixed, and latent (Desmet 1992; Venkatanarasimha et al. 2011). Portal hypertension can present in infancy and adulthood, with splenomegaly, hypersplenism, and pancytopenia as possible presenting features. Also, bleeding from gastroesophageal varices is a frequent presentation. Hepatopulmonary syndrome may present as an advanced finding. The pathogenesis of portal hypertension has been related to the compression of portal vein ramifications by periportal fibrosis and to abnormal development of portal vein branches, with hypoplastic small branches (Desmet 1992; Kerr et al. 1961). Patients with the cholangitic form of disease present mainly with cholestasis and recurrent episodes of cholangitis. As with other chronic cholestatic diseases, the risk for intrahepatic stones and cholangiocarcinoma development is increased (Summerfield et al. 1986). The mixed form of the disease represents simultaneous portal hypertensive and cholangitic findings; the latent form represents asymptomatic patients who are diagnosed incidentally during adulthood or later stages in life (Desmet 1992; Veigel et al. 2009).

Therapy is dependent on the manifestations of the disease. Variceal bleeding from portal hypertension can be treated with endoscopic procedures with sclerotherapy or ligation (Drenth et al. 2010; Shneider and Magid 2005). Elective surgical or percutaneous portosystemic shunt creation is an option in patients with gastroesophageal varices. Acute cholangitis can be treated with antibiotics and percutaneous procedures, if drainage is needed. Liver transplantation is also an option, mainly in patients with advanced hepatic disease or recurrent hemorrhagic or cholangitic complications (Shneider and Magid 2005). If Caroli syndrome is present, therapeutic interventions directed to cyst complications may be needed, as explained previously in this chapter.

5.2   Imaging Findings

The imaging findings in CHF are generally not specific. Atrophy of the right liver lobe and hypertrophy of the lateral left and caudate lobes may be found, mimicking chronic liver disease from other causes (Santiago et al. 2012; Mamone et al. 2019). However, the left medial segments (IVa and IVb) may remain with normal volume, or be even enlarged (Zeitoun et al. 2004). The typical findings of portal hypertension, including portosystemic shunts (splenorenal and gastro-esophageal, as the most typical), splenomegaly, and increased portal vein diameter, can be observed with ultrasound, CT, or MRI. The liver has a coarse texture in these imaging modalities. Periportal fibrosis can be identified as hyper-echoic portal branches on ultrasound or high signal intensity in T2-weighted images along portal branches (Mamone et al. 2019; Veigel et al. 2009). Large regenerative hepatic nodules may appear in the course of portal hypertension; a hypervascular behavior due to increased arterial vascular supply has been demonstrated in contrast-enhanced studies (Brancatelli et al. 2005). These benign nodules are entirely similar to focal nodular hyperplasia in imaging studies. Vascular complications of portal hypertension can be initially assessed by ultrasound, and further identified on contrast-enhanced CT or MRI. MRCP can clearly depict the irregular caliber of intrahepatic bile ducts. In the presence of Caroli syndrome, the typical liver cysts will be a major imaging finding, as described previously.

6   Biliary Hamartomas (von Meyenburg Complexes)

6.1   Epidemiology, Clinical Features, and Management

Biliary hamartomas are clinically silent lesions, also known as von Meyenburg complexes, usually found incidentally in imaging studies (von Meyenburg 1918). These are dispersed throughout the liver parenchyma, as focal collections of dilated bile ducts, lined by biliary epithelium and surrounded by fibrous stroma (Mamone et al. 2019; Principe et al. 1997). The lesions are usually smaller than 10 mm and represent failure of involution of embryonic bile ducts, with a reported incidence of 5.6% in adult patients (Santiago et al. 2012; Zheng et al. 2005; Redston and Wanless 1996). The patients are asymptomatic and liver function is normal; direct complications of cystic lesions are not usual. However, reports of intrahepatic cholangiocarcinoma in patients with biliary hamartomas suggest an increased risk for the development of this tumor (Xu et al. 2009; Yang et al. 2017; Song et al. 2008; Jain et al. 2000).

6.2   Imaging Findings

As previously stated, these lesions are incidentally identified in imaging studies. In ultrasound studies, a typical presentation is with numerous hypoechoic or hyperechoic foci with comet-tail artifacts (Fig. 8a, b) (Santiago et al. 2012; Mamone et al. 2019; Zheng et al. 2005). On CT, the lesions are usually presented as disperse hypoattenuating foci (Fig. 8c, d) (Brancatelli et al. 2005). In MRI, the lesions are hyperintense in T2-weighted images (Fig. 8e) and hypointense in T1-weighted images. MRCP has a characteristic "starry-sky" appearance, with multiple foci of hyperintense cystic lesions dispersed throughout the liver parenchyma (Esseghaier et al. 2017; Giambelluca et al. 2018). The lesions do not enhance with the administration of intravenous contrast agents; however a peripheral rim enhancement has been described to represent compressed liver parenchyma (Semelka et al. 1999). As the cysts do not communicate with the biliary tree, they do not enhance in hepatobiliary phase of hepatospecific contrast agents. A differential diagnosis with multiple metastases may arise, and the characteristic findings of "starry sky" in MRCP (Fig. 8f) and comet-tail artifacts (arrow in Fig. 8b) in ultrasound help in this regard.

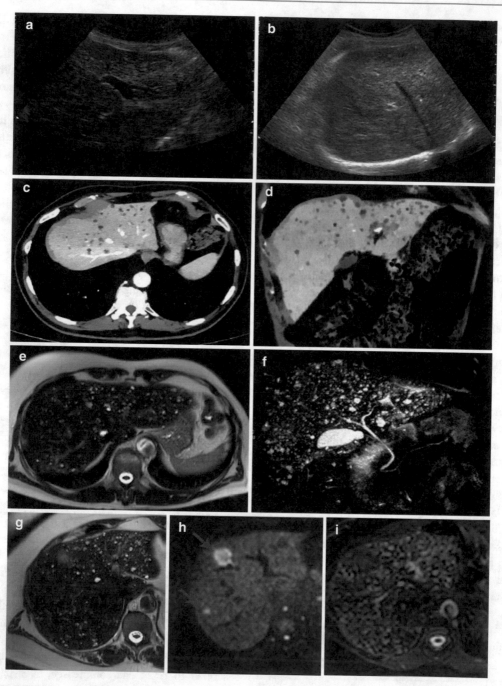

Fig. 8 Biliary hamartomas. Biliary hamartomas present on ultrasound as small (<15 mm) hyperechoic or anechoic lesions, depending on the amount of fluid content (**a**, **b**), sometimes with posterior acoustic enhancement causing the characteristic comet-tail artifact (arrow in **b**). On CT, they are usually hypoattenuating and non-enhancing (**c**: axial, portal venous phase post-contrast image; **d**: coronal oblique minimum intensity projection). The lesions are hyperintense on T2-weighted imaging (**e**) and particularly visible on heavily T2-weighted MRCP images, in which, when numerous, a "starry-sky" appearance is typical (**f**). Biliary hamartomas may obscure the detection of other liver lesions. In such cases, high b-value diffusion-weighted imaging may be particularly useful, highlighting solid, highly cellular, restricting lesions. (**g–i**) Depict a case of a patient with biliary hamartomas and two colorectal cancer liver metastases (arrows in **h**) as observed in T2-weighted imaging (**g**), b900 diffusion-weighted imaging (**h**), and corresponding ADC map (**i**)

7   Conclusion

The fibropolycystic liver diseases include several distinct pathological entities, with a common origin in developmental disorders of the ductal plate. Their management and therapeutic options are quite distinct; therefore a correct diagnosis must be performed. Imaging studies are critical in this regard and the findings described in this chapter represent the most important diagnostic features.

A short summary is present in Table 1.

Table 1 Key imaging findings diagnostic for each fibropolycystic liver disease

Fibropolycystic disease	Key imaging findings
Simple hepatic cyst	– Well-defined lesion, without solid or enhancing components – Anechoic in ultrasound – Water density in CT – Hyperintense in T2WI/hypointense in T1WI
Caroli disease and syndrome	– Saccular and fusiform dilatation of intrahepatic bile ducts – Intrahepatic biliary sludge and stones – Central dot sign in CT and MRI – Intracystic gadolinium with hepatospecific contrast agents
ADPLD	– No significant kidney disease – Liver enlargement – Multiple liver cysts with varying dimensions – Complicated cysts appear heterogeneous in ultrasound, high density in CT, and heterogeneous signal in MRI – Peripheral calcifications may appear in previously complicated cysts – Hepatospecific contrast agents show no intracystic gadolinium
ADPKD	– Kidney involvement with multiple cysts – Liver enlargement – Multiple liver cysts with varying dimensions – Complicated cysts appear heterogeneous in ultrasound, high density in CT, and heterogeneous signal in MRI – Peripheral calcifications may appear in previously complicated cysts – Hepatospecific contrast agents show no intracystic gadolinium
ARPKD	– Similar to CHF – Findings related to portal hypertension – Coarse liver texture – Portal tracts echogenic in ultrasound and hyperintense in T2WI – MRCP depicts the intrahepatic bile ducts' irregular caliber – Atrophy of the right liver lobe and hypertrophy of the lateral left and caudate with left medial segments with normal/enlarged volume – Large regenerative hepatic nodules
CHF	– Similar to ARPKD – Findings related to portal hypertension – Coarse liver texture – Portal tracts echogenic in ultrasound and hyperintense in T2WI MRI – MRCP depicts the intrahepatic bile ducts' irregular caliber – Atrophy of the right liver lobe and hypertrophy of the lateral left and caudate with left medial segments with normal/enlarged volume – Large regenerative hepatic nodules
Biliary hamartomas	– Ultrasound with hypo/hyperechoic foci with comet-tail artifacts – Hyperintense tiny foci in T2WI – MRCP with "starry-sky" appearance

References

Ando H (2010) Embryology of the biliary tract. Dig Surg 27:87–89

Bergmann C, Senderek J, Windelen E, Küpper F, Middeldorf I, Schneider F, Dornia C, Rudnik-Schöneborn S, Konrad M, Schmitt CP, Seeman T, Neuhaus TJ, Vester U, Kirfel J, Büttner R, Zerres K (2005) Clinical consequences of PKHD1 mutations in 164 patients with autosomal-recessive polycystic kidney disease (ARPKD). Kidney Int 67: 829–848

Besse W, Dong K, Choi J, Punia S, Fedeles SV, Choi M, Gallagher AR, Huang EB, Gulati A, Knight J, Mane S, Tahvanainen E, Tahvanainen P, Sanna-Cherchi S, Lifton RP, Watnick T, Pei YP, Torres VE, Somlo S (2017) Isolated polycystic liver disease genes define effectors of polycystin-1 function. J Clin Invest 127:3558

Bloustein PA (1977) Association of carcinoma with congenital cystic conditions of the liver and bile ducts. Am J Gastroenterol 67:40–46

Brancatelli G, Federle MP, Vilgrain V, Vullierme MP, Marin D, Lagalla R (2005) Fibropolycystic liver disease: CT and MR imaging findings. Radiographics 25:659–670

Caroli J, Couinaud C, Soupault R et al (1958) Une affection nouvelle, sans doutecongénitale, des voies-biliaires: la dilatation cystiqueunilobaire des canaux-hépatiques. Sem Hop Paris 34:136–142

Cnossen WR, Drenth JP (2014) Polycystic liver disease: an overview of pathogenesis, clinical manifestations and management. Polycystic liver disease: an overview of pathogenesis, clinical manifestations and management. Orphanet J Rare Dis 9:69

Cnossen WR, teMorsche RH, Hoischen A, Gilissen C, Chrispijn M, Venselaar H, Mehdi S, Bergmann C, Veltman JA, Drenth JP (2014) Whole-exome sequencing reveals LRP5 mutations and canonical Wnt signaling associated with hepatic cystogenesis. Proc Natl Acad Sci U S A 111:5343–5348

Crawford JM (2002) Development of the intrahepatic biliary tree. Semin Liver Dis 22:213–226

Dell KM (2011) The spectrum of polycystic kidney disease in children. Adv Chronic Kidney Dis 18: 339–347

Desmet VJ (1992) What is congenital hepatic fibrosis? Histopathology 20:465–477

Desmet VJ (2005) Cystic diseases of the liver: from embryology to malformations. Gastroenterol Clin Biol 9:858–860

Drenth JP, Chrispijn M, Bergmann C (2010) Congenital fibrocystic liver diseases. Best Pract Res Clin Gastroenterol 24:573–584

Drenth JP, Tahvanainen E, teMorsche RH, Tahvanainen P, Kääriäinen H, Höckerstedt K, van de Kamp JM, Breuning MH, Jansen JB (2004) Abnormal hepatocystin caused by truncating PRKCSH mutations leads to autosomal dominant polycystic liver disease. Hepatology 39:924–931

Elsayes KM, Narra VR, Yin Y, Mukundan G, Lammle M, Brown JJ (2005) Focal hepatic lesions: diagnostic value of enhancement pattern approach with contrast-enhanced 3D gradient-echo MR imaging. Radiographics 25:1299–1320

Esseghaier S, Aidi Z, Toujani S, Daghfous MH (2017) A starry sky: multiple biliary hamartomas. Presse Med 46:787–788

Gabow PA (1993) Autosomal dominant polycystic kidney disease. N Engl J Med 329:332–342

Gaines PA, Sampson MA (1989) The prevalence and characterization of simple hepatic cysts by ultrasound examination. Br J Radiol 62:335–337

Gevers TJ, Hol JC, Monshouwer R, Dekker HM, Wetzels JF, Drenth JP (2015) Effect of lanreotide on polycystic liver and kidneys in autosomal dominant polycystic kidney disease: an observational trial. Liver Int 35:1607–1614

Giambelluca D, Caruana G, Cannella R, Lo Re G, Midiri M (2018) The starry sky liver: multiple biliary hamartomas on MR cholangiopancreatography. Abdom Radiol 43:2529–2530

Guay-Woodford LM, Desmond RA (2003) Autosomal recessive polycystic kidney disease: the clinical experience in North America. Pediatrics 111: 1072–1080

Gunay-Aygun M, Gahl WA, Heller T (2008) Congenital hepatic fibrosis overview [Updated 2014 Apr 24]. In: Adam MP, Ardinger HH, Pagon RA et al (eds) GeneReviews® [Internet]. University of Washington, Seattle (WA). 1993–2019

Hogan MC, Masyuk TV, Page LJ, Kubly VJ, Bergstralh EJ, Li X, Kim B, King BF, Glockner J, Holmes DR 3rd, Rossetti S, Harris PC, LaRusso NF, Torres VE (2010) Randomized clinical trial of long-acting somatostatin for autosomal dominant polycystic kidney and liver disease. J Am Soc Nephrol 21:1052–1061

Horton KM, Bluemke DA, Hruban RH, Soyer P, Fishman EK (1999) CT and MR imaging of benign hepatic and biliary tumors. Radiographics 19:431–451

Jain D, Sarode VR, Abdul-Karim FW, Homer R, Robert ME (2000) Evidence for the neoplastic transformation of von Meyenburg complexes. Am J Surg Pathol 24:1131–1139

Jordon D, Harpaz N, Thung SN (1989) Caroli's disease and adult polycystic kidney disease: a rarely recognized association. Liver 9:30–35

Jung G, Benz-Bohm G, Kugel H, Keller KM, Querfeld U (1999) MR cholangiography in children with autosomal recessive polycystic kidney disease. Pediatr Radiol 29:463–466

Kassahun WT, Kahn T, Wittekind C, Mössner J, Caca K, Hauss J, Lamesch P (2005) Caroli's disease: liver resection and liver transplantation. Experience in 33 patients. Surgery 138:888–898

Kerr DN, Harrisson CV, Sherlock S, Walker RM (1961) Congenital hepatic fibrosis. Q J Med 30:91–117

Lazaridis KN, Strazzabosco M, Larusso NF (2004) The cholangiopathies: disorders of biliary epithelia. Gastroenterology 127:1565–1577

Lendoire J, Barros Schelotto P, Alvarez Rodríguez J, Duek F, Quarin C, Garay V, Amante M, Cassini E, Imventarza O (2007) Bile duct cyst type V (Caroli's disease): surgical strategy and results. HPB 9:281–284

Lendoire JC, Raffin G, Grondona J, Bracco R, Russi R, Ardiles V, Gondolesi G, Defelitto J, de Santibañes E, Imventarza O (2011) Caroli's disease: report of surgical options and long-term outcome of patients treated in Argentina. Multicenter study. J Gastrointest Surg 15:1814–1819

Lewis S, Vasudevan P, Chatterji M, Besa C, Jajamovich G, Facciuto M, Taouli B (2016) Comparison of gadoxetic acid to gadobenate dimeglumine for assessment of biliary anatomy of potential liver donors. Abdom Radiol 41:1300–1309

Lonergan GJ, Rice RR, Suarez ES (2000) Autosomal recessive polycystic kidney disease: radiologic-pathologic correlation. Radiographics 20:837–855

Mamone G, Carollo V, Cortis K, Aquilina S, Liotta R, Miraglia R (2019) Magnetic resonance imaging of fibropolycystic liver disease: the spectrum of ductal plate malformations. Abdom Radiol 44:2156–2171

Mehta L, Jim B (2017) Hereditary renal diseases. Semin Nephrol 37:354–361

Meijer E, Visser FW, van Aerts RMM, Blijdorp CJ, Casteleijn NF, D'Agnolo HMA, Dekker SEI, Drenth JPH, de Fijter JW, van Gastel MDA, Gevers TJ, Lantinga MA, Losekoot M, Messchendorp AL, Neijenhuis MK, Pena MJ, Peters DJM, Salih M, Soonawala D, Spithoven EM, Wetzels JF, Zietse R, Gansevoort RT, DIPAK 1 Investigators (2018) Effect of lanreotide on kidney function in patients with autosomal dominant polycystic kidney disease: the DIPAK 1 randomized clinical trial. JAMA 320:2010–2019

Morgan DE, Lockhart ME, Canon CL, Holcombe MP, Bynon JS (2006) Polycystic liver disease: multimodality imaging for complications and transplant evaluation. Radiographics 26:1655–1668

Neijenhuis MK, Wijnands TFM, Kievit W, Ronot M, Gevers TJG, Drenth JPH (2019) Symptom relief and not cyst reduction determines treatment success in aspiration sclerotherapy of hepatic cysts. Eur Radiol 29:3062–3068

O'Brien K, Font-Montgomery E, Lukose L, Bryant J, Piwnica-Worms K, Edwards H, Riney L, Garcia A, Daryanani K, Choyke P, Mohan P, Heller T, Gahl WA, Gunay-Aygun M (2012) Congenital hepatic fibrosis and portal hypertension in autosomal dominant polycystic kidney disease. J Pediatr Gastroenterol Nutr 54:83–89

Paul BM, VandenHeuvel GB (2014) Kidney: polycystic kidney disease. Wiley Interdiscip Rev Dev Biol 3:465–487

Perugorria MJ, Masyuk TV, Marin JJ, Marzioni M, Bujanda L, LaRusso NF, Banales JM (2014) Polycystic liver diseases: advanced insights into the molecular mechanisms. Nat Rev Gastroenterol Hepatol 11:750–761

Principe A, Lugaresi ML, Lords RC, D'Errico A, Polito E, Gallö MC, Bicchierri I, Cavallari A (1997) Bile duct hamartomas: diagnostic problems and treatment. Hepatogastroenterology 44:994–997

Ramond MJ, Huguet C, Danan G, Rueff B, Benhamou JP (1984) Partial hepatectomy in the treatment of Caroli's disease. Report of a case and review of the literature. Dig Dis Sci 29:367–370

Redston MS, Wanless IR (1996) The hepatic von Meyenburg complex: prevalence and association with hepatic and renal cysts among 2843 autopsies. Mod Pathol 9:233–237

Rogers TN, Woodley H, Ramsden W, Wyatt JI, Stringer MD (2007) Solitary liver cysts in children: not always so simple. J Pediatr Surg 42:333–339

Russell RT, Pinson CW (2007) Surgical management of polycystic liver disease. World J Gastroenterol 13:5052–5059

Santiago I, Loureiro R, Curvo-Semedo L, Marques C, Tardáguila F, Matos C, Caseiro-Alves F (2012) Congenital cystic lesions of the biliary tree. Am J Roentgenol 198:825–835

Sayma M, Walters HR, Hesford C, Tariq Z, Nakhosteen A (2019) Rapidly enlarging, giant hepatic cyst growing pseudomonas. BMJ Case Rep 1:12

Semelka RC, Hussain SM, Marcos HB, Woosley JT (1999) Biliary hamartomas: solitary and multiple lesions shown on current MR techniques including gadolinium enhancement. J Magn Reson Imaging 10:196–201

Shneider BL, Magid MS (2005) Liver disease in autosomal recessive polycystic kidney disease. Pediatr Transplant 9:634–639

Song JS, Lee YJ, Kim KW, Huh J, Jang SJ, Yu E (2008) Cholangiocarcinoma arising in von Meyenburg complexes: report of four cases. Pathol Int 58:503–512

Srinath A, Shneider BL (2012) Congenital hepatic fibrosis and autosomal recessive polycystic kidney disease. J Pediatr Gastroenterol Nutr 54:580–587

Summerfield JA, Nagafuchi Y, Sherlock S, Cadafalch J, Scheuer PJ (1986) Hepatobiliary fibropolycystic diseases. A clinical and histological review of 51 patients. J Hepatol 2:141–156

Torres VE, Harris PC, Pirson Y (2007) Autosomal dominant polycystic kidney disease. Lancet 369:1287–1301

Turkbey B, Ocak I, Daryanani K, Font-Montgomery E, Lukose L, Bryant J, Tuchman M, Mohan P, Heller T, Gahl WA, Choyke PL, Gunay-Aygun M (2009) Autosomal recessive polycystic kidney disease and congenital hepatic fibrosis (ARPKD/CHF). Pediatr Radiol 39:100–111

van de Laarschot LFM, Drenth JPH (2018) Genetics and mechanisms of hepatic cystogenesis. Biochim Biophys Acta Mol Basis Dis 1864:1491–1497

van Keimpema L, de Koning DB, Strijk SP, Drenth JP (2008) Aspiration-sclerotherapy results in effective control of liver volume in patients with liver cysts. Dig Dis Sci 53:2251–2257

van Keimpema L, Nevens F, Vanslembrouck R, van Oijen MG, Hoffmann AL, Dekker HM, de Man RA, Drenth JP (2009) Lanreotide reduces the volume of polycystic liver: a randomized, double-blind, placebo-controlled trial. Gastroenterology 137:1661–1668. e1–2

Veigel MC, Prescott-Focht J, Rodriguez MG, Zinati R, Shao L, Moore CA, Lowe LH (2009) Fibropolycystic liver disease in children. Pediatr Radiol 39:317–327

Venkatanarasimha N, Thomas R, Armstrong EM, Shirley JF, Fox BM, Jackson SA (2011) Imaging features of ductal plate malformations in adults. Clin Radiol 66:1086–1093

von Meyenburg H (1918) Uber die cystenliber. Beitr Pathol Anat 64:477e532

Willey CJ, Blais JD, Hall AK, Krasa HB, Makin AJ, Czerwiec FS (2017) Prevalence of autosomal dominant polycystic kidney disease in the European Union. Nephrol Dial Transplant 32:1356–1363

Xu AM, Xian ZH, Zhang SH, Chen XF (2009) Intrahepatic cholangiocarcinoma arising in multiple bile duct hamartomas: report of two cases and review of the literature. Eur J Gastroenterol Hepatol 21: 580–584

Yang XY, Zhang HB, Wu B, Li AJ, Fu XH (2017) Surgery is the preferred treatment for bile duct hamartomas. Mol Clin Oncol 7:649–653

Yoshida H, Onda M, Tajiri T, Mamada Y, Taniai N, Mineta S, Hirakata A, Futami R, Arima Y, Inoue M, Hatta S, Kishimoto A (2003) Infected hepatic cyst. Hepato-Gastroenterology 50:507–509

Zeitoun D, Brancatelli G, Colombat M, Federle MP, Valla D, Wu T, Degott C, Vilgrain V (2004) Congenital hepatic fibrosis: CT findings in 18 adults. Radiology 231:109–116

Zerres K, Mücher G, Becker J, Steinkamm C, Rudnik-Schöneborn S, Heikkilä P, Rapola J, Salonen R, Germino GG, Onuchic L, Somlo S, Avner ED, Harman LA, Stockwin JM, Guay-Woodford LM (1998) Prenatal diagnosis of autosomal recessive polycystic kidney disease (ARPKD): molecular genetics, clinical experience, and fetal morphology. Am J Med Genet 76:137–144

Zheng RQ, Zhang B, Kudo M, Onda H, Inoue T (2005) Imaging findings of biliary hamartomas. World J Gastroenterol 11:6354–6359

Inflammatory Liver Diseases

İlkay S. İdilman, Deniz Akata,
and Muşturay Karçaaltıncaba

Contents

Abstract

Liver inflammation may be acute or chronic form which leads to fibrosis and cirrhosis. The diagnosis depends on histopathologic evaluation which can be confounding especially in cases with heterogeneous involvement. In this chapter, we reviewed inflammatory liver diseases such as autoimmune hepatitis, overlap syndromes, sarcoidosis, drug disease, Wilson's disease, alfa 1 antitripsin deficiency, and radiation injury with imaging findings.

Several etiological factors cause liver inflammation that is characterized by acute or chronic inflammatory cell accumulation within the liver. Liver inflammation may be in acute or chronic form that leads to fibrosis and cirrhosis. The diagnosis of liver inflammation primarily depends on liver biopsy and histopathologic evaluation. However, imaging findings may guide both clinician and pathologist especially in cases with confounding laboratory or pathologic findings. In this chapter, we review inflammatory liver diseases such as autoimmune hepatitis, overlap syndromes, sarcoidosis, drug disease, Wilson's disease, alpha-1 antitrypsin deficiency, and radiation injury with imaging findings.

İ. S. İdilman · D. Akata · M. Karçaaltıncaba (✉)
Liver Imaging Team, Department of Radiology,
Hacettepe University School of Medicine,
Ankara, Turkey

© Springer Nature Switzerland AG 2021
E. Quaia (ed.), *Imaging of the Liver and Intra-hepatic Biliary Tract*,
Medical Radiology, Diagnostic Imaging, https://doi.org/10.1007/978-3-030-38983-3_12

1   Autoimmune Hepatitis

Autoimmune hepatitis (AIH) is a chronic liver disease that is seen in all ages and races with a female predominance (Manns et al. 2015). Genetic susceptibility with an exposure to a trigger environmental agent such as herbs, microbes, immunization, and drugs is a blamed factor in the etiopathogenesis of AIH. In general, AIH present with an episode of acute hepatitis with subsequent chronic course. Clinical manifestation of AIH may vary such as mildly elevated liver function tests in asymptomatic patient, acute fulminant hepatitis, or cirrhosis. The diagnosis of the disease primarily depends on clinical, laboratory, and liver histology findings. Interface hepatitis with lymphoplasmocytic infiltrates and varying degrees of lobular inflammation is a histopathologic finding in AIH (Manns et al. 2015).

Imaging findings of AIH may change according to the severity of the disease. Ultrasonography (US) may reveal no abnormal finding in the early stage of the disease as well as features of chronic liver disease such as coarsening of hepatic echotexture, nodularity, and volume redistribution (Malik and Venkatesh 2017). The main role of US in AIH is HCC surveillance. Transient US elastography was shown to be a reliable method for estimation of hepatic fibrosis in AIH (Obara et al. 2008). Computed tomography may reveal normal findings or findings associated with chronic liver disease. Benign hypervascular nodules can be observed in AIH that may enhance after contrast administration, some with delayed washout (Qayyum et al. 2004). Nonspecific findings such as hepatic surface nodularity, ascites, and splenomegaly were found to be the most common findings on CT (Sahni et al. 2010).

Magnetic resonance imaging (MRI) may demonstrate similar findings as CT. Hepatic surface nodularity that is associated with fibrosis is the most common finding observed in AIH on MRI (Bilaj et al. 2005; Sahni et al. 2010) (Fig. 1). Reticular fibrosis that is defined as fine lines that had low signal intensity at out-of-phase MR images with prominent enhancement on post-contrast images is another finding observed on MRI (Bilaj et al. 2005). Global atrophy was the

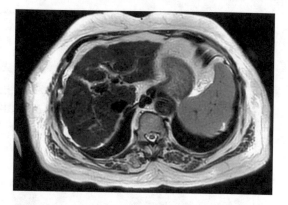

Fig. 1 A 70-year-old female patient with autoimmune hepatitis. T2W imaging demonstrates hepatic surface nodularity, which is the most common imaging finding

main volumetric change observed in AIH (Obara et al. 2008). Lymphadenopathy is not common as other autoimmune liver diseases such as primary sclerosing cholangitis (PSC) and primary biliary cholangitis (PBC). MR elastography is a promising method in the evaluation of fibrosis in patients with AIH. It was shown that a liver stiffness threshold of >4.1 kPa predicted advanced fibrosis with 89.5% sensitivity and 100% specificity, and a threshold of >4.5 kPa predicted cirrhosis with 92% sensitivity and 96% specificity (Wang et al. 2017).

1.1   Overlap Syndromes

Overlap syndromes are variant forms of autoimmune liver diseases, which share histological, biochemical, serological, and imaging characteristics of AIH, primary biliary cholangitis (PBC), and primary sclerosing cholangitis (PSC). It was reported that 7–13% of patients with AIH have overlapping features of PBC and 6–11% of patients have features of PSC (Czaja 2013). Biochemical and imaging findings of overlap syndromes may vary according to the difference of coexistence disease.

AIH-PBC overlap syndrome presents with serum liver tests typically showing a hepatitic pattern in AIH and a cholestatic pattern with predominant elevation of alkaline phosphatase (ALP) and gamma-glutamyl transferase (GGT) and only mild elevation of serum transaminases in PBC. Primary biliary cirrhosis is a slow progressive disease with destruction of small intrahepatic bile ducts ending up with chronic cholestasis and cirrhosis. Imaging findings of PBC include heterogeneous attenuating parenchyma and segmental atrophy on CT (Blachar et al. 2001). Atrophy or hypertrophy may be observed as well as smooth or nodular liver contour (Blachar et al. 2001). Findings of portal hypertension are commonly seen in advanced PBC. Lymphadenopathy is an expected finding in PBC with most commonly in portacaval region and porta hepatis (Blachar et al. 2001). Conspicuous low signal intensity around portal vein branches on T1 and T2 images was defined for MRI finding of PBC (Wenzel et al. 2001). "Periportal halo sign" was described as a finding of PBC consisting of a rounded lesion centered on a portal venous branch 5 mm–1 cm in size, and numerous lesions involving all hepatic segments, with low signal intensity on T1- and T2-weighted images, and no mass effect (Fig. 2) (Wenzel et al. 2001). In AIH-PBC overlap, imaging findings may be consistent with either isolated AIH or isolated PBC (Hyslop et al. 2010).

AIH-PSC overlap syndrome is diagnosed with characteristic changes in biliary tree observed in imaging such as strictures and segmental dilatations in a patient with AIH. PSC is a chronic inflammatory large duct cholangiopathy, which results with fibrotic biliary duct strictures, cholestasis, and biliary cirrhosis. Diffuse involvement of both intrahepatic and extrahepatic bile ducts is the commonest form (75%) followed by isolated intrahepatic bile duct involvement (15%) and isolated extrahepatic bile duct involvement (10%) (Tischendorf et al. 2007). Central lobe enlargement with left lateral hypertrophy predominates in PSC (Bilaj et al. 2005). Imaging findings in AIH-PSC overlap syndrome on MRI include central macroregenerative nodules, peripheral atrophy, biliary ductal obstruction, and biliary ductal beading (Hyslop et al. 2010). The presence of macroregenerative nodules, peripheral atrophy, and biliary ductal irregularity, alone or in combination, had 100% specificity for PSC-type overlap syndrome.

2 Sarcoidosis

Sarcoidosis is a multisystem disease characterized with noncaseating granulomas in affected organs. The prevalence of the disease is 2–60 per 100,000 people with a predominance in African American populations (Baughman and Lower 2008). The etiopathogenesis of the disease remains unclear with blamed genetic susceptibility and environmental factors. Liver is one of the most affected organs after lung and lymph node involvement. The disease may involve all compartments of the liver and results in various patterns of liver injury such as portal and lobular inflammation of hepatocytes, biliary involvement with cholestasis, or sinusoidal dilatation as a result of compressive effect of granulomas (Deutsch-Link et al. 2018). The majority of patients with hepatic involvement are asymptomatic. Clinical symptoms include fatigue, abdominal pain, and fever (Tadros et al. 2013). The diagnosis generally depends on clinical and radiological findings with histopathological sarcoid granuloma identification.

Imaging findings are not evident in most of the cases. The most common imaging feature of hepatic sarcoidosis is hepatomegaly that is seen in more than 50% of the patients (Warshauer et al. 1995). Increased parenchymal echogenicity

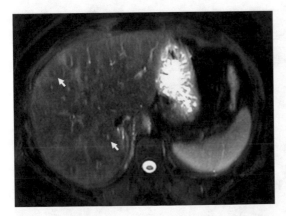

Fig. 2 A 48-year-old female patient with overlap syndrome (autoimmune hepatitis—primary biliary cholangitis). T2W images show periportal halo sign (arrows)

may be observed in US examination. Heterogeneous echogenicity and coarse echo pattern may be detected in diffuse parenchymal involvement (Karaosmanoğlu et al. 2015). Contour irregularity and parenchymal calcifications are also expected findings in diffuse hepatic involvement (Kessler et al. 1993). Focal lesions that are consistent with granulomas are detected as well-defined hypoechoic or hyperechoic nodules in the liver (Gezer et al. 2015).

Cross-sectional imaging findings may demonstrate similar findings with US. The appearance of the liver may range from normal to chronic parenchymal liver disease in diffuse hepatic sar-

coidosis. It was reported that both macroregenerative nodules and wedge-shaped peripheral atrophy presence may suggest the diagnosis of hepatic sarcoidosis in a patient with chronic parenchymal liver disease (Ferreira et al. 2013). Periportal thickening that is best seen on T2-weighted images can be observed in sarcoidosis. Imaging findings consistent with portal hypertension can be seen as a result of cirrhosis or compression effect of portal lymphadenopathies. Focal nodules in hepatic sarcoidosis are typically seen as hypo-attenuating subcentimeter focal lesions on CT (Fig. 3). On MR imaging, these are seen as T1 hypo-isointense and T2 hypointense foci with no evident contrast enhancement (Fig. 4).

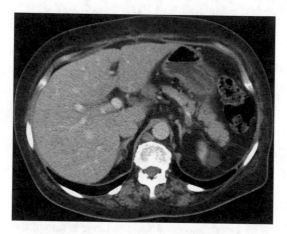

Fig. 3 A 54-year-old female patient with diagnosis of sarcoidosis. On contrast-enhanced CT images, multiple millimetric hypoattenuating nodules are seen

3 Drug Disease

Drug-induced liver injury (DILI) is an important cause of mortality around the world caused by various mechanisms causing liver injury. Hundreds of drugs have been identified causing DILI such as antibiotics (amoxicillin-clavulanate, isoniazid, doxycycline), diclofenac, acetaminophen, atorvastatin, and carbamazepine that are the commonest ones (Alempijevic et al. 2017). Besides, herbals and dietary supplements are used increasingly and cause increase in HDS-induced liver injury proportionally (Navarro et al.

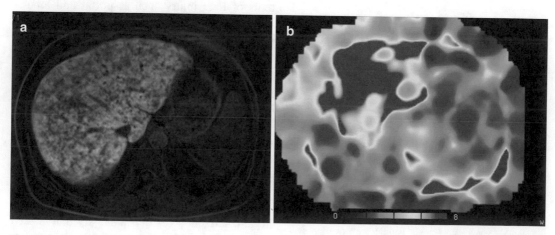

Fig. 4 A 47-year-old female patient with sarcoidosis. Postcontrast T1W MR images demonstrate heterogeneous enhancement of the liver (**a**). Liver stiffness was 9.9 kPa on MR elastography consistent with involvement (**b**)

2017). Acute and chronic hepatitic, acute and chronic cholestatic, and mixed hepatitis-cholestatic types are the most common forms of DILI within various histopathologic categories (Kleiner et al. 2014).

Imaging findings may vary according to the type of injury. Hepatic steatosis, which is defined as excessive triglyceride accumulation in the hepatocytes, is one of the possible mechanisms of DILI. Chemotherapeutic agents such as 5-fluorouracil, irinotecan, and methotrexate and amiodarone, tamoxifen, corticosteroids, and antipsychotics are frequently associated with steatosis or steatohepatitis (McGettigan et al. 2016). Increased echogenicity of the liver in US examination and decreased attenuation at CT are imaging findings of hepatic steatosis. Signal drop on out-of-phase image relative to in-phase image is present at MRI. Drugs such as immunosuppressive cyclosporine, the antibiotic trimethoprim-sulfamethoxazole, and the antipsychotic chlorpromazine cause cholestatic injury that predominantly affects bile ducts (Bhamidimarri and Schiff 2013; Padda et al. 2011). US and CT imaging have no specific finding in cholestatic injury and may demonstrate nonspecific findings of inflammation such as heterogeneous contrast enhancement or hepatomegaly (Fig. 5). Imaging modalities such as cholangiography and MRCP may demonstrate small bile ducts diminished in number (ElSayed et al. 2013; Gossard 2014, p. 1). Sclerosing cholangitis like changes such as

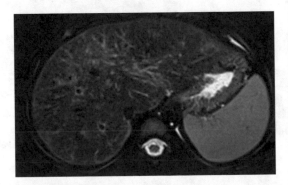

Fig. 5 Heterogeneous liver parenchyma and periportal thickening on T2W image are seen in a 2-year-old male patient with Wilms' tumor after chemotherapy. Follow-up MRI demonstrated resolution of the findings

intrahepatic and common hepatic duct strictures on MRCP was also defined in patients with DILI (Ahmad et al. 2019).

4 Wilson's Disease

Wilson's disease is an autosomal recessively inherited disease with approximately 1/30,000 prevalence (Gitlin 2003). There is a defect in copper homeostasis which leads to accumulation of copper in different tissues such as liver, brain, and cornea. Liver is the main regulator of copper metabolism by storing both the copper and biliary excretion of this metal. There are different mutations reported in the ATP7G gene which give rise to dysfunction of the corresponding ATPase that transfers copper into the secretory pathway by incorporation into apoccruloplasmin and excretion into the bile (Lutsenko and Petris 2003; Schaefer and Gitlin 1999). This results in intrahepatocellular copper accumulation with resultant copper-mediated oxidative damage and activation of cell death pathways (Strand et al. 1998). Early diagnosis of Wilson's disease is important for complete recovery which might be fatal otherwise. Affected individuals mainly present with liver disease which may mimic different acute or chronic liver diseases. The presence of Kayser–Fleischer rings, decreased serum ceruloplasmin, and hepatic or neuropsychiatric symptoms are sufficient for the diagnosis of Wilson's disease.

There are different imaging findings of Wilson's disease according to the disease course. US is one of the most preferred imaging modalities for Wilson's disease. Increased hepatic echogenicity due to fatty change or fibrosis can be observed in individuals with Wilson's disease which is also the main US finding of nonalcoholic fatty liver disease and may be confusing (Akhan et al. 2009; Akpinar and Akhan 2007). Parenchymal heterogeneity was reported to be detected in most of the patients in Wilson's disease (Akhan et al. 2009). This heterogeneity can be diffuse or associated with multiple hypoechoic nodules or multiple hypoechoic and hyperechoic nodules (Akhan et al. 2009). Contour irregularity and increased periportal thickness are other US findings seen in Wilson's disease. Perihepatic fat layer that is recognized by perihepatic hyper-echogenic zone in US is a possible finding in Wilson's disease (Akhan et al. 2002, 2009; Akpinar and Akhan 2007). Cholelithiasis may be observed in individuals with Wilson's disease as a coexisting disease.

Diffuse increased hepatic attenuation due to copper accumulation on computed tomography (CT) can be detected in Wilson's disease. This may not be noticed due to opposing effect of fat deposition that decreases the attenuation on CT. Parenchymal heterogeneity and contour irregularity are other possible findings in Wilson's disease. Unenhanced CT generally reveals hyperdense nodules that will be hypodense on contrast-enhanced CT images and

become more apparent on portal venous phase images (Akpinar and Akhan 2007; Li et al. 2011). The hyperdense nodules on unenhanced CT are seen hyperintense on T1W images and hypointense on T2W MR images due to para-magnetic effect of copper. Honeycomb pattern is defined as hyperdense nodules with hypodense septa on unenhanced CT with enhancement of septa after contrast administration (Li et al. 2011). This pattern is detected as hypointense nodules with surrounding hyperintense septa on T2W images (Fig. 6). Honeycomb pattern is pro-posed as the most sensitive imaging finding for Wilson's disease (Vargas et al. 2016). Perihepatic fat layer can also be observed as perihepatic hypodense zone on CT and hyperintense on MR images. In advanced stages of the disease, find-ings consistent with portal hypertension would

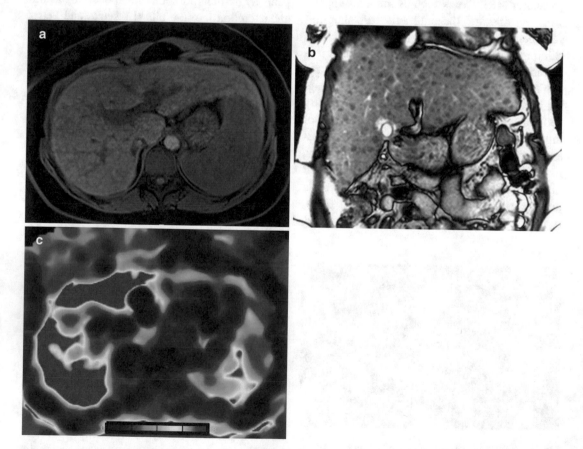

Fig. 6 A 34-year-old female patient with diagnosis of Wilson. T1W images demonstrate hypointense nodules (**a**) and T2W coronal image demonstrates hypointense nodules with surrounding hyperintense septa (**b**). MR elastography demonstrates severe fibrosis in this patient with liver stiffness value of 8 kPa (**c**)

be evident. Contrary to other chronic liver diseases, caudate lobe hypertrophy is not an expected finding and normal caudate-to-right lobe ratio is reported as a diagnostic finding in Wilson's disease (Akpinar and Akhan 2007). Wilson's disease complicated by hepatocellular carcinoma is not an infrequent finding and should be evaluated in follow-up imaging.

5 Alpha-1 Antitrypsin Deficiency

Alpha-1 antitrypsin deficiency (AATD) is a rare hereditary disease with decreased production of alpha-1 antitrypsin that results in serious lung and/or liver disease. Aggregation of alpha-1 antitrypsin polymers within the endoplasmic reticulum of liver cells promotes hepatocyte injury and forms periodic acid-Schiff-positive inclusions, which are hallmark biopsy feature in AATD-related liver disease (Edgar et al. 2017). Phenotypic expression may vary based on genetic and environmental factors in both lung and liver diseases in AATD. The clinical course of AATD-related liver disease is poorly understood that affects about 10% of the patients with AATD (Townsend et al. 2018). There is no specific imaging finding defined for AATD-related liver disease in the literature. Imaging findings of chronic liver disease and portal hypertension may be detected in advanced liver disease. In recent studies, it was shown that elastography techniques performed with MRI and US have the potential to detect AATD-related liver fibrosis before development of cirrhosis (Kim et al. 2016; Reiter et al. 2018).

6 Radiation Injury

Radiation-induced liver disease (RILD), in other words radiation hepatitis, is a form of veno-occlusive disease with fibrous obliteration of hepatic venules. It is a complication of radiotherapy and is characterized with anicteric ascites, hepatomegaly, and elevated liver enzymes within 2–8 weeks after radiotherapy. Imaging finding characteristically demonstrates a sharp line of demarcation between normal and abnormal parenchyma compatible with radiation port (Fig. 7). Hypodense area at unenhanced CT and hypo- or hyperdense area at enhanced CT reveal RILD (Unger et al. 1987). In patients with hepatic steatosis, irradiated zone may demonstrate higher attenuation than fatty liver. Affected area appears hypointense on T1W images and hyperintense on T2-weighted images due to edema on MRI. Imaging findings usually regress within 4–6 months and atrophy of the irradiated area and compensatory hypertrophy of the remaining liver can be observed (Federle 2004).

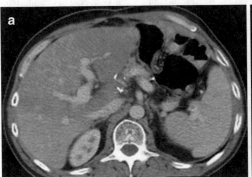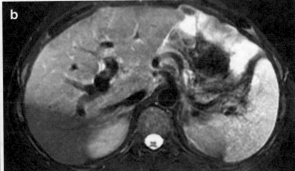

Fig. 7 A patient with breast carcinoma with a history of radiation therapy. A well-demarcated hypodense area on contrast-enhanced CT image (**a**) and hyperintense area on T2W image (**b**) that are consistent with radiation port are seen

References

Ahmad J, Rossi S, Rodgers SK et al (2019) Sclerosing cholangitis-like changes on magnetic resonance cholangiography in patients with drug induced liver injury. Clin Gastroenterol Hepatol 17:789–790

Akhan O, Akpinar E, Karcaaltincaba M et al (2009) Imaging findings of liver involvement of Wilson's disease. Eur J Radiol 69:147–155

Akhan O, Akpinar E, Oto A et al (2002) Unusual imaging findings in Wilson's disease. Eur Radiol 12:66–69

Akpinar E, Akhan O (2007) Liver imaging findings of Wilson's disease. Eur J Radiol 61:25–32

Alempijevic T, Zec S, Milosavljevic T (2017) Drug-induced liver injury: do we know everything? World J Hepatol 9:491–502

Baughman RP, Lower EE (2008) Sarcoidosis. In: Harrison's principles of internal medicine. McGraw-Hill, Medical Publishing Division, New York, pp 2135–2142

Bhamidimarri KR, Schiff E (2013) Drug-induced cholestasis. Clin Liver Dis 17:519–531

Bilaj F, Hyslop WB, Rivero H et al (2005) MR imaging findings in autoimmune hepatitis: correlation with clinical staging. Radiology 236:896–902

Blachar A, Federle MP, Brancatelli G (2001) Primary biliary cirrhosis: clinical, pathologic, and helical CT findings in 53 patients. Radiology 220:329–336

Czaja AJ (2013) The overlap syndromes of autoimmune hepatitis. Dig Dis Sci 58:326–343

Deutsch-Link S, Fortuna D, Weinberg EM (2018) A comprehensive review of hepatic sarcoid. Semin Liver Dis 38:284–297

Edgar RGPM, Bayliss S, Crossley D et al (2017) Treatment of lung disease in alpha-1 antitrypsin deficiency: a systematic review. Int J Chron Obstruct Pulmon Dis 12:1295–1308

ElSayed EY, El Maati AA, Mahfouz M (2013) Diagnostic value of magnetic resonance cholangiopancreatography in cholestatic jaundice. Egypt J Radiol Nucl Med 44:137–146

Federle MP (2004) Diagnostic imaging: abdomen, 1st edn. Amyrsis. II-I-p 148

Ferreira A, Ramalho M, de Campos ROP et al (2013) Hepatic sarcoidosis: MR appearances in patients with chronic liver disease. Magn Reson Imaging 31:432–438

Gezer NS, Basara I, Altay C et al (2015) Abdominal sarcoidosis: cross-sectional imaging findings. Diagn Interv Radiol 21:111–117

Gitlin JD (2003) Wilson disease. Gastroenterology 125:1868–1877

Gossard AA (2014) Diagnosis of cholestasis. In: Carey EJ, Lindor KD (eds) Cholestatic liver disease, 2nd edn. Springer, New York, NY, pp 1–12

Hyslop WB, Kierans AS, Leonardou P et al (2010) Overlap syndrome of autoimmune chronic liver diseases: MRI findings. J Magn Reson Imaging 31:383–389

Karaosmanoğlu AD, Onur MR, Saini S et al (2015) Imaging of hepatobiliary involvement in sarcoidosis. Abdom Imaging 40:3330–3337

Kessler A, Mitchell DG, Israel HL et al (1993) Hepatic and splenic sarcoidosis: ultrasound and MR imaging. Abdom Imaging 18:159–163

Kim RG, Nguyen P, Bettencourt R et al (2016) Magnetic resonance elastography identifies fibrosis in adults with alpha-1 antitrypsin deficiency liver disease: a prospective study. Aliment Pharmacol Ther 44:287–299

Kleiner DE, Chalasani NP, Lee WM et al (2014) Hepatic histological findings in suspected drug-induced liver injury: systematic evaluation and clinical associations. Hepatology 59:661–670

Li W, Zhao X, Zhan Q et al (2011) Unique CT imaging findings of liver in Wilson's disease. Abdom Imaging 36:69–73

Lutsenko S, Petris MJ (2003) Function and regulation of the mammalian copper-transporting ATPases: insights from biochemical and cell biological approaches. J Membr Biol 191:1–12

Malik N, Venkatesh SK (2017) Imaging of autoimmune hepatitis and overlap syndromes. Abdom Radiol (NY) 42:19–27

Manns MP, Lohse AW, Vergani D (2015) Autoimmune hepatitis—update 2015. J Hepatol 62(1 Suppl):S100–S111

McGettigan MJ, Menias CO, Gao ZJ et al (2016) Imaging of drug-induced complications in the gastrointestinal system. Radiographics 36:71–87

Navarro VJ, Khan I, Björnsson E et al (2017) Liver injury from herbal and dietary supplements. Hepatology 65:363–373

Obara N, Ueno Y, Fukushima K et al (2008) Transient elastography for measurement of liver stiffness measurement can detect early significant hepatic fibrosis in Japanese patients with viral and nonviral liver diseases. J Gastroenterol 43:720–728

Padda MS, Sanchez M, Akhtar AJ et al (2011) Drug-induced cholestasis. Hepatology 53:1377–1387

Qayyum A, Graser A, Westphalen A et al (2004) CT of benign hypervascular liver nodules in autoimmune hepatitis. Am J Roentgenol 183:1573–1576

Reiter R, Wetzel M, Hamesch K et al (2018) Comparison of non-invasive assessment of liver fibrosis in patients with alpha-1-antitrypsin deficiency using magnetic resonance elastography (MRE), acoustic radiation force impulse (ARFI) quantification, and 2D-shear wave elastography (2D-SWE). PLoS One 13:e0196486

Sahni VA, Raghunathan G, Mearadji B et al (2010) Autoimmune hepatitis: CT and MR imaging features with histopathological correlation. Abdom Imaging 35:75–84

Schaefer M, Gitlin JD (1999) Genetic disorders of membrane transport. IV. Wilson's disease and Menkes disease. Am J Phys 276:311–314

Strand S, Hofmann WJ, Grambihler A et al (1998) Hepatic failure and liver cell damage in acute Wilson's disease involve CD95 (APO-1/Fas) mediated apoptosis. Nat Med 4:588–593

Tadros M, Forouhar F, Wu GY (2013) Hepatic sarcoidosis. J Clin Transl Hepatol 1:87–93

Tischendorf JJ, Hecker H, Krüger M et al (2007) Characterization, outcome, and prognosis in 273 patients with primary sclerosing cholangitis: a single center study. Am J Gastroenterol 102:107–114

Townsend SA, Edgar RG, Ellis PR et al (2018) Systematic review: the natural history of alpha-1 antitrypsin deficiency, and associated liver disease. Aliment Pharmacol Ther 47:877–885

Unger EC, Lee JK, Weyman PJ (1987) CT and MR imaging of radiation hepatitis. J Comput Assist Tomogr 11:264–268

Vargas O, Faraoun SA, Dautry R et al (2016) MR imaging features of liver involvement by Wilson disease in adult patients. Radiol Med 121:546–556

Wang J, Malik N, Yin M et al (2017) Magnetic resonance elastography is accurate in detecting advanced fibrosis in autoimmune hepatitis. World J Gastroenterol 23:859–868

Warshauer DM, Molina PL, Hamman SM et al (1995) Nodular sarcoidosis of the liver and spleen: analysis of 32 cases. Radiology 195:757–762

Wenzel JS, Donohoe A, Ford KL 3rd et al (2001) Primary biliary cirrhosis: MR imaging findings and description of MR imaging periportal halo sign. AJR Am J Roentgenol 176:885–889

Liver Steatosis and NAFLD

Manuela França and João Mota Louro

Contents

M. França (✉)
Radiology Department, Centro Hospitalar e
Universitário do Porto, Oporto, Portugal

Instituto de Ciências Biomédicas de Abel Salazar,
Universidade do Porto, Oporto, Portugal

i3S, Instituto de Investigação e Inovação em Saúde,
Universidade do Porto, Oporto, Portugal
e-mail: manuelafranca.radiologia@chporto.
min-saude.pt

J. M. Louro
Radiology Department, Centro Hospitalar e
Universitário do Porto, Oporto, Portugal

Abstract

Liver steatosis is the hallmark of non-alcoholic fatty liver disease (NAFLD), the most frequent chronic liver disease in the western countries. NAFLD ranges from simple steatosis to non-alcoholic steatohepatitis (NASH) and cirrhosis. Steatosis is also common in other diffuse liver diseases. Regardless the etiology, liver fat accumulation induces liver damage, being associated with poor outcomes of chronic liver diseases. Liver biopsy is the gold standard for diagnosis and stratification of NAFLD, and also for distinguishing simple steatosis from NASH and staging fibrosis. However, liver biopsy is invasive and subject to substantial variability. Therefore, over the last years, the global burden of NALFD and the potential clinical impact of early detection

© Springer Nature Switzerland AG 2021
E. Quaia (ed.), *Imaging of the Liver and Intra-hepatic Biliary Tract*,
Medical Radiology, Diagnostic Imaging, https://doi.org/10.1007/978-3-030-38983-3_13

and monitoring of hepatic steatosis has fostered the use of non-invasive imaging modalities for the assessment of steatosis and the search for imaging biomarkers of fat. In this chapter, we will review the role of different imaging modalities in the detection and quantification of liver steatosis, highlighting the role of imaging biomarkers of steatosis.

1   Introduction

Steatosis consists of the accumulation of fatty vacuoles in >5% of hepatocytes, resulting from the disruption of hepatic lipid metabolism. It is the hallmark of nonalcoholic fatty liver disease (NAFLD), which is now the most frequent chronic liver disease in the Western countries, being considered the hepatic manifestation of the metabolic syndrome (Younossi et al. 2016).

NAFLD encompasses three stages: simple steatosis, nonalcoholic steatohepatitis (NASH), and cirrhosis. The prognosis is variable, but up to 40% of the patients will develop inflammatory activity and fibrosis. Cirrhosis and its known complications may ensue, namely hepatocellular carcinoma and portal hypertension (McPherson et al. 2015). Fibrosis is the key factor for determining long-term prognosis, with those in advanced stages (F3–F4) estimated to have a >3-fold increased risk of all-cause mortality (Ekstedt et al. 2015; Angulo et al. 2015). Recent guidelines recommend lifestyle changes for NAFLD patients but those patients with NASH may benefit from pharmacotherapy. Nevertheless, although promising trials are underway, no specific drug has yet been approved (EASL–EASD–EASO 2016).

Besides NAFLD, steatosis is also common in other diffuse liver diseases, such as alcoholic liver disease, viral hepatitis, drug toxicity, and hemochromatosis (Chalasani et al. 2012). Regardless of the etiology, intracellular fat induces liver damage and has been associated to poor outcomes in liver diseases (Leandro et al. 2006; Hwang and Lee 2011). Additionally, it reduces the response to antiviral treatment in viral hepatitis (Hwang and Lee 2011) and worsens the prognosis of patients undergoing liver

surgery or transplant (Ploeg et al. 1993; de Meijer et al. 2010).

Liver biopsy is the gold standard for diagnosis and stratification of NAFLD, and also for distinguishing simple steatosis from NASH and staging fibrosis (Yeh and Brunt 2014). The most used semiquantitative method to grade liver steatosis relies on a visual score based on the percentage of liver parenchyma containing steatotic hepatocytes: 6–33%, 33–66%, or >66% (Kleiner et al. 2005; Yeh and Brunt 2014). Although promising semiautomated and automated methods have been developed (Nativ et al. 2014; Vanderbeck et al. 2014), liver biopsy is still subject to substantial inter- and intra-reader variability (Villeneuve et al. 1996; Ratziu et al. 2005; Brunt and Tiniakos 2010). Furthermore, it is an invasive procedure and suffers from sampling variability (Bravo et al. 2001; Rockey et al. 2009). Therefore, over the last years, the global burden of NALFD and the potential clinical impact of early detection and monitoring of hepatic steatosis have fostered the use of noninvasive imaging modalities for the assessment of steatosis and the search for imaging biomarkers of fat.

2   Ultrasound (US)

Ultrasound (US) is an inexpensive and widely available imaging tool for the initial screening of steatosis. Normal liver echogenicity is similar to the renal cortex and the spleen's parenchyma. Hepatic steatosis, on the other hand, results in increased echogenicity of the liver's parenchyma, and is commonly graded as mild, moderate (loss of vein and portal wall definition), or severe (acoustic attenuation hampering the observation of the deepest hepatic regions and the diaphragm contour) (Idilman et al. 2016) (Fig. 1).

US findings and histological results may differ, as the same amount of fat distributed in several microvesicles will result in a higher echogenicity than if present in few macrovesicles. Another limitation of this technique is that the coexistence of fibrosis can also affect its performance, as fibrosis might also increase the parenchyma's echogenicity (Ma et al. 2009; Idilman

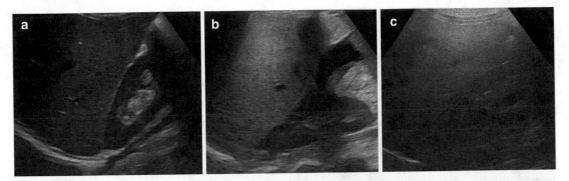

Fig. 1 US images from different patients demonstrating cases of mild (**a**), moderate (**b**), and severe (**c**) diffuse steatosis

et al. 2016). US is also limited for being an operator-dependent technique, with associated intra- and interobserver variability and for its reduced accuracy for detecting mild steatosis (Strauss et al. 2007; Hernaez et al. 2011). Nevertheless, US is still the preferred first-line diagnostic procedure for imaging of NAFLD, especially in primary care, as it is more widely available and cheaper than other imaging techniques (5).

To improve US diagnostic performance, several quantitative US-based methods have been recently introduced, such as the Hepatorenal Index (HRI), Acoustic Structure Quantification (ASQ), and Controlled Attenuation Parameter (CAP). HRI is a computerized parameter defined as the ratio between the brightness level in a region of interest (ROI) in the liver and the right kidney, with a good reported accuracy (Webb et al. 2009; Marshall et al. 2012; Borges et al. 2013; Shiralkar et al. 2015). In the liver, the ROI has to be far from vessels or bile ducts whereas in the kidney it should be located in the cortical area between the pyramids. On the other hand, ASC analyzes the echo amplitude of the US beam within a ROI, which is strongly correlated with hepatic fat fraction (Kuroda et al. 2012; Karlas et al. 2015; Son et al. 2016; Lee et al. 2017). Finally, CAP is an application of transient elastography, an US-based method that is commonly used in clinical practice for quantifying liver stiffness and staging fibrosis. CAP has been developed to quantify hepatic steatosis by assessing the degree of US beam attenuation by the intracellular fat vacuoles, with results being expressed as decibels per meter (dB/m), ranging from 100 to 400 dB/m (Stern and Castera 2017). Although these new US-based quantitative techniques have been gathering promising results, they are still on the research field and further validation is needed before they start to being used in clinical practice (Shi et al. 2014; Karlas et al. 2017; Lee 2017).

3 Computed Tomography (CT)

The parenchyma of the normal liver appears homogeneous at unenhanced CT, with attenuation ranging from 55 to 65 Hounsfield Units (HU), slightly exceeding the spleen's density by about 10 HU. The presence of fatty hepatocytes lowers the attenuation of liver parenchyma, with steatosis being defined at unenhanced CT scans by hepatic attenuation values under 40 HU or a spleen-to-liver attenuation difference (CT_{L-S}) of at least 10 HU (Lee 2017). Rarely, the liver's attenuation might be near 0 HU or even negative in the most severe cases (Boll and Merkle 2009) (Fig. 2). It has been reported that the portal venous phase CT images have comparable diagnostic performance to the unenhanced CT images for detecting steatosis. Nevertheless, the latter is preferred, as different injection protocols and delay times can affect the attenuation values of the liver's parenchyma (Kim et al. 2010; Lawrence et al. 2012). Furthermore, due to differences between CT scanners and reconstruction algorithms, CT_{L-S} is the preferred parameter to determine steatosis, as it uses the spleen, which does not accumulate fat, as an internal control (Birnbaum et al. 2007; Pickhardt et al. 2012; Lee and Park 2014). CT_{L-S} has demon-

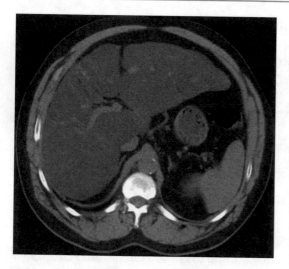

Fig. 2 Diffuse and severe hepatic steatosis on unenhanced CT, with negative spontaneous attenuation (−15 Hounsfield Units) of the liver parenchyma and a CT_{L-S} of 60

strated to provide good diagnostic performance in the detection of moderate-to-severe steatosis, but not of mild steatosis (Lee et al. 2010). Also, relying uniquely on attenuation measurements can be deceiving since iron deposition (as occurs in hemochromatosis, hemosiderosis, or chronic liver diseases, including NAFLD) or iodine deposition (as in patients taking amiodarone) can increase the attenuation of the liver parenchyma, misleading the assessment of steatosis (Patrick et al. 1984; Park et al. 2011; Pickhardt et al. 2012). Although dual-energy CT could have the potential to provide better diagnostic performance in the detection and quantification of hepatic steatosis, this was not confirmed so far (Mendler et al. 1998; Artz et al. 2012; Kramer et al. 2017).

Thus, the use of ionizing radiation, the lack of accuracy for detecting mild steatosis, and the fact that other disorders may affect the liver attenuation make CT an unsuitable method for screening, staging, or monitoring NAFLD patients (Stern and Castera 2017).

4 Magnetic Resonance (MR) Imaging

MR imaging has a unique capability to detect the presence of fat within the tissues. Both water and fat contain hydrogen protons: a water molecule contains two protons, whereas a triglyceride molecule contains multiple protons in several different chemical configurations, including those of terminal methyl (CH_3), methylene (CH_2), and methine (CH=CH) groups. Due to their chemical configuration, protons in water and fat resonate at different frequencies, a phenomenon known as "chemical shift": fat protons resonate at a slightly lower frequency than water protons, at a rate proportional to the magnetic field strength (Yokoo and Browning 2014). By exploiting these different chemical shifts of fat and water protons, MR imaging can detect fat in tissues where water and fat coexist, such as the liver.

4.1 MR Sequences for Detecting Hepatic Steatosis

Chemical shift-based gradient-echo (GRE) sequences take advantage of the different chemical shifts of water and fat, allowing to separate the MR signal into its water and fat components by acquiring images at two or more echo times (TEs) after signal excitation: the first TE when water and fat protons are "out of phase" (OP), and the second TE when both water and fat are "in phase" (IP). The TE corresponding to the OP and IP images depends on the magnetic field strength: fat and water protons are OP every 2.3 (at 1.5-T) or 1.15 ms (at 3-T), and IP every 4.6 ms (at 1.5-T) or 2.3 ms (at 3-T).

For several years, T1 dual-echo "chemical shift" GRE sequences have been widely used in clinical practice for the visual detection of liver steatosis. The liver signal intensity (SI) on the IP images results from water plus fat signals while on the OP images the liver SI results from the difference between water and fat signals. Therefore, steatosis is depicted as a liver SI dropout on the OP image with respect to the IP image (Fig. 3). Nevertheless, these MR sequences are only accurate in cases of isolated steatosis, as fat detection may be confounded by coexistence of hepatic iron deposits. As iron is a paramagnetic substance, its presence increases the T2* signal decay (Sirlin and Reeder 2010), resulting in low SI of the liver parenchyma on the second (IP)

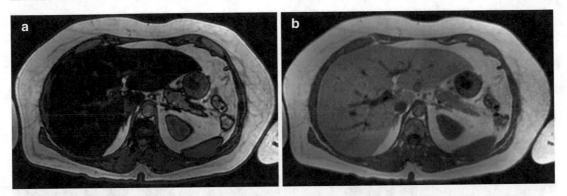

Fig. 3 Severe and homogeneously diffuse hepatic steatosis, with marked signal dropout on T1 chemical shift OP images (**a**) relative to IP images (**b**)

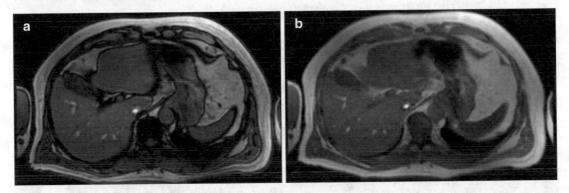

Fig. 4 Hepatic steatosis and siderosis in a patient with abnormal liver enzymes and hyperferritinemia. On T1 chemical shift GRE, there is no apparent SI change between the OP (**a**) and IP (**b**) images. However, this patient has both liver steatosis and siderosis (please refer to Fig. 14). The coexistence of fat and iron biases fat detection on T1 dual-echo images, underestimating the liver fat content

image as compared to the first (OP) echo image. Therefore, when fat and iron coexist, as may occur in NAFLD and other chronic liver diseases, the effect of iron may obscure the effect of liver steatosis on the SI of the liver parenchyma. This will result in less or no apparent liver SI change between the OP and IP images, which may lead to misinterpretation and to underestimation of liver fat content (Westphalen et al. 2007) (Fig. 4).

Fat has a high SI on T2-weighted images. Therefore, *turbo spin-echo (TSE) T2-weighted images* can also be used to detect hepatic steatosis, by acquiring two sets of images. Because fat has a high SI on T2-weighted images, steatosis can be depicted by acquiring two sets of TSE T2-weighted images, with and without fat suppression. If there is hepatic steatosis, the SI of the liver parenchyma will be higher on the nonfat-suppressed images than on the fat-suppressed images (Fig. 5). These sequences are less sensitive to iron deposits than GRE sequences, but they may still be confounded by the presence of moderate-to-severe iron overload. Additionally, T2-weighted TSE sequences are also dependent on the B0 magnetic field homogeneity (Sirlin and Reeder 2010; Martí-Bonmatí et al. 2012).

4.1.1 Imaging Patterns of Hepatic Steatosis

Different imaging patterns of hepatic steatosis can be recognized on the MR images. The most common imaging pattern of hepatic steatosis is a diffuse and homogenous fatty infiltration (Figs. 3 and 5). Nevertheless, other patterns can appear, such as diffuse and heterogeneous deposition (Fig. 6), diffuse deposition with

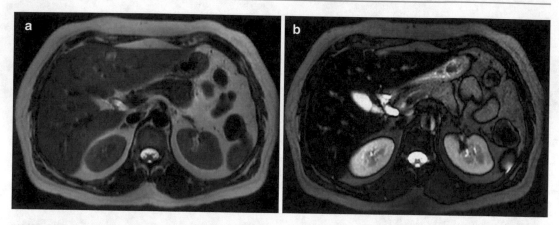

Fig. 5 Diffuse severe hepatic steatosis. On TSE T2-weighted images, there is signal loss of the liver parenchyma on the fat-suppressed images (**b**) when compared to the non-suppressed images (**a**)

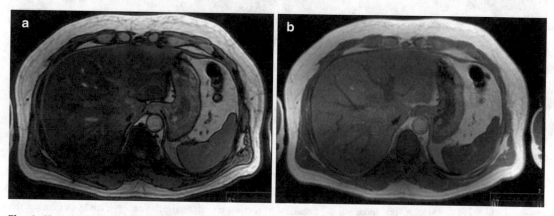

Fig. 6 Hepatic steatosis with heterogeneous distribution. T1-weighted chemical shift GRE images show patchy and heterogeneous signal dropout of the liver parenchyma on the OP images (**a**) relative to the IP images (**b**)

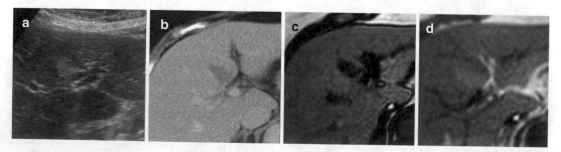

Fig. 7 Focal fat deposition on segment IV, demonstrated as a hyperechogenic area on US (**a**) and hypodense on CT (**b**). On T1-weighted chemical shift GRE MR sequences, there is signal dropout on the OP images (**c**) relative to the IP images (**d**)

areas of focal sparing, or focal, multifocal, perilesional, subcapsular, and perivascular steatosis (Idilman et al. 2016). In some of these cases, steatosis can mimic other lesions, and other imaging findings should be looked for, namely iso-enhancement compared to the remaining parenchyma, absence of mass effect or displacement of vascular structures, and stability on follow-up examinations (Hamer et al. 2006).

Focal fat deposition or, on the other hand, focal fat sparing in a diffusely steatotic liver, usually appears in typical shapes (e.g., geographic or wedge shaped) and areas of the liver parenchyma (e.g., adjacent to the falciform ligament, the liver hilum, and/or the gallbladder fossa) (Figs. 7 and 8). The reason for this distri-bution is not fully understood, although it has been attributed to variant venous inflow and oxy-gen pressure imbalances (Yoshikawa et al. 1987; Hashimoto et al. 2002; Yves Menu 2005). Multifocal steatosis appears as multiple small (0.5–2 cm) fatty nodules, often distributed throughout the liver parenchyma, that may

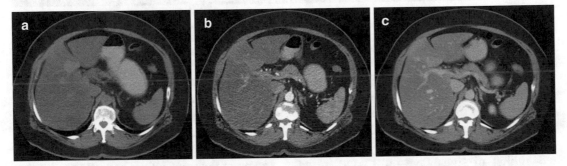

Fig. 8 Focal spared area on segment IV in a diffuse hepatic steatosis. The liver parenchyma has very low density on CT images and the focal spared area appears as a hyperdense area on unenhanced CT (**a**) that enhances comparably to the remaining liver parenchyma in the arterial (**b**) and portal venous phase (**c**) images

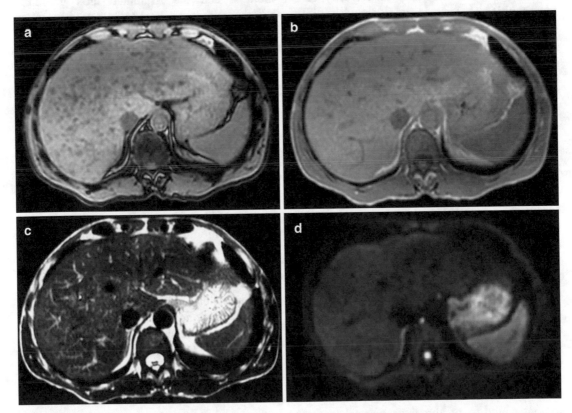

Fig. 9 Multifocal steatosis. Multiple small fatty nodules are seen throughout the liver parenchyma, showing signal dropout on T1 GRE OP (**a**) relative to the IP (**b**) image, signal hyperintensity on T2 TSE (**c**), and absence of diffusion restriction on the diffusion weighted image ($b = 1000$) (**d**)

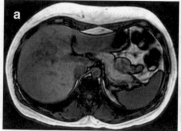 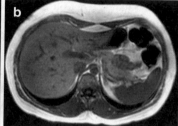 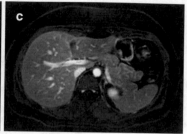

Fig. 10 Nodular steatosis. On T1-weighted chemical shift sequence, a fatty nodular area is recognized on the OP image (**a**) but not seen on the IP image (**b**), not displacing the vascular structures and showing iso- enhancement on the portal venous phase (**c**). This focal nodular deposition of fat is a pseudolesion and should not be misdiagnosed as a true focal liver lesion

coalesce. This form is often seen in oncological patients after chemotherapy, either as new-appearing lesions or in the location of metastasis, probably due to fatty necrosis. The recognition of signal loss on T1 OP images, absence of restriction to diffusion on diffusion weighted images, and iso-enhancement on contrast-enhanced MR help to correctly diagnose multifocal steatosis and distinguish it from liver metastasis (Figs. 9 and 10).

Subcapsular fatty infiltration is commonly observed in patients who receive insulin within their peritoneal dialysate. Insulin diffuses through the Glisson's sheath, stimulating the conversion of glucose to fatty acids in hepatocytes (Khalili et al. 2003). The same mechanism explains the perilesional fat deposition that is usually seen around liver metastases from pancreatic insulinoma (Fregeville et al. 2005).

Another pattern that can be recognized mainly in association with alcohol intake or oral corticosteroids is perivascular steatosis. This pattern is characterized by a halo of fat surrounding the hepatic veins and/or the portal veins, and it can have a similar appearance to edema, fibrosis, perfusion abnormalities, or even lymphoma (Lawson et al. 1993; Hamer et al. 2005; Karcaaltincaba et al. 2007).

It is important to be aware that some focal or diffuse abnormalities may, in turn, mimic hepatic steatosis on imaging studies. For example, radiation-induced liver disease can lead to hypoattenuation of the liver parenchyma on CT, hypo- or hyperechogenicity at US, and hypointensity on T1- and hyperintensity on T2-weighted MR images, similar to steatosis. Differential diagnosis can be made by the sharp borders with lack of anatomic correspondence of the irradiated area, as the radiation beam geometry does not follow vascular or segmental territories. Also, findings of radiation-induced liver disease usually regress in 4–6 months, and the irradiated area gradually shrinks, with compensatory hypertrophy of the remaining liver (Kwek et al. 2006; Maturen et al. 2013). Liver metastasis from fat-containing primary tumors such as teratomas, liposarcomas, Wilms' tumors, and renal cell carcinomas may also mimic steatosis (Bartolozzi et al. 2001). Usually, other imaging findings, namely on contrast-enhanced and diffusion wieghted MR images, help to establish the correct diagnosis. Confluent hepatic fibrosis appears hypodense on unenhanced CT, isodense or slightly hypodense on contrast-enhanced CT, and hyperintense on T2-weighted images (Ohtomo et al. 1993) and, therefore, can also mimic hepatic steatosis. Nevertheless, confluent fibrosis is usually seen as wedge-shaped areas, usually extending from the hilum to the periphery, affecting the medial and anterior segments and causing capsular retraction, and without signal dropout on OP T1-weighted images (Fig. 11). Perfusion anomalies may also morphologically resemble fat deposition, but they are visible only during the arterial and portal venous phases after contrast agent administration, and they are not detectable on unenhanced or equilibrium phase images (Hamer et al. 2005).

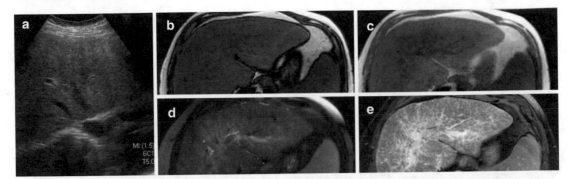

Fig. 11 Confluent liver fibrosis in a patient with liver cirrhosis. The liver parenchyma is hyperechoic and heterogeneous on US (**a**). On MR images, there is signal drop out of the liver parenchyma on the T1 GRE OP image (**b**) indicating liver steatosis. Furthermore, the T1 GRE IP image (**c**) shows a hypointense ill-defined perihilar area, without signal dropout on the OP image (**b**), which is hypertintense on the fat supressed T2-weighted image (d), corresponding to confluent fibrosis. Fibrosis has progressive enhancement on contrast-enhanced T1 images (**e**)

4.2 Quantification of Hepatic Steatosis with MR Spectroscopy and MR Imaging

As liver biopsy is not feasible for diagnosing or monitoring the large number of patients with NAFLD and NASH, there was a need for developing noninvasive accurate imaging biomarkers. Both MR spectroscopy (MRS) and advanced MR imaging sequences take advantage of the different chemical shifts of water and fat protons to quantify fat. The best imaging biomarker of hepatic steatosis is proton density fat fraction (PDFF), and it is now being used in research studies and clinical trials with new drugs tailored for NASH.

4.2.1 MR Spectroscopy

Knowing *a priori* the chemical shift of the water and fat protons allows measuring their concentrations directly from the hepatic spectral signal acquired by MR spectroscopy, as the amplitude of each peak is related with its proton density (Yokoo and Browning 2014). As mentioned in chapter "Magnetic Resonance Imaging of the Liver: Technical Considerations", proton density of fat is the sum of the multiple frequency components of fat molecules. Thus, PDFF can be determined as a ratio between the sum of the fat peaks (fat proton density, FPD) and water proton density (WPD): PDFF (%) = FPD/WPD.

PDFF determined by MR spectroscopy is closely correlated with the molecular density of fat, therefore being considered the imaging gold standard for hepatic fat quantification (Reeder et al. 2011). Nevertheless, it is not widely available on MR scanners, it needs dedicated software tools, and it is time consuming, being only available in specialized hospital or research centers (Reeder et al. 2011; Yokoo and Browning 2014).

4.2.2 Chemical Shift-Encoded MR Sequences

To overcome the limitations of MR spectroscopy, chemical shift-based advanced MR imaging sequences were developed for PDFF quantification. These sequences can be easily implemented on every MR equipment being used in clinical practice.

As explained before, on T1-weighted "dual-echo" sequences, the liver SI on IP images results from the water plus fat signals, while on OP images, liver signal intensity results from the difference between the water and fat signal components. Thus, theoretically, hepatic fat fraction could be calculated as $(S_{IP} - S_{OP})/2S_{IP}$, where S_{IP} corresponds to liver/spleen signal intensity measured on the IP image, and S_{OP} represents the relative signal measured on the OP image, with the spleen being used for internal signal normalization (Martí-Bonmatí et al. 2012). However, these fat fraction measurements are based on fat

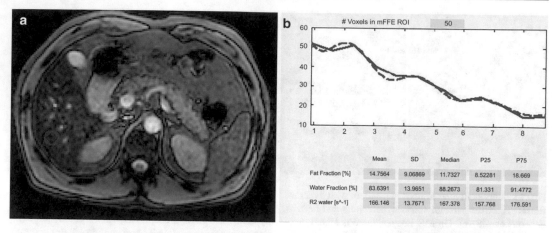

Fig. 12 Multi-echo chemical shift-encoded GRE sequence for fat (PDFF) and iron (R2*) quantification. (**a**) Axial phase image demonstrating a ROI in the segment VI, avoiding the vessels. (**b**) The signal decay is modeled as a function of TE for PDFF and iron quantification

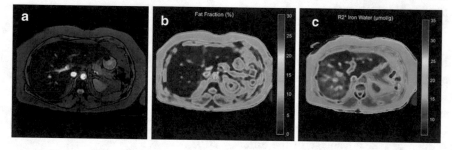

Fig. 13 Severe diffuse hepatic steatosis (same patient as in Fig. 3). Multi-echo chemical shift-encoded GRE MR sequence for fat and iron quantification estimated severe hepatic steatosis (PDFF 27%), also with mild elevation of R2* (160 s^{-1}): Phase image (**a**), fat parametric map (**b**), and iron parametric map (**c**)

and water SI, rather than on its proton densities. The "signal" fat fraction is influenced by numerous biological, physical, and technical factors, such as the T1 bias and the T2* decay bias, and also the spectral complexity of the fat spectrum, J-coupling, noise bias, or eddy currents. Thus, the "signal" fat fraction is not a precise measure and the "classic" dual-echo chemical shift sequences should not be used for quantification of hepatic steatosis (Reeder and Sirlin 2010). Nevertheless, if these confounding factors are corrected or attenuated, the "signal" fat fraction will be similar to the PDFF, as estimated by MR spectroscopy. For this purpose, multi-echo chemical shift-based GRE sequences have been recently developed. For precise quantification of PDFF, these sequences must consider the effect of T1

and T2* decay, and the spectral complexity of fat (also refer to chapter "Magnetic Resonance Imaging of the Liver: Technical Considerations"). By using multiple OP and IP echoes, water and fat signals are separated, allowing the estimation of fat fraction (Fig. 12). At the same time, for each echo, the T2* decay (or R2*) is estimated, which will be used to correct the effect of T2* decay on PDFF quantification. This T2* correction is particularly important when fat and iron coexist in the liver parenchyma, as can be often seen in patients with NAFLD and other chronic liver diseases (Sirlin and Reeder 2010). Moreover, because T2* decay estimation is closely related to iron content, it can be used for simultaneously estimating the hepatic iron burden (Yokoo and Browning 2014; França et al. 2017a, b) (Fig. 12).

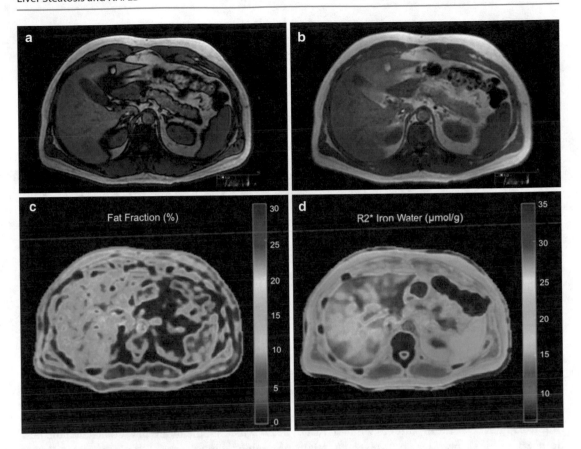

Fig. 14 Patient with excessive alcoholic consumption and hyperferritinemia, with coexistence of hepatic steatosis and siderosis. There is a slight increase on liver SI on OP (**a**) images when compared to IP (**b**) images, suggesting iron deposition. Multiparametric maps of fat (**c**) and iron (**d**), obtained with a multi-echo chemical shift-encoded sequence, allow to recognize heterogeneous deposition of both fat and iron throughout the liver parenchyma: mean PDFF is 10% (mild steatosis); mean R2* is 150 s^{-1}

These sequences are very fast, being acquired during one or two breath-hold acquisitions, and can be performed with commercially available tools or using in-house advanced methods, both on 1.5-T and 3.0-T equipment. Then, fat measurements can be presented in parametric maps, demonstrating the hepatic PDFF values, pixel by pixel, with the advantage of demonstrating the distribution of fat throughout the parenchyma (Figs. 13, 14, and 15).

Multi-echo chemical shift-encoded sequences are accurate for quantification of hepatic steatosis (Tang et al. 2013; Idilman et al. 2013; França et al. 2017a) and have an excellent linearity and precision across different manufacturers, field strengths, and reconstruction methods (Yokoo and Browning 2014).

Although PDFF threshold values have been proposed to diagnose liver steatosis and to differentiate histological grades of steatosis (Permutt et al. 2012; Tang et al. 2013, 2015; Idilman et al. 2013; França et al. 2017a), they still need further validation in large cohorts of patients before they become standardized. Besides, when interpreting PDFF measurements, it should be remembered that PDFF and histologically estimated steatosis percentages are highly correlated, but they are not equivalent, as they express different metrics: the percentage of hepatocytes with macrovesicles of fat is evaluated on liver biopsy,

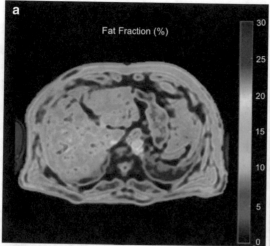

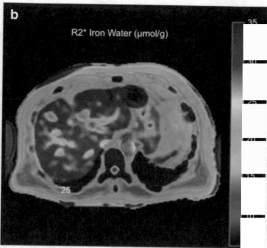

Fig. 15 Patient with abnormal liver enzymes and hyperferritinemia (same patient as in Fig. 4). By using a multiecho chemical shift-encoded sequence, estimated PDFF (**a**) is 14% (moderate steatosis). The hepatic R2* (**b**) is mildly elevated (180 s⁻¹). The coexistence of fat and iron biases fat detection on the T1 dual-echo MR images, underestimating the liver fat content, but can be accurately quantified by multi-echo chemical shift MR sequences

while PDFF measures the density of mobile fat protons within the hepatocytes.

Multi-echo chemical shift-encoded MR sequences are now being used for longitudinal monitoring of liver fat in patients with NAFLD, both in clinical practice and research trials (Oscarsson et al. 2018; Noureddin et al. 2013; Caussy et al. 2018; Eriksson et al. 2018; Loomba et al. 2018; Chalasani et al. 2018). They were considered to be even more precise than liver biopsy for therapy monitoring in patients with NASH (Reeder et al. 2011; Noureddin et al. 2013). Other applications for PDFF measurements are the evaluation of living liver donors (Satkunasingham et al. 2018), assessment of steatosis related with chemotherapy in oncologic patients (Corrias et al. 2018), and pre- and postoperative assessment of fatty liver disease in patients undergoing bariatric surgery (Luo et al. 2018; Pooler et al. 2018).

5   Conclusion

Hepatic steatosis is the hallmark of NAFLD but it can also be present in many other diffuse chronic liver diseases, being associated with the development of liver fibrosis. Although moderate-to-severe steatosis can be depicted with US or CT, MR imaging is the best technique to accurately detect and quantify steatosis. MR-determined PDFF measurements are now considered the best imaging biomarker of hepatic steatosis, being widely available on MR equipment, and are being used for diagnosing and monitoring steatosis in NAFLD patients, in both clinical practice and research trials.

Different patterns of fat deposition can be recognized on imaging examinations. Radiologists should be aware of them and should not misinterpret them as other liver abnormalities or focal lesions.

References

Angulo P, Kleiner DE, Dam-Larsen S et al (2015) Liver fibrosis, but no other histologic features, is associated with long-term outcomes of patients with nonalcoholic fatty liver disease. Gastroenterology 149:389–397 .e10. https://doi.org/10.1053/j.gastro.2015.04.043

Artz NS, Hines CDG, Brunner ST et al (2012) Quantification of hepatic steatosis with dual-energy computed tomography: comparison with tissue reference standards and quantitative magnetic resonance imaging in the ob/ob mouse. Invest Radiol 47:603–610. https://doi.org/10.1097/RLI.0b013e318261fad0

Bartolozzi C, Cioni D, Donati F, Lencioni R (2001) Focal liver lesions: MR imaging-pathologic correlation. Eur Radiol 11:1374–1388. https://doi.org/10.1007/s003300100845

Birnbaum BA, Hindman N, Lee J, Babb JS (2007) Multi-detector row CT attenuation measurements: assessment of intra- and interscanner variability with an anthropomorphic body CT phantom. Radiology 242:109–119. https://doi.org/10.1148/radiol.2421052066

Boll DT, Merkle EM (2009) Diffuse liver disease: strategies for hepatic CT and MR imaging. Radiographics 29:1591–1614. https://doi.org/10.1148/rg.296095513

Borges VF, de AE DALD, Cotrim HP et al (2013) Sonographic hepatorenal ratio: a noninvasive method to diagnose nonalcoholic steatosis. J Clin Ultrasound 41:18 25. https://doi.org/10.1002/jcu.21994

Bravo AA, Sheth SG, Chopra S (2001) Liver biopsy. N Engl J Med 344:495–500. https://doi.org/10.1056/NEJM200102153440706

Brunt EM, Tiniakos DG (2010) Histopathology of non-alcoholic fatty liver disease. World J Gastroenterol 16:5286. https://doi.org/10.3748/wjg.v16.i42.5286

Caussy C, Alquiraish MH, Nguyen P et al (2018) Optimal threshold of controlled attenuation parameter with MRI-PDFF as the gold standard for the detection of hepatic steatosis. Hepatology 67:1348–1359. https://doi.org/10.1002/hep.29639

Chalasani N, Vuppalanchi R, Rinella M et al (2018) Randomised clinical trial: a leucine-metformin-sildenafil combination (NS-0200) vs placebo in patients with non-alcoholic fatty liver disease. Aliment Pharmacol Ther 47:1639–1651. https://doi.org/10.1111/apt.14674

Chalasani N, Younossi Z, Lavine JE et al (2012) The diagnosis and management of non-alcoholic fatty liver disease: Practice Guideline by the American Association for the Study of Liver Diseases, American College of Gastroenterology, and the American Gastroenterological Association. Hepatology 55:2005–2023. https://doi.org/10.1002/hep.25762

Corrias G, Krebs S, Eskreis-Winkler S et al (2018) MRI liver fat quantification in an oncologic population: the added value of complex chemical shift-encoded MRI. Clin Imaging 52:193–199. https://doi.org/10.1016/j.clinimag.2018.08.002

de Meijer VE, Kalish BT, Puder M, IJzermans JNM (2010) Systematic review and meta-analysis of steatosis as a risk factor in major hepatic resection. Br J Surg 97:1331–1339. https://doi.org/10.1002/bjs.7194

Ekstedt M, Hagström H, Nasr P et al (2015) Fibrosis stage is the strongest predictor for disease-specific mortality in NAFLD after up to 33 years of follow-up. Hepatology 61:1547–1554. https://doi.org/10.1002/hep.27368

Eriksson JW, Lundkvist P, Jansson P-A et al (2018) Effects of dapagliflozin and n-3 carboxylic acids on non-alcoholic fatty liver disease in people with type 2 diabetes: a double-blind randomised placebo-controlled study. Diabetologia 61:1923–1934. https://doi.org/10.1007/s00125-018-4675-2

EASL–EASD–EASO (2016) Clinical practice guidelines for the management of non-alcoholic fatty liver disease. J Hepatol 64:1388–1402. https://doi.org/10.1016/j.jhep.2015.11.004

França M, Alberich-Bayarri Á, Martí-Bonmatí L (2017b) Use Case VI: imaging biomarkers in diffuse liver disease. Quantification of fat and iron. In: Imaging biomarkers. Springer International Publishing, Cham, pp 279–294

França M, Alberich-Bayarri A, Martí-Bonmatí L et al (2017a) Accurate simultaneous quantification of liver steatosis and iron overload in diffuse liver diseases with MRI. Abdom Radiol 42:1434–1443

Fregeville A, Couvelard A, Paradis V et al (2005) Metastatic insulinoma and glucagonoma from the pancreas responsible for specific peritumoral patterns of hepatic steatosis secondary to local effects of insulin and glucagon on hepatocytes. Gastroenterology 129:1150–1365. https://doi.org/10.1053/j.gastro.2005.08.033

Hamer OW, Aguirre DA, Casola G, Sirlin CB (2005) Imaging features of perivascular fatty infiltration of the liver: initial observations. Radiology 237:159–169. https://doi.org/10.1148/radiol.2371041580

Hamer OW, Aguirre DA, Casola G et al (2006) Fatty liver: imaging patterns and pitfalls. Radiographics 26:1637–1653. https://doi.org/10.1148/rg.266065004

Hashimoto M, Heianna J, Tate E et al (2002) Small veins entering the liver. Eur Radiol 12:2000–2005. https://doi.org/10.1007/s00330-002-1321-6

Hernaez R, Lazo M, Bonekamp S et al (2011) Diagnostic accuracy and reliability of ultrasonography for the detection of fatty liver: a meta-analysis. Hepatology 54:1082–1090. https://doi.org/10.1002/hep.24452

Hwang S-J, Lee S-D (2011) Hepatic steatosis and hepatitis C: still unhappy bedfellows? J Gastroenterol Hepatol 26(Suppl 1):96–101. https://doi.org/10.1111/j.1440-1746.2010.06542.x

Idilman IS, Aniktar H, Idilman R et al (2013) Hepatic steatosis: quantification by proton density fat fraction with MR imaging versus liver biopsy. Radiology 267:767–775. https://doi.org/10.1148/radiol.13121360

Idilman IS, Ozdeniz I, Karcaaltincaba M (2016) Hepatic steatosis: etiology, patterns, and quantification. Semin Ultrasound, CT MRI 37:501–510. https://doi.org/10.1053/j.sult.2016.08.003

Karcaaltincaba M, Haliloglu M, Akpinar E et al (2007) Multidetector CT and MRI findings in periportal space pathologies. Eur J Radiol 61:3–10. https://doi.org/10.1016/j.ejrad.2006.11.009

Karlas T, Berger J, Garnov N et al (2015) Estimating steatosis and fibrosis: comparison of acoustic structure quantification with established techniques. World J Gastroenterol 21:4894–4902. https://doi.org/10.3748/wjg.v21.i16.4894

Karlas T, Petroff D, Sasso M et al (2017) Individual patient data meta-analysis of controlled attenuation parameter (CAP) technology for assessing steatosis. J Hepatol 66:1022–1030. https://doi.org/10.1016/j.jhep.2016.12.022

Khalili K, Lan FP, Hanbidge AE et al (2003) Hepatic subcapsular steatosis in response to intraperitoneal insulin delivery: CT findings and prevalence. Am J Roentgenol 180:1601–1604. https://doi.org/10.2214/ajr.180.6.1801601

Kim DY, Park SH, Lee SS et al (2010) Contrast-enhanced computed tomography for the diagnosis of fatty liver: prospective study with same-day biopsy used as the reference standard. Eur Radiol 20:359–366. https://doi.org/10.1007/s00330-009-1560-x

Kleiner DE, Brunt EM, Van Natta M et al (2005) Design and validation of a histological scoring system for nonalcoholic fatty liver disease. Hepatology 41:1313–1321. https://doi.org/10.1002/hep.20701

Kramer H, Pickhardt PJ, Kliewer MA et al (2017) Accuracy of liver fat quantification with advanced CT, MRI, and ultrasound techniques: prospective comparison with MR spectroscopy. Am J Roentgenol 208:92–100. https://doi.org/10.2214/AJR.16.16565

Kuroda H, Kakisaka K, Kamiyama N et al (2012) Non-invasive determination of hepatic steatosis by acoustic structure quantification from ultrasound echo amplitude. World J Gastroenterol 18:3889–3895. https://doi.org/10.3748/wjg.v18.i29.3889

Kwek J-W, Iyer RB, Dunnington J et al (2006) Spectrum of imaging findings in the abdomen after radiotherapy. Am J Roentgenol 187:1204–1211. https://doi.org/10.2214/AJR.05.0941

Lawrence DA, Oliva IB, Israel GM (2012) Detection of hepatic steatosis on contrast-enhanced CT images: diagnostic accuracy of identification of areas of presumed focal fatty sparing. Am J Roentgenol 199:44–47. https://doi.org/10.2214/AJR.11.7838

Lawson TL, Thorsen MK, Erickson SJ et al (1993) Periportal halo: a CT sign of liver disease. Abdom Imaging 18:42–46

Leandro G, Mangia A, Hui J et al (2006) Relationship between steatosis, inflammation, and fibrosis in chronic hepatitis C: a meta-analysis of individual patient data. Gastroenterology 130:1636–1642. https://doi.org/10.1053/j.gastro.2006.03.014

Lee DH (2017) Imaging evaluation of non-alcoholic fatty liver disease: focused on quantification. Clin Mol Hepatol:290–301. https://doi.org/10.3350/cmh.2017.0042

Lee DH, Lee JY, Lee KB, Han JK (2017) Evaluation of hepatic steatosis by using acoustic structure quantification US in a rat model: comparison with pathologic examination and MR spectroscopy. Radiology 285:445–453. https://doi.org/10.1148/radiol.2017161923

Lee SS, Park SH (2014) Radiologic evaluation of non-alcoholic fatty liver disease. World J Gastroenterol 20:7392–7402. https://doi.org/10.3748/wjg.v20.i23.7392

Lee SS, Park SH, Kim HJ et al (2010) Non-invasive assessment of hepatic steatosis: prospective comparison of the accuracy of imaging examinations. J Hepatol 52:579–585. https://doi.org/10.1016/j.jhep.2010.01.008

Loomba R, Kayali Z, Noureddin M et al (2018) GS-0976 Reduces hepatic steatosis and fibrosis markers in patients with nonalcoholic fatty liver disease. Gastroenterology 155:1463–1473 . e6. https://doi.org/10.1053/j.gastro.2018.07.027

Luo RB, Suzuki T, Hooker JC et al (2018) How bariatric surgery affects liver volume and fat density in NAFLD patients. Surg Endosc 32:1675–1682. https://doi.org/10.1007/s00464-017-5846-9

Ma X, Holalkere N-S, Mino-Kenudson M, Hahn PF, Sahani DV (2009) Imaging-based quantification of hepatic fat: methods and clinical applications. Radiographics 29:1253–1277. https://doi.org/10.1148/rg.295085186

Marshall RH, Eissa M, Bluth EI et al (2012) Hepatorenal index as an accurate, simple, and effective tool in screening for steatosis. Am J Roentgenol 199:997–1002

Martí-Bonmatí L, Alberich-Bayarri A, Sánchez-González J (2012) Overload hepatitides: quanti-qualitative analysis. Abdom Imaging 37:180–187. https://doi.org/10.1007/s00261-011-9762-5

Maturen KE, Feng MU, Wasnik AP et al (2013) Imaging effects of radiation therapy in the abdomen and pelvis: evaluating "Innocent Bystander" tissues. Radiographics 33:599–619. https://doi.org/10.1148/rg.332125119

McPherson S, Hardy T, Henderson E et al (2015) Evidence of NAFLD progression from steatosis to fibrosing-steatohepatitis using paired biopsies: implications for prognosis and clinical management. J Hepatol 62:1148–1155. https://doi.org/10.1016/j.jhep.2014.11.034

Mendler MH, Bouillet P, Le Sidaner A et al (1998) Dual-energy CT in the diagnosis and quantification of fatty liver: limited clinical value in comparison to ultrasound scan and single-energy CT, with special reference to iron overload. J Hepatol 28:785–794

Nativ NI, Chen AI, Yarmush G et al (2014) Automated image analysis method for detecting and quantifying macrovesicular steatosis in hematoxylin and eosin-stained histology images of human livers. Liver Transpl 20:228–236. https://doi.org/10.1002/lt.23782

Noureddin M, Lam J, Peterson MR et al (2013) Utility of magnetic resonance imaging versus histology for quantifying changes in liver fat in nonalcoholic fatty liver disease trials. Hepatology 58:1930–1940. https://doi.org/10.1002/hep.26455

Ohtomo K, Baron RL, Dodd GD et al (1993) Confluent hepatic fibrosis in advanced cirrhosis: evaluation with MR imaging. Radiology 189:871–874. https://doi.org/10.1148/radiology.189.3.8234718

Oscarsson J, Önnerhag K, Risérus U et al (2018) Effects of free omega-3 carboxylic acids and fenofibrate on liver fat content in patients with hypertriglyceridemia and non-alcoholic fatty liver disease: a double-blind, randomized, placebo-controlled study. J Clin Lipidol 12:1390–1403. e4. https://doi.org/10.1016/j.jacl.2018.08.003

Park YS, Park SH, Lee SS et al (2011) Biopsy-proven nonsteatotic liver in adults: estimation of reference range for difference in attenuation between the liver and the spleen at nonenhanced CT. Radiology 258:760–766. https://doi.org/10.1148/radiol.10101233

Patrick D, White FE, Adams PC (1984) Long-term amiodarone therapy: a cause of increased hepatic attenuation on CT. Br J Radiol 57:573–576. https://doi.org/10.1259/0007-1285-57-679-573

Permutt Z, Le T-A, Peterson MR et al (2012) Correlation between liver histology and novel magnetic resonance imaging in adult patients with non-alcoholic fatty liver disease—MRI accurately quantifies hepatic steatosis in NAFLD. Aliment Pharmacol Ther 36:22–29. https://doi.org/10.1111/j.1365-2036.2012.05121.x

Pickhardt PJ, Park SH, Hahn L et al (2012) Specificity of unenhanced CT for non-invasive diagnosis of hepatic steatosis: implications for the investigation of the natural history of incidental steatosis. Eur Radiol 22:1075–1082. https://doi.org/10.1007/s00330-011-2349-2

Ploeg RJ, D'Alessandro AM, Knechtle SJ et al (1993) Risk factors for primary dysfunction after liver transplantation—a multivariate analysis. Transplantation 55:807–813

Pooler BD, Wiens CN, McMillan A et al (2019) Monitoring fatty liver disease with MRI following bariatric surgery: a prospective, dual-center study. Radiology 290(3):682–690. https://doi.org/10.1148/radiol.2018181134

Ratziu V, Charlotte F, Heurtier A et al (2005) Sampling variability of liver biopsy in nonalcoholic fatty liver disease. Gastroenterology 128:1898–1906

Reeder SB, Cruite I, Hamilton G, Sirlin CB (2011) Quantitative assessment of liver fat with magnetic resonance imaging and spectroscopy. J Magn Reson Imaging 34:729–749. https://doi.org/10.1002/jmri.22580

Reeder SB, Sirlin CB (2010) Quantification of liver fat with magnetic resonance imaging. Magn Reson Imaging Clin N Am 18:337–357

Rockey DC, Caldwell SH, Goodman ZD et al (2009) Liver biopsy. Hepatology 49:1017–1044. https://doi.org/10.1002/hep.22742

Satkunasingham J, Nik HH, Fischer S et al (2018) Can negligible hepatic steatosis determined by magnetic resonance imaging-proton density fat fraction obviate the need for liver biopsy in potential liver donors? Liver Transpl 24:470–477. https://doi.org/10.1002/lt.24965

Shi K-Q, Tang J-Z, Zhu X-L et al (2014) Controlled attenuation parameter for the detection of steatosis severity in chronic liver disease: a meta-analysis of diagnostic accuracy. J Gastroenterol Hepatol 29:1149–1158. https://doi.org/10.1111/jgh.12519

Shiralkar K, Johnson S, Bluth EI et al (2015) Improved method for calculating hepatic steatosis using the hepatorenal index. J Ultrasound Med 34:1051–1059

Sirlin CB, Reeder SB (2010) Magnetic resonance imaging quantification of liver iron. Magn Reson Imaging Clin N Am 18:359–381. https://doi.org/10.1016/j.mric.2010.08.014

Son J-Y, Lee JY, Yi N-J et al (2016) Hepatic steatosis: assessment with acoustic structure quantification of US imaging. Radiology 278:257–264. https://doi.org/10.1148/radiol.2015141779

Stern C, Castera L (2017) Non-invasive diagnosis of hepatic steatosis. Hepatol Int 11:70–78. https://doi.org/10.1007/s12072-016-9772-z

Strauss S, Gavish E, Gottlieb P, Katsnelson L (2007) Interobserver and intraobserver variability in the sonographic assessment of fatty liver. Am J Roentgenol 189:W320–W323

Tang A, Desai A, Hamilton G et al (2015) Accuracy of MR imaging–estimated proton density fat fraction for classification of dichotomized histologic steatosis grades in nonalcoholic fatty liver disease. Radiology 274:416–425. https://doi.org/10.1148/radiol.14140754

Tang A, Tan J, Sun M et al (2013) Nonalcoholic fatty liver disease: MR imaging of liver proton density fat fraction to assess hepatic steatosis. Radiology 267:422–431. https://doi.org/10.1148/radiol.12120896

Vanderbeck S, Bockhorst J, Komorowski R et al (2014) Automatic classification of white regions in liver biopsies by supervised machine learning. Hum Pathol 45:785–792. https://doi.org/10.1016/j.humpath.2013.11.011

Villeneuve JP, Bilodeau M, Lepage R et al (1996) Variability in hepatic iron concentration measurement from needle-biopsy specimens. J Hepatol 25.172–177

Webb M, Yeshua H, Zelber-Sagi S et al (2009) Diagnostic value of a computerized hepatorenal index for sonographic quantification of liver steatosis. Am J Roentgenol 192:909–914

Westphalen ACA, Qayyum A, Yeh BM et al (2007) Liver fat: effect of hepatic iron deposition on evaluation with opposed-phase MR imaging. Radiology 242:450–455. https://doi.org/10.1148/radiol.2422052024

Yeh MM, Brunt EM (2014) Pathological features of fatty liver disease. Gastroenterology 147:754–764. https://doi.org/10.1053/j.gastro.2014.07.056

Yokoo T, Browning JD (2014) Fat and iron quantification in the liver: past, present, and future. Top Magn Reson Imaging 23:73–94. https://doi.org/10.1097/RMR.0000000000000016

Yoshikawa J, Matsui O, Takashima T et al (1987) Focal fatty change of the liver adjacent to the falciform ligament: CT and sonographic findings in five surgically confirmed cases. Am J Roentgenol 149:491–494. https://doi.org/10.2214/ajr.149.3.491

Younossi ZM, Koenig AB, Abdelatif D et al (2016) Global epidemiology of nonalcoholic fatty liver disease—meta-analytic assessment of prevalence, incidence, and outcomes. Hepatology 64:73–84. https://doi.org/10.1002/hep.28431

Yves Menu CG (2005) Radiologic-pathologic correlations in diffuse liver diseases. In: Radiologic-Pathologic correlations from head to toe: understanding the manifestations of disease. Springer, Berlin, Heidelberg, pp 391–407

Liver Increased Iron Deposition and Storage Diseases

Manuela França and João Pinheiro Amorim

Contents

M. França (✉)
Radiology Department, Centro Hospitalar e
Universitário do Porto, Oporto, Portugal

Instituto de Ciências Biomédicas de Abel Salazar,
Universidade do Porto, Oporto, Portugal

i3S, Instituto de Investigação e Inovação em Saúde,
Universidade do Porto, Oporto, Portugal
e-mail: manuelafranca.radiologia@chporto.
min-saude.pt

J. P. Amorim
Radiology Department, Centro Hospitalar e
Universitário do Porto, Oporto, Portugal

Escola de Medicina, Universidade do Minho,
Braga, Portugal

ICVS/3B's, Life and Health Sciences Research
Institute, Universidade do Minho, Braga, Portugal

Abstract

Hepatic iron overload may be found in several disorders, such as hereditary hemochromatosis, secondary hemochromatosis and chronic liver disease. Because hepatic iron concentration is a surrogate of total body iron stores, assessment and quantification of hepatic iron overload is important to select those patients who will benefit from specific treatments and also to accurately monitor the therapy. Over the last decades, MR imaging has become an important tool for evaluating iron overload disorders and for non-invasively quantifying hepatic iron concentration.

In this chapter, we review the current state-of-the-art of advanced MR imaging techniques used for imaging and quantification of hepatic iron overload. Furthermore, the imaging findings of other liver storage disorders are also presented.

© Springer Nature Switzerland AG 2021
E. Quaia (ed.), *Imaging of the Liver and Intra-hepatic Biliary Tract*,
Medical Radiology, Diagnostic Imaging, https://doi.org/10.1007/978-3-030-38983-3_14

1 Introduction

The liver serves as an important storage for many substances, particularly when they are in excess. The paradigmatic example of this is hepatic iron accumulation in the setting of iron-overload disorders, in which the liver is the main storage organ and the first one to accumulate the excess of circulating iron.

Over the last decades, MR imaging has become an important tool for evaluating iron-overload disorders and other hepatic deposition diseases, and a growing cohort of patients are now being referred for assessing hepatic iron, fat, and fibrosis. In fact, technological developments have made MR imaging an indispensable tool in the evaluation of these diseases, not only providing information on diffuse liver parenchymal abnormalities, but also showing multifocal involvement in multiorgan and systemic diseases.

Knowledge of imaging findings related with hepatic deposition disorders is important for abdominal imagers as they can be the first ones to incidentally discover these diseases.

2 Iron-Overload Disorders

2.1 Pathophysiology of Iron Overload

Iron is a double-edge nutrient: while it is crucial for many cellular functions and proliferation, it can become toxic when in excess, inducing oxidative stress and cellular damage (Steinbicker and Muckenthaler 2013; Pietrangelo 2016). Dietary iron is absorbed at the duodenum and exported by ferroportin. Then, it bonds to transferrin in order to circulate in the bloodstream, for finally being used in cellular metabolism and erythropoiesis. Iron recycling results from the destruction of aged or damaged red blood cells that are phagocytized by the mononuclear phagocytic system in the spleen (Ganz 2008). Only a small amount of iron is lost due to bleeding, skin desquamation, or urinary excretion. Because there is no regulated pathway to eliminate excess iron, incoming of iron is crucial, which is controlled by hepcidin, the hormone that regulates the expression of ferroportin (the iron exporter) in the enterocytes, macrophages, and hepatocytes (Ganz 2008). When there is excess of iron, it is stored as ferritin within the hepatocytes and also at the mononuclear phagocytic system within the liver (the Kupffer cells) and spleen. Nevertheless, when the ferritin storage capacity is exceeded, nonbonded iron induces oxidative stress and cellular damage, ultimately leading to fibrosis and organ dysfunction. The clinical manifestations will depend on the pattern and severity of organ iron deposition, which are related with the etiology of iron overload (Piperno 1998). Increased liver iron deposition can result from either genetic hemochromatosis or transfusional hemosiderosis (secondary hemochromatosis), but it is also increasingly recognized in association with chronic liver diseases and metabolic diseases.

Hereditary hemochromatosis is caused by mutations in the genes involved in the iron metabolism and trafficking. Most of the patients are homozygous for the p.C282Y variant of the HFE gene (EASL 2010), resulting in deficient synthesis of hepcidin, which leads to increased plasma iron concentration and transferrin saturation. Iron will accumulate mainly in the liver but also in other organs with transferrin receptors, such as the pancreas and the heart (Pietrangelo 2015). Clinical manifestations include liver cirrhosis, diabetes, and heart failure. In these patients, the excess of iron is efficiently treated through periodic phlebotomies.

Secondary hemochromatosis results from an oversupply of either endogenous or exogenous iron in cases of iron-loading anemias (e.g., thalassemia, sickle cell, or sideroblastic anemias) or in patients with multiple blood transfusions, with increased erythrophagocytosis leading to excess of iron (Piperno 1998). Consequently, iron will accumulate in the mononuclear phagocytic system in the spleen, bone marrow, and also liver, and then in the parenchyma of the pancreas, heart, and endocrine glands. Because these patients usually have anemia, they cannot be treated with phlebotomies, but, instead, iron chelates are used in order to prevent organ toxicity.

Chronic liver diseases, such as alcoholic liver disease, nonalcoholic fatty liver disease, viral hepatitis, and end-stage liver disease, can present hepatic iron overload but usually at a lower level than in primary or secondary hemo-chromatosis. Interestingly, iron coexistence with other hepatotoxins, such as concomitant steatosis or viral hepatitis, may have a synergetic effect on the progression of the underlying liver disease, and this appears to happen even with low-grade overload (Pietrangelo 2016). Progression of liver fibrosis and increased risk of hepatocellular carcinoma have also been associated with iron overload in chronic liver diseases (Pietrangelo 2009; Corradini and Pietrangelo 2012; Kew 2014).

Finally, **dysmetabolic iron overload syndrome** is another condition associated with hepatic iron overload, being defined as hepatic iron overload in association with one or more metabolic abnormality related with insulin resistance, such as obesity, dyslipidemia, or abnormal glucose metabolism (Moirand et al. 1997). It is the major cause for hyperferritinemia in the outpatient setting, being much more common than hereditary hemochromatosis (Mendler et al. 1999). Even though the iron excess is usually mild, in some cases it can be as high as in hereditary hemochromatosis (Deugnier and Turlin 2007). Furthermore, associated liver steatosis and steatohepatitis are common findings in these patients (Turlin et al. 2001; Riva et al. 2008).

2.2 Markers of Iron Overload

The **total body iron stores (TBIS)** can be estimated through quantitative phlebotomies, because the amount of iron in the removed blood can be measured. Nevertheless, phlebotomies should only be used if they provide therapeutic benefit (EASL 2010) and, therefore, TBIS cannot be estimated by blood depletion in every iron-overload disorder.

Serum ferritin is widely used as a serum marker of iron overload. Nevertheless, it is not specific, since it is an acute-phase reactant, being frequently elevated in acute and chronic inflammatory conditions, and also in malignancy or in liver diseases with hepatocellular necrosis (Wang et al. 2010; Wood 2014a, b).

Liver iron concentration (LIC) has been demonstrated to be directly correlated with the TBIS and, therefore, it is considered as a surrogate marker of TBIS (Brissot et al. 1981; Angelucci et al. 2000). Therefore, liver core biopsy with biochemical determination of LIC, performed by atomic absorption spectrometry of liver tissue, has been considered the reference standard for the quantification of hepatic iron overload and for assessment of body iron stores (Barry 1974). However, spectrophotometry is not widely available (Wood 2014a, b). Furthermore, besides operator dependency and other important disadvantages related to the invasive nature of liver biopsy, such as pain or hemorrhagic complications, there are also important concerns related to its sampling variability (Villeneuve et al. 1996; Emond et al. 1999). In fact, only a small sample of the liver parenchyma is analyzed and the variability of iron deposition throughout the liver parenchyma can be very high, particularly in cases of cirrhosis (Hernando et al. 2014).

In this scenario, imaging techniques have been explored as noninvasive alternatives for iron detection and quantification.

Ultrasonography (US) and **computed tomography (CT)** are not useful in the detection of hepatic iron overload. Iron overload is usually associated with an increased attenuation of the liver parenchyma on CT images but this finding is not accurate (Wood 2014a, b). Even though dual-energy CT has been shown to be more accurate for detecting and quantifying liver iron content than monoenergetic CT (Luo et al. 2015), it still needs further validation. Besides, CT uses radiation, hampering its use in the long-term follow-up of iron-reducing therapies, particularly in young patients.

On the other hand, **magnetic resonance imaging** (MRI) has a unique ability to detect the presence of iron within tissues and it has been increasingly used as an alternative to liver biopsy, allowing both detection and quantification of iron overload. In fact, MRI is now considered the standard of care, even being more precise than liver biopsy for assessing LIC and TBIS (Wood et al. 2015). Furthermore, MRI enables the detection and quantification of iron deposition in other tissues besides the liver, depicting different distribution patterns of iron overload.

2.3 MR Imaging for Iron Detection and Assessment of Distribution Patterns of Iron Overload

MRI depicts the paramagnetic effect of iron on the neighborhood protons, accelerating the T2 relaxation and mainly the T2* signal decay, resulting in a recognizable signal loss on T2- and T2*-weighted images, which is proportional to the iron content (Sirlin and Reeder 2010). Thus, the presence of liver iron overload can be recognized by the low signal intensity (SI) of the liver on T2- and T2*-weighted images (Fig. 1). Moreover, on chemical shift (dual echo) gradient-

echo (GRE) T1-weighted sequences, iron over-load is recognized by decreased SI on the in-phase images (second echo images) as compared with out-of-phase images (first echo images) (Fig. 2).

Certain **distribution patterns** of iron accumulation may be recognized on abdominal MR images of different iron-overload diseases, according to their different physiopathology. For example, iron deposits within the liver and pancreas, depicted as low SI of these organs on T2-weighted images, are most commonly observed in patients with severe hereditary hemochromatosis, usually sparing the spleen and bone marrow (Fig. 3). On the other hand, a pattern of low SI of the liver, spleen, and bone marrow is related to iron accumulation inside the cells of the mononuclear phagocytic system (Fig. 4), being classically attributed to transfusional hemosiderosis or hemolytic anemias. Nevertheless, with time, these patients can also accumulate iron in the pancreas (Fig. 5). Autosplenectomy is also frequently seen in hemolytic anemias and, particularly in sickle cell anemia, iron overload may also be depicted in the renal cortex, due to accumulation of hemoglobin during renal filtration (Fig. 4) (Schein et al. 2008). On the other hand, the presence of isolated hepatic iron deposition is classically associated to iron overload in the setting of chronic liver diseases but can also be recognized on milder forms of hereditary hemochromatosis (Fig. 1) (Queiroz-Andrade et al. 2009; Gourtsoyiannis 2011).

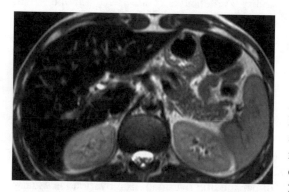

Fig. 1 TSE T2-weighted TSE image in a patient with hereditary hemochromatosis, with low SI of liver parenchyma due to iron overload. The pancreas and spleen have normal SI. This pattern is usually present in milder forms of hemochromatosis but can also be seen in chronic liver diseases

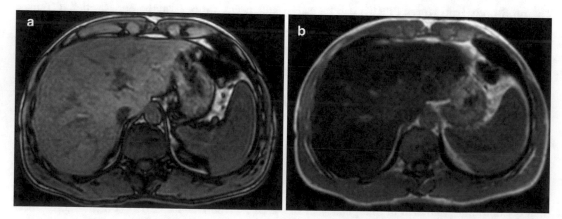

Fig. 2 Hepatic iron overload recognized on chemical shift T1-weighted MR images. The liver intensity is lower on the second echo in-phase image (**b**) in comparison to the first echo (opposed phase) image (**a**), due to iron T2* decay effect

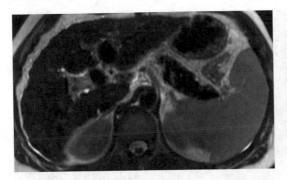

Fig. 3 T2-weighted TSE image of a patient with hereditary hemochromatosis and liver cirrhosis, with low SI of the liver and pancreas parenchyma, and normal SI in the spleen

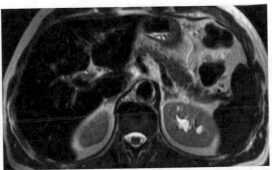

Fig. 6 T2-weighted TSE image of a patient with alcoholic chronic liver disease and predominant iron deposition in the mononuclear phagocytic system, showing low SI in the liver, spleen, and bone marrow. The pancreas has normal SI

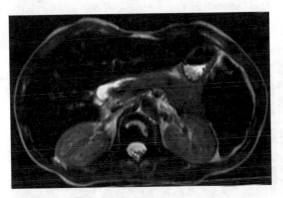

Fig. 4 T2-weighted image of a patient with sickle cell anemia and long-term treatment with blood transfusions. There is marked low SI of the liver, spleen, and bone marrow, sparing the pancreatic parenchyma, related with iron overload in the mononuclear phagocytic system. Also, low SI is seen in the renal cortex due to iron deposition

These distribution patterns can help abdominal imagers to recognize iron-overload diseases but, nevertheless, many variants can be seen in clinical practice and, thus, these patterns of iron distribution should be interpreted with caution. For example, iron deposition in the liver, spleen and bone marrow is also frequent in patients with chronic diffuse liver diseases (Fig. 6) (França et al. 2018a, b), whereas iron overload in the liver and pancreas can be depicted in non-hereditary hemochromatosis liver cirrhosis (Fig. 7) (Abu Rajab et al. 2014).

2.4 MR Imaging Techniques for Iron Quantification

In the last decade, MRI techniques for iron quantification have become available in clinical practice and, nowadays, noninvasive MR imaging biomarkers of hepatic iron are being used for the diagnosis of iron-overload disorders and also to monitor iron-reducing therapies (Wood 2015). Furthermore, for patients referred for hyperferritinemia, MR imaging can be performed for diagnosing iron overload and for assessing the severity and distribution of iron deposition.

MRI methods developed for liver iron quantification can be divided into signal intensity ratio (SIR) methods and relaxometry methods, and all of these methods have been validated against LIC determined from biopsies (Sirlin and Reeder 2010; Labranche et al. 2018).

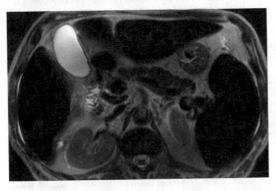

Fig. 5 T2-weighted TSE image of a patient with myelodysplastic syndrome, treated with multiple blood transfusions. The liver parenchyma, spleen, and bone marrow have low SI, as well as the pancreas. This is related with long-standing mononuclear phagocytic system iron accumulation, with iron overflow to the pancreas

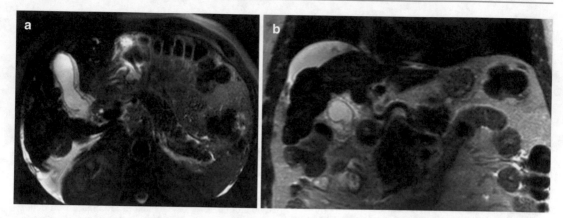

Fig. 7 Axial (**a**) and coronal (**b**) TSE T2-weighted images of a male patient with liver cirrhosis with hyperferritinemia but normal transferrin saturation. Low SI of the parenchyma of the liver and pancreas was seen, as well as ascites. Although liver cirrhosis with hepatic and pancreatic iron overload is the usual pattern in non-treated hereditary hemochromatosis, this was excluded by genetic tests. Iron overload related with liver cirrhosis can also be associated with iron accumulation in other organs, mimicking hereditary hemochromatosis

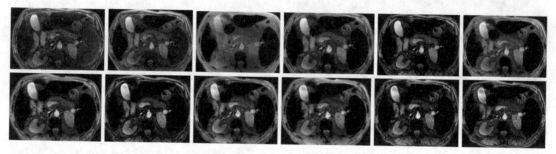

Fig. 8 Iron overload in a patient with myelodysplastic syndrome. Magnitude images from a multiecho chemical shift-encoded GRE sequence with 12 different TEs demonstrating severe liver signal dropout with increasing TEs, which is related to iron overload. The mean R2* was 1700 s^{-1}. The presence of concomitant iron overload in the pancreas and spleen can also be observed

Signal intensity ratio (SIR) methods measure the liver-to-muscle SI ratio: the decrease of liver SI, due to iron-related T2* shortening, is compared to the SI of a reference tissue that does not accumulate iron, usually the skeletal muscle. The most widely used SIR method was first published in 2004 (Gandon et al. 2004), requiring five in-phase GRE sequences, with constant TR but with different flip angles and increasing TE, acquired with a body coil. This was an easy method, as a free online worksheet provided by the University of Rennes allowed to estimate LIC (μmol Fe/g) from SI determined from ROIs placed within the liver and paraspinal muscles. However, this technique has low diagnostic accuracy (around 60%), with a tendency to overestimate overload, particularly in cases of mild-to-moderate overload (Castiella et al. 2011). Moreover, it could be confounded by coexisting hepatic steatosis and/or muscle fatty infiltration, since fat increases the tissue's SI, and it is also affected by B0 and B1 signal inhomogeneity (Sirlin and Reeder 2010). Therefore, this protocol was recently updated, now providing a free available Java application that allows to calculate LIC from both SIR and T2*, and also on 3.0 T (Paisant et al. 2017; https://imagemed.univ-rennes1.fr/en/mrquantif/).

Relaxometry methods measure relaxation time constants after acquiring a series of images with increasing TEs, usually with more than six echoes, and can be performed with surface coils (Fig. 8). The liver SI is modeled as a function of TE (Fig. 9) and signal decay constants are then

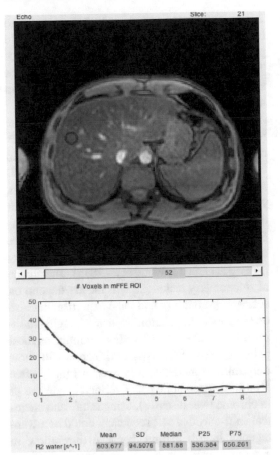

Fig. 9 R2* relaxometry, using a multiecho GRE sequence with 12 TEs. Using a dedicated software for quantification of hepatic R2*, the plot of mean SI within a circular ROI is modeled as a function of TE, as a bi-exponential decay curve. The estimated R2* is 603 s⁻¹

calculated (Sirlin and Reeder 2010): T2 or T2* values (measured in ms) or their mathematical inverses, R2 or R2* (measured in s^{-1} or Hertz), depending on whether a spin-echo or a GRE-based sequence is performed, respectively. Hepatic T2 and T2* are closely related to LIC: the greater the LIC, the higher the relaxation rates (R2 or R2*) and the lower the relaxation times (T2 or T2*) (Wood 2014a, b).

The most known **R2 relaxometry method** (St. Pierre 2005) is currently available as a commercial service ("FerriScan®"), which has been approved by the Food and Drug Administration (FDA) in the USA. After calibration, MR images are acquired with five T2-weighted sequences,

during free breathing, and then are forwarded for centralized image data analysis and R2 measurements. This method has shown a low inter-exam variability and good inter-machine reproducibility (Wood et al. 2005; St Pierre et al. 2014). However, it requires additional costs and longer examination time, being prone to motion artifact and also being affected by hepatic steatosis.

R2* relaxometry methods, on the other hand, are performed with fast GRE multi-echo sequences; thus they require shorter acquisition time and are easier to implement. The liver R2* is calculated either on a voxel-by-voxel basis or by averaging the measured signal within a ROI (Hernando et al. 2014), using either in-house-developed (Fig. 9) or commercially available software.

The most used R2* relaxometry method was described by Wood et al. (2005), in a 1.5-T equipment, demonstrating a linear strong relationship between R2* and biopsy-based LIC measurements.

R2* relaxometry can be performed at both 1.5 and 3.0 T but relaxation rates are dependent on the magnetic field strength. Therefore, calibration curves obtained at one magnetic field strength cannot be directly transposed to another field strength: the R2* values at 3.0 T are twice the R2* at 1.5 T (Storey et al. 2007; Meloni et al. 2012). Although assessment of T2*/R2* is feasible at 3.0 T, the faster signal decay lowers the accuracy for detecting heavy-to-moderate liver iron burden (Meloni et al. 2012) and reduces the upper limit of measurable iron concentration (Fig. 10). Ultrashort-TE sequences, with TE as low as 0.1 ms, have been developed for allowing R2* quantification in patients with high iron overload (Krafft et al. 2017). However, these sequences still need further validation and, meanwhile, 1.5-T equipment should be preferentially used in patients with severe iron overload.

R2* relaxometry methods have shown good reproducibility across different scanners and centers, as also good interobserver reproducibility (Kirk et al. 2010). Nevertheless, more recently, other authors have also derived calibration curves to transform R2* values into LIC values (mg Fe/g or μmol Fe/g) (Hankins et al. 2009; Anderson

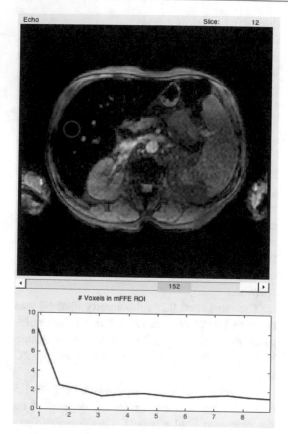

Fig. 10 R2* relaxometry in severe iron overload, on a 3-T MR equipment. In this case of severe iron overload, the signal decay is even faster on 3.0 T, and most of the MRI signal has irreversibly disappeared by the time of first or second image acquisition, which may hamper accurate iron quantification

et al. 2001; Garbowski et al. 2014; d'Assignies et al. 2018), with some small discrepancies between these methods (Garbowski et al. 2014). These differences are most probably due to the sampling bias related to the heterogeneous distribution of iron within the liver, but also with variability in biopsy handling and processing (Wood et al. 2015).

While most of the validation studies compared R2* measurements against biopsy-determined LIC, which is a biomarker of TBIS, more recently, R2* measurements were directly compared with TBIS, determined as the amount of mobilized iron by quantitative phlebotomies, in patients with hereditary hemochromatosis (França et al.

2018a, b). Liver and pancreas R2* were shown to be good predictors of TBIS, and, therefore, could potentially be used to estimate the severity of TBIS at the time of diagnosis and, consequently, the expected duration of intensive treatment in hereditary hemochromatosis.

Although there is still no consensus on the recommended acquisition parameters for R2* relaxometry, R2* measurements can be used in clinical practice, as long as validated methods and acquisition protocols are used (St Pierre et al. 2014; Wood 2015; Meloni et al. 2012), either for diagnosing or for monitoring iron-reducing therapies (Fig. 11). In fact, R2* measurements were considered to be more precise than liver biopsy (Zhang et al. 2013; Wood et al. 2015). The choice of relaxometry technique will mostly depend on software availability and local expertise, but also on the patient population requiring imaging monitoring (Wood et al. 2015). For example, as most patients referred for hyperferritinemia will show only mild-to-moderate iron overload (as is often seen in dysmetabolic iron overload syndrome or in chronic liver diseases), using multiecho chemical shift-encoded MR sequences could be advantageous in this setting, because they allow to simultaneously quantify hepatic iron and steatosis (Figs. 12, 13, and 14 from chapter "Liver Steatosis and NAFLD") (França et al. 2017, Donato et al. 2017). Quite important, if fat and iron coexist in the liver parenchyma, fat will introduce signal oscillations as water and fat signals become in and out of phase, and the T2* signal decay will no longer be monoexponential (chapter "Liver Steatosis and NAFLD," Fig. 11). Thus, if this effect of fat on T2* signal decay is not taken into account, iron quantification could be biased by steatosis (Hernando et al. 2014, França et al. 2017).

3 Liver Storage Diseases

Glycogen storage disorders are a group of genetic diseases related to the deficient processing of glycogen, due to the lack of different enzymes involved in glycogen storage or breakdown. Up to 12 types of disease have been

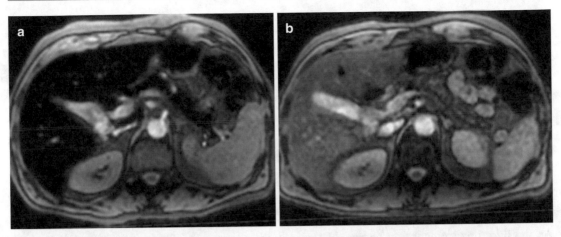

Fig. 11 TSE T2-weighted images of a patient with hereditary hemochromatosis, by the time of diagnosis (**a**) and after intensive treatment with weekly phlebotomies (**b**). On the first MR examination (**a**), the mean hepatic R2* was 635 s⁻¹ and biopsy-estimated LIC value was 101 μmol/g dry liver. On the second MR examination, the mean hepatic R2* was 69 s⁻¹ and the biopsy-estimated LIC value was 16 μmol/g dry liver. The increase on hepatic and pancreatic SI can be recognized, related with the iron-reducing therapy

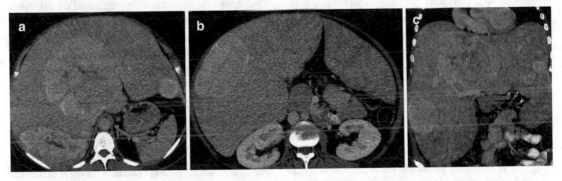

Fig. 12 Axial (**a, b**) and coronal (**c**) contrast-enhanced CT images demonstrate hepatomegaly and multiple liver adenomas in a patient with glycogen storage disease type Ia

described and only some of these have been associated with liver disease, including types I, III, and IV, which can result in severe liver disease (Matern et al. 1999; Ozen 2007).

Imaging features of liver disease include hepatomegaly and hyperechogenicity of the parenchyma, similar to fat deposition on US examinations. Chemical-shift T1 GRE sequences can be quite useful, distinguishing fat deposition in these patients (Pozzato et al. 2007). Nevertheless, the main role of imaging in glycogen storage disease is not for diagnosis, which is usually done biochemically or genetically, neither for staging the severity of the disease. Instead, imaging plays an important role in assessing cirrhosis, hepatic adenomas, or hepato-

cellular carcinoma, which can develop in these patients (Fig. 12) (Hope et al. 2014).

Wilson's disease, also called hepatolenticular degeneration, is a rare genetic disorder of copper metabolism with autosomal recessive inheritance, being characterized by abnormal accumulation of copper in the liver and other organs such as the brain, cornea, or kidneys. Therefore, patients with Wilson's disease may present clinical manifestations related with liver disease but also with neurological symptoms and kidney stones.

The diagnosis is most often during childhood or in young adults, and is usually confirmed with low serum ceruloplasmin and elevated 24-h urinary copper excretion. The Kayser-Fleischer rings in the cornea are another distinctive feature associated with the disease. Nevertheless, in patients with inconclusive tests, liver biopsy may be needed for copper quantification (Ferenci et al. 2005).

Regarding the liver, copper accumulation results in oxidative stress that leads to cellular damage, steatosis, inflammation, and fibrosis. Thus, histopathological findings can be quite similar to those found with other diffuse liver diseases, including fatty liver disease, acute hepatitis, chronic active hepatitis, cirrhosis, and even fulminant hepatic necrosis (Davies et al. 1989). As the liver involvement may be variable, comprehending steatosis, hepatitis, fibrosis, and cirrhosis (Merle et al. 2007), comprehensibly the imaging features of Wilson's disease are nonspecific and cannot distinguish Wilson's disease from other chronic diffuse liver diseases. Furthermore, copper concentration cannot be determined by imaging examinations. Therefore, the main role of liver imaging is to depict signs of liver disease and to rule out liver cirrhosis.

Liver steatosis has been described in more than 50% of patients (Merle et al. 2007) and can be easily recognized on US, CT, or MR imaging. Other common imaging findings are the heterogenicity of the liver parenchyma on US images (Fig. 13), and the presence of a perihepatic fat layer. In fact, it has been suggested that Wilson's disease should be suspected in non-overweight children or young patients with liver steatosis, parenchymal heterogenicity, and a perihepatic fat layer. Parenchymal heterogenicity is often associated with multiple nodules, which can be hypoechoic or hyperechoic on US, and are usually hyperdense on non-enhanced CT and hypodense on contrast-enhanced CT. On MR imaging, parenchymal nodules are commonly hypointense on T2-weighted image and hyperintense on T1-weighted images, probably due to the focal accumulation of copper (Cheon et al. 2010). A honeycomb pattern may be seen due to the presence of fibrotic septa surrounding the nodules. These fibrotic septa are hyperintense on T2-weighted images and hyperintense on contrast-enhanced images (Fig. 14).

As the liver disease progresses to cirrhosis, structural changes can be recognized on different imaging modalities, such as irregular liver surface contours, widening of the liver fissures and gallbladder fossa, and enlargement of the hilar periportal space (Figs. 14 and 15). Nevertheless, in Wilson's disease, usually there is no hypertrophy of the caudate lobe and the caudate-to-right lobe ratio is normal (Figs. 14 and 15), contrary to liver cirrhosis from other causes. Therefore, Wilson's disease should be considered as a leading diagnosis in young adults with liver cirrhosis and absence of caudate lobe hypertrophy (Akhan et al. 2009).

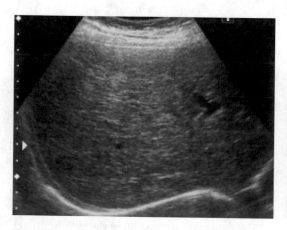

Fig. 13 US showing parenchymal heterogenicity and multiple tiny hypoechoic nodules, in a patient with Wilson's disease. The presence of a perihepatic fat layer is also noted

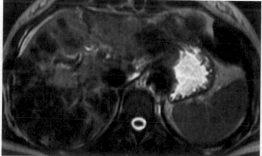

Fig. 14 TSE T2-weighted MR image of a patient with Wilson's disease and liver cirrhosis, showing hyperintense septa and areas of confluent fibrosis. The absence of caudate lobe hypertrophy should also be noted

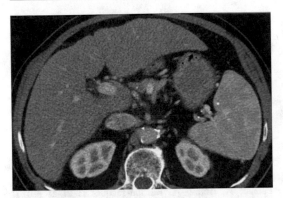

Fig. 15 Axial contrast-enhanced CT image in a patient with Wilson's disease and liver cirrhosis, showing structural changes of cirrhosis but with absence of caudate lobe hypertrophy

4 Conclusion

MRI is a valuable tool for assessing patients with iron-overload diseases, being used for diagnosing and quantifying iron overload, and for monitoring iron-reducing therapies. Liver iron quantification by MRI should be performed with validated methods, either with relaxometry or SIR methods. While there is no standardization nor consensus regarding different methods, the choice also depends on the available tools at each institution.

Imaging findings in liver storage diseases, such as glycogen storage disease and Wilson's disease, are not specific. Nevertheless, Wilson's disease should be suspected in young non-overweight patients with liver steatosis, parenchymal heterogenicity, and perihepatic fat layer, or with liver cirrhosis without caudate lobe hypertrophy.

References

Abu Rajab M, Guerin L, Lee P, Brown KE (2014) Iron overload secondary to cirrhosis: a mimic of hereditary haemochromatosis? Histopathology 65:561–569. https://doi.org/10.1111/his.12417

Akhan O, Akpinar E, Karcaaltincaba M et al (2009) Imaging findings of liver involvement of Wilson's disease. Eur J Radiol 69:147–155. https://doi.org/10.1016/j.ejrad.2007.09.029

Anderson LJ, Holden S, Davis B et al (2001) Cardiovascular T2-star (T2*) magnetic resonance for the early diagnosis of myocardial iron overload. Eur Heart J 22:2171–2179

Angelucci E, Brittenham GM, McLaren CE et al (2000) Hepatic iron concentration and total body iron stores in thalassemia major. N Engl J Med 343:327–331. https://doi.org/10.1056/NEJM200008033430503

Barry M (1974) Liver iron concentration, stainable iron, and total body storage iron. Gut 15:411–415

Brissot P, Bourel M, Herry D et al (1981) Assessment of liver iron content in 271 patients: a reevaluation of direct and indirect methods. Gastroenterology 80:557–565

Castiella A, Alústiza JM, Emparanza JI et al (2011) Liver iron concentration quantification by MRI: are recommended protocols accurate enough for clinical practice? Eur Radiol 21:137–141. https://doi.org/10.1007/s00330-010-1899-z

Cheon J-E, Kim I-O, Seo JK et al (2010) Clinical application of liver MR imaging in Wilson's disease. Korean J Radiol 11:665–672. https://doi.org/10.3348/kjr.2010.11.6.665

Corradini E, Pietrangelo A (2012) Iron and steatohepatitis. J Gastroenterol Hepatol 27(Suppl 2):42–46. https://doi.org/10.1111/j.1440-1746.2011.07014.x

d'Assignies G, Paisant A, Bardou-Jacquet E et al (2018) Non-invasive measurement of liver iron concentration using 3-Tesla magnetic resonance imaging: validation against biopsy. Eur Radiol 28.2022–2030. https://doi.org/10.1007/s00330-017-5106-3

Davies SE, Williams R, Portmann B (1989) Hepatic morphology and histochemistry of Wilson's disease presenting as fulminant hepatic failure: a study of 11 cases. Histopathology 15:385–394

Deugnier Y, Turlin B (2007) Pathology of hepatic iron overload. World J Gastroenterol 13:4755–4760

Donato H, França M, Candelária I, Caseiro-Alves F (2017) Liver MRI: from basic protocol to advanced techniques. Eur J Radiol 93:30–39. https://doi.org/10.1016/j.ejrad.2017.05.028

Emond MJ, Bronner MP, Carlson TH et al (1999) Quantitative study of the variability of hepatic iron concentrations. Clin Chem 45:340–346

European Association for the Study of the Liver (2010) EASL clinical practice guidelines for HFE hemochromatosis. J Hepatol 53:3–22. https://doi.org/10.1016/j.jhep.2010.03.001

Ferenci P, Steindl-Munda P, Vogel W et al (2005) Diagnostic value of quantitative hepatic copper determination in patients with Wilson's disease. Clin Gastroenterol Hepatol 3:811–818

França M, Alberich-Bayarri Á, Martí-Bonmatí L et al (2017) Accurate simultaneous quantification of liver steatosis and iron overload in diffuse liver diseases with MRI. Abdom Radiol (New York) 42:1434–1443. https://doi.org/10.1007/s00261-017-1048-0

França M, Martí-Bonmatí L, Porto G et al (2018a) Tissue iron quantification in chronic liver diseases using MRI shows a relationship between iron accumulation in liver, spleen, and bone marrow. Clin Radiol 73:215. e1–215.e9. https://doi.org/10.1016/j.crad.2017.07.022

França M, Martí-Bonmatí L, Silva S et al (2018b) Optimizing the management of hereditary haemochromatosis: the value of MRI R2* quantification to predict and monitor body iron stores. Br J Haematol 183:491–493. https://doi.org/10.1111/bjh.14982

Gandon Y, Olivié D, Guyader D et al (2004) Non-invasive assessment of hepatic iron stores by MRI. Lancet (London, England) 363:357–362. https://doi.org/10.1016/S0140-6736(04)15436-6

Ganz T (2008) Iron homeostasis: fitting the puzzle pieces together. Cell Metab 7:288–290. https://doi.org/10.1016/j.cmet.2008.03.008

Garbowski MW, Carpenter J-P, Smith G et al (2014) Biopsy-based calibration of T2* magnetic resonance for estimation of liver iron concentration and comparison with R2 Ferriscan. J Cardiovasc Magn Reson 16:40. https://doi.org/10.1186/1532-429X-16-40

Gourtsoyiannis NC (2011) Clinical MRI of the abdomen. Berlin, Heidelberg

Hankins JS, McCarville MB, Loeffler RB et al (2009) R2* magnetic resonance imaging of the liver in patients with iron overload. Blood 113:4853–4855. https://doi.org/10.1182/blood-2008-12-191643

Hernando D, Levin YS, Sirlin CB, Reeder SB (2014) Quantification of liver iron with MRI: state of the art and remaining challenges. J Magn Reson Imaging 40:1003–1021. https://doi.org/10.1002/jmri.24584

Hope TA, Ohliger MA, Qayyum A (2014) MR imaging of diffuse liver disease: from technique to diagnosis. Radiol Clin N Am 52:709–724. https://doi.org/10.1016/j.rcl.2014.02.016

Kew MC (2014) Hepatic iron overload and hepatocellular carcinoma. Liver Cancer 3:31–40. https://doi.org/10.1159/000343856

Kirk P, He T, Anderson LJ et al (2010) International reproducibility of single breath-hold T2* MR for cardiac and liver iron assessment among five thalassemia centers. J Magn Reson Imaging 32:315–319. https://doi.org/10.1002/jmri.22245

Krafft AJ, Loeffler RB, Song R et al (2017) Quantitative ultrashort echo time imaging for assessment of massive iron overload at 1.5 and 3 Tesla. Magn Reson Med 78:1839–1851. https://doi.org/10.1002/mrm.26592

Labranche R, Gilbert G, Cerny M et al (2018) Liver iron quantification with MR imaging: a primer for radiologists. Radiographics 38:392–412. https://doi.org/10.1148/rg.2018170079

Luo XF, Xie XQ, Cheng S et al (2015) Dual-energy CT for patients suspected of having liver iron overload: can virtual iron content imaging accurately quantify liver iron content? Radiology 277:95–103. https://doi.org/10.1148/radiol.2015141856

Matern D, Starzl TE, Arnaout W et al (1999) Liver transplantation for glycogen storage disease types I, III, and IV. Eur J Pediatr 158(Suppl 2):S43–S48

Meloni A, Positano V, Keilberg P et al (2012) Feasibility, reproducibility, and reliability for the T*2 iron evaluation at 3 T in comparison with 1.5 T. Magn Reson Med 68:543–551. https://doi.org/10.1002/mrm.23236

Mendler MH, Turlin B, Moirand R et al (1999) Insulin resistance-associated hepatic iron overload. Gastroenterology 117:1155–1163

Merle U, Schaefer M, Ferenci P, Stremmel W (2007) Clinical presentation, diagnosis and long-term outcome of Wilson's disease: a cohort study. Gut 56:115–120. https://doi.org/10.1136/gut.2005.087262

Moirand R, Mortaji AM, Loréal O et al (1997) A new syndrome of liver iron overload with normal transferrin saturation. Lancet (London, England) 349:95–97. https://doi.org/10.1016/S0140-6736(96)06034-5

Ozen H (2007) Glycogen storage diseases: new perspectives. World J Gastroenterol 13:2541–2553

Paisant A, Boulic A, Bardou-Jacquet E et al (2017) Assessment of liver iron overload by 3 T MRI. Abdom Radiol (New York) 42:1713–1720. https://doi.org/10.1007/s00261-017-1077-8

Pietrangelo A (2009) Iron in NASH, chronic liver diseases and HCC: how much iron is too much? J Hepatol 50:249–251. https://doi.org/10.1016/j.jhep.2008.11.011

Pietrangelo A (2015) Genetics, genetic testing, and management of hemochromatosis: 15 years since hepcidin. Gastroenterology 149:1240–1251. https://doi.org/10.1053/j.gastro.2015.06.045

Pietrangelo A (2016) Mechanisms of iron hepatotoxicity. J Hepatol 65:226–227. https://doi.org/10.1016/j.jhep.2016.01.037

Piperno A (1998) Classification and diagnosis of iron overload. Haematologica 83:447–455

Pozzato C, Dall'asta C, Radaelli G et al (2007) Usefulness of chemical-shift MRI in discriminating increased liver echogenicity in glycogenosis. Dig Liver Dis 39:1018–1023. https://doi.org/10.1016/j.dld.2007.06.008

Queiroz-Andrade M, Blasbalg R, Ortega CD et al (2009) MR imaging findings of iron overload. Radiographics 29:1575–1589. https://doi.org/10.1148/rg.296095511

Riva A, Trombini P, Mariani R et al (2008) Revaluation of clinical and histological criteria for diagnosis of dysmetabolic iron overload syndrome. World J Gastroenterol 14:4745–4752

Schein A, Enriquez C, Coates TD, Wood JC (2008) Magnetic resonance detection of kidney iron deposition in sickle cell disease: a marker of chronic hemolysis. J Magn Reson Imaging 28:698–704. https://doi.org/10.1002/jmri.21490

Sirlin CB, Reeder SB (2010) Magnetic resonance imaging quantification of liver iron. Magn Reson Imaging Clin N Am 18:359–381. https://doi.org/10.1016/j.mric.2010.08.014

St Pierre TG, El-Beshlawy A, Elalfy M et al (2014) Multicenter validation of spin-density projection-assisted R2-MRI for the noninvasive measurement of liver iron concentration. Magn Reson Med 71:2215–2223. https://doi.org/10.1002/mrm.24854

St. Pierre TG (2005) Noninvasive measurement and imaging of liver iron concentrations using proton magnetic resonance. Blood 105:855–861. https://doi.org/10.1182/blood-2004-01-0177

Steinbicker AU, Muckenthaler MU (2013) Out of balance--systemic iron homeostasis in iron-related disorders. Nutrients 5:3034–3061. https://doi.org/10.3390/nu5083034

Storey P, Thompson AA, Carqueville CL et al (2007) R2* imaging of transfusional iron burden at 3T and comparison with 1.5T. J Magn Reson Imaging 25:540–547. https://doi.org/10.1002/jmri.20816

Turlin B, Mendler MH, Moirand R et al (2001) Histologic features of the liver in insulin resistance-associated iron overload. A study of 139 patients. Am J Clin Pathol 116:263–270. https://doi.org/10.1309/WWNE-KW2C-4KTW-PTJ5

Villeneuve JP, Bilodeau M, Lepage R et al (1996) Variability in hepatic iron concentration measurement from needle-biopsy specimens. J Hepatol 25:172–177

Wang W, Knovich MA, Coffman LG et al (2010) Serum ferritin: Past, present and future. Biochim Biophys Acta 1800:760–769. https://doi.org/10.1016/j.bbagen.2010.03.011

Wood JC (2014a) Guidelines for quantifying iron overload. Hematol Am Soc Hematol Educ Progr 2014:210–215. https://doi.org/10.1182/asheducation-2014.1.210

Wood JC (2014b) Use of magnetic resonance imaging to monitor iron overload. Hematol Oncol Clin North Am 28(747–64):vii. https://doi.org/10.1016/j.hoc.2014.04.002

Wood JC (2015) Estimating tissue iron burden: current status and future prospects. Br J Haematol 170:15–28. https://doi.org/10.1111/bjh.13374

Wood JC, Enriquez C, Ghugre N et al (2005) MRI R2 and R2* mapping accurately estimates hepatic iron concentration in transfusion-dependent thalassemia and sickle cell disease patients. Blood 106:1460–1465. https://doi.org/10.1182/blood-2004-10-3982

Wood JC, Zhang P, Rienhoff H et al (2015) Liver MRI is more precise than liver biopsy for assessing total body iron balance: a comparison of MRI relaxometry with simulated liver biopsy results. Magn Reson Imaging 33:761–767. https://doi.org/10.1016/j.mri.2015.02.016

Zhang P, Rienhoff HY, Abi-Saab W, Neufeld EJ (2013) Liver MRI Is better than biopsy for assessing total body iron balance: validation by simulation. Blood 122:958

Chronic Hepatitis and Liver Fibrosis/Cirrhosis

Sara Mehrabi, Enza Genco, Mariacristina Maturi, and Mirko D'Onofrio

Contents

Abstract

Liver fibrosis constitutes a potentially reversible significant health problem worldwide, and its identification is fundamental to prevent evolution and to identify complications.

Its most common causes include viral hepatitis, chronic alcoholism and nonalcoholic steatohepatitis (NASH); all these conditions increase scar tissue deposition inside the liver, with a progressive process resulting in cirrhosis.

Liver biopsy represents the gold standard for fibrosis identification, although this technique is not free from possible complications and sampling limitations. Together with biopsy, noninvasive imaging techniques are acquiring an increasingly important role to diagnosis and monitoring of liver fibrosis.

S. Mehrabi · E. Genco · M. Maturi · M. D'Onofrio (✉)
Istituto di Radiologia, Policlinico GB Rossi,
Università di Verona, Verona, Italy
e-mail: mirko.donofrio@univr.it

© Springer Nature Switzerland AG 2021
E. Quaia (ed.), *Imaging of the Liver and Intra-hepatic Biliary Tract*,
Medical Radiology, Diagnostic Imaging, https://doi.org/10.1007/978-3-030-38983-3_15

US and CT-based imaging methods depicts morphologic changes of end-stage liver fibrosis, but are limited in evaluating patients with earlier stages of liver disease. Conventional MR imaging scores well in advanced phases of fibrosis, while latest advances in MRI techniques may revolutionize how we image patients with early stage fibrosis.

In addition, Elastosonography assessment of the stiffness of liver parenchyma is a useful tool to identify and evaluate presence and evolution of liver fibrosis.

1 Introduction

Liver fibrosis is a significant health problem with a worldwide mortality attributable to cirrhosis and primary liver cancer (Shaheen et al. 2006). Liver fibrosis precedes and coexists with many chronic liver diseases, and its early identification is fundamental to prevent the evolution of cirrhosis and hepatocellular carcinoma. The extent of liver fibrosis is therefore one of the most important factors in determining the prognosis and need for active treatment in chronic liver disease (Friedman and Bansal 2006). Liver biopsy is the gold standard investigation for diagnosis of fibrosis. This technique, however, represents an invasive investigation, expensive, with possible complications and with the risk of not scouring all the liver parenchyma. Imaging techniques are acquiring an increasingly important role, in order to identify noninvasive, accurate, reproducible, and less expensive methods for the diagnosis and monitoring of liver fibrosis. Noninvasive tests reduce but do not abolish the need for liver biopsy; they should be used as an integrated system. US and CT-based imaging methods can demonstrate the morphologic alterations of cirrhosis, but they are limited in evaluating patients with earlier stages of liver disease. Advances in MR imaging, with its unique and intrinsic imaging capabilities, have provided the opportunity to revolutionize how we image and evaluate patients with liver fibrosis.

2 Definition

Liver fibrosis is a progressive process determined by excess deposition of collagen, proteoglycans, and other macromolecules in the extracellular matrix in response to chronic liver injury from various causes (Wallace et al. 2008). The result is a diffuse disorganization of hepatic morphology and architecture, which leads to cirrhosis and end-stage liver disease in 20–30% of patients (Friedman and Bansal 2006). Liver cirrhosis is one of the leading causes of death and morbidity within the European Union; an early diagnosis is therefore necessary to delay its progression.

3 Etiology and Epidemiology

The most common causes of liver fibrosis/cirrhosis are hepatitis B and C virus infection and chronic alcoholism; in a lesser number of cases liver fibrosis/cirrhosis is the result of metabolic diseases, autoimmune hepatitis, primary biliary cirrhosis, primary sclerosing cholangitis, hereditary hemochromatosis, Wilson disease, congenital hepatic fibrosis, α1-antitrypsin deficiency, and cystic fibrosis (Schuppan and Afdhal 2008). Alcoholic liver disease, nonalcoholic steatohepatitis (NASH), and hepatitis C are the most common causes in developed countries, whereas hepatitis B is the prevailing cause in most parts of Asia and sub-Saharan Africa. The prevalence of chronic liver disease is thought to be underestimated, as many patients are unaware of it and are diagnosed incidentally (Parkin et al. 2002).

4 Clinical Presentation

Clinically, patients with liver fibrosis remain asymptomatic or have only mild, nonspecific symptoms until the development of cirrhosis. Liver fibrosis usually progresses slowly over decades. Cirrhotic patients may present with accidental increase in transaminases or various sequelae of hepatic decompensation, including jaundice, splenomegaly, variceal hemorrhage, ascites, hepatic encephalopathy, and hepatic and renal failure (Afdhal and Nunes 2004).

5 Pathogenesis and Pathological Anatomy

Liver fibrosis is a potentially reversible disorder, in which vascularized scar tissue bridges together portal triads and central veins (Faria et al. 2009). Cirrhosis is the advanced stage of liver fibrosis that is associated with distortion of the hepatic vasculature. The hepatic sinusoids are lined by fenestrated endothelia that rest on a sheet of permeable connective tissue in the space of Disse, which also contains hepatic stellate cells and some mononuclear cells. In fibrosis, the space of Disse is filled with scar tissue and endothelial fenestrations are lost, a process known as sinusoidal capillarization (Wallace et al. 2008). The major consequence of this process is an increased intrahepatic resistance with portal hypertension; this leads to increase of hepatic arterial flow (Schuppan and Afdhal 2008; Marcellin et al. 2002). Liver parenchyma responds to these injuries with hepatocyte proliferation and regenerative nodule formation, a characteristic aspect of cirrhosis. Depending on the causes, the fibrous pattern can change: in viral hepatitis fibrosis originates from the portal triad and extends to the surrounding parenchyma; instead, in alcoholic hepatitis and in NASH, fibrosis originates from the centrilobular vein and thus extends to the portal triad (Schuppan and Afdhal 2008).

6 Staging of Fibrosis

Currently the gold standard for staging liver fibrosis is percutaneous liver biopsy. For histological evaluation of liver fibrosis, three scoring methods are in widest use: the Ishak score (Ishak et al. 1995), the METAVIR score (for viral and autoimmune hepatitis) (Imbert-Bismut et al.

2001), and the Desmet/Scheuer staging system (Desmet et al. 1999). All these systems are based on the following qualitative parameters to assess the stage of the disease: the degree of fibrous portal tract expansion, fibrous portal-portal linking, portal-central fibrous bridges, and formation of fibrous septa and parenchymal nodules (Standish et al. 2006). The histological stages range from normal portal triads with no signs of fibrosis (METAVIR stage F0) to early-stage disease with portal fibrous expansion (stage F1) or thin fibrous septa emanating from portal triads (stage F2); as the disease progresses, histology may reveal fibrous septa bridging portal triads and central veins (stage F3), or established cirrhosis with the presence of regenerative nodules (stage F4). Disadvantages of staging with liver biopsy are mainly represented by intra- and inter-observer variability and sample variability; in order to avoid under- or over-staging of disease, adequate samples must be obtained, with >20 mm in length or >11 portal triads (Colloredo et al. 2003; Bedossa et al. 2003). Moreover, due to its invasiveness, biopsy presents complications such as hemorrhage, hospitalization, and a fatality rate of 0.03% and is therefore not performed routinely (Terjung et al. 2003; Ito and Mitchell 2004). The risk of complications is of the order of 1%, and the risk of mortality has been put at between 0.1% and 0.01% (Standish et al. 2006).

7 Diagnosis

The gold standard for the diagnosis and staging of liver fibrosis is liver biopsy. Noninvasive hepatic fibrosis diagnosis can be achieved through imaging methods such as US and CT or through elastographic methods (some of which have imaging support), which estimate hepatic deformability as an indirect measure of fibrosis such as elastosonography, in particular point shear-wave elastography such as acoustic radiation force impulse (ARFI), transient elastography (TE), and MR elastography (MRE) (De Robertis et al. 2014). In early-stage fibrosis, US and CT examination may reveal a normal liver or only subtle changes of liver morphology. As the disease progresses, atrophy of right liver and enlargement of caudate and left lobe are often observed, as well as micro- and macro-regenerative nodules (Talwalkar 2006). Among various US techniques, ARFI is a dynamic technique that uses ultrasound-induced radiation force impulses to obtain qualitative and quantitative measure of liver displacement and measure of shear wave speed (ARFI quantification) (Wong et al. 2010; D'Onofrio et al. 2010). High variability in normal values for this methodic has been reported; this represents a useful tool to differentiate between the two extremes of the grading scale (distinction between non-cirrhotics and cirrhotic parenchyma). However ARFI results can be partially affected by the presence of necroinflammation.

7.1 Imaging MRI

7.1.1 MRI Technique

Field-strength magnets of 1.5 Tesla or greater are recommended to obtain high-quality liver imaging with protocols that include T2-weighted turbo spin-echo sequences (with and without fat suppression), T1 gradient echo-weighted in- and opposed-phase sequences, DWI sequences with ADC map, and contrast-enhanced T1 gradient echo sequences with fat suppression (Agnello et al. 2016). For better identification and characterization of liver lesions the use of contrast agent with biliary excretion is recommended, such as gadolinium ethoxybenzyl diethylenetriamine pentaacetic acid (gadoxetic acid; Eovist/Primovist; Bayer-Healthcare, Leverkusen, Germany) and gadobenate dimeglumine (MultiHance, Bracco, Italy). Both agents are distributed in the extracellular-interstitial space immediately after intravenous administration. Subsequently, the agents are taken up by functional hepatocytes and the compounds are excreted into the bile.

The biliary excretion rate of gadobenate dimeglumine is approximately 3–5%, whereas the biliary excretion rate of gadoxetic acid is up to 50%. In addition, gadoxetic acid has an advantage in terms of obtaining its hepatobiliary phase as early as 20 min following contrast injection, while gadobenate dimeglumine-enhanced MRI is performed >60 min following injection (Yulri et al. 2010).

The biliary excretion phase allows a better characterization of focal liver lesions, identifying those with nonfunctioning hepatocytes (HCC) or non-hepatocyte cell lesions. The early arterial phase is acquired after 15–20 s from the highlight of the aorta visualized with a fluoroscopic system and eventually the late arterial phase is acquired a few seconds away. After 50–70 s the venous phase is acquired. Starting from 90 s the transitional phase begins, and the contrast medium passes from the interstitium to the hepatocytes by anion transporter. Subsequently, the biliary excretion phase is acquired, which begins 20 min after the administration of gadoxetic acid and not before 60–180 min after administration of gadobenate dimeglumine. Pathological hepatocytes or non-hepatocyte cells do not have the ability to take contrast agent from the interstitium and this results in less excretion of the contrast agent in the hepatobiliary phase: so HCC and non-hepatocyte lesions such as cholangiocarcinoma, hemangioma, and metastasis appear hypointense. In liver fibrosis/cirrhosis several factors influence the dynamics of the contrast agent: the hepatobiliary phase is slower because the hepatocytes are altered so it is necessary to make a delayed phase not earlier than 180 min (Tamada et al. 2011a); furthermore, cirrhotic vascular shunts as well as steatosis, fibrosis, and martial accumulation reduce the blood flow of contrast agent and its hepatic retention. Brighter signal intensity of the liver parenchyma compared with the portal vein and kidney indicates an adequate hepatobiliary phase (Tamada et al. 2011b); opacification of the biliary tree shows no correlation with the severity

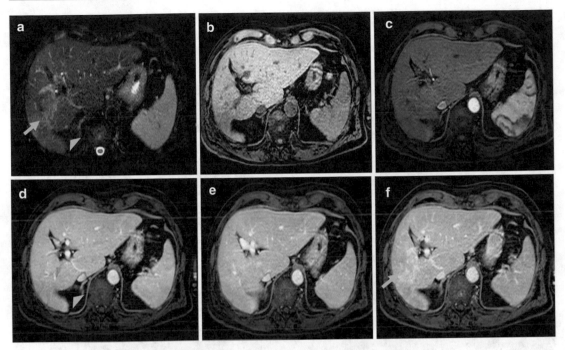

Fig. 1 Patient 54 years old with HCV infection. (**a**) Axial T2-weighted image with fat suppression and (**b**) unenhanced axial T1-weighted image: liver with sinuous margins, enlargement of the left lobe, and inhomogeneous parenchymal signal intensity. Deep incision along inferior-posterior margin of the right lobe ("posterior notch sign," arrowhead). Thin fibrous septa in the IV hepatic segment (arrow), hyperintense on T2-W image (**a**) and hypointense on T1-W image (**b**). Images **c**, **d**, **e**, **f**: axial T1-weighted images after intravenous contrast medium administration; arterial phase (**c**), venous phase (**d**), late phases (**e**, **f**). Progressive post-contrastographic enhancement of the septa, particularly in the late phase, at 5 min from the administration of contrast medium (**f**, arrow)

of cirrhosis and cannot be used alone to evaluate the adequacy of the hepatobiliary phase (Annet et al. 2003).

7.1.2 Conventional MRI

At MR imaging, cirrhotic livers show changed morphologic features, which may include irregular contours, atrophy of the right lobe, and relative enlargement of the lateral segments of the left lobe and caudate lobe, with expansion of the gallbladder fossa. In particular, atrophy of right liver is mostly seen in alcoholic cirrhosis, while enlargement of caudate and left lobe is more often observed in viral forms. Useful indicators for morphologic changes are "caudate-right lobe ratio" and its newer variant "modified caudate-right lobe ratio" indicators that correlate well with the assessment of fibro-

sis (Awaya et al. 2002; Harbin et al. 1980). Other often visualized morphologic changes are the "posterior notch sign," a sharp notch in the posterior surface of the liver (Fig. 1), and the "expanded gallbladder fossa sign," an enlargement of the peri-cholecystic space (Fig. 2), bounded laterally by the right hepatic lobe and medially by the left lateral segment; their presence correlates with advanced fibrosis (Ito et al. 1999).

In advanced stages, alteration of the hepatic profile is almost always present, due to the development of micro- and macro-regenerative nodules. Micronodular cirrhosis is defined as nodules less than 0.3 cm in diameter, whereas macronodular cirrhosis is defined as nodules larger than 0.3 cm. Micronodular cirrhosis is generally associated with uniform and diffuse liver injury (alco-

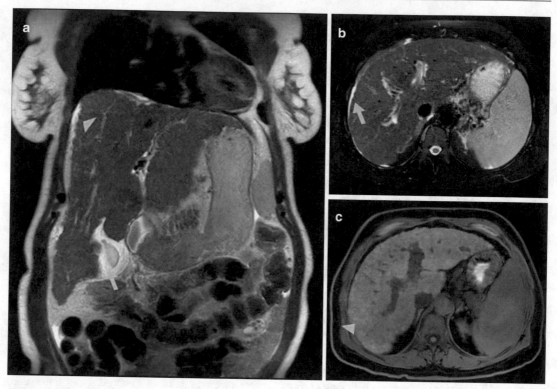

Fig. 2 Patient 49 years old with primary biliary cirrhosis. (**a**) Coronal T2-weighted image: liver markedly increased in volume, with irregular margins (arrowhead), multinodular appearance, and enlargement of the gallbladder fossa (arrow). (**b**) Axial T2-weighted image with fat suppression: increased liver volume with ascites along the margin of the right lobe (arrow). (**c**) Unenhanced axial T1-weighted image: innumerable hyperintense regenerative nodules throughout the liver, more evident on the right lobe (arrowhead)

hol, other hepatotoxic agents, and metabolic disorders) (Fig. 3); processes where hepatocellular regeneration plays a significant role such as chronic hepatitis (particularly hepatitis B) and autoimmune disease are more often associated with macronodular cirrhosis (Fig. 4) (Thiese et al. 2006; Banerjee et al. 2014).

Nevertheless, these aspects remain as morphological characteristics, not specific for determining the cause of the cirrhosis and in general not clinically useful. These signs have high specificity for cirrhosis but low sensitivity for earlier stages of liver disease and are not suitable for staging liver fibrosis over its entire spectrum (Ito and Mitchell 2004). Compared to the morphologic alterations associated with cirrhosis, early fibrosis itself is not well visualized with conventional MR imaging. In patients with early-stage liver fibrosis (pre-cirrhotic stages), the liver parenchyma usually has a normal MR imaging appearance or may only show nonspecific heterogeneity (Martin 2002). Conversely, in patients with advanced fibrosis, unenhanced MR imaging may depict fibrotic septa and reticulation with low signal intensity on T1-weighted images and high signal intensity on T2-weighted images, due to high water content of advanced fibrosis (Talwalkar et al. 2008; Hshiao et al. 2012). The reticulations surround regenerative nodules, which typically have ill-defined margins and intermediate-to-high signal intensity on unenhanced T1-weighted images and intermediate-to-low signal intensity on T2-weighted images (Figs. 5 and 6).

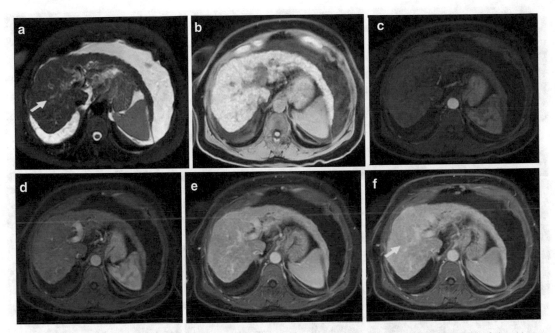

Fig. 3 Patient 59 years old with chronic alcoholism. (**a**) Axial T2-weighted image with fat suppression. (**b**) Unenhanced axial T1-weighted image. (**c–f**) Axial T1-weighted images after intravenous contrast medium administration. Atrophy of right liver (typical features of alcoholic cirrhosis), lobulated margins, and micronodular appearance of hepatic parenchyma; discrete ascites coexist. In the central parts of the right lobe some small fibrotic septa are appreciated, hyperintense on T2-weighted image (**a**, arrow) and hypointense on unenhanced T1-weighted image (**b**). On axial T1-weighted unenhanced sequence multiple small nodules, poorly defined and softly hyperintense, are also shown (**b**). After intravenous contrast medium administration fibrotic septa show late enhancement (**f**, arrow)

When fibrosis is an inherent part of hepatic cirrhosis, it can be typically detected as patchy fibrosis, as a lacelike pattern, or as a confluent mass. Lacelike fibrosis is seen in one-third of patients with primary biliary cirrhosis (Fig. 7) (Dodd 3rd et al. 1999).

Focal confluent fibrosis is observed in 15% of patients with end-stage liver disease and it appears as cuneiform broad fibrotic scar that irradiates from the hilum to the peripheral regions (to segment IV, V, or VII) with or without capsule retraction and a "mass-like" appearance at imaging.

Regenerative nodules may show heterogeneous appearance in the T1-weighted images in relation to their content of iron or intracellular fat. After contrast medium administration, most gadolinium-based contrast agent formulations freely equilibrate with the extracellular compartment and accumulate in tissues with large extracellular volumes such as liver fibrosis. Therefore, on T1-weighted images there is progressive enhancement of the reticulations which peaks during the late venous and equilibrium phases. The fibrosis is usually not well visualized during the arterial phase, contrary to primary liver cancer (HCC) (Fig. 8); this feature, together with other more typical ones, allows differentiation between the two entities. In association with the described liver changes, in advanced fibrosis/cirrhosis it is possible to detect secondary signs of liver disease such as enlarged hepatic hilar lymph nodes, splenomegaly, portal hypertension with portosystemic shunts, varices, and ascites (Fig. 9) (Brancatelli et al. 2007).

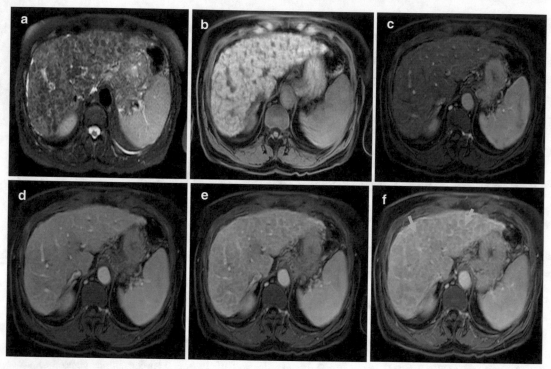

Fig. 4 Patient 69 years old with primary biliary cholangitis. (**a**) Axial T2-weighted image with fat suppression. (**b**) Unenhanced axial T1-weighted image. (**c–f**) Axial T1-weighted images after intravenous contrast medium administration. Liver parenchyma subverted by several nodules ("macronodular appearance") and septa. The reticulations surround regenerative nodules, which have low signal intensity on T2-weighted image (**a**) and high signal intensity on unenhanced T1-weighted image (**b**). The fibrotic septa are hyperintense on T2-weighted image (**a**) and hypointense on (**b**) unenhanced T1-weighted image, showing progressive post-contrastographic impregnation, more pronounced in the late phases (**e**, **f** arrows)

7.1.3 Diffusion-Weighted MRI

Diffusion-weighted MRI (DWI) is a technique that measures diffusion of water molecules "in vivo," calculating the apparent diffusion coefficient (ADC) (Le Bihan 1990). In the presence of fibrosis, the diffusion of water molecules is restricted, and several studies have shown a correlation between decrease in hepatic ADC and hepatic fibrosis (Mehmet et al. 2013; Cece et al. 2013). However, correlation with the stage of fibrosis is only partially reliable in DWI due to overlap of values between different stages of fibrosis; advanced fibrosis presents decreased values of ADC, while early fibrosis remains hard to identify (Taouli et al. 2007). Moreover, despite technical improvements, DWI remains sensitive to susceptibility and motion-related artifacts, as well as many confounding factors such as perfusion effects, hepatic steatosis, hepatic iron, and liver inflammation (Bülow et al. 2013).

7.1.4 MR Elastography

MR elastography (MRE) provides a noninvasive qualitative and quantitative imaging of liver stiffness by analyzing the propagation of mechanical waves through tissue, with specific MRI sequences (De Robertis et al. 2014). The application of this technique for assessing liver fibrosis is based on the biologic concept that

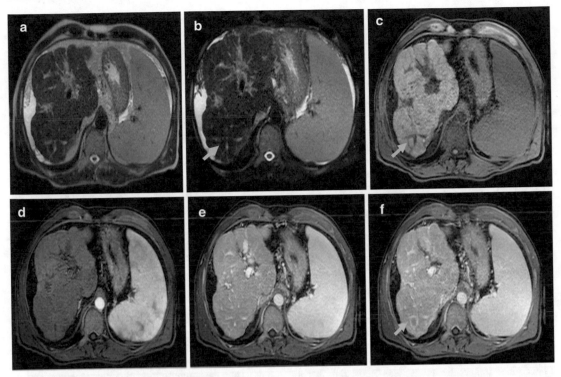

Fig. 5 Patient 49 years old with HBV infection. (**a**) Axial T2-weighted image and axial T2-weighted image with fat suppression. (**c**) Unenhanced axial T1-weighted image. (**d–f**) Axial T1-weighted images after intravenous contrast medium administration. Liver with atrophy of the right lobe, enlargement of the caudate lobe, and irregular contours; splenomegaly and ascites are also visible. In the posterior sectors of the right lobe thin reticulations are appreciated surrounding regenerative nodule (arrow) typically hypointense on T2-weighted image (**a, b**) and hyperintense on unenhanced T1-weighted image (**c**). After intravenous contrast medium administration we do not recognize altered nodule enhancement (regenerative nodule) and progressive impregnation of the fibrotic septa is visualized (**f**, arrow)

stiffness of hepatic parenchyma increases as fibrosis advances, due to progressive deposition of interconnecting collagen fibers. The results are elaborated to generate quantitative maps ("elastograms"). Several studies proved that the differences in stiffness between patients with early stages of fibrosis are small and there is overlap between different groups, but the differences between groups with higher stages are consistent (Venkatesh et al. 2013; Yin et al. 2007). Thus, MRE can be a useful noninvasive tool for evaluating advanced fibrosis. Besides MRE is more accurate than any noninvasive technique, is suitable for patients with obesity or ascites, and can be included in standard protocols, providing a comprehensive evaluation of the liver (Rustogi et al. 2012).

7.2 Elastosonography

Virtual touch tissue quantification is a point shear-wave elastographic technique able to evaluate liver stiffness to diagnose cirrhosis. Ultrasonography and virtual touch tissue quantification for liver stiffness assessment can be used in a single step. It is difficult to determine the definitive impact of ARFI in the early diagnosis

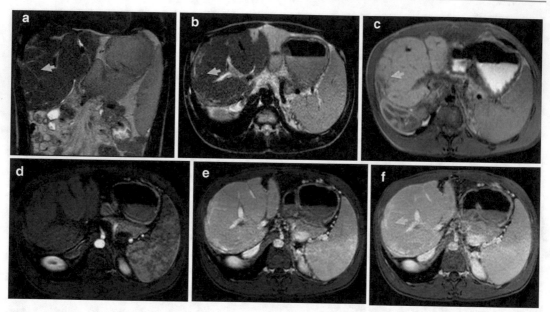

Fig. 6 Patient 51 years old, with biliary atresia. (**a, b**) T2-weighted images: liver with lobulated contours and hyperintense septa (arrow) with retraction of the right hepatic lobe capsule. Absence of the bile vessels. (**c**) Axial T1-weighted image: the reticulations on the right hepatic lobe are hypointense. (**d–f**) Axial T1-weighted images after intravenous contrast medium administration: in the arterial phase (**a**) there is no significant enhancement of the septa. Progressive post-contrastographic impregnation of the reticulations, more evident in the late phase, at 5 min from the administration of contrast medium (**f**)

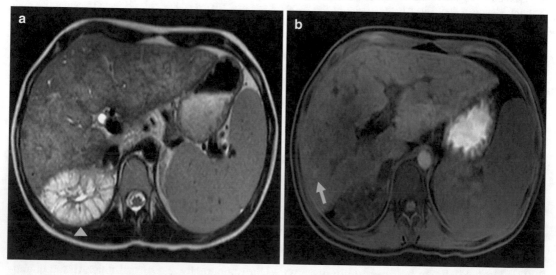

Fig. 7 Patient 17 years old with congenital hepatic fibrosis associated with polycystic kidney disease (PKD). (**a**) Axial T2-weighted image: liver with sinuous contours and enlargement of the lateral segments of the left lobe. Diffuse and heterogeneous hyperintensity of the hepatic parenchyma, with "lacelike" fibrosis. Right kidney is subverted by the presence of multiple cystic formations (arrowhead). (**b**) Axial T1-weighted image: inhomogeneous hypointensity of fibrosis areas on unenhanced sequences. Note the presence of a small hyperintense nodule in the VII segment, compatible with regenerative nodule (arrow)

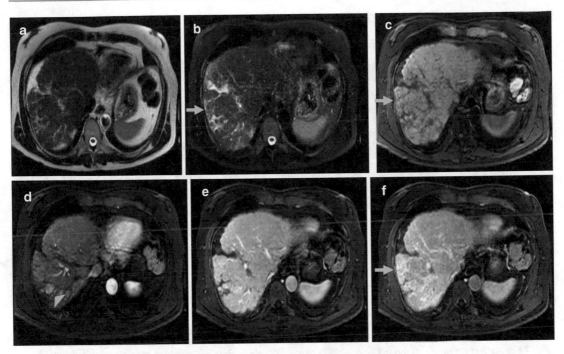

Fig. 8 Patient 66 years old with alcoholic and dysmetabolic cirrhosis. (**a**) Axial T2-weighted image and axial T2-weighted image with fat suppression. (**c**) Unenhanced axial T1-weighted image. (**d–f**) Axial T1-weighted images after intravenous contrast medium administration. Multiple fibrotic septa of the right hepatic lobe, hyperintense on T2-weighted image (**a**, **b** arrow) and hypointense on unenhanced T1-weighted image (**c** arrow), with progressive post-contrastographic enhancement on T1-weighted images after intravenous contrast medium administration (**d–f**, arrow). Hypervascular nodule with washout in the venous and late phases, suspected for HCC (d, e, f, arrowhead)

of hepatic fibrosis (Fierbinteanu-Braticevici et al. 2009). According to Fierbinteanu-Braticevici, there is a value overlap between F0-F1 and F2 fibrosis stages. The increased velocity is more important between stages F2 and F3 than between F1 and F2 owing to the fact that the increase in fibrous tissue is basically more important between stages F2 and F3 than between F1 and F2. Moreover there is a range of variability of normal and pathological values in the literature. So what is absolutely important is to give the correct task to this ultrasonographic technique that needs to be based on the true possibility of this system to detect changes in liver stiffness related to the development of different amounts of fibrosis in liver diseases. Absolutely the overestimation of pathology diagnosing inconsistent diseases should be avoided: the normal cutoff values must

not be too strict and have to be adapted in relation to clinical and technical setting related to the examination and obtained measurements (D'Onofrio et al. 2013).

Several studies about ARFI application in diffuse liver pathology have been made, and most of them state that ARFI itself can be used in the study of the liver with similar accuracy than transient elastography in diagnosing significant fibrosis or cirrhosis. The optimal cutoff value in predicting cirrhosis (stage F4) was 1.94 m/s with a sensitivity of 100% and a specificity of 98.1%. ARFI has some advantages in respect to TE: does not require separate equipment, an examination not necessary in addition to conventional US, saves time and costs, and quantification measurements can be successfully carried out in every patient by selecting the areas on B-mode ultrasound images.

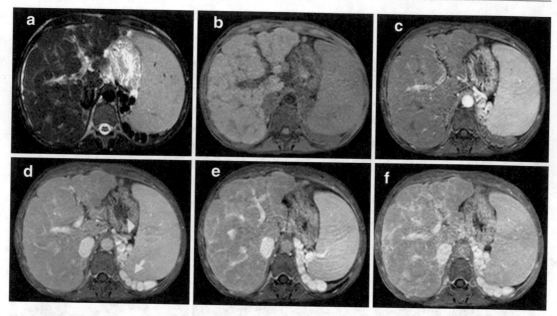

Fig. 9 Patient 24 years old with cystic fibrosis. (**a**) Axial T2-weighted image with fat suppression. (**b**) Unenhanced axial T1-weighted image. (**c–f**) Axial T1-weighted images after intravenous contrast medium administration. Liver enlarged in size, with sinuous margins and multiple fibrous shoots with retraction of the hepatic capsule. The fibrous septa are hyperintense on T2-weighted image and hypointense on unenhanced T1-weighted image, with a more marked post-contrast enhancement in the late phases (**f**, late phase at 5 min). Note splenic posterior venous varices (arrow) and splenomegaly (arrowhead)

References

Afdhal NH, Nunes D (2004) Evaluation of liver fibrosis: a concise review. Am J Gastroenterol 99(6):1160–1174

Agnello F, Dioguardi Burgio M, Picone D et al (2016) Magnetic resonance imaging of the cirrhotic liver in the era of gadoxetic acid. World J Gastroenterol 22(1):103–111

Annet L, Materne R, Danse E et al (2003) Hepatic flow parameters measured with MR imaging and Doppler US: correlations with degree of cirrhosis and portal hypertension. Radiology 229:409–441

Awaya H, Mitchell DG, Kamishima T et al (2002) Cirrhosis: modified caudate-right lobe ratio. Radiology 224(3):769–774

Banerjee R, Pavlides M, Tunnicliffe EM et al (2014) Multiparametric magnetic resonance for the noninvasive diagnosis of liver disease. J Hepatol 60:69–77

Bedossa P, Dargère D, Paradis V (2003) Sampling variability of liver fibrosis in chronic hepatitis C. Hepatology 38:1449–1457

Brancatelli G, Federle MP, Ambrosini R et al (2007) Cirrhosis: CT and MR imaging evaluation. Eur J Radiol 61:57–69

Bülow R, Mensel B, Meffert P et al (2013) Diffusion-weighted magnetic resonance imaging for staging liver fibrosis is less reliable in the presence of fat and iron. Eur Radiol 23:1281–1128

Cece H, Ercan A, Yıldız S et al (2013) The use of DWI to assess spleen and liver quantitative ADC changes in the detection of liver fibrosis stages in chronic viral hepatitis. Eur J Radiol 82:e307–e312

Colloredo G, Guido M, Sonzogni A, Leandro G (2003) Impact of liver biopsy size on histological evaluation of chronic viral hepatitis: the smaller the sample, the milder the disease. J Hepatol 39(2):239–244

D'Onofrio M, Gallotti A, Pozzi Mucelli R (2010) Tissue quantification with acoustic radiation force impulse imaging: measurement repeatability and normal values in the healthy liver. Am J Roentgenol 195:132–136

D'Onofrio M, Crosara S, De Robertis R et al (2013) Acoustic radiation force impulse of the liver. World J Gastroenterol 19(30):4841–4849

De Robertis R, D'Onofrio M, Demozzi E et al (2014) Noninvasive diagnosis of cirrhosis: a review of different imaging modalities. World J Gastroenterol 20(23):7231–7241

Desmet VJ, Gerber M, Hoofnagle JH et al (1999) Classification of chronic hepatitis: diagnosis, grading and staging. Hepatology 19(6):1513–1520

Dodd GD 3rd, Baron RL, Oliver JH 3rd, Federle MP (1999) Spectrum of imaging findings of the liver in end-stage cirrhosis: part I gross morphology and diffuse abnormalities. AJR 173(4):1031–1036

Faria SC, Ganesan K, Mwangi I et al (2009) MR imaging of liver fibrosis: current state of the art. Radiographics 29:1615–1635

Fierbinteanu-Braticevici C, Andronescu D, Usvat R et al (2009) Acoustic radiation force imaging sonoelastography for noninvasive staging of liver fibrosis. World J Gastroenterol 15:5525–5532

Friedman SL, Bansal MB (2006) Reversal of hepatic fibrosis - fact or fantasy? Hepatology 43:S82–S88

Harbin WP, Robert NJ, Ferrucci JT Jr (1980) Diagnosis of cirrhosis based on regional changes in hepatic morphology: a radiological and pathological analysis. Radiology 135(2):273–283

Hshiao MH, Chen PC, Jao JC et al (2012) Quantifying liver cirrhosis by extracting significant features from MRI T2 image. Scientific World Journal 2012:343847

Imbert-Bismut F, Ratziu V, Pieroni L et al (2001) Biochemical markers of liver fibrosis in patients with hepatitis C virus infection: a prospective study. Lancet 357(9262):1069–1075

Ishak K, Baptista A, Bianchi L et al (1995) Histological grading and staging of chronic hepatitis. J Hepatol 22(6):696–699

Ito K, Mitchell DG, Gabata T, Hussain SM (1999) Expanded gallbladder fossa: simple MR imaging sign of cirrhosis. Radiology 211:723–726

Ito K, Mitchell DG (2004) Imaging diagnosis of cirrhosis and chronic hepatitis. Intervirology 47(3–5):134–143

Le Bihan D (1990) Diffusion/perfusion MR imaging of the brain: from structure to function. Radiology 177:328–329

Marcellin P, Asselah T, Boyer N (2002) Fibrosis and disease progression in hepatitis C. Hepatology 36:S47–S56

Martin DR (2002) Magnetic resonance imaging of diffuse liver diseases. Top Magn Reson Imaging 13(3):151–163

Mehmet RO, Ahmet KP, Pinar GB et al (2013) Diffusion weighted MRI in chronic viral hepatitis: correlation between ADC values and histopathological scores. Insights Imaging 4:339–345

Parkin MD, Bray F, Ferlay J et al (2002) Global cancer statistics. CA Cancer J Clin 55:74–108

Rustogi R, Horowitz J, Harmath C et al (2012) Accuracy of MR elastography and anatomic MR imaging features in the diagnosis of severe hepatic fibrosis and cirrhosis. J Magn Reson Imaging 35(6):1356–1364

Schuppan D, Afdhal NH (2008) Liver cirrhosis. Lancet 371:838–851

Shaheen NJ, Hansen RA, Morgan DR et al (2006) The burden of gastrointestinal and liver diseases. Am J Gastroenterol 101:2128–2138

Standish RA, Cholongitas E, Dhillon A et al (2006) An appraisal of the histopathological assessment of liver fibrosis. Gut 55:569–578

Venkatesh SK, Yin M, Ehman RL (2013) Magnetic resonance elastography of liver: technique, analysis and clinical applications. J Magn Reson Imaging 37(3):544–555

Talwalkar JA (2006) Shall we bury the sword? Imaging of hepatic fibrosis. Gastroenterology 131:1669–1167

Talwalkar JA, Yin M, Fidler JL et al (2008) Magnetic resonance imaging of hepatic fibrosis: emerging clinical applications. Hepatology 47:332–342

Tamada T, Ito K, Higaki A et al (2011a) Gd-EOB-DTPA-enhanced MR imaging: evaluation of hepatic enhancement effects in normal and cirrhotic livers. Eur J Radiol 80:e311–e316

Tamada T, Ito K, Sone T et al (2011b) Gd-EOBDTPA enhanced MR imaging: evaluation of biliary and renal excretion in normal and cirrhotic livers. Eur J Radiol 80:207–211

Taouli B, Tolia AJ, Losada M et al (2007) Diffusion-weighted MRI for quantification of liver fibrosis: preliminary experience. AJR 189(4):799–806

Terjung B, Lemnitzer I, Dumoulin FL et al (2003) Bleeding complications after percutaneous liver biopsy. An analysis of risk factors. Digestion 67:138–145

Thiese ND, Bodenheimer HC, Ferrell LD (2006) Acute and chronic viral hepatitis. In: Burt AD, Portmann BC, Ferrell LD (eds) MacSween's pathology of the liver. Chapter 8, 5th edn. Churchill Livingstone, Edinburgh, Scotland

Wallace K, Burt AD, Wright MC (2008) Liver fibrosis. Biochem Genet 411(1):1–18

Wong VW, Vergniol J, Wong GL et al (2010) Diagnosis of fibrosis and cirrhosis using liver stiffness measurement in nonalcoholic fatty liver disease. Hepatology 51:454–462

Yin M, Talwalkar JA, Glaser KJ et al (2007) A preliminary assessment of hepatic fibrosis with magnetic resonance elastography. Clin Gastroenterol Hepatol 5(10):1207–1213

Yulri P, Seong Hyun K, Seung Hoon K et al (2010) Gadoxetic acid (Gd-EOB-DTPA)-enhanced MRI versus gadobenate dimeglumine (Gd-BOPTA)-enhanced MRI for preoperatively detecting hepatocellular carcinoma: an initial experience. Korean J Radiol 11(4):433–440

Vascular Liver Diseases

Manuela França and Joana Pinto

Contents

M. França (✉)
Radiology Department, Centro Hospitalar e
Universitário do Porto, Oporto, Portugal

Instituto de Ciências Biomédicas de Abel Salazar,
Universidade do Porto, Oporto, Portugal

i3S, Instituto de Investigação e Inovação em Saúde,
Universidade do Porto, Oporto, Portugal
e-mail: manuelafranca.radiologia@chporto.
min-saude.pt

J. Pinto
Radiology Department, Centro Hospitalar e
Universitário do Porto, Oporto, Portugal

Abstract

Hepatic vascular diseases may affect the vascular inflow, vascular outflow or flow at the sinusoidal level, most of them resulting in decreased portal venous perfusion and increased arterialization of the liver parenchyma. The underlying physiopathological mechanisms lead to key imaging findings that should be promptly recognized by radiologists, in order to provide an accurate diagnosis. Hepatic vascular impairment can be due to primary vascular disease or secondary to hepatocellular liver diseases, as

© Springer Nature Switzerland AG 2021
E. Quaia (ed.), *Imaging of the Liver and Intra-hepatic Biliary Tract*,
Medical Radiology, Diagnostic Imaging, https://doi.org/10.1007/978-3-030-38983-3_16

occurs in liver cirrhosis. This chapter will focus mainly on primary hepatic vascular diseases, describing the main imaging findings and differentials of each condition.

1   Introduction

The liver is the only organ in the body that has a dual blood supply, receiving blood from the portal vein (PV) (70–80%) and a minor part from the hepatic artery (HA) (20–30%). Blood from these vessels ("vascular inflow") conveys at the sinusoids but it also communicates at the peribiliary venous plexus that is composed of small branches of the PV and HA. These communications between both systems allow reciprocal supporting mechanisms of blood supply, explaining the compensatory response of increasing the arterial blood supply when there is a decrease in the PV blood supply, as occurs in the setting of PV obstruction. In addition, there is a "third vascular inflow" to the liver, referring to splanchnic venous flow that is not drained by the PV, but instead enters the liver and flows into the sinusoids, independently from the PV. These small veins may originate from a digestive organ (e.g., cholecystic vein and parabiliary venous system) or from systemic veins (epigastric-paraumbilical venous system) (Kobayashi et al. 2010). Finally,

blood from sinusoids is then drained to the hepatic veins and inferior vena cava, and then to the heart ("vascular outflow").

These unique characteristics of blood supply can be observed on contrast-enhanced imaging studies. As explained in Chapters "Embryology and Development of the Liver" and "Liver Anatomy", a spectrum of vascular variants can involve the liver and these should be promptly recognized by radiologists, as they may result in areas of enhancement or pseudolesions on contrast-enhanced imaging studies that can mimic hepatocellular lesions or vascular diseases.

Regional changes in the balance between hepatic arterial, portal venous, and third inflow are frequently seen on contrast-enhanced CT or MRI examinations, as transient hepatic attenuation differences (THAD) or transient hepatic intensity differences (THID). These perfusion changes are recognized as segmental wedge-shaped areas of enhancement during the hepatic arterial phase and become isoattenuating or isointense in the portal venous or equilibrium phases (Fig. 1). They are not visualized in the pre-contrast phase, which also helps to differentiate them from true vascular lesions. Usually, THAD/THID result from small arterioportal shunts secondary to an increase in hepatic arterial inflow, in response to decreased portal venous flow. Moreover, they may also result from extrinsic compression (Fig. 2) or surgical liga-

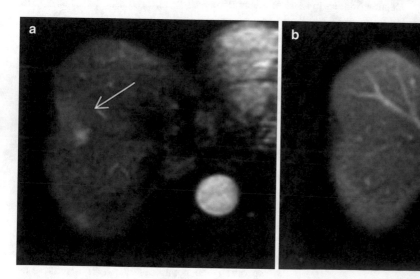

Fig. 1 Transient hepatic intensity difference (THID). Axial post-contrast T1-weighted images in the hepatic arterial (**a**) and portal venous phase (**b**) show an ill-defined subcapsular area of hyperenhancement in the arterial phase (arrow) that becomes isointense in the venous phase, recognized as a functional THID of the liver parenchyma

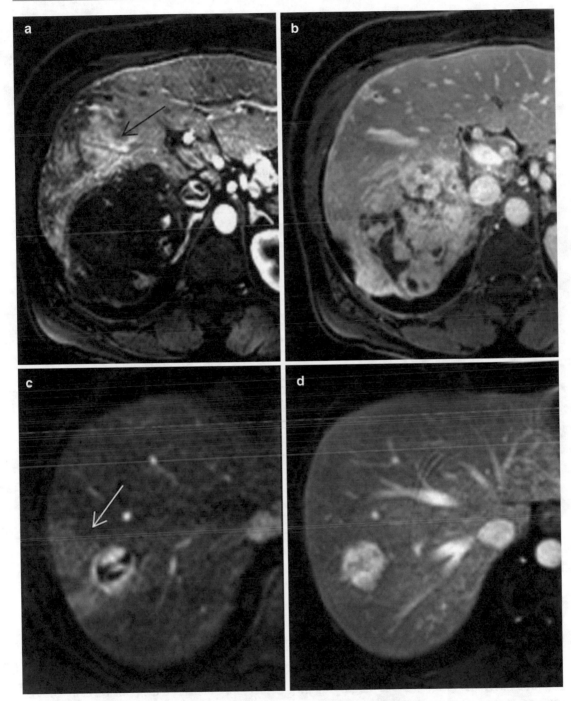

Fig. 2 THID associated to focal liver lesions. Axial post-contrast T1-weighted MR images in the arterial (**a**) and portal venous phase (**b**) demonstrate a wedge-shaped area of hyperenhancement in the arterial phase (black arrow) which becomes isointense in the portal venous phase. An adjacent large hemangioma is seen, occupying almost all of the VI and VII hepatic segments. Contrast-enhanced T1-weighted MR images of another patient, in the hepatic arterial (**c**) and portal venous phases (**d**), show wedge-shaped area of hyperenhancement in the hepatic arterial phase (white arrow) that becomes isointense on the portal venous phase, representing a THID adjacent to a hepatic hemangioma

tion, as well as from conditions related to increased arterial flow, such as shunts or liver parenchyma hyperemia associated with inflammation of the biliary ducts or gallbladder (Desser 2009).

Although rare, vascular disorders of the liver represent an important health problem worldwide because most of them can lead to noncirrhotic portal hypertension, therefore being associated with high morbidity and mortality (Garcia-Pagán et al. 2016). Most vascular diseases result from the obstruction at the vascular inflow, sinusoids, or vascular outflow. Hepatic vascular impairment can be due to primary vascular disease or secondary to hepatocellular liver diseases, as occurs, for example, in liver cirrhosis with the development of microvascular changes and consequent portal hypertension. This chapter focuses mainly on primary hepatic vascular diseases, describing the main imaging findings and differentials of each condition.

2 Vascular Inflow Diseases

2.1 Hepatic Artery Obstruction

The obstruction of the HA is the most common liver complication after liver transplantation (Pareja et al. 2010), occurring most frequently within the first 4 months after transplantation, and often requires retransplantation (Ishigami et al. 2004). The initial diagnosis is usually made with ultrasound (US), demonstrating the absence of color and spectral Doppler flow in the HA due to thrombus. An intraluminal filling defect is evident at post-contrast CT or MR imaging, accompanied by a peripheral wedge-shaped hypointensity area in liver parenchyma, extending to the capsular surface (Fig. 3). At angiographic images, it appears as an arterial cutoff. Infarct of the liver parenchyma is rare because the hepatic blood supply can be maintained by the PV inflow. Nevertheless, as the main blood supply of the biliary ducts is dependent on the HA, bile lakes may be seen as a late complication of large infarcts due to ischemic necrosis of bile duct epithelium.

2.2 Aneurysm/Pseudoaneurysm of the Hepatic Artery

True aneurysms of the HA are rare and represent the second most common visceral aneurysm after splenic artery aneurysms (Lu et al. 2015). Most patients are asymptomatic and HA aneurysms are usually an incidental finding at imaging studies. Extrahepatic aneurysms are three times more frequent than intrahepatic and are usually solitary, being associated with conditions as atherosclerosis, arterial fibrodysplasia vasculitis, polyarteritis nodosa, or systemic lupus (Dolapci et al. 2003). A clear association between size and rupture was not established. On the other hand, HA aneurysms developed in patients without atherosclerotic disease are known to have an increased risk for rupture (Abbas et al. 2003). Endovascular treatment is indicated for symptomatic aneurysms larger than 2 cm because of an elevated risk of rupture and high mortality rate (Erben et al. 2015; Elsayes et al. 2017).

Pseudoaneurysms may also be classified as intrahepatic or extrahepatic, with the latter being the commonest type. Extrahepatic pseudoaneurysms typically result from local infection or inflammation and frequently involve the right hepatic artery. Unlike true HA aneurysms, patients usually present with symptoms as acute abdominal pain, gastrointestinal bleeding, jaundice, or fever. Intrahepatic pseudoaneurysms may result from blunt trauma or iatrogenic injury, complicating percutaneous interventional procedures, such as biopsy or biliary stent placement (Lu et al. 2015). On color and spectral Doppler US, a characteristic bidirectional flow with a "yin-yang" pattern is usually seen. Contrast-enhanced CT and MRI confirm the diagnosis, revealing the focal dilatation of the HA, frequently accompanied by calcification or adjacent hematoma on non-contrast-enhanced CT (Dolapci et al. 2003).

2.3 Hereditary Hemorrhagic Telangiectasia (HHT)

Hereditary hemorrhagic telangiectasia (HHT) or Osler-Weber-Rendu disease is an autosomal dominant vascular disorder characterized by telangi-

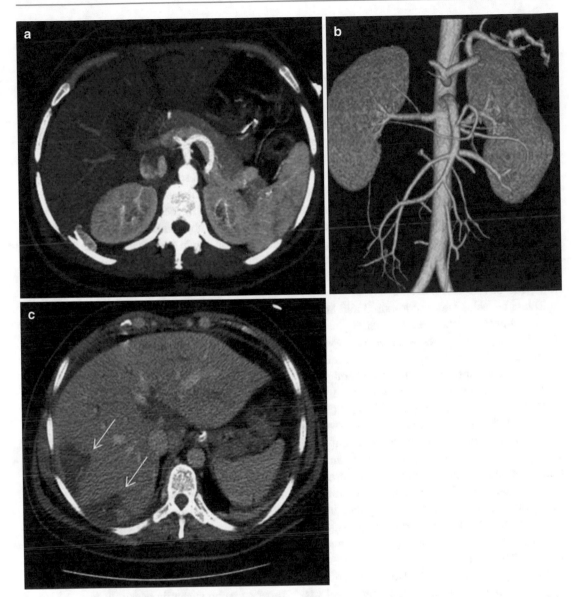

Fig. 3 Hepatic artery obstruction after liver transplantation. Axial maximum intensity projection in the arterial phase (**a**) and volume-rendered reconstruction CT (**b**) demonstrate an abrupt occlusion of the common hepatic artery secondary to a thrombus. Axial contrast- enhancement in portal venous phase (**c**) shows two peripheral wedge-shaped hypointensity areas in segment VII, extending to the capsular surface due to hypoperfusion (arrows)

ectasias and arteriovenous malformations (AVMs) with a multisystemic involvement, including mucocutaneous tissue and visceral organs such as the liver and lungs. Telangiectasia is the elementary lesion of HHT resulting from the dilatation of a postcapillary venule that joins directly with an arteriole, bypassing the capillary system (Buscarini et al. 2018). The diagnosis is based on the presence of mucocutaneous telangiectasias, spontaneous and recurrent episodes of epistaxis, and evidence of visceral involvement, along with a family history of this disease. The prevalence of HHT is estimated at 1/5000, with the liver affected in up to 74% of the patients (Siddiki et al. 2008). Hepatic involvement is usually diffuse, and small telangiectasias to large AVM may develop, with diverse stages of severity, depending on the number, type, and location of telangiectasias or AVMs

(Mahmoud et al. 2010). There are three different types of intrahepatic shunting, which often occur concomitantly: HA to PV, HA to hepatic vein, and/or PV to hepatic vein. Arterio-portal shunts are seen in 65% of the cases (Elsayes et al. 2017). Hepatic involvement can be asymptomatic or, because of shunting, can present as high-output cardiac failure, hepatic encephalopathy, portal hypertension, and biliary or mesenteric ischemia (Garcia-Tsao et al. 2000).

Doppler US evaluation demonstrates dilated common HA, intrahepatic arterial hypervascularization, and flow abnormalities of hepatic vessels. In fact, Doppler US criteria have been suggested to grade the disease severity, based on a combination of hepatic vessel abnormalities and abnormal flow patterns (Buscarini et al. 2004).

Telangiectasias and arterio-portal and arterio-venous shunts are observed on arterial phase CT or MR images (Fig. 4) whereas porto-venous shunts are seen on portal venous phase images. Telangiectasias appear as small peripheral perfusion abnormalities, sometimes better recognized on maximum intensity projection images (Torabi et al. 2008). Arterio-portal and arteriovenous shunts are observed as multiple prominent intra- and extrahepatic arterial branches, with an early filling of portal or hepatic venous branches (Ianora et al. 2004; Wu et al. 2006). Therefore, the liver enhancement on the arterial phase images can be quite heterogeneous, due to AVMs, telangiectasias, perfusion abnormalities, and multiple THAD/THID (Fig. 4a–c). Dilation of HA, PV, and/or hepatic veins can also be often seen. Moreover, imaging studies frequently reveal vascular malformations in other organs, such as the pancreas or lungs, or cardiomegaly and prominent central pulmonary arteries (Fig. 4d) (Buscarini et al. 2004; Siddiki et al. 2008).

Perfusion abnormalities may increase the hepatocellular regenerative activity, with the development of focal nodular hyperplasia (FNH) or nodular regenerative hyperplasia (Buscarini et al. 2018). In fact, the prevalence of FNH is 100× greater in HHT than in general population (Buscarini et al. 2004), and a confident diagnosis can usually be established with the classic imaging features of FNH on contrast-enhanced CT or MR imaging, without the need of liver biopsy (Garcia-Pagán et al. 2016; Vilgrain et al. 2018).

On the other hand, hepatocellular carcinoma is rather exceptional in HHT (Lee et al. 2011a).

2.4 Portal Vein Aneurysm

Aneurysms of the PV represent 3% of all aneurysms of the venous system (López-Machado et al. 1998), with the extrahepatic PV being the commonest involved segment (Elsayes et al. 2017). In the majority of the cases, PV aneurysms are asymptomatic and an incidental imaging finding. When symptomatic, abdominal pain is the commonest presentation. Some complications like thrombosis, rupture, and compression of the biliary tree or duodenum have been reported (Sfyroeras et al. 2009). Contrast-enhanced CT or MR may confirm the diagnosis, but color Doppler US is usually the most helpful imaging technique for diagnosing PV aneurysms, as a fusiform or saccular dilation of the PV greater than 2 cm in diameter, and further workup may not be necessary (Atasoy et al. 1998; Gallego et al. 2002; Elsayes et al. 2017) (Fig. 5).

2.5 Portal Vein Obstruction

Portal vein thrombosis (PVT) has a high incidence in general population (Tardáguila Montero 2016) and it can occur in up to 30% of adult patients with portal hypertension (Ögren et al. 2006). Thrombosis can be caused by multiple conditions, either local or systemic (Table 1), with the myeloproliferative syndrome being the most common systemic cause. In fact, the onset of a PVT in a young, apparently healthy patient may be the first manifestation of a myeloproliferative syndrome (Denninger et al. 2000). Clinical manifestations may be variable and depend on the degree of obstruction and on the duration of thrombosis (acute versus chronic PVT). Imaging diagnosis is based on the recognition of the thrombus, as well on the associated perfusion abnormalities in the liver parenchyma.

2.5.1 Acute PVT

In acute PVT, abdominal pain is the major symptom, being present in 90% of the patients (Garcia-Pagán et al. 2016). Involvement of the superior mesenteric vein was reported in 5% of

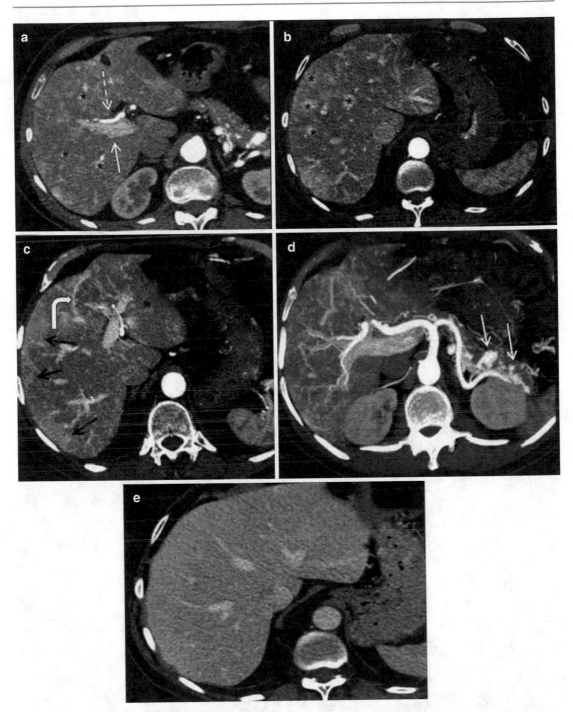

Fig. 4 Liver involvement in hereditary hemorrhagic telangiectasia (HHT). Contrast-enhanced CT images in the hepatic arterial phase (**a**, **b**) and the maximum intensity projection images (**c**, **d**) demonstrate a prominent HA (dashed arrow) and early enhancement of the PV branches (white arrow) due to multiple arteriovenous malformations between the HA and the PV. THAD is also seen, as wedge-shaped areas of hyperenhancement at the periphery of the liver (black arrows). Multiple telangiectasias can be recognized as small peripheral hypervascular areas (asterisk). Vascular shunts are better recognized on maximum intensity projection images (curved arrow). Moreover, multiple vascular malformations are also depicted in the pancreas (white arrows in **d**). The portal venous phase image (**e**) shows homogenization of the liver parenchyma, with telangiectasias becoming isodense with the surrounding hepatic tissue

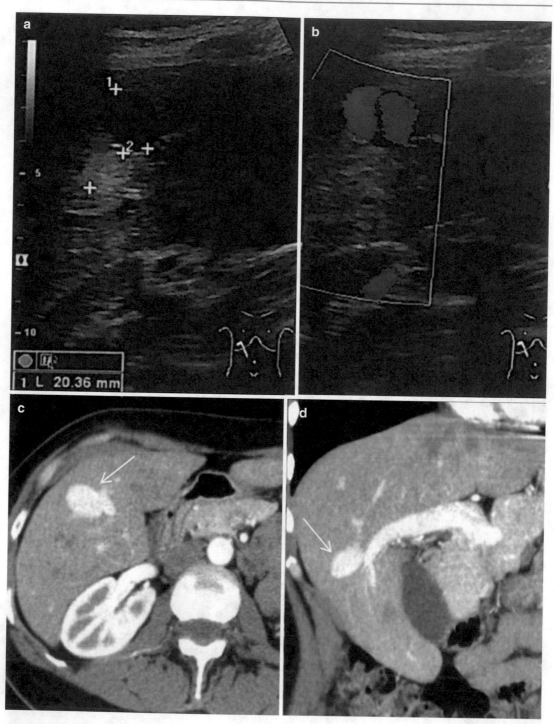

Fig. 5 Portal vein aneurysm. B mode US (**a**) and color Doppler US (**b**) images show an aneurysm of the right branch of the PV, an incidental finding. On Doppler US, the multidirectional flow ("yin-yang sign") is characteristic. Axial (**c**) and coronal (**d**) contrast-enhanced CT images in portal venous phase confirm the presence of a saccular aneurysm (arrows) of the right portal vein branch (US images are a courtesy of Jorge Pinto, MD, Oporto, Portugal)

Table 1 Systemic and local factors associated to portal vein thrombosis

Local factors	Systemic factors
Mass:	**Hereditary factors:**
– Any abdominal tumour	– Factor V Leiden mutation
Abdominal infection:	– Factor II mutation
– Diverticulitis	– Protein C deficiency
– Appendicitis	– Protein S deficiency
– Pancreatitis	– Antithrombin deficiency
– Duodenal ulcer	
– Cholecystitis	
– Inflammatory Bowel Disease	
– Hepatitis	
– Neonatal Omphalitis	
– …	
Portal venous system injury:	**Aquired factors:**
– Splenectomy	– Myeloproliferative syndrome
– Colectomy	– Antiphospholipid syndrome
– Gastrectomy	– Paroxysmal nocturnal hemoglobinuria
– Cholecystectomy	– Oral contraceptive
– Liver Transplant	– Pregnancy
– Abdominal Trauma	– Hyperhomocysteinemia
– TIPS	– Cancer
– …	
Cirrhosis	

the cases and may lead to bowel infarction (Plessier et al. 2007).

Doppler US is the first-line imaging modality and it detects the hyperechoic thrombus and the absence of flow within the PV. Contrast-enhanced CT is usually performed to confirm the diagnosis and to evaluate the extension of thrombosis (Garcia-Pagán et al. 2016). On portal venous phase images, the PVT is recognized by the lack of enhancement of the PV lumen (Fig. 6). Furthermore, CT images are important for assessing the extension of thrombosis to the mesenteric veins and arches and the presence of a local factor, such as cirrhosis, inflammation, or tumor, and also to look for signs of bowel ischemia. Bowel dilation, bowel wall thickening, abnormal or absent wall enhancement, pneumatosis, ascites, and portal venous gas are worrisome features of bowel ischemia (Fig. 7), and surgical exploration must be considered in these cases.

When PVT is due to infection ("pylephlebitis"), clinical manifestations are often unspecific. Therefore, imaging is extremely important to report PV thrombophlebitis and to depict the primary cause of infection (Lee et al. 2011b), as any intra-abdominal infection process, such as

appendicitis, diverticulitis, or pancreatitis, can complicate with pylephlebitis. A low-attenuation thrombus within the portal venous system along with portal edema and hepatic abscesses is one of the early hepatic findings at post-contrast CT.

The mainstay of treatment for acute PVT is anticoagulation therapy, and recanalization of the portal vein is expected to occur in up to 6 months. Therefore, a CT scan should be performed at 6–12 months to confirm PV recanalization (Garcia-Pagán et al. 2016).

2.5.2 Chronic PVT

In the absence of recanalization, the obliteration of the PV lumen leads to the development of porto-portal collaterals, connecting the patent portion of the vein upstream from the thrombus to the patent portion downstream. Consequently, the obstructed PV is replaced by a network of porto-portal collateral veins ("cavernoma"), this process being called cavernomatous transformation of the PV. In chronic PVT, the patients can be asymptomatic and portal thrombosis an incidental finding, or it can be discovered because of manifestations of portal hypertension such as hypersplenism or gas-

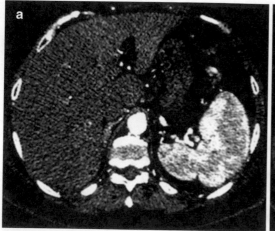
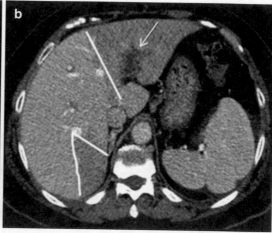

Fig. 6 Acute PV thrombosis in a patient with acute pancreatitis. Contrast-enhanced CT images on the hepatic arterial phase (**a**) and portal venous phase (**b**) show thrombosis of the PV left branch (arrow). Segmental hyperenhancement on the hepatic arterial phase ("segmental staining") is related with the HA buffer response, to compensate the decreased PV flow. On the portal venous phase, there is decreased parenchymal enhancement of the left lobe segments in comparison to the right lobe, due to PV thrombosis. There is also another perfusion abnormality in the right lobe (between lines) related to thrombosis of a small intrahepatic branch of the right PV branch (not shown)

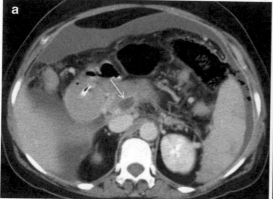
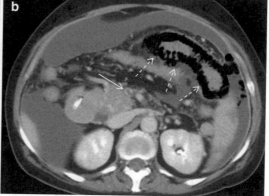

Fig. 7 Acute PV in a patient with myeloproliferative syndrome, complicated by small-bowel ischemia. Contrast-enhanced portal venous phase CT images (**a**, **b**) show acute thrombosis of the PV, extending to the mesenteric vein (white arrow). There are dilation and ischemia (pneumatosis intestinalis) of small-bowel loops (dashed arrows), pneumoperitoneum, and ascites. The patient was promptly operated for resection of the ischemic bowel

trointestinal bleeding. Ascites and encephalopathy are uncommon (DeLeve et al. 2009).

Extrahepatic portal vein obstruction (EHPVO) is considered a primary vascular disorder, characterized by chronic PVT with normal liver function. It is more frequent in the Eastern countries and in children (Khanna and Sarin 2014). These patients present portal cavernoma and signs of portal hypertension (splenomegaly and portosystemic collaterals) in the presence of a normal-looking liver with normal smooth contours.

The diagnosis of chronic PVT is based on Doppler US or contrast-enhanced CT or MR imaging, by recognizing the absence of visible PV lumen and the presence of portal cavernoma, which appears as multiple serpiginous vessels in porta hepatis (Figs. 8 and 9). On unenhanced CT, small or linear calcifications may be seen

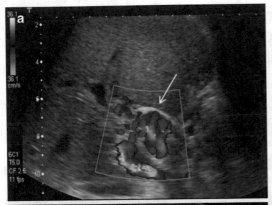

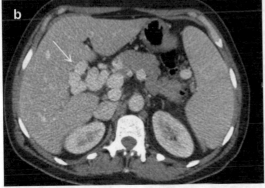

Fig. 8 Portal cavernoma. Color Doppler US (**a**) and axial (**b**) contrast-enhanced CT images in the portal venous phase revealing porto-portal serpiginous collaterals corresponding to cavernous transformation of the PV (cavernoma) (arrow)

(Gallego et al. 2002). On arterial phase, as described for THAD/THID, an increased enhancement may be observed in the parenchyma of the liver segments supplied by the occluded PV, due to the compensatory arterial inflow by the peribiliary plexus (Fig. 9). On the other hand, on portal venous phase, there is decreased parenchymal enhancement in these liver segments due to decreased PV perfusion (Gallego et al. 2002). Sometimes, portal cavernoma appears as a uniform mass-like structure in the porta hepatis, surrounding the bile duct and enhancing at the portal venous phase, and porto-portal collaterals cannot be individualized. This mass-like appearance cavernoma should not be mistaken with cholangiocarcinoma, and the absence of diffusion restriction on ADC map helps to exclude the diagnosis of malignancy (Condat et al. 2003; Kalra et al. 2014) (Fig. 10).

The portal cavernoma can cause compression or deformation of intra- and extrahepatic bile ducts, this being designated as portal cholangiopathy. Most of the patients are asymptomatic, although abnormal liver analysis might be present in >50% of the patients. Symptomatic portal cholangiopathy may develop in 19% of patients after 5 years of an acute PVT (Llop et al. 2011) and, rarely, progressive cholestatic disease or recurrent bacterial cholangitis may occur (Garcia-Pagán et al. 2016; Khuroo et al. 2016). MR cholangiography should be performed in patients with persistent cholestasis or biliary tract abnormalities (Shin et al. 2007; Garcia-Pagán et al. 2016). Suggestive imaging findings of portal cholangiopathy include smooth extrinsic indentations and narrowing of the extra- and/or the intrahepatic biliary tree, or displacement of the common bile duct (Condat et al. 2003; Shin et al. 2007; Walser et al. 2011; Rajesh et al. 2018) (Figs. 9 and 10).

Other clues for chronic PVT on CT or MR images are a mosaic pattern of parenchymal enhancement (increased enhancement of the peripheral parts of the liver at arterial phase followed by homogeneous enhancement at portal venous phase images), a dysmorphic liver with a smooth surface, hypertrophy of caudate lobe, atrophy of right lobe and left lateral segments, a normal or enlarged segment IV ("atrophy-hypertrophy complex") (Figs. 9 and 11), and presence of a dilated hepatic artery (Vilgrain et al. 2006). Therefore, some features resemble those of cirrhosis, such as the hypertrophy of caudate lobe and right lobe atrophy, splenomegaly, varices, and collateral veins. However, on the other hand, left lateral segment atrophy is observed in the majority of patients with portal cavernoma, unlike in patients with cirrhosis, in whom this segment is usually enlarged. Also, patients with portal cavernoma usually have a normal or hypertrophied segment IV and smooth liver surface, while atrophy of segment IV and nodular surface is a characteristic of cirrhosis (Fig. 12). Moreover, biliary dilatation is very rare in patients with cirrhosis (Vilgrain et al. 2006).

Nevertheless, portal cavernoma can be superimposed on liver cirrhosis or obliterative portal

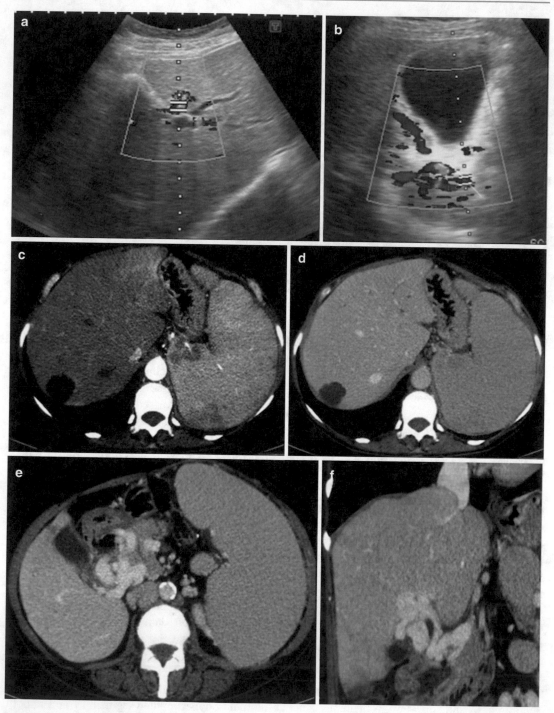

Fig. 9 Portal cavernoma and biliary cholangiopathy, same patients as in Fig. 7. Three years after the acute PV thrombosis, there was no repermeabilization of the PV and the Doppler US (**a, b**) shows multiple serpiginous collaterals in the porta hepatis (cavernoma) and dilated intrahepatic bile ducts. Contrast-enhanced CT images (**c–f**) show THAD in the hepatic arterial phase (**c**) that becomes homogenous at the portal venous phase (**d**). The presence of cavernoma is confirmed (**e, f**) as well as small dilation of the intrahepatic bile ducts (**b**). Also note severe splenomegaly

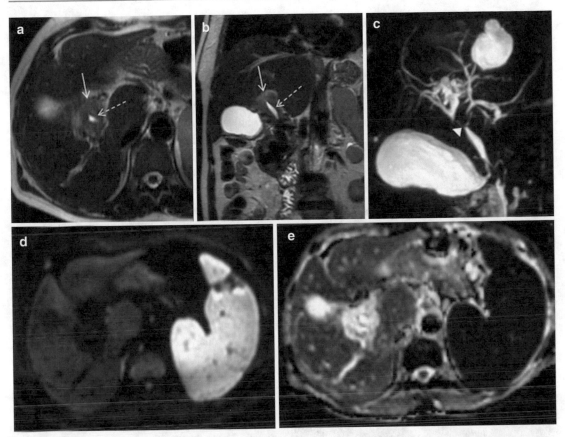

Fig. 10 Portal cavernoma and biliary cholangiopathy, same patients as in Figs. 7 and 9, 5 years after the acute PV thrombosis. Axial (**a**) and coronal (**b**) T2-weighted images show a hyperintense mass-like cavernoma (strain arrow) with encasement of the common biliary duct (dashed arrow). MRCP (**c**) demonstrates a stenosis of the main biliary duct and hepatic duct bifurcation (arrow- head) due to extrinsic compression from cavernoma, with upstream dilatation. The absence of restriction on DWI images (**d**, b1000) and ADC map (**e**) help to distinguish a tumorlike cavernoma from cholangiocarcinoma. The appearance of the cavernoma did not change on 6-year follow-up MR examination (not shown)

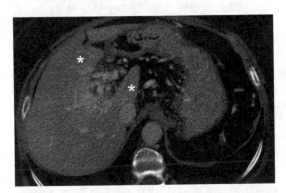

Fig. 11 Portal cavernoma and liver dysmorphic changes. Axial contrast-enhanced CT in portal venous phase demon- strates a cavernoma and related liver morphological changes, as hypertrophy of caudate lobe, atrophy of right lobe and left lateral segments, and enlargement of segment IV

venopathy and, therefore, imaging features of these conditions should be looked for and liver biopsy may be required in patients with abnormal liver tests and/or a dysmorphic liver (Garcia- Pagán et al. 2016).

2.6 Idiopathic Non-cirrhotic Portal Hypertension, or Porto-Sinusoidal Vascular Disease

Idiopathic non-cirrhotic portal hypertension is defined as intrahepatic pre-sinusoidal hyperten- sion in the absence of cirrhosis or other causes of

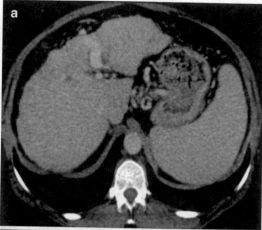

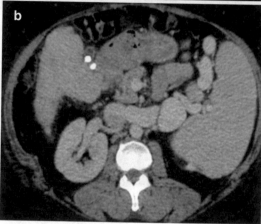

Fig. 12 PV thrombosis and portal hypertension associated with liver cirrhosis. Axial contrast-enhanced CT in portal venous phase (**a**, **b**) exhibits signs of portal hypertension, as splenomegaly and splenic varices. Also, a dysmorphic liver is seen, with hypertrophy of left lateral segments and atrophy of segment IV. The liver surface is nodular and irregular. These signs indicate liver cirrhosis and are different from the characteristic signs of non-cirrhotic portal hypertension

liver disease (Nakanuma et al. 2001). The nomenclature is ambiguous, and it can also be referred as obliterative portal venopathy, idiopathic portal hypertension, incomplete septal cirrhosis, or nodular regenerative hyperplasia. Recently, the term porto-sinusoidal vascular disease (PSVD) was proposed (Gottardi et al. 2019). The etiology remains undetermined in half of the cases, and autoimmune disorders, infections, hypercoagulable factors, and infection with human immunodeficiency virus are some of the implicated causative factors (Rajesh et al. 2018).

Most commonly, patients present with gastrointestinal hemorrhage and splenomegaly, whereas ascites and hepatic encephalopathy are rare. The diagnosis of PSVD should be considered in patients with portal hypertension without any cause for liver disease, and it requires exclusion of hepatic cirrhosis or other causes of non-cirrhotic portal hypertension. Therefore, the diagnosis of PSVD requires liver biopsy and it must fulfill the following five criteria: clinical signs of portal hypertension (e.g., gastroesophageal varices, portocaval collaterals, splenomegaly); exclusion of cirrhosis on liver biopsy; exclusion of chronic liver disease causing cirrhosis or non-cirrhotic portal hypertension; exclusion conditions causing non-cirrhotic portal hypertension (e.g., schistosomiasis, congenital hepatic fibrosis, and sarcoidosis); and patent portal and hepatic veins (Garcia-Pagán et al. 2016). Histologically, PSVD is characterized by phlebosclerosis and obliteration of small intrahepatic PV branches, nodular regeneration, sinusoidal dilatation, and periportal and perisinusoidal fibrosis (Hillaire et al. 2002; Schouten et al. 2012). The liver function is commonly normal at presentation (Garcia-Pagán et al. 2016) and, unlike cirrhotic portal hypertension, it usually remains normal except in very advanced stages. Moreover, hepatic decompensation and development of hepatocellular carcinoma are rare (Rajesh et al. 2018). Overall, the disease course is indolent, and the long-term prognosis is better than cirrhotic portal hypertension (Khanna and Sarin 2014). Due to its rarity, this disease is often misdiagnosed as hepatic cirrhosis on imaging examinations (Hillaire et al. 2002; Schouten et al. 2012).

On US examinations, marked splenomegaly and patent splenoportal axis are recognized, and the liver usually has a normal-looking smooth surface. The portal vein may have mural thickening due to periportal fibrosis (Rajesh et al. 2018). US elastography may help to differentiate PSVD from cirrhosis, as it has been demonstrated that patients with PSVD usually have normal lower liver stiffness and high splenic stiffness, while cirrhotic patients have higher liver stiffness and relatively low splenic stiffness (Seijo et al. 2012; Furuichi et al. 2013).

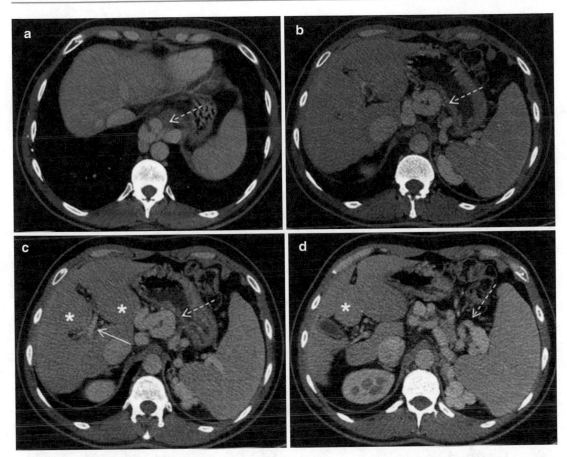

Fig. 13 Porto-sinusoidal vascular disease. Axial contrast-enhanced CT in portal venous phase (**a–d**) demonstrates imaging signs of portal hypertension, such as splenomegaly and varices (dashed arrows). The liver is dysmorphic (*), with hypertrophy of segment IV and caudate lobe and atrophy of the right lobe and left lateral segments. However, the liver surface is smooth and non-nodular. Also, the PV is narrow, although permeable (white arrow). These findings suggest non cirrhotic portal hypertension, which was confirmed by liver biopsy

Contrast-enhanced CT or MR imaging display morphological, vascular, and perfusional abnormalities that raise the possibility of PSVD (Fig. 13). The most common findings are intra- and extrahepatic PV abnormalities, namely the abrupt tapering or pruning of the medium-size PV branches and intraluminal filling defects. Intrahepatic portal abnormalities, as well as extrahepatic PV mural thickening, calcifications, PVT, or portal cavernoma, are more frequent than in cirrhotic patients (Glatard et al. 2012). Perfusional abnormalities can be recognized by the heterogeneous and decreased enhancement of the liver periphery, due to portal hypoperfusion, accompanied by compensatory increased arterialization, manifested by increased arterial perfusion of the periphery and dilation of the hepatic artery (Arora and Sarin 2015; Rajesh et al. 2018). Morphologically, the liver contour is firstly smooth, although, with the progression of the disease, it may become nodular and difficult to distinguish from cirrhosis. Like cirrhosis, usually there is atrophy of the right hepatic lobe and hypertrophy of the caudate lobe. However, like in chronic PVT or EHPVO, patients with PSVD usually have hypertrophy of segment IV while cirrhotic patients usually present atrophy of segment IV (Vilgrain et al. 2006; Glatard et al. 2012; Rajesh et al. 2018). Furthermore, splenomegaly is usually massive and greater in PSVD than in cirrhotic patients (Furuichi et al. 2013) (Fig. 14). Because there is increased arterialization of the liver, focal nodular hyperpla-

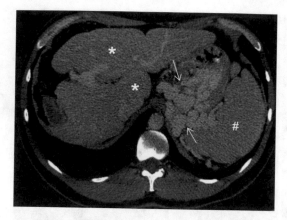

Fig. 14 Porto-sinusoidal vascular disease. Axial contrast-enhanced CT on the portal venous phase shows a dysmorphic liver, with atrophy of right liver lobe and hypertrophy of segment IV and caudate lobe (*), with smooth contours. The PV is patent but there are signs of portal hypertension, such as gastroesophageal varices (arrow) and splenomegaly (#)

sia-like nodules can be recognized on dynamic CT or MR imaging as hypervascular nodules (Glatard et al. 2012; Vilgrain et al. 2018).

3 Vascular Outflow Obstruction

3.1 Cardiac or Pericardial Disease

Liver passive congestion is secondary to the impairment of hepatic venous outflow. Several cardiovascular disorders (as tricuspid regurgitation or stenosis, cardiomyopathy, constrictive pericarditis, cor pulmonale, and left heart failure) with consequent right-sided cardiac failure result in parenchymal congestion and subsequently liver injury. Once severe heart disease induces poor cardiac output, hepatic perfusion may also be compromised. Therefore, a combination of congestive hepatopathy with liver ischemia may occur (Koehne de Gonzalez and Lefkowitch 2017). Symptoms are usually related to cardiac failure and, rarely, patients may present with mild jaundice or right upper quadrant pain. Hepatomegaly and hepatojugular reflux may be detected at physical examination, but splenomegaly is not a common finding (Giallourakis et al. 2002; Myers et al. 2003).

On US evaluation, hepatic vein dilatation is observed, and abnormal echogenicity of the liver parenchyma may be observed due to edema or fibrosis. When using spectral Doppler, the normal hepatic venous waveform ("triphasic" pattern) is lost because of right-sided heart failure (Moreno et al. 1984). On contrast-enhanced CT and MR imaging, an early enhancement of dilated IVC and central hepatic veins, due to the reflux of contrast material from the right atrium into the IVC, is usually seen (Fig. 15) (Gore et al. 1994). Decreased portal venous inflow associated with poor cardiac output leads to a delayed bolus arrival to the liver. Heterogeneous parenchyma enhancement showing reticular regions of low attenuation, particularly at the periphery of the liver, is highly suggestive of congestive hepatopathy (Fig. 16) and has been described as "nutmeg liver" (Kiesewetter et al. 2007; Elsayes et al. 2017).

3.2 Budd-Chiari Syndrome

Budd-Chiari syndrome (BCS) is a rare disease, secondary to partial or complete obstruction of hepatic venous outflow, which can occur at any level from the small hepatic venules up to the entrance of the inferior vena cava into the right atrium (Garcia-Pagán et al. 2016). Hepatic venous outflow obstruction will lead to increased intrahepatic sinusoidal pressure and congestion, decreasing the hepatic perfusion, resulting in hepatocyte necrosis and evolving to centrilobular fibrosis, nodular regenerative hyperplasia, and cirrhosis (Valla 2009). Furthermore, the blockage of hepatic venous outflow will lead to the development of extrahepatic collateral vessels and portal hypertension. While primary BCS is usually associated with prothrombotic conditions, secondary BCS results from vascular extrinsic compression associated with hepatic abscesses and benign or malignant tumors, or from vascular invasion by malignant tumors. Clinical manifestations of BCS depend on the stage of the disease, ranging from asymptomatic and incidentally discovered disease to an acute or fulminant presentation (Langlet et al. 2003), with abrupt onset of ascites, abdominal pain and liver, and kidney failure. Subacute or chronic forms are the most fre-

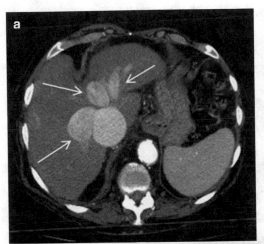

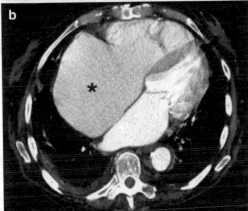

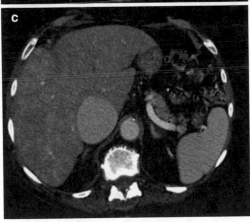

Fig. 15 Hepatic congestion related to right heart failure. Axial contrast-enhanced CT in arterial phase (**a** and **b**) shows early enhancement of a dilated IVC and central hepatic veins (**a**) secondary to the reflux of contrast material from the right atrium into the IVC. Cardiomegaly with severe dilation of the right atrium (*) is also observed (**b**). Axial contrast-enhanced CT in the portal venous phase (**c**) demonstrates abnormal parenchymal enhancement with reticular regions of low attenuation at the periphery of the liver, related with hepatic congestion

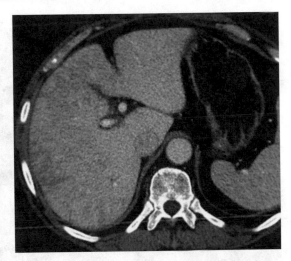

Fig. 16 Hepatic congestion. Axial contrast-enhanced portal venous phase CT image demonstrates a heterogeneous parenchyma enhancement with linear areas of poor enhancement, mainly at the peripheric regions of the liver, described as "nutmeg" appearance or mosaic pattern, related with congestive hepatopathy

quent presentations (Langlet et al. 2003), with indolent development of symptoms related to an impairment of liver function and portal hypertension.

Imaging findings will also depend on the stage of the disease. Doppler US and contrast-enhanced MR or CT examinations play an important role for diagnosing BCS, and biopsy is usually not necessary (Van Wettere et al. 2018). Although CT can also demonstrate the thrombosed hepatic veins, these are usually more evident at US or MR imaging.

Doppler US is the first-line modality for suspected BCS (Ralls et al. 1992; Cura et al. 2009) demonstrating the absence of venous flow or a focal acceleration of blood velocities at the level of stenosis (Fig. 17). The absence of normal triphasic spectrum of the hepatic veins can also be recognized but it is not specific, as it can be present in cirrhosis or chronic hepatitis. The evidence of at least one of the following imaging features at B-mode US is sufficient to make the diagnosis: endoluminal vein hypoechoic material (Fig. 18); venous stenosis with upstream dilatation; and fibrous hyperechoic cord replacing the vein or an intraluminal thrombus (Van Wettere et al. 2018). In the acute phase, hepatomegaly and ascites are commonly present (Fig. 17) while

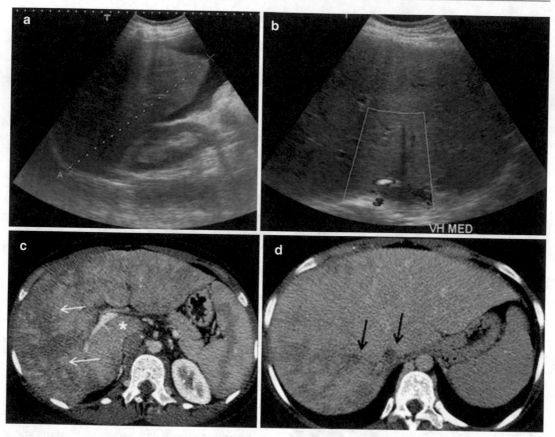

Fig. 17 Acute Budd-Chiari syndrome. Doppler US examination (**a**, **b**) shows ascites, hepatomegaly, and absence of flow within the right and middle hepatic veins. Contrast-enhanced axial CT images (**c**, **d**) show hyperenhancement of the central portions of the liver, including the caudate lobe (*), and decreased enhancement at the periphery (white arrow) on the hepatic arterial phase (**c**). On the venous phase (**d**), there is no enhancement of the right and middle hepatic veins (black arrow)

in subacute or chronic BCS, an important finding for the diagnosis is the observation of hepatic venous collateral circulation (Valla 2003), draining blood from the liver segments with obstructed vein into the patent veins. Other imaging findings include hypertrophy of the caudate lobe, presence of a vein draining the caudate lobe greater than or equal to 3 mm in caliber (Bargalló et al. 2006), and dilation of the HA and splenomegaly. Doppler US also demonstrates slow hepatofugal flow at the portal vein (Brancatelli et al. 2007). Furthermore, PV thrombosis can be found in approximately 15% of the cases and it might be related to prothrombotic state or portal hypertension (Murad et al. 2006).

On contrast-enhanced CT or MR images, hepatomegaly, ascites, and splenomegaly are the main findings in acute BCS, along with occlusion of the hepatic veins (Figs. 17, 18, and 19). Other characteristic findings are the delayed and decreased enhancement, particularly at the periphery of the liver parenchyma, and an early strong enhancement of the central portions of the liver and caudate lobe (Fig. 19). Because of edema and congestion, hyperintensity of the liver parenchyma can be seen on T2-weighted images, especially in subcapsular areas.

On the other hand, on subacute or chronic BCS, morphological changes of the liver are often seen, with peripheric parenchymal atrophy along with hypertrophy of the central liver and caudate lobe (Fig. 20). Furthermore, an enlargement of the hepatic artery and portosystemic and intrahepatic collateral vessels are frequently rec-

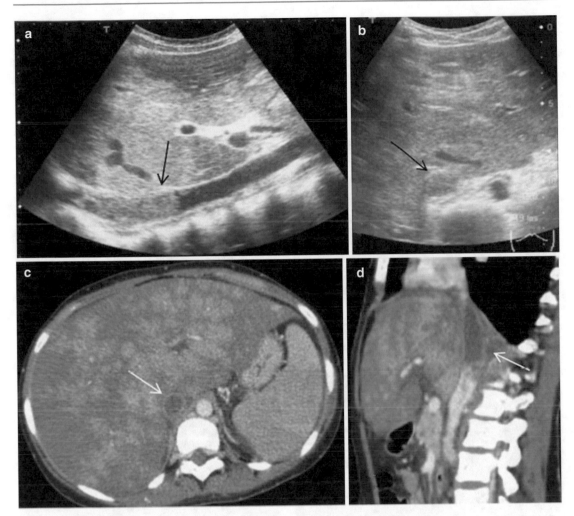

Fig. 18 Acute Budd-Chiari syndrome. Longitudinal (**a**) and transversal (**b**) B-mode US shows hepatomegaly with heterogeneous echogenicity of the parenchyma, and a prominent echogenic thrombus (black arrow) within the intrahepatic portion of the IVC. Axial (**c**) and sagittal (**d**) contrast-enhanced CT in portal venous phase confirmed the acute BCS diagnosis demonstrating the thrombus in the IVC lumen as a non-enhanced filling defect (white arrow). Note also the heterogeneous enhancement of the liver parenchyma, with increased enhancement of the central regions and decreased enhancement of the liver periphery

ognized (Figs. 20 and 21). The latter are considered to be the most sensitive feature and a key to chronic BCS diagnosis (Valla 2003). A "mosaic" pattern of enhancement of the liver parenchyma is commonly observed (Fig. 20), which appears as a reticulated enhancement on arterial and/or venous phases, with complete or partial homogenization on delayed phases. This heterogeneous enhancement is more evident at the liver periphery and it is a sign of sinusoidal dilatation. Thus, a mosaic enhancement may also be found in other conditions such as hepatic congestion sec-

ondary to cardiac dysfunction (Fig. 16), or more infrequently due to chronic/acute systemic inflammatory states (Ronot et al. 2016).

In chronic BCS, the development of multiple regenerative nodules is very frequent due to hyperarterialization of the liver parenchyma in response to PV hypoperfusion. In most of the cases, these nodules are multiple (more than 10), with a diameter ranging from 0.5 to 4.0 cm (Vilgrain et al. 1999; Brancatelli et al. 2007; Vilgrain et al. 2018). Typically, these regenerative nodules are markedly and homogenously

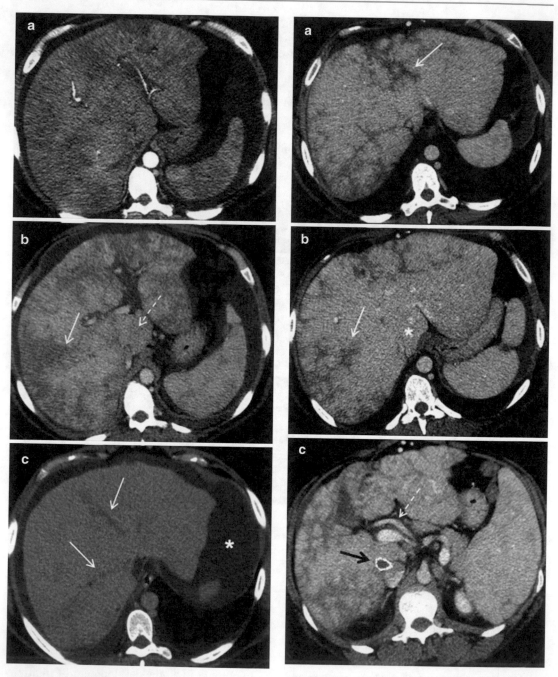

Fig. 19 Acute BCS. Axial contrast-enhanced CT in arterial phase (a) shows markedly heterogeneous enhancement of the liver parenchyma, still evident on portal venous phase (b), with a notable decreased peripheral enhancement (white arrow) and a stronger enhancement of the central portion. The caudate lobe is enlarged and shows increased enhancement (dashed arrow). Axial contrast-enhanced CT in delayed phase (c) shows occlusion of the hepatic veins (arrows). This enhancement pattern in association with obstructed hepatic veins is characteristic of acute BCS. Ascites (*) is also present

Fig. 20 Chronic BCS, same patient as in Fig. 19. Axial contrast-enhanced CT in portal venous phase (a, b, and c) demonstrates atrophy of the periphery and hypertrophy of the central portions of the liver, with the typical zonal perfusion and patchy enhancement of the parenchyma (white arrows), also referred to as the mosaic pattern. The caudate lobe is normally enlarged and homogenously enhanced (*). An enlarged HA is usually present in the chronic cases (dashed arrow) due to hyperarterialization, to compensate the decreased portal flow. A TIPS is observed (black arrow) which is occluded. Also, there is splenomegaly due to portal hypertension

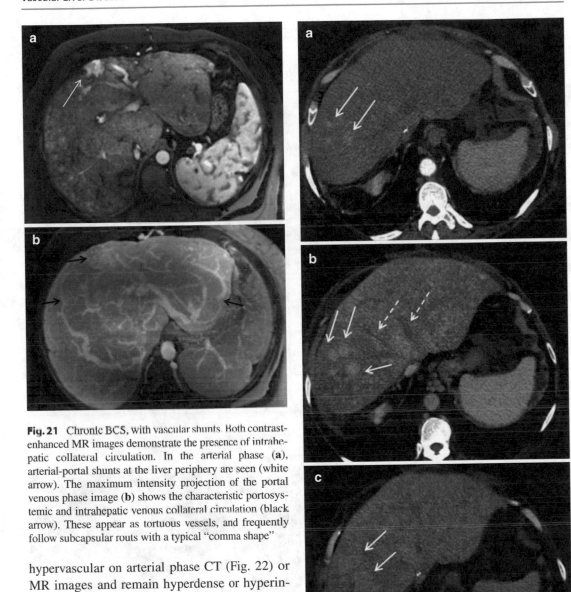

Fig. 21 Chronic BCS, with vascular shunts. Both contrast-enhanced MR images demonstrate the presence of intrahepatic collateral circulation. In the arterial phase (**a**), arterial-portal shunts at the liver periphery are seen (white arrow). The maximum intensity projection of the portal venous phase image (**b**) shows the characteristic portosystemic and intrahepatic venous collateral circulation (black arrow). These appear as tortuous vessels, and frequently follow subcapsular routs with a typical "comma shape"

Fig. 22 Chronic BCS, with benign hypervascular nodules. Axial contrast-enhanced CT in arterial (**a**), portal venous (**b**), and delayed (**c**) phase demonstrating multiple hypervascular peripheral nodules (white arrows) with no washout on either portal venous or delayed phase. Obstruction of the middle hepatic vein is visible (dashed arrows)

hypervascular on arterial phase CT (Fig. 22) or MR images and remain hyperdense or hyperintense on portal venous and delayed phase, and also at the hepatobiliary phase, if a hepatospecific contrast agent is used. Largest lesions often contain a central scar, like FNH (Vilgrain et al. 2018). Furthermore, these nodules are usually hyperdense on unenhanced CT images, and usually show high signal on T1-weighted and iso- to low signal on T2-weighted MR images, without restriction on diffusion-weighted MR images (Vilgrain et al. 2018) (Table 2). Nevertheless, some regenerative nodules may present washout on delayed phases and they may also increase in size and/or number, making them difficult to be differentiated from hepatocellular carcinoma

(Vilgrain et al. 2018). Moreover, patients with BCS are at risk of developing hepatocellular carcinoma. In fact, the incidence of hepatocellular carcinoma in BSC is similar to that observed in other chronic liver diseases, although it is seldom observed in Western countries, probably because BCS is a rare disease (Van Wettere et al. 2018). Hepatocellular carcinoma is usually solitary and larger, and usually shows delayed wash-out (Fig. 23). Serum alpha-fetoprotein is specific for hepatocellular carcinoma (Vilgrain et al. 2018). Nevertheless, because the diagnosis of hypervascular lesions is not always straightforward in patients with BCS, if nodules are large (> 3 cm) or solitary, with atypical imaging features or with significant changes over time, a liver biopsy should be performed (Vilgrain et al. 2018).

Table 2 Different characteristics of BCS nodules on CT and MRI

Unenhanced CT	T1	T2	Arterial phase	PVP	HBP
Hyper	Hyper	Hyper ISO/HYPO	Hyper	Hyper	Hyper

PVP portal venous phase, *HBP* hepatobiliary phase

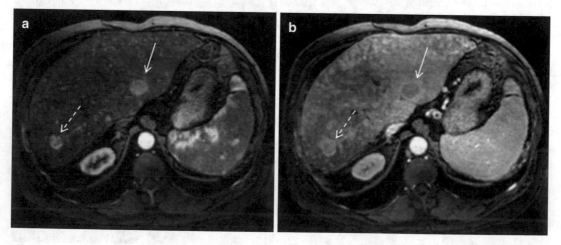

Fig. 23 Hepatocellular carcinoma in chronic BCS. This patient with BCS presented multiple hypervascular nodules on follow-up MR examinations (**a**, arterial phase; **b**, portal venous phase image), most of them with no washout on delayed phase (dashed arrow). However, one of these nodules (solid arrow) showed progressive enlargement regarding the previous examinations and further-more showed washout and a pseudocapsule (white arrow) on delayed phase (**b**). This nodule was suspicious for hepatocellular carcinoma. Due to rapidly progressive liver failure, the patient underwent a liver transplantation and the presence of hepatocellular carcinoma was confirmed on the explanted liver

4 Sinusoidal Obstruction

4.1 Sinusoidal Obstruction Syndrome

Hepatic sinusoidal obstruction syndrome (SOS), previously known as veno-occlusive disease, is a vascular disease characterized by endothelial sinusoidal damage due to toxin exposure with consequent sinusoidal congestion and centrilobular necrosis, leading to sinusoidal and central hepatic vein obstruction, while large hepatic vein continues to be patent (Elsayes et al. 2017; Brancatelli et al. 2018). There are several well-recognized causes for this sinusoidal injury, such as cytoreductive therapy before hematopoietic stem cell transplantation, use of pyrrolizidine alkaloid-containing herbal remedies, use of azathioprine in immunosuppression for solid organ transplant or inflammatory bowel disease, and chemotherapy drugs with platinum (Hubert et al. 2013; Fan and Crawford 2014). In the acute stage, the clinical symptoms are abdominal pain and ascites while in the subacute phase, the patients usually present with recurrent ascites, hepatosplenomegaly, and jaundice. Chronically, the clinical and histology findings will be similar to those of cirrhosis (Elsayes et al. 2017).

As the imaging features of SOS are nonspecific, a relevant clinical history is important to raise the suspicion of SOS. On contrast-enhanced CT and MRI images, a patchy and irregular enhancement of the liver enhancement is seen, mainly at the periphery, with mosaic appearance, resembling the imaging finding of BCS, but with patent hepatic veins (Figs. 24 and 25). Gallbladder wall thickening, hepatomegaly, portal edema, splenomegaly, and ascites may also be observed. On gadoxetic acid contrast-enhanced MR, a reticular hypointense parenchymal pattern, mainly in the peripheral areas of the liver, is highly specific for SOS (Shin et al. 2012). Resolution of the imaging findings is expected to occur once the causative agent is suspended (Han et al. 2015; Garcia-Pagán et al. 2016; Brancatelli et al. 2018).

4.2 Hepatic Peliosis

Hepatic peliosis is a rare benign vascular condition characterized by sinusoidal dilation and multiple

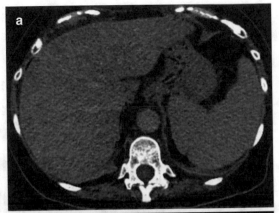

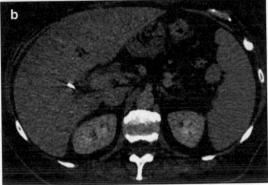

Fig. 24 Sinusoidal obstruction syndrome in a patient treated with oxaliplatin chemotherapy for colorectal cancer. Axial contrast-enhanced CT in the portal venous phase (**a** and **b**) shows patchy and irregular enhancement of the liver, essentially at the periphery, with a mosaic pattern. This patient had also peri-hepatic ascites

blood-filled cystic lesions, with loss of endothelium. Several causes have been suggested, such as steroids, oral contraceptives, tamoxifen methotrexate or toxins, hematological or infectious diseases, and even pregnancy, but it is often idiopathic (Elsayes et al. 2017; Brancatelli et al. 2018). Although patients with hepatic peliosis are generally asymptomatic and incidentally diagnosed, symptoms related to portal hypertension or hepatic rupture with hemoperitoneum may also be present (Cimbanassi et al. 2015; Elsayes et al. 2017).

On post-contrast CT, the peliotic lesions can have different appearances depending on the presence of afferent vessels or thrombotic tissue. The lesions may show a central hyperenhancement on arterial phase (target sign) with centrifugal enhancement during the venous phase, although enhancement may also be centripetal (Elsayes et al. 2017). On delayed images, hyperenhancement is usually observed. Nevertheless, throm-

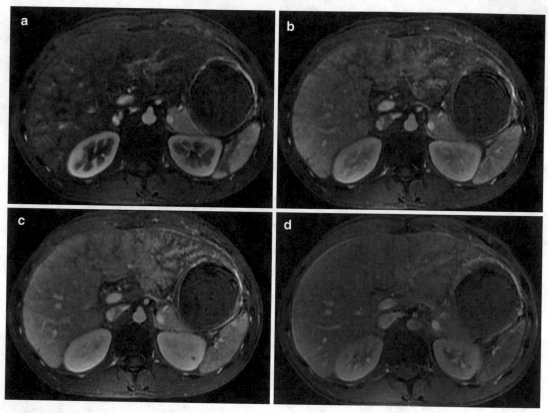

Fig. 25 Sinusoidal obstruction syndrome in a patient treated with immunosuppression after liver transplant. Axial dynamic contrast-enhanced MR images (**a–d**) show patchy and irregular enhancement of the liver, in a mosaic pattern, mainly at the periphery of the left lobe. Images are courtesy of Luis Martí-Bonmatí, MD PhD, Valencia, Spain

bosed lesions may not enhance and lesions smaller than 1 cm are often too small to be depicted. On MR images, peliotic lesions are usually hyperintense on T2-weighted images (Fig. 26). Differential diagnosis includes hepatic hemangioma or hypervascular metastasis, and the absence of mass effect on adjacent hepatic vessels may help to differentiate these lesions from hepatic tumors (Ferrozzi et al. 2001). Peliosis may resolve after cessation of the causative agent or adequate treatment of the underlying cause (Elsayes et al. 2017).

4.3   Nonobstructive Sinusoidal Dilation

Nonobstructive hepatic sinusoidal dilation may be observed in association with acute inflammatory or infectious diseases (such as pyelonephri-tis, cholecystitis, pneumonia, and pancreatitis) or oral contraceptives (Ronot et al. 2016; Brancatelli et al. 2018). Imaging findings are nonspecific and similar to those of sinusoidal obstruction or venous outflow obstruction, with a mosaic enhancement pattern on the periphery of the liver parenchyma (Brancatelli et al. 2018).

5   Hepatic Nodules in Liver Vascular Diseases

The majority of liver vascular diseases are associated with hepatocellular tumors, most of them being hypervascular on enhanced CT or MR images. Most of these nodules are benign, and the size and number of these nodules may increase over time. FNH-like nodules are the most common type, but focal nodular regenera-

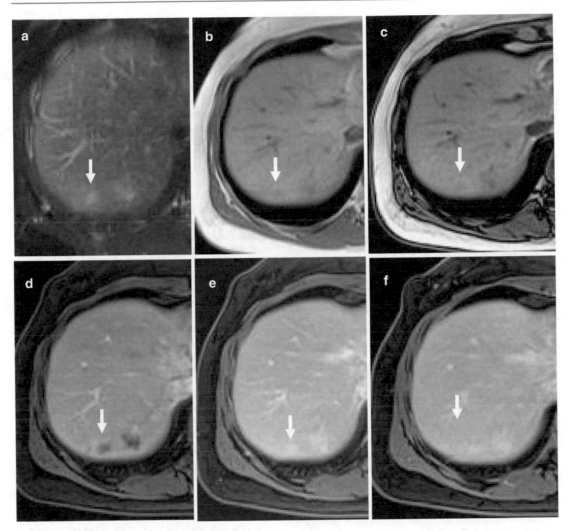

Fig. 26 48-year-old woman with peliosis hepatis. Patient had renal transplantation 4 years before and, presently, has diabetes and Hodgkin lymphoma. Lesion (arrow) appears mildly hyperintense on fat suppressed T2-w MRI sequence (**a**) and hypointense on T1-w in-phase (**b**) and out-of-phase (**c**) MRI sequence. (**d**) In arterial phase of contrast enhancement, lesion shows peripheral rim-like enhancement. In portal venous (**e**) and equilibrium phase (**f**), lesion enhancement is isointense to liver parenchyma. Note centripetal progression of contrast enhancement, which simulates hemangioma. Peliotic lesions have typically centrifugal progression of contrast enhancement, but centripetal enhancement can also be observed (Courtesy of Prof. Luigi Grazioli, Brescia)

tive hyperplasia and hepatocellular adenoma may also be found (Sempoux et al. 2015; Vilgrain et al. 2018). Contrast-enhanced CT and MR, especially with hepatospecific contrast agents, are very important for the diagnosis. Nevertheless, imaging findings are not pathognomonic and liver biopsy may be needed for a definite diagnosis. Hepatocellular carcinoma is rare except in patients with BCS, who should be followed over time (Vilgrain et al. 2018).

6 Conclusion

Hepatic vascular diseases may affect the vascular inflow, vascular outflow, or flow at the sinusoidal level, most of them resulting in decreased portal perfusion and increased arterialization of the parenchyma. The underlying physiopathological mechanisms lead to key imaging findings that should be promptly recognized by radiologists, in order to provide an accurate diagnosis.

References

Abbas MA, Fowl RJ, Stone WM et al (2003) Hepatic artery aneurysm: factors that predict complications. J Vasc Surg 38:41–45

Arora A, Sarin SK (2015) Multimodality imaging of obliterative portal venopathy: what every radiologist should know. Br J Radiol 88:20140653

Atasoy KÇ, Fitoz S, Akyar G et al (1998) Aneurysms of the portal venous system: gray-scale and color Doppler ultrasonographic findings with CT and mri correlation. Clin Imaging 22:414–417

Bargalló X, Gilabert R, Nicolau C et al (2006) Sonography of Budd-Chiari syndrome. AJR Am J Roentgenol 187:W33–W41

Brancatelli G, Vilgrain V, Federle MP et al (2007) Budd-Chiari syndrome: spectrum of imaging findings. AJR Am J Roentgenol 188:W168–W176

Brancatelli G, Furlan A, Calandra A, Dioguardi Burgio M (2018) Hepatic sinusoidal dilatation. Abdom Radiol 43:2011–2022

Buscarini E, Danesino C, Olivieri C et al (2004) Doppler ultrasonographic grading of hepatic vascular malformations in hereditary hemorrhagic telangiectasia - results of extensive screening. Ultraschall der Medizin 25:348–355

Buscarini E, Gandolfi S, Alicante S et al (2018) Liver involvement in hereditary hemorrhagic telangiectasia. Abdom Radiol 43:1920–1930

Cimbanassi S, Aseni P, Mariani A et al (2015) Spontaneous hepatic rupture during pregnancy in a patient with peliosis hepatis. Ann Hepatol 14:553–558

Condat B, Vilgrain V, Asselah T et al (2003) Portal cavernoma-associated cholangiopathy: a clinical and MR cholangiography coupled with MR portography imaging study. Hepatology 37:1302–1308

Cura M, Haskal Z, Lopera J (2009) Diagnostic and interventional radiology for Budd-Chiari syndrome. Radiographics 29:669–681

DeLeve LD, Valla D, Garcia-Tsao G (2009) Vascular disorders of the liver. Hepatology 49:1729–1764

Denninger MH, Chaït Y, Casadevall N et al (2000) Cause of portal or hepatic venous thrombosis in adults: the role of multiple concurrent factors. Hepatology 31:587–591

Desser TS (2009) Understanding transient hepatic attenuation differences. Semin Ultrasound CT MRI 30:408–417

Dolapci M, Ersoz S, Kama NA (2003) Hepatic artery aneurysm. Ann Vasc Surg 17:214–216

Elsayes KM, Shaaban AM, Rothan SM et al (2017) A comprehensive approach to hepatic vascular disease. Radiographics 37:813–836

Erben Y, De Martino RR, Bjarnason H et al (2015) Operative management of hepatic artery aneurysms. J Vasc Surg 62:610–615

Fan CQ, Crawford JM (2014) Sinusoidal obstruction syndrome (hepatic veno-occlusive disease). J Clin Exp Hepatol 4:332–346

Ferrozzi F, Tognini G, Zuccoli G et al (2001) Peliosis hepatis with pseudotumoral and hemorrhagic evolution: CT and MR findings. Abdom Imaging 26:197–199

Furuichi Y, Moriyasu F, Taira J et al (2013) Noninvasive diagnostic method for idiopathic portal hypertension based on measurements of liver and spleen stiffness by ARFI elastography. J Gastroenterol 48:1061–1068

Gallego C, Velasco M, Marcuello P et al (2002) Congenital and acquired anomalies of the portal venous system. Radiographics 22:141–159

Garcia-Pagán JC, Buscarini E, HLA J et al (2016) EASL Clinical Practice Guidelines: Vascular diseases of the liver. J Hepatol 64(1):179

Garcia-Tsao G, Korzenik JR, Young L et al (2000) Liver disease in patients with hereditary hemorrhagic telangiectasia. N Engl J Med 343:931–936

Giallourakis C, Rosenberg P, Friedman L (2002) The liver in heart failure. Clin Liver Dis 6:947–967

Glatard AS, Hillaire S, D'Assignies G et al (2012) Obliterative portal venopathy: findings at CT imaging. Radiology 263:741–750

Gore RM, Mathieu DG, White EM et al (1994) Passive hepatic congestion: cross-sectional imaging features. AJR Am J Roentgenol 162:71–75

Gottardi A, Rautou PE, Schouten J et al (2019) Porto-sinusoidal vascular disease: proposal and description of a novel entity. Lancet Gastroenterol Hepatol 4:399–411

Han NY, Park BJ, Kim MJ et al (2015) Hepatic parenchymal heterogeneity on contrast-enhanced CT scans following oxaliplatin-based chemotherapy: natural history and association with clinical evidence of sinusoidal obstruction syndrome. Radiology 276:766–774

Hillaire S, Bonte E, Denninger MH et al (2002) Idiopathic non-cirrhotic intrahepatic portal hypertension in the West: a re-evaluation in 28 patients. Gut 51:275–280

Hubert C, Sempoux C, Humblet Y et al (2013) Sinusoidal obstruction syndrome (SOS) related to chemotherapy for colorectal liver metastases: factors predictive of severe SOS lesions and protective effect of bevacizumab. HPB 15:858–864

Ianora AAS, Memeo M, Sabbà C et al (2004) Hereditary hemorrhagic telangiectasia: multi-detector row helical CT assessment of hepatic involvement. Radiology 230:250–259

Ishigami K, Zhang Y, Rayhill S et al (2004) Does variant hepatic artery anatomy in a liver transplant recipient increase the risk of hepatic artery complications after transplantation? AJR Am J Roentgenol 183:1577–1584

Kalra N, Shankar S, Khandelwal N (2014) Imaging of portal cavernoma cholangiopathy. J Clin Exp Hepatol 4:S44–S52

Khanna R, Sarin SK (2014) Non-cirrhotic portal hypertension - diagnosis and management. J Hepatol 60:421–441

Khuroo MS, Rather AA, Khuroo NS, Khuroo MS (2016) Portal biliopathy. World J Gastroenterol 22:7973–7982

Kiesewetter CH, Sheron N, Vettukattill JJ et al (2007) Hepatic changes in the failing Fontan circulation. Heart 93:579–584

Kobayashi S, Gabata T, Matsui O (2010) Radiologic manifestation of hepatic pseudolesions and pseudotumors in the third inflow area. Imaging Med 2:519–528

Koehne de Gonzalez AK, Lefkowitch JH (2017) Heart disease and the liver: pathologic evaluation. Gastroenterol Clin N Am 46:421–435

Langlet P, Escolano S, Valla D et al (2003) Clinicopathological forms and prognostic index in Budd-Chiari syndrome. J Hepatol 39:496–501

Lee JH, Lee YS, Kim PN et al (2011a) Osler-Weber-Rendu disease presenting with hepatocellular carcinoma: radiologic and genetic findings. Korean J Hepatol 17:313–318

Lee WK, Chang SD, Duddalwar VA et al (2011b) Imaging assessment of congenital and acquired abnormalities of the portal venous system. Radiographics 31:905–926

Llop E, De Juan C, Seijo S et al (2011) Portal cholangiopathy: radiological classification and natural history. Gut 60:853–860

López-Machado E, Mallorquín-Jiménez F, Medina-Benítez A et al (1998) Aneurysms of the portal venous system: ultrasonography and CT findings. Eur J Radiol 26:210–214

Lu M, Weiss C, Fishman E et al (2015) Review of visceral aneurysms and pseudoaneurysms. J Comput Assist Tomogr 39:1–6

Mahmoud M, Allinson KR, Zhai Z et al (2010) Pathogenesis of arteriovenous malformations in the absence of endoglin. Circ Res 106:1425–1433

Moreno FL, Hagan AD, Holmen JR et al (1984) Evaluation of size and dynamics of the inferior vena cava as an index of right-sided cardiac function. Am J Cardiol 53:579–585

Murad SD, Valla DC, De Groen PC et al (2006) Pathogenesis and treatment of Budd-Chiari syndrome combined with portal vein thrombosis. Am J Gastroenterol 101:83–90

Myers RP, Cerini R, Sayegh R et al (2003) Cardiac hepatopathy: clinical, hemodynamic, and histologic characteristics and correlations. Hepatology 37:393–400

Nakanuma Y, Tsuneyama K, Makoto O, Katayanagi K (2001) Pathology and pathogenesis of idiopathic portal hypertension with an emphasis on the liver. Pathol Res Pract 197:65–76

Ögren M, Bergqvist D, Björck M et al (2006) Portal vein thrombosis: prevalence, patient characteristics and lifetime risk: a population study based on 23796 consecutive autopsies. World J Gastroenterol 12:2115–2119

Pareja E, Cortes M, Navarro R et al (2010) Vascular complications after orthotopic liver transplantation: hepatic artery thrombosis. Transplant Proc 42:2970–2972

Plessier A, Darwish-Murad S, Hernandez-Guerra M, et al (2007) A prospective multicentric follow-up study on 105 patients with acute portal vein thrombosis (PVT): results from the european network for vascular disorders of the liver. In: Hepatology

Rajesh S, Mukund A, Sureka B et al (2018) Non-cirrhotic portal hypertension: an imaging review. Abdom Radiol 43:1991–2010

Ralls PW, Johnson MB, Radin DR et al (1992) Budd-Chiari syndrome: detection with color Doppler sonography. AJR Am J Roentgenol 159:113–116

Ronot M, Kerbaol A, Rautou PE et al (2016) Acute extrahepatic infectious or inflammatory diseases are a cause of transient mosaic pattern on CT and MR imaging related to sinusoidal dilatation of the liver. Eur Radiol 26:3094–3101

Schouten JNL, Nevens F, Hansen B et al (2012) Idiopathic noncirrhotic portal hypertension is associated with poor survival: results of a long-term cohort study. Aliment Pharmacol Ther 35:1424–1433

Seijo S, Reverter E, Miquel R et al (2012) Role of hepatic vein catheterisation and transient elastography in the diagnosis of idiopathic portal hypertension. Dig Liver Dis 44:855–860

Sempoux C, Paradis V, Komuta M et al (2015) Hepatocellular nodules expressing markers of hepatocellular adenomas in Budd-Chiari syndrome and other rare hepatic vascular disorders. J Hepatol 63:1173–1180

Sfyroeras GS, Antoniou GA, Drakou AA et al (2009) Visceral venous aneurysms: clinical presentation, natural history and their management: a systematic review. Eur J Vasc Endovasc Surg 38:498–505

Shin SM, Kim S, Lee JW et al (2007) Biliary abnormalities associated with portal biliopathy: evaluation on MR cholangiography. AJR Am J Roentgenol 188:W341–W347

Shin NY, Kim MJ, Lim JS et al (2012) Accuracy of gadoxetic acid-enhanced magnetic resonance imaging for the diagnosis of sinusoidal obstruction syndrome in patients with chemotherapy-treated colorectal liver metastases. Eur Radiol 22:864–871

Siddiki H, Doherty MG, Fletcher JG et al (2008) Abdominal findings in hereditary hemorrhagic telangiectasia: pictorial essay on 2D and 3D findings with isotropic multiphase CT. Radiographics 28:171–184

Tardáguila Montero F (ed) (2016) Serie de monografías virtuales - avances en imagen hepática. Colegio Interamericano de Radiología

Torabi M, Hosseinzadeh K, Federle MP (2008) CT of nonneoplastic hepatic vascular and perfusion disorders. Radiographics 28:1967–1982

Valla DC (2003) The diagnosis and management of the Budd-Chiari syndrome: consensus and controversies. Hepatology 38:793–803

Valla DC (2009) Primary Budd-Chiari syndrome. J Hepatol 50:195–203

Van Wettere M, Bruno O, Rautou PE et al (2018) Diagnosis of Budd–Chiari syndrome. Abdom Radiol 43:1896–1907

Vilgrain V, Lewin M, Vons C et al (1999) Hepatic nodules in Budd-Chiari syndrome: imaging features. Radiology 210:443–450

Vilgrain V, Condat B, Bureau C et al (2006) Atrophy-hypertrophy complex in patients with cavernous transformation of the portal vein: CT evaluation. Radiology 241:149–155

Vilgrain V, Paradis V, Van Wettere M et al (2018) Benign and malignant hepatocellular lesions in patients with vascular liver diseases. Abdom Radiol 43:1968–1977

Walser EM, Runyan BR, Heckman MG et al (2011) Extrahepatic portal biliopathy: proposed etiology on the basis of anatomic and clinical features. Radiology 258:146–153

Wu JS, Saluja S, Garcia-Tsao G et al (2006) Liver involvement in hereditary hemorrhagic telangiectasia: CT and clinical findings do not correlate in symptomatic patients. AJR Am J Roentgenol 187:W399–W405

Imaging of Liver Trauma

Stefania Romano, Tomas Andrasina,
Hana Petrasova, Luca Tarotto, Gianluca Gatta,
Alfonso Ragozzino, and Vlastimil Valek

Contents

Abstract

Abdominal traumas represent a frequent conditions in Emergency Department, with liver lesions commonly observed. This Chapter will be focused on the role of the diagnostic methods in evaluating liver traumas, especially CT with management correlations considered.

S. Romano (✉) · A. Ragozzino
Department of Diagnostic Imaging, Santa Maria delle Grazie Hospital, Pozzuoli, Italy

T. Andrasina · H. Petrasova · V. Valek
Department of Radiology and Nuclear Medicine, Masaryk University of Brno, Brno, Czech Republic

L. Tarotto
Department of Advanced Biomedical Sciences, Federico II University, Naples, Italy

G. Gatta
Institute of Radiology, "Luigi Vanvitelli" University, Naples, Italy

1 Introduction

Abdominal traumas represent a common emergency condition, with liver injuries frequently observed (Badger et al. 2009; Feliciano 1989; Fodor et al. 2018; Raza et al. 2013; Tarchouli et al. 2018). The role of diagnostic imaging in the evaluation of patients with blunt or penetrating lesions is crucial and essential in the emergency department. The mortality rate in liver traumatic damages depends on the extension and degree of the lesions as well as on the association with other organ injuries (Tarchouli et al. 2018). Because the management of hepatic traumatic lesions has changed in the last decades with a preferred nonsurgical management in hemodynamically stable subjects, to avoid all postoperative potential complications from organ resections in emergency (Raza et al. 2013; Tarchouli et al. 2018) the laparotomy with perihepatic packing and the use of the interventional

© Springer Nature Switzerland AG 2021
E. Quaia (ed.), *Imaging of the Liver and Intra-hepatic Biliary Tract*,
Medical Radiology, Diagnostic Imaging, https://doi.org/10.1007/978-3-030-38983-3_17

radiologic procedure when indicated led to a decrease in mortality rates (Tarchouli et al. 2018). The grading scale for the liver trauma is represented by the American Association for Surgery of Trauma (AAST) score that indicates six levels of injuries based on the anatomical description of the alterations (Raza et al. 2013; Moore et al. 1989; Moore and Moore 2010), with the reported lesions from I to III predominantly treated conservatively, whereas the major extended of grade IV, V, or VI requesting surgery, although if a nonoperative management could be evoked in specialized centers for hemodynamically stable patients (Raza et al. 2013; Piper and Peitzman 2010). The imaging grading scale of the liver injuries to assess lesion severity and to help the clinical management of the organ traumas plays an important although if sometimes a discussed role (Raza et al. 2013; Moore and Moore 2010). Classic classification of CT graded the scale of liver injures varying from capsular avulsion to major parenchymal damage and vascular injury (Mirvis et al. 1989; Raza et al. 2013; Yoon et al. 2005); however the AAST grading scale includes several criteria that could not be assessed with CT, with potential differences and discrepancies between the imaging and the intraoperative findings (Yoon et al. 2005), often underestimating the lesion severity (Yoon et al. 2005). The evidence of hemodynamic instability more than the degree severity at CT seems to represent the best predictor for the surgery in patients with blunt liver trauma (Yoon et al. 2005; Poletti et al. 2002; Delgado Millan and Deballon 2001).

2 Diagnostic Imaging

CT is the imaging modality of choice to evaluate hemodynamically stable patients suffering from blunt abdominal trauma (Shanmuganathan and Mirvis 1995; Shanmuganathan 2004), showing a spectrum of diagnostic findings useful in the characterization of hemorrhage as well as in the planning of the injury management (Shanmuganathan and Mirvis 1995; Shanmuganathan 2004). Multi-detector row computed tomography (MDCT) enables fast and thin acquisition of the abdominal anatomy (Aschoff 2006). Acquisition in subisotropic voxel allows maximizing efficiency in evaluating patients with blunt polytrauma not just with axial but in multiple planes using coronal and sagittal reformatting images (Dreizin and Munera 2012).

Administration of intravenous contrast medium is essential in emergency and almost crucial in polytrauma imaging: in the evaluation of severe trauma patients multiphase CT scanning protocols are frequently used in most institions (arterial, venous, and delayed phase), but in literature other experiences regarding the contrast administration protocol have been reported. A split bolus contrast protocol had been shown to reduce the radiation exposure and the number of passes in young population (Beenen et al. 2015), whereas other authors proposed a triphasic injection single-pass whole-body imaging protocol that appeared to be superior to the conventional multiphase protocol allowing a better vascular and abdominal parenchymal imaging with reduction in radiation dose and image overload (Loupatatzis et al. 2008; Yaniv et al. 2013).

In a study comparing a low-dose polytrauma multiphase whole-body CT protocol on a 258-slice multi-detector CT (MDCT) scanner with advanced dose reduction techniques to a single-phase polytrauma whole-body CT protocol on a 64-slice MDCT scanner, it has been shown that the low-dose multiphase CT protocol could improve diagnostic accuracy and image quality at markedly reduced radiation, but with an increased examination time that could reduce workflow in acute emergency situations (Alagic et al. 2017). Rising numbers of computed tomography (CT) examinations worldwide have led to a focus on dose reduction in the latest developments in CT technology. Iterative reconstruction (IR) models bear the potential to effectively reduce dose while maintaining adequate image quality (Graves et al. 2017).

There are still challenges in CT imaging of the polytrauma individual including time restraints, diagnostic errors, radiation dose effects, and bridging the gap between anatomy and physiology: possible solutions could be offered by the unique design of the dual-source CT scanner (Nicolaou et al. 2008).

Dual-energy CT improves the detection and the contrast-to-noise ratio of the hypovascular lesions of the abdominal organ, so that in case of hepatic laceration, the contrast between the hypovascular laceration and the liver parenchyma increases on low-kilovolt peak and low-kiloelectron volt images (Wortman et al. 2018).

In the evaluation of the traumatized patient, diagnostic imaging modalities including radiographs, ultrasound, and computed tomography have demonstrated utility in injury detection (long). Many centers routinely utilize whole-body CT trauma (WBCT) based on the premise that this test will improve mortality (Long et al. 2017). However, WBCT may increase radiation and incidental findings when used without considering pretest probability of actionable traumatic injuries (Long et al. 2017). Studies supporting WBCT are predominantly retrospective and incorporate trauma scoring systems, which have significant design weaknesses (Long et al. 2017). The REACT-2 trial randomized trauma patients with high index of suspicion for actionable injuries to WBCT versus selective imaging and found no mortality difference (Long et al. 2017). Additional prospective trials evaluating WBCT in specific trauma subgroups (e.g., polytrauma) are probably needed to evaluate the effective benefit (Long et al. 2017). In the interim, the available data suggests that clinicians should adopt a selective imaging strategy driven by history and physical examination (Long et al. 2017). While observational data suggests an association between WBCT and a benefit in mortality and ED length of stay, randomized controlled data suggests no mortality benefit to this diagnostic tool (Long et al. 2017). The literature would benefit from confirmatory studies of the use of WBCT in trauma subgroups to clarify its impact on mortality for patients with specific injury patterns (Long et al. 2017).

A study to assess the accuracy of the trauma team leader's clinical suspicion of injury in patients who have undergone whole-body computed tomography (WBCT) for suspected polytrauma and to assess the frequency of unsuspected injuries and specific patterns of injury at WBCT was published in 2015 (Shannon et al. 2015). The authors concluded that clinical suspicion of injury correlates poorly with findings at WBCT, with a high proportion of uninjured body areas (Shannon et al. 2015). The number of unsuspected injuries found at WBCT was low, but the majority of these were serious injuries, possibly masked by distracting injury to other body areas (Shannon et al. 2015). The use of a WBCT protocol is recommended for suspected polytrauma, but the authors suggested a regular monitoring of WBCT findings and regular feedback of the results to emergency physicians to help inform their selection of patients for trauma WBCT (Shannon et al. 2015).

Independently from any consideration regarding the indication to WBCT in major trauma patients, the emergency radiologist must be able to accurately and rapidly identify the range of CT manifestations of the traumatized body (Graves et al. 2017) and the findings of liver injury. Contrast CT should be considered in the management algorithm for hepatic trauma, particularly in the setting of blunt injury (Kutcher et al. 2015), to detect the evidence of injury and the degree, and also in order to help clinician to select those who could benefit from a nonoperative management. Nonoperative management of common intra-abdominal solid organ injuries relies increasingly on computed tomographic findings and other clinical factors, including patient age, presence of concurrent injuries, and serial clinical assessments (Kokabi et al. 2014).

CT examination appears to play an important role in the management setting of suspected liver trauma (Figs. 1–8). Moreover, some patients explored for abdominal injury could have persistent hepatic bleeding on postoperative computed tomography (CT) and/or angiography, either not identified or not manageable at initial laparotomy (Kutcher et al. 2015). To identify patients at risk for ongoing hemorrhage and guide triage to angiography, some authors investigated the relationship of early postoperative CT scan with outcomes in operative hepatic trauma (Kutcher et al. 2015). They assessed that early postoperative CT scan after laparotomy for hepatic trauma

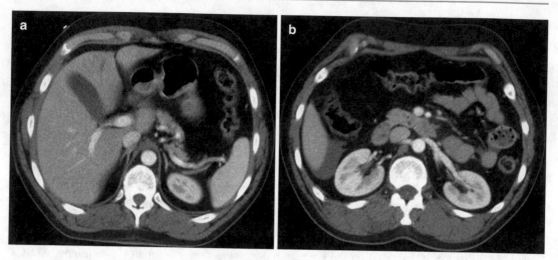

Fig. 1 (**a**, **b**) Contrast-enhanced CT scan in patient with blunt abdominal trauma: small linear hypodensity of the fourth hepatic segment from contusion (**a**); small amount of perihepatic fluid (**b**)

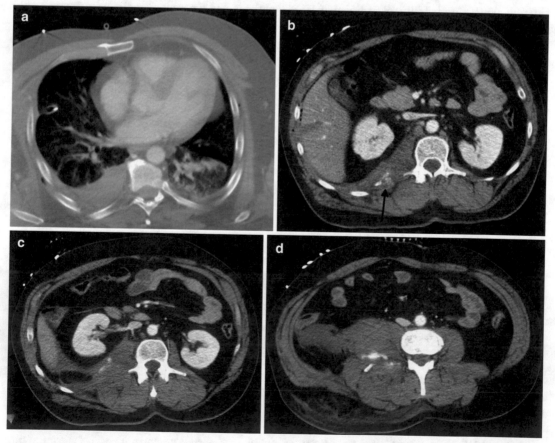

Fig. 2 (**a–d**) Contrast-enhanced CT in polytrauma patient: inferior lobe lung contusion, pleural effusion, and right costal fractures (**a**); small peripheral laceration of the right hepatic lobe (**b**); note the homolateral active poste-rior intercostal bleeding (black arrow in b), caudally extended in a retroperitoneal hematoma with multiple signs of active bleeding from right lumbar contusion and transverse process fractures (**c**, **d**)

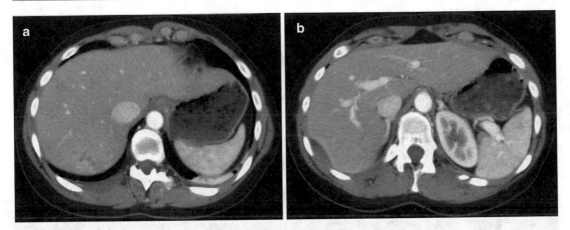

Fig. 3 (**a**, **b**) Contrast-enhanced CT images of small lacerative contusion of the right hepatic lobe (**a**), associated to a lenticular inhomogeneous subcapsular hypodensity from hematoma (**b**)

identifies clinically relevant ongoing bleeding and is sufficiently sensitive and specific to guide triage to angiography (Kutcher et al. 2015).

However, nonoperative management in some cases could lead to delayed complication and appropriate follow-up is therefore crucial (Mebert et al. 2018): in the reviewed literature, it was shown that routine imaging follow-up CT scans may not be indicated in asymptomatic patients with lower grade blunt hepatic injuries, whereas contrast-enhanced ultrasound (CEUS) appeared to be a promising alternative imaging modality for the follow-up of these patients (Mebert et al. 2018).

In the evaluation of the traumatized patient with suspected abdominal lesions, there are a large number of papers dealing with FAST (focused assessment with sonography in trauma) which, in practice, is the definition for detection of free fluid in the abdomen (Thorelius 2004). However, contrast-enhanced ultrasound (CEUS) has been reported to be an effective tool in the evaluation of blunt hepatic trauma, being more sensitive than baseline sonography and better correlating with CT findings (Catalano et al. 2005). Moreover, other authors assessed that CEUS is more accurate than US and nearly as accurate as CT, and CEUS could therefore be proposed for the initial evaluation of patients with blunt abdominal trauma (Valentino et al. 2010), in expert hands. In fact, CEUS greatly

improves the visualization and characterization of hepatic, renal, and splenic injuries compared to conventional ultrasound and appears to correlate well with CT (Clevert et al. 2008). This imaging technique could detect even minor blood flow and is able to depict vascular structures in detail (Clevert et al. 2008). Owing to its bedside availability, CEUS provides a good alternative to CT especially in patients with contraindications to CT contrast agents (e.g., due to renal failure or severe allergy) and in hemodynamically compromised patients (Clevert et al. 2008).

The use of contrast-enhanced ultrasound (CEUS) improves the accuracy of the sonography in the diagnosis and assessment of the extent of parenchymal lesions (Cagini et al. 2013). The CEUS could then be used in the follow-up of traumatic injuries of abdominal parenchymal organs (liver, spleen, and kidneys), especially in young people or children (Cagini et al. 2013). In the literature it has been noted that CEUS and serum liver enzyme measurement exhibited high consistency with contrast-enhanced CT for both detection and grading of intraparenchymal lesions in blunt liver trauma (Zhao et al. 2017) and these techniques may allow a more accurate diagnosis of liver trauma (Zhao et al. 2017). Contrast-enhanced sonography has also been reported to be able to play a role in the detection of pseudoaneurysms (Poletti et al. 2004) in solid organ injury from blunt trauma.

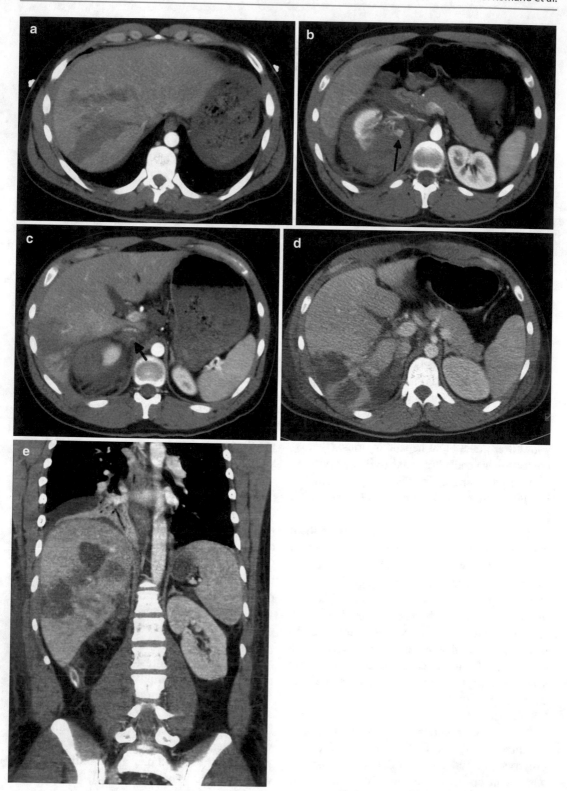

Fig. 4 (**a–e**) Major "bear-claw" lacerative contusion of the right hepatic lobe (**a**) with hemoperitoneum (**a–c**), evidence of right adrenal gland hematoma (arrow in **c**) and right perirenal hematoma (**b, c**) from major renal trauma with vascular peduncle involvement and active bleeding sign (arrow in **b**). Post-right nephrectomy CT control 48 h later (**d, e**): note the more defined hypodensity areas from lacerocontusive injuries of the right hepatic lobe and the appearance of the adrenal right hematoma in the axial (**d**) and coronal views (**e**)

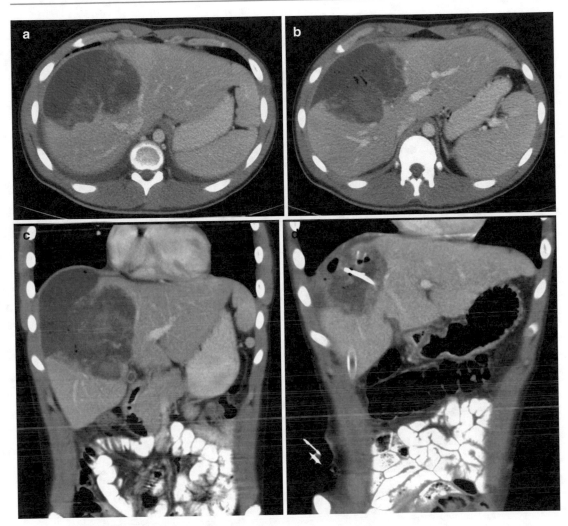

Fig. 5 (**a–d**) Liver trauma with large parenchymal hematoma (**a**) complicated with subcapsular biloma with some bubble of gas from sign of infection (**b, c**), successfully treated with percutaneous drainage (**d**)

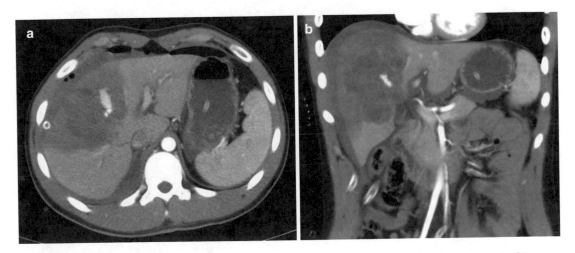

Fig. 6 (**a, b**) Major liver trauma involving the right lobe with hyperdensity from active bleeding findings (**a, b**)

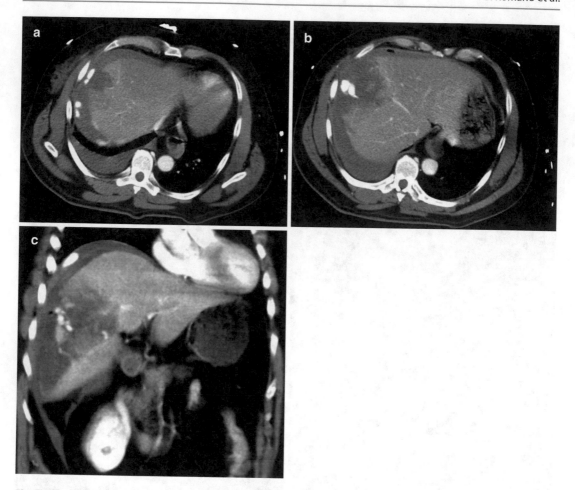

Fig. 7 (a–c) Right hepatic lobe fracture with blood pool hyperdensity from active bleeding (a–c)

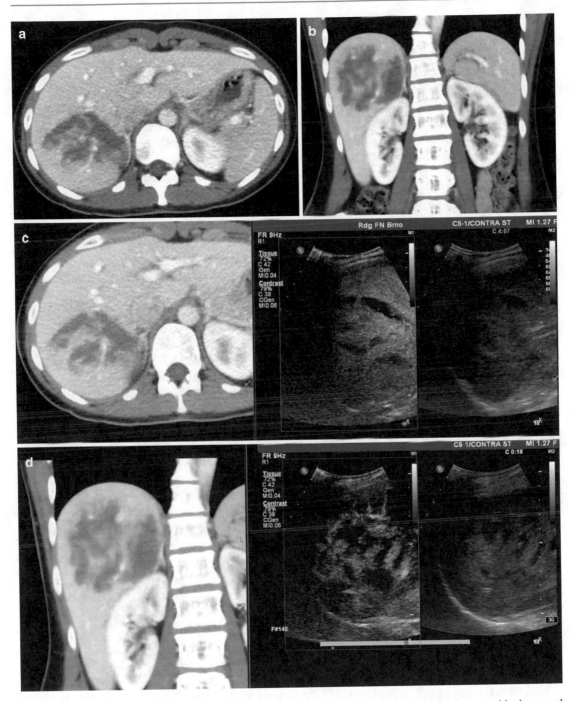

Fig. 8 (**a–d**) Lacerative contusion of the right hepatic lobe (**a**, **b**); note the correlative follow-up images with ultrasound and contrast-enhanced sonography (**c**, **d**)

3   Essential Findings

In emergency, radiologist plays an important role in making the diagnosis of hepatic traumatic lesions (Figs. 1, 2, 3, 4, 5, 6, 7, and 8). At the initial evaluation with ultrasound, the evidence of peritoneal free fluid, anechoic or corpusculated, as well as the visualization of any alteration in echogenicity of the abdominal organs and structures is basilar as a first step. The CT examination in case of supportive suspicion for liver trauma forms the basic examination eventually performed; even in all cases in which the clinical conditions and noted symptoms are directly suggestive for injury, this diagnostic tool represents the gold standard method. Mirvis classification (Mirvis et al. 1989) considers a grading of hepatic injuries varying from capsular avulsion, superficial laceration(s), subcapsular hematoma <1 cm and periportal tracking, and typical CT findings of grade 1 lesion to parenchymal fragmentation and devascularization of grade 5 hepatic injury. Whereas CT protocol could vary depending on the machine and equipment available at the institution, it should include back reconstructions with thickness <1 mm to allow an optimal multiplanar postprocessing and contrast-enhanced multiphase scans. Essential findings related to liver trauma that could be noted in the liver traumatic injuries are periportal tracking, contusion, subcapsular/central hematoma, streaking or complex lacerations, fragmentation, active hemorrhage, and avulsion of the vascular hepatic peduncle (Mirvis et al. 1989; Moore et al. 1989; Croce et al. 1991; Yoon et al. 2005). In traumatic injury of the liver, periportal tracking has been described as low attenuation density especially at the level of right hepatic lobe (63% of cases), due to evidence of blood in periportal tissue (Yokota and Sugjmoto 1994). In other cases, this finding is related to distension of periportal lymphatics and lymphedema associated with elevated central venous pressure produced by rapid expansion of intravascular volume during vigorous intravenous fluid resuscitation (Lawson et al. 1993; Cox et al. 1990; Lee Molina et al. 1998; Schanmuganathan et al. 1993). Contusion

appears at CT as a low hypodense area due to interstitial bleeding, with irregular margins, rarely appreciable as isolated finding and often associated to lacerations and hematomas (Romano et al. 2004). Hematomas are caused by bleeding into a tissue laceration and may present rounded margins; CT features are of hyperdense areas in unenhanced scans. Superficial lacerations usually cause a subcapsular hematoma, a very common hepatic traumatic lesion that appears as a biconvex collection imprinting the hepatic parenchyma (Romano et al. 2004). Laceration is a typical lesion that appears as a linear streaking area, single or multiple, interesting parenchymal areas contiguous to intrahepatic portal vascular branches and suprahepatic veins (Romano et al. 2004). Deeper lacerations present more frequent complications such as biliary duct involvement (bilomas, hemobilia) (Romano et al. 2004). In lacerations, the margins of the lesions are irregular and opened, with blood collection between edges (Romano et al. 2004). Multiple lacerations and fragmentation of the liver parenchyma as well as the avulsion of the vascular pedicle represent major traumatic lesions to the organ. The CT examination should be correctly and adequately performed from a technical point of view in order to support the emergency radiologist in detecting the presence of the active bleeding in liver trauma, allowing to visualize the site and the entity of the vascular damage in order to help clinicians to plan the patient management, if any interventional or surgical procedures should be done.

4   Considerations

In the traumatized patient, isolated hepatic lesions are rare and in a high percentage of cases, the involvement of other organs could be observed (Romano et al. 2004; Anderson and Ballinger 2006). The most voluminous part of liver parenchyma is represented by the right lobe, frequently the site of traumatic injuries (Romano et al. 2004). Moreover, the posterior-superior hepatic segments are close to fixed anatomical structures (ribs, spine) that may play an important role in determining the traumatic lesion (Romano et al. 2004); also the coronal ligament insertion in this parenchymal region may enhance the effect of acceleration-deceleration mechanism (Romano et al. 2004). Frequently associated lesions are the right costal fractures, right inferior pulmonary lobe laceration or contusion, hemothorax, pneumothorax, and renal and/or adrenal lesions (Shanmuganathan and Mirvis 1995; Romano et al. 2004). Traumatic lesions of left hepatic lobe are rare and usually associated with a direct impact on the superior abdomen, as it happens in the car crashes when the wheel causes a compressive effect on the thoracic and abdominal anatomical compartments (Romano et al. 2004; Shanmuganathan and Mirvis 1995). Associated lesions to left hepatic lobe injuries could be the sternal fractures and injuries to the pancreas, myocardium, or gastrointestinal tract (Romano et al. 2004). Lesions of the caudal lobe are uncommon, usually not isolated and associated with other major hepatic lesions (Romano et al. 2004). The institution of specialized trauma centers and the technical progress in the imaging methodology in the last couple of decades allowed a great reduction in mortality rate for traumas (Romano et al. 2004). Modern diagnostic methodologies contributed to reduce the number of negative laparotomies, improving the possibility of conservative treatment in numerous traumatic lesions (Romano et al. 2004). Computed tomography certainly represents a large impact on the diagnosis and management of patients with lesions from blunt abdominal traumas (Romano et al. 2004). Other kinds of traumatic injury such as the gunshot wounds to the liver have a high morbidity and mortality rate (Sachwani-Daswani et al. 2016): it has been reported that survivors should have a follow-up CT scan performed within 7 days, to allow detection and intervention for complications, as this seems to dramatically decrease the overall morbidity rate (Sachwani-Daswani et al. 2016). In case of surgically treated hepatic lesions from trauma, complications that could be observed are represented by fluid collections, hemorrhage, vascular disease, hematoma, abscesses, or intrahepatic biloma (Romano et al.

2005; Choudhary et al. 2011). If a biliary leak is suspected, MR cholangiopancreatography presents the added advantage of being able to localize the bile leak, which can help determine if endoscopic management could be sufficient or if a surgical management is requested (Melamud et al. 2014). Endoscopic retrograde cholangiopancreatography may provide a diagnostic confirmation and concurrent therapy when nonsurgical management is pursued (Melamud et al. 2014). Among all other diagnostic methods and procedures, the central role of the CT examination, from the initial assessment of the trauma to the follow-up control in case of suspected complications and not conclusive findings from other imaging methods, seems to be well established for a comprehensive evaluation of the liver parenchyma and associated abdominal findings.

References

Alagic Z, Eriksson A, Drageryd E et al (2017) A new low-dose multi-phase trauma CT protocol and its impact on diagnostic assessment and radiation dose in multi-trauma patients. Emerg Radiol 24(5):509–518

Anderson CB, Ballinger WF (2006) Abdominal injuries. In: Zuidema GD et al (eds) The management of trauma, 4th edn. Saunders, Philadelphia, PA

Aschoff AJ (2006) MDCT of the abdomen. Eur Radiol 16(Suppl 7):M54–M57

Badger SA, Barclay R, Campbell P et al (2009) Management of liver trauma. World J Surg 33:2522–2537

Beenen LF, Sierink JC, Kolkman S et al (2015) Split bolus technique in polytrauma: a prospective study on scan protocols for trauma analysis. Acta Radiol 56(7):873–880

Cagini L, Gravante S, Malaspina CM et al (2013) Contrast enhanced ultrasound (CEUS) in blunt abdominal trauma. Crit Ultrasound J 5(Suppl 1):S9

Catalano O, Lobianco R, Raso MM, Siani A (2005) Blunt hepatic trauma: evaluation with contrast-enhanced sonography: sonographic findings and clinical application. J Ultrasound Med 24(3):299–310

Choudhary N, Duseja A, Kalra N, Chawla Y (2011) Hepatobiliary and pancreatic: intrahepatic biloma after blunt abdominal trauma. J Gastroenterol Hepatol 26(8):1342

Clevert DA, Weckbach S, Minaifar N et al (2008) Contrast-enhanced ultrasound versus MS-CT in blunt abdominal trauma. Clin Hemorheol Microcirc 39(1–4):155–169

Cox JF, Friedman AC, Radecki PD, Lev-Toaff AS, Caroline DF (1990) Periportal lymphedema in trauma patients. AJR 154:1124–1125

Croce MA, Fabian TC, Kudsk KA, Baum SL, Payne LW, Mangiante LC, Britt LG (1991) AAST organ injury scale: correlation of CT graded liver injuries and operative findings. J Trauma 31(6):806–812

Delgado Millan MA, Deballon PO (2001) Computed tomography, angiography and endoscopic retrograde cholangiopancreatography in the management of hepatic and splenic trauma. World J Sur 25: 1397–1402

Dreizin D, Munera F (2012) Blunt polytrauma: evaluation with 64-section whole body CT angiography. Radiographics 32(3):609–632

Feliciano DV (1989) Surgery for liver trauma. Surg Clin North Am 69:273–284

Fodor M, Primavesi F, Morell-Hofert D et al (2018) Non-operative management of blunt hepatic and splenic injuries-practical aspects and value of radiological scoring systems. Eur Surg 50(6):285–298

Graves JA, Hanna TN, Herr KD (2017) Pearls and pitfalls of hepatobiliary and splenic trauma: what every trauma radiologist needs to know. Emerg Radiol 24(5):557–568

Kokabi N, Shuaib W, Xing M et al (2014) Intra-abdominal solid organ injuries: an enhanced management algorithm. Can Assoc Radiol J 65(4):301–309

Kutcher ME, Weis JJ, Siada SS (2015) The role of computed tomographic scan in ongoing triage of operative hepatic trauma: a Western Trauma Association multicenter retrospective study. J Trauma Acute Care Surg 79(6):951–956; discussion 956

Lawson TL, Thorsen MK, Erickson SJ, Perret RS, Quiroz FA, Foley WD (1993) Periportal halo: a CT sign of liver disease. Abdom Imaging 18(1):42–46

Lee Molina PL, Warshauer DM, Lee JKT (1998) Computed tomography of thoracoabdominal trauma: 1275–1341. In: Computed body tomography with MRI correlation, 3rd edn. Lippincott-Raven Press, Philadelphia, PA/NewYork

Long B, April MD, Summers S et al (2017) Whole body CT versus selective radiological imaging strategy in trauma: an evidence-based clinical review. Am J Emerg Med 35(9):1356–1362

Loupatatzis C, Schindera S, Gralla J et al (2008) Whole-body computed tomography for multiple traumas using a triphasic injection protocol. Eur Radiol 18(6):1206–1214

Mebert RV, Schnüriger B, Candinas D, Haltmeier T (2018) Follow-up imaging in patients with blunt splenic or hepatic injury managed nonoperatively. Am Surg 84(2):208–214

Melamud K, LeBedis CA, Anderson SW et al (2014) Biliary imaging: multimodality approach to imaging of biliary injuries and their complications. Radiographics 34(3):613–623

Mirvis SE, Whitley NO, Vainwright JR et al (1989) Blunt hepatic trauma in adults: CT-based classification and correlation with prognosis and treatment. Radiology 171(1):27–32

Moore EE, Moore FA (2010) American Association for the Surgery of Trauma Organ Injury Scaling: 50th anniversary review article of the journal of trauma. J Trauma 69(6):1600–1601

Moore EE, Shackford SR, Pachter HL, McAninch JW, Browner BD, Champion HR et al (1989) Organ injury scaling: spleen, liver, and kidney. J Trauma 29(12):1664–1666

Nicolaou S, Eftekhari A, Sedlic T et al (2008) The utilization of dual source CT in imaging of polytrauma. Eur J Radiol 68(3):398–408

Piper GL, Peitzman AB (2010) Current management of hepatic trauma. Surg Clin North Am 90(4): 775–785

Poletti PA, Wintermark M, Scchnyer P, Backer CD (2002) Traumatic injuries: role of imaging in the management of the polytrauma victim. Eur Radiol 12:969–978

Poletti PA, Platon A, Becker CD et al (2004) Blunt abdominal trauma: does the use of a second-generation sonographic contrast agent help to detect solid organ injuries? AJR Am J Roentgenol 183(5): 1293–1301

Raza M, Abbas Y, Devi V, Prasad KV, Rizk KN, Nair PP (2013) Non operative management of abdominal trauma—a 10 years review. World J Emerg Surg 8:14

Romano L, Giovine S, Guidi G et al (2004) Hepatic trauma: CT findings and considerations based on our experience in emergency diagnostic imaging. Eur J Rad 50(1):59–66

Romano S, Tortora G, Scaglione M et al (2005) MDCT imaging of post interventional liver: a pictorial essay. Eur J Radiol 53(3):425–432

Sachwani-Daswani G, Dombrowski A, Shetty PC, Carr JA (2016) The role of computed tomography in determining delayed intervention for gunshot wounds through the liver. Eur J Trauma Emerg Surg 42(2): 219–223

Schanmuganathan K, Mirvis SE, Amoroso M (1993) Periportal low density on CT in patient with blunt trauma: association with elevated venous pressure. AJR 160:279–283

Shanmuganathan K (2004) Multi-detector row CT imaging of blunt abdominal trauma. Semin Ultrasound CT MR 25(2):180–204

Shanmuganathan K, Mirvis SE (1995) CT evaluation of the liver with acute blunt trauma. Crit Rev Diagn Imaging 36:73–113

Shannon L, Peachey T, Skipper N et al (2015) Comparison of clinically suspected injuries with injuries detected at whole-body CT in suspected multi-trauma victims. Clin Radiol 70(11):1205–1211

Tarchouli M, Elabsi M, Njoumi N et al (2018) Liver trauma: What current management? Hepatobiliary Pancreatic Dis Int 17(1):39–44

Thorelius L (2004) Contrast-enhanced ultrasound in trauma. Eur Radiol 14(Suppl 8):P43–P52

Valentino M, De Luca C, Galloni SS et al (2010) Contrast-enhanced US evaluation in patients with blunt abdominal trauma. J Ultrasound 13(1):22–27

Wortman JR, Uyeda JW, Fulwadkva UP, Sodickson AD (2018) Dual energy CT for abdominal and pelvic trauma. Radiographics 38(2):586–602

Yaniv G, Portnoy O, Simon D et al (2013) Revised protocol for whole-body CT for multi-trauma patients applying triphasic injection followed by a single-pass scan on a 64-MDCT. Clin Radiol 68(7):668–675

Yokota J, Sugjmoto T (1994) Clinical significance of periportal tracking on computed tomographic scan in patients with blunt liver trauma. Am J Surg 168(3):247–250

Yoon W, Jeong YY, Kim JK et al (2005) CT in blunt liver trauma. Radiographics 25(1):87–104

Zhao DW, Tian M, Zhang LT et al (2017) Effectiveness of contrast-enhanced ultrasound and serum liver cnzyme measurement in detection and classification of blunt liver trauma. J Int Med Res 45(1):170–181

Non-tumoral Pathology of the Intrahepatic Biliary Tract

Jelena Kovač

Contents

J. Kovač (✉)
Center for Radiology and Magnetic Resonance
Imaging, Clinical Center of Serbia, Belgrade, Serbia

© Springer Nature Switzerland AG 2021
E. Quaia (ed.), *Imaging of the Liver and Intra-hepatic Biliary Tract,*
Medical Radiology, Diagnostic Imaging, https://doi.org/10.1007/978-3-030-38983-3_18

Abstract

Cholestatic liver diseases include a wide variety of entities, characterized by impaired hepatobiliary production and excretion of bile, leading to cholestasis. Primary biliary cirrhosis (PBC) and primary sclerosing cholangitis (PSC) are the two most common chronic cholestatic liver diseases, caused by immune-mediated cholangiocytes injury, through a complex interaction with environmental factors. PBC is characterized by small bile duct lymphocytic cholangitis occurring mainly in women, with a good response to ursodeoxycholic acid. PSC is characterized by inflammation, fibrosis, and stricture of the large bile ducts, affecting young men, still without effective therapy. Besides PBC and PSC, cholestatic liver diseases include also secondary sclerosing cholangitis with identifiable causes of bile duct injury. Secondary sclerosing cholangitis is large group of diseases which include immunoglobulin G4-related sclerosing disease, recurrent pyogenic cholangitis, ischemic cholangitis, acquired immunodeficiency syndrome-related cholangitis, and eosinophilic cholangitis. In addition to clinical and laboratory findings, the recognition of typical imaging features on computed tomography and magnetic resonance (MR) imaging with MR cholangiography is essential for differential diagnosis among cholestatic liver diseases.

1   Introduction

Cholestatic liver diseases include a wide variety of entities, characterized by impaired hepatobiliary production and excretion of bile, leading to cholestasis. Primary biliary cirrhosis (PBC) and primary sclerosing cholangitis (PSC) are the two most common chronic cholestatic liver diseases, caused by immune-mediated cholangiocyte injury, through a complex interaction with environmental factors (Hirschfield et al. 2010). PBC is characterized by small bile duct lymphocytic cholangitis mainly in women, and has a good response to ursodeoxycholic acid (UDCA). On the other hand, classic PSC is a large duct cholangiopathy affecting young men, still without effective therapy (Hirschfield et al. 2009). Ultimately, both diseases result in biliary fibrosis, cirrhosis, and hepatic failure.

Unlike PSC, where exact etiopathogenesis is still not known, secondary sclerosing cholangitis (SSC) is a group of chronic cholestatic disorders, which are clinically and radiologically similar to PSC, but have an identifiable underlying pathologic cause (Abdalian and Heathcote 2006). In contrast to PSC, a known pathologic process in secondary sclerosing cholangitis leads to inflammation, obliterative fibrosis of the bile ducts, stricture formation, progressive destruction of the intrahepatic bile ducts, and at the end biliary cirrhosis (Gossard et al. 2005). The most common causes underlying SSC are immunologic, infective, obstructive, and ischemic processes (Abdalian and Heathcote 2006). Although these different entities present with similar symptoms, the prognosis and clinical outcome are quite different (Abdalian and Heathcote 2006). Thus, acquired immune deficiency syndrome (AIDS) cholangiopathy and sclerosing cholangitis in critically ill patients are associated with poor prognosis, while IgG4-related sclerosing cholangitis shows good response to steroids, and a favorable prognosis (Imam et al. 2013). In the appropriate clinical setting, imaging findings are usually sufficient for accurate diagnosis.

2 Primary Biliary Cirrhosis

PBC is a slowly progressive cholestatic liver disease, with immune-mediated destruction of small intrahepatic bile ducts, leading to chronic cholestasis and cirrhosis (Trivedi and Hirschfield 2016). It usually occurs in middle-aged women, with prevalence ranging from 1.9 to 40.2 per 100,000 people (Kaplan and Gershwin 2005). Although causes and underlying pathophysiology are not clearly understood, it is stated that environmental factors trigger autoimmune response in genetically susceptible individuals (Trivedi and Hirschfield 2016). The association of PBC and high titer of circulating anti-mitochondrial antibodies (AMA) has been shown in the majority of patients. Moreover, coexistence with other autoimmune diseases has been observed in 33% of patients (Jones 2007). PBC is characterized by chronic, nonsuppurative, lymphocytic cholangitis that predominantly affects small, interlobular bile ducts in the portal triads leading to vanishing bile duct syndrome (Crosignani et al. 2008). It develops slowly, through four stages, with only periportal inflammation in stage 1. There is focal destruction of small septal and interlobular bile ducts, leading to ductopenia in stage 2. The fibrous septa formation connecting the adjacent portal triads (bridging fibrosis) is a predominant feature in stage III, whereas micro- or macronodular cirrhosis is evident in stage 4 (Ludwig et al. 1978).

2.1 Diagnosis and Imaging Findings

The diagnosis of PBC is usually based on a combination of clinical findings, cholestatic biochemical pattern persisting for more than 6 months, and presence of detectable AMA in serum (Nguyen et al. 2010). Liver biopsy is considered the standard reference procedure for grading of liver fibrosis, but it is not routinely required for PBC diagnosis, except in AMA-negative patients (Bizzaro et al. 2012). Currently, there are also noninvasive methods for the assessment of liver fibrosis, such as transient elastography (TE) and magnetic resonance imaging (MRI) including diffusion-weighted imaging (DWI)

(Kovač et al. 2012a, b; Corpechot et al. 2006). These methods allow whole-liver examination, as well as repetitive measurements for monitoring disease progression and treatment response (Kovač et al. 2012a, b; Corpechot et al. 2006). However, the main role of MRI is in long-term follow-up, with early detection of complications such as hepatocellular carcinoma (HCC) and portal hypertension (Kobayashi et al. 2005).

Even though the end stage of all chronic liver diseases is cirrhosis, there are some MRI features which favor the diagnosis of PBC. T2-weighted periportal hyperintensity is frequently seen in PBC patients, as it has been reported in 87% in early stage and 66.7% in advanced stages of disease (Fig. 1a) (Kovač et al. 2012a, b). This sign represents periportal edema, inflammatory cell infiltration, and dilatation of lymph vessels in portal triads (Kobayashi et al. 2005; Kovač et al. 2012a, b). However, while periportal hyperintensity occurs also in other inflammatory liver conditions, "periportal halo sign" is considered a pathognomonic MRI feature for PBC. It is seen as an area of hypointensity on both T1- and T2-weighted MR images, 5 mm–1 cm in size, around portal venous branches, without mass effect (Fig. 1b) (Wenzel et al. 2001). This sign is most commonly observed in advanced disease, as a result of fibrous tissue deposition, and hepatocellular parenchymal extinction around the portal triads (Kovač et al. 2012a, b; Wenzel et al. 2001). However, due to the inhomogeneous distribution of liver fibrosis, both periportal hyperintensity and periportal halo signs could be seen in the same patient (Kovač et al. 2012a, b). Abdominal lymphadenopathy (enlarged lymph nodes in porta hepatis, gastrohepatic ligament, and upper retroperitoneal space) is a frequent finding in PBC patients, observed in up to 88% of cases of all histological stages (Blachar et al. 2001). Concerning morphological liver changes, diffuse hepatomegaly is the most common pattern, which can also be found in the end-stage disease (Haliloglu et al. 2009). Patients with PBC usually develop micronodular or lacelike fibrosis, as was observed in the study by Ito et al. (Fig. 2a) (Ito et al. 2002).

Magnetic resonance cholangiopancreatography (MRCP) findings in PBC patients are not characteristic, and could be normal in the early

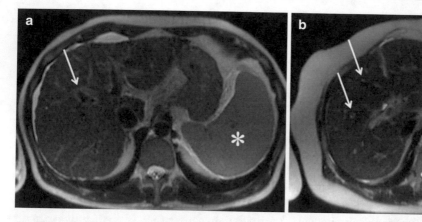

Fig. 1 Primary biliary cirrhosis. (**a**) Axial T2-weighted image shows periportal hyperintensity around medium-sized portal triads (*solid arrow*). (**b**) Axial T2-weighted image in another patient shows periportal halo sign as hypointense areas around portal veins (*solid arrow*). Note also splenomegaly (*asterisks*) (**a, b**)

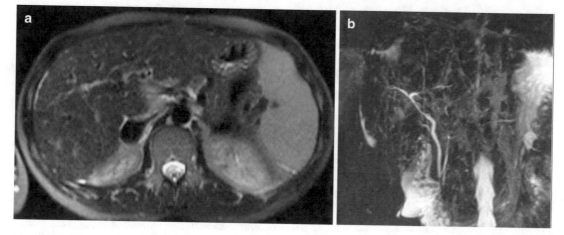

Fig. 2 MRI findings in a 58-year-old woman with primary biliary cirrhosis. (**a**) Axial T2-weighted image shows lacelike fibrosis in end-stage liver PBC. (**b**) MRCP in the same patient shows reduction and obliteration of peripheral intrahepatic ducts as a sign of vanishing bile duct syndrome

stage of disease. With disease progression, reduction of peripheral intrahepatic bile ducts is seen, together with decrease in the caliber of medium-size bile ducts, leading to vanishing bile duct syndrome (Fig. 2b) (Reau and Jensen 2008). Although MRCP is not a necessary diagnostic procedure for PBC patients, it can help in the differential diagnosis from PSC, since clinically both entities show chronic cholestatic features.

2.2 Complications

The signs of portal hypertension (ascites, splenomegaly, portosystemic collaterals, and portal vein thrombosis) are a frequent finding in PBC, since portal hypertension occurs early in the course of disease (Kobayashi et al. 2005). In addition, patients with PBC may present with severe splenomegaly even in noncirrhotic stage of disease, probably due to immunological disorders and prolonged portal hypertension (Terayama et al. 1994).

Hepatocellular carcinoma (HCC) in PBC is rare, with male predominance in end-stage disease. The high incidence of HCC in male PBC patients could be explained by common comorbidities like alcoholism, smoking, and viral hepatitis (Rong et al. 2015). As far as the development of HCC is concerned, all PBC patients who have reached stage IV disease should undergo regular surveillance, like other cirrhotic patients according to published guidelines for the HCC management (Shibuya et al. 2002).

2.3 Treatment of Primary Biliary Cirrhosis

PBC is a slowly progressive disease that advances variably among individuals and can span over several decades (Carey et al. 2015; Lindor et al. 2009). Without effective therapy, the disease progresses to cirrhosis in 4–6 years (Lindor et al. 2009). Currently, the primary pharmacotherapy for PBC is UDCA which demonstrates anti-cholestatic and anti-fibrotic effects. UDCA delays or even prevents the need for transplantation, and improves 10-year survival (Pares et al. 2006). Patients who respond have laboratory improvement within 6–9 months (Lammert et al. 2014). Incomplete biochemical response to UDCA is seen in about 40% of patients, and these patients have a higher risk for disease progression (Lammert et al. 2014). Liver transplantation remains the only definite treatment for patients with advanced PBC. One-, 5-, and 10-year survival rates for PBC in Europe are 86%, 80%, and 72%, respectively, which are higher than those for patients transplanted for hepatitis B, hepatitis C, alcoholic cirrhosis, or other autoimmune liver diseases (MacQuillan and Neuberger 2003). Recurrence of PBC after liver transplantation has been described in 9–30% of patients, with usually a mild course under immunosuppressive treatment (Silveira et al. 2010).

3 Primary Sclerosing Cholangitis

PSC is a chronic inflammatory cholestatic disease, characterized by affection of large bile ducts (Lewin et al. 2009; Eksteen 2016; Hirschfield et al. 2013; Cullen et al. 2001). PSC typically occurs in young and middle-aged men

with an age of onset of 30–40 years (male-to-female ratio of 2:1) (Lewin et al. 2009). A strong association exists between PSC and inflammatory bowel disease (IBD) (Eksteen 2016). Approximately 70–80% of patients with PSC develop IBD during their life, of which 87% have ulcerative colitis and 13% have Crohn's disease, whereas the incidence of PSC in IBD patients is 4% (Eksteen 2016). PSC is a slowly progressive disease leading to biliary cirrhosis. The long-standing PSC is associated with serious complications, like development of dominant bile duct strictures, recurrent cholangitis, and disease-associated malignancies, including cholangiocarcinoma (Hirschfield et al. 2013).

Although the exact etiopathogenesis of PSC is still not known, it is postulated that complex interaction of different autoimmune, genetic, and environmental factors is responsible for changes in PSC (Cullen and Chapman 2001). There is a 100-fold increased risk for developing PSC in first-degree relatives and siblings, indicating the important role of genetic factors (Cullen and Chapman 2001). Association of PSC with other autoimmune-related diseases, elevated serum levels of immunoglobulins, and circulating immune complexes is highly suggestive of the major role of autoimmunity in the pathogenesis of PSC. Histologically, medium- and large-size bile ducts are damaged with typical concentric periductal fibrosis (onion skinning) and minimal inflammatory cells (Grant et al. 2002). Nevertheless, this finding is observed in <20% of patients, and may also be found in secondary sclerosing cholangitis (Ludwig et al. 1978). Therefore, liver biopsy is not sufficient for PSC diagnosis and must be evaluated in combination with clinical and radiological findings.

3.1 Diagnosis and Imaging Features

The diagnosis of PSC is made on the basis of clinical, biochemical, and cholangiographic findings (Gotthardt et al. 2011). Sclerosing cholangitis can be called "primary" only in cases when there is no previous history of bile duct surgery (except simple cholecystectomy) and/or choledocholithiasis, before the development of symptoms. PSC might be discovered in asymptomatic patients during routine examination, after detection of cholestatic laboratory findings with alkaline phosphatase levels more than three times higher than normal. Both the American Association for the Study of Liver Diseases and European Association of the Study of the Liver guidelines recommend MRCP as the first-line modality for investigating bile duct abnormalities in clinically suspected cases (Chapman et al. 2010; European Association for the Study of the Liver 2009). MRCP has high sensitivity and specificity, reaching 88% and 99%, respectively (Dave et al. 2010). In contrast to MRCP, endoscopic retrograde cholangiopancreatography (ERCP) is at the same time a therapeutic procedure with balloon dilatation or stenting possibilities, but with postprocedural complications ranging from 3 to 8%. Currently, ERCP is recommended when there is clinical suspicion with negative or nondiagnostic MRCP findings (Cohen et al. 1996). Liver biopsy is not a necessary procedure for the diagnosis of PSC, except when the small bile duct type of PSC is suspected. This rare variant accounts for 5% of all PSC, and

yields better prognosis (Björnsson et al. 2008). This diagnosis should be suspected when a patient with IBD presents with cholestatic disease, but shows normal cholangiogram and a negative antimitochondrial antibody profile (Björnsson et al. 2008).

The most common cholangiographic findings in PSC are diffuse, multifocal band-like strictures, alternating with normal or mildly dilated ducts, giving rise to a "beaded" appearance (Fig. 3). Both intrahepatic and extrahepatic bile duct involvement is the most common finding, seen in 75% of patients. Isolated intrahepatic bile duct involvement is observed in 15% of patients, while only extrahepatic bile duct manifestation is the least common pattern (10% of cases) (Tischendorf et al. 2007). Occasionally, strictures and a slight dilatation might also be seen in the main pancreatic duct and cystic duct. As the disease progresses, and strictures worsen, small peripheral ducts can become completely obliterated, showing a "pruned-tree" appearance (Fig. 4) (Bader et al. 2003). In addition, the angles among peripheral and central bile ducts become obtuse. The most important finding suggestive of PSC is subtle duct dilatation, although there are many strictures (Kovač et al.

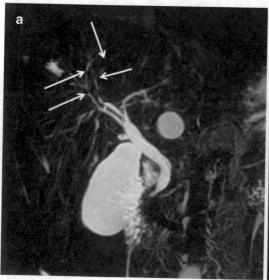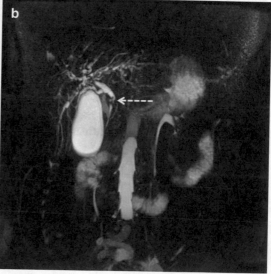

Fig. 3 Primary sclerosing cholangitis. (**a**) MRCP shows multiple short band-like strictures and slight luminal dilatation in a 35-year-old man (*solid arrows*). (**b**) PSC in another 36-year-old patient reveals classical "beaded appearance" of bile ducts—multiple short segmental and annular strictures with slightly dilated bile ducts in between. Note also the stricture of the middle third of common bile duct (*dotted arrow*)

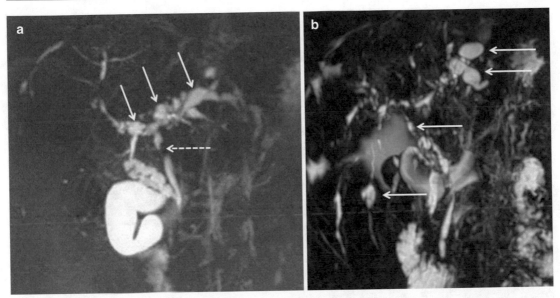

Fig. 4 Advanced primary sclerosing cholangitis. (**a**) MRCP shows obliterated peripheral bile ducts resulting in "pruned-tree" appearance and multiple diverticular outpouchings (*solid arrows*). Note also the stricture of the common hepatic duct (*dotted arrow*). (**b**) MRCP in 44-year-old patient with primary sclerosing cholangitis shows very irregular bile ducts and multiple strictures in combination with diverticular biliary dilatation (*solid arrows*)

2013). The possible explanation is the fact that periductal inflammation and fibrosis prevent significant dilatation (Hirschfield et al. 2013). Development of prominent proximal biliary dilatation must raise suspicion of other processes, like bacterial cholangitis or cholangiocellular carcinoma. Another characteristic finding in PSC is diverticular outpouchings, seen in up to 27% of cases (Fig. 4) (Ito et al. 1999). Less frequent cholangiographic features include webs and pigmented stones (Ito et al. 1999). Webs are defined as focal 1–2 mm thick area of incomplete circumferential narrowing.

Besides ductal changes, computed tomography (CT) and MRI also show associated parenchymal liver changes in PSC. Spherical liver shape, observed due to caudate lobe hypertrophy and left lateral and right posterior segment atrophy, is considered pathognomonic for PSC (Fig. 5a) (Ito et al. 1999; Düşünceli et al. 2005). The most common type of liver cirrhosis in PSC patients is macronodular cirrhosis, with large regenerative nodules usually located in central liver parts. A wedge-shaped or reticular heterogeneous area of increased T2-weighted signal intensity, with peripheral distribution, is also commonly seen in PSC patients (Fig. 5a) (Revelon et al. 1999). Frequently, these areas show increased enhancement on arterial phase contrast-enhanced MR (Fig. 5b), which persists on delayed phases in a patchy or segmental pattern (Fig. 5c). These findings could be explained by vascular or lymphatic drainage impairment, caused by periductal inflammation of segmental bile ducts and parenchymal edema. Hilar lymphadenopathy can be detected in up to 33% of PSC patients (Ito et al. 1999). In addition, periportal hyperintensity representing edema and inflammation in periportal space is commonly present (Bader et al. 2003; Kovač et al. 2013; Ito et al. 1999). Nevertheless, these findings are not specific for PSC but are also seen in cirrhosis of other etiologies.

3.2 Differential Diagnosis

Differential diagnosis of PSC includes IgG4-sclerosing cholangitis (IgG4-SC), ischemic cholangitis, and AIDS cholangitis (Hirschfield et al. 2013; Gotthardt et al. 2011; Chapman et al. 2010). Younger age, association with IBD,

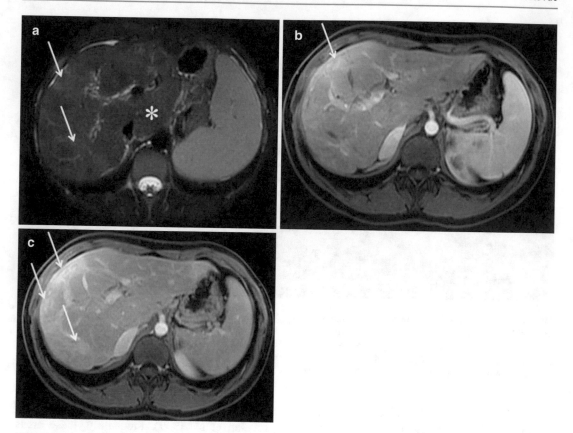

Fig. 5 Primary sclerosing cholangitis in 44-year-old man. (**a**) Axial T2-weighted image shows increased signal in peripheral, atrophic regions in the right liver lobe, corresponding to areas of parenchymal inflammation, and increased water content (*solid arrows*). Note also the enlarged caudate lobe (*asterisks*). Axial T1-weighted image in the same patient obtained after intravenous administration of gadolinium chelates during arterial (**b**) and portal venous phase (**c**) shows increased and persistent enhancement of peripheral areas of liver representing intrahepatic perfusion abnormalities (*solid arrows*)

characteristic cholangiographic findings of band-like strictures, a beaded or "pruned-tree" appearance, and diverticulum-like outpouchings favor the diagnosis of PSC (Bader et al. 2003). In contrast, long segmental strictures with prestenotic dilation and strictures of the lower common bile duct are significantly more common in IgG4-SC (Tokala et al. 2014). Additionally, IgG4-SC occurs mostly in elderly men and is associated with autoimmune pancreatitis in majority of patients (Zen and Nakanuma 2012). In cases where papillary stenosis is prominent, AIDS cholangitis should be suspected (Devarbhavi et al. 2010). Ischemic cholangitis is usually characterized with strictures of middle third of common bile duct and hilar part of biliary tree (Azizi

et al. 2012). Differential diagnosis among PSC and ischemic cholangitis is possible on the basis of imaging features compatible with ischemic injury and evidence of a compromised arterial supply.

Infiltrative processes such as histiocytosis X, sarcoidosis, amyloidosis, cirrhosis, and metastatic liver disease can mimic cholangiographic features of PSC (Azizi et al. 2012). In these conditions, compression of nodules or multiple focal lesions on bile ducts creates cholangiographic appearance similar to PSC (Katabathina et al. 2014). However, characteristic MR findings on conventional sequences in abovementioned conditions are usually sufficient for differential diagnosis with PSC.

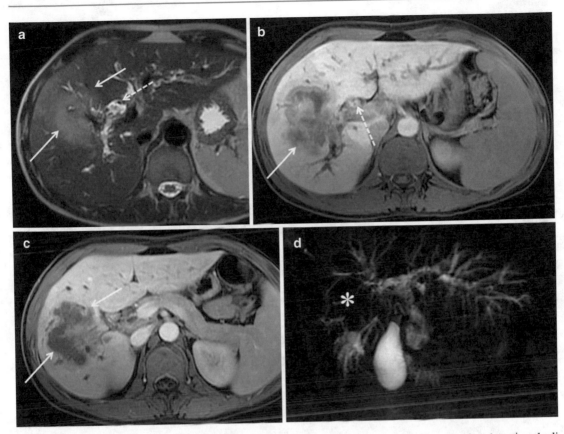

Fig. 6 Cholangiocellular carcinoma complicating long-standing primary sclerosing cholangitis in a 52-year-old male patient. (**a**) Axial T2-weighted image shows large irregular moderately hyperintense mass in right liver (*solid arrows*). Bile ducts are irregularly dilatated in both lobes due to primary disease. Multiple intrahepatic calculi are also present (*dotted arrows*). (**b**) Axial T1-weighted fat-saturated image shows hypointense mass with central necrotic part (*solid arrow*). Note also intrahepatic calculi as hyperintense lesions in dilated bile ducts (*dotted arrow*). (**c**) On portal venous phase T1-weighted fat-saturated image tumor is seen as hypovascular centrally necrotic lesion (*solid arrows*). (**d**) Thick-slab MRCP demonstrates multifocal alternating strictures of intrahepatic bile ducts with loss of bile duct visualization in segment V corresponding to tumor infiltration (*asterisks*)

3.3 Complications

Cholangiocellular carcinoma (CCC) is the most serious complication of long-standing PSC, present in up to 10–15% of patients (Claessen et al. 2009). The tumor is usually seen as an ill-defined hypovascular mass with progressive delayed enhancement on imaging (Fig. 6) (Abbas and Lindor 2009). Nevertheless, the findings could be more subtle when there is no identifiable mass. In such cases, stricture with prominent wall thickening, in association with marked proximal biliary dilatation, is suggestive of CCC (Abbas and Lindor 2009). In this regard, MRI should be routinely performed, since it is superior to CT in detecting small hilar and intrahepatic periductal growing tumors. In order to detect CCC at early stage, regular screening of PSC patients is proposed with CA 19–9 measurements every 6 months, and MRCP every year. The elevation of CA 19–9 has high diagnostic accuracy, with the sensitivity of 75% and specificity of 80% for a cutoff value of 100 U/ml, but normal levels do not exclude the diagnosis (Bonato et al. 2015). If the symptoms in PSC patient worsen at sudden with cholestasis and weight loss, CCC should be suspected. Unfortunately, development of CCC in the setting of PSC has a very poor prognosis, even after resection or liver transplantation, with 3-year survival ranging from 0% to 39% (Abbas

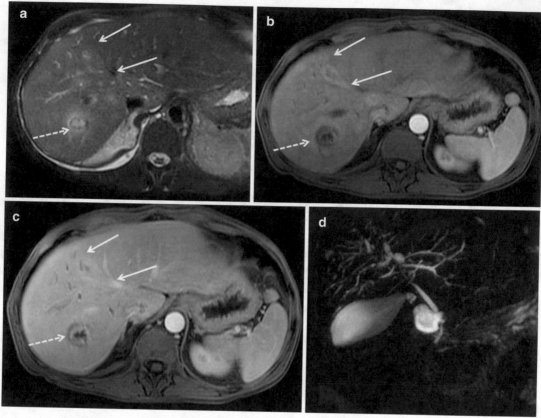

Fig. 7 Primary sclerosing cholangitis in 55-year-old man complicated with acute bacterial cholangitis. (**a**) Axial T2-weighted fat-saturated image shows slight parenchymal hyperintensity of right lobe (*solid arrows*) in association with abscess in segment VII (*dotted arrow*). Arterial (**b**) and portal venous phases (**c**) demonstrate perfusion abnormalities in affected segments (*solid arrows*), slight biliary dilatation, and hypointense lesion with thick wall corresponding to liver abscess (*dotted arrows*). (**d**) MRCP in the same patient reveals multiple short segmental strictures with slight luminal dilatation between creating characteristic cholangiographic findings for PSC

and Lindor 2009; Bonato et al. 2015). Moreover, CCC has a marked tendency to recur.

In long-standing PSC acute ascending cholangitis can occur as a complication of bile stasis, and superimposed biliary sepsis (Fig. 7) (Azizi et al. 2012).

3.4 Treatment of Primary Sclerosing Cholangitis

Medical therapy for PSC, including ursodeoxycholic acid, corticosteroids, and immune therapy, usually has only limited value (Yimam and Bowlus 2014). Liver transplantation remains the only curative treatment approach for patients with end-stage PSC, with 5-year posttransplant survival of 75–85% (Cullen and Chapman 2006). Recurrence of PSC occurs in up to 25% of patients, with follow-up period of 5–10 years after liver transplantation (Chapman et al. 2010). The diagnosis of recurrent PSC after liver transplantation is challenging, since there are a variety of causes responsible for posttransplant biliary strictures, including ischemia, rejection, allograft reperfusion injury, recurrent biliary sepsis, ABO incompatibility, or technically flawed biliary reconstruction (Gautam et al. 2006; Vera et al. 2002). The diagnosis of recurrent PSC is possible only in case of detecting non-anastomotic stricture occurring 3 months after liver transplantation, with confirmed PSC diagnosis in the native liver, and after exclusion of all other causes of biliary strictures (Fig. 8) (Brandsaeter et al. 2005;

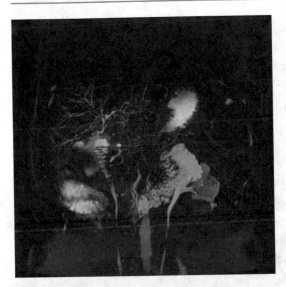

Fig. 8 Recurrent primary sclerosing cholangitis in a 43-year-old patient 3 years after liver transplantation. Thick-slab MRCP demonstrates multiple diffuse segmental bile duct strictures with moderate luminal dilatation

Campsen et al. 2008). Nevertheless, differential diagnosis among chronic rejection and recurrence is still challenging. In this regard, certain imaging features have been previously described (Sheng et al. 1996). In patients with recurrent PSC, liver is enlarged with slightly nodular contour, while in chronic rejection it is usually normal in size. Additionally, MRCP in recurrent disease reveals multiple non-anastomotic strictures with slightly dilated bile ducts among them, while cholangiogram in patients with chronic rejection depicts pruning of the peripheral biliary tree due to peripheral arterial insufficiency and chronic ischemia (Sheng et al. 1996). Hilar lymphadenopathy could be seen in recurrent PSC similar to native PSC, while it is uncommon in chronic rejection (Sheng et al. 1996). Liver biopsy is suggested in cases where noninvasive differential diagnosis cannot be made.

4 IgG4-Related Sclerosing Cholangitis

IgG4-related sclerosing cholangitis is the biliary manifestation of IgG4-related systemic disease (IgG4-RD), characterized histologically by abundant lymphoplasmacytic infiltration, storiform interstitial fibrosis, and obliterative phlebitis (Bjornsson et al. 2007; Zen and Nakanuma 2012). IgG4-SC typically occurs in men in their 60s or older, with a male-to-female ratio of approximately 4:1 (Bjornsson et al. 2007). In the majority of patients, IgG4 cholangiopathy is associated with type 1 autoimmune pancreatitis (AIP), while other organs can also be involved (Stone et al. 2012; Kamisawa et al. 2015).

4.1 Diagnosis and Imaging Features

Patients with IgG4-SC present with obstructive jaundice, since hilar and intrapancreatic parts of common bile duct are most commonly affected (Okazaki et al. 2014; Bjornsson et al. 2007). Other nonspecific symptoms such as abdominal pain, pruritus, and fatigue are also frequently seen (Okazaki et al. 2014). Ultrasound evaluation usually shows only bile duct dilatation without identifiable cause of obstruction (Zen and Nakanuma 2012). Further CT and MRI demonstrate symmetric, marked thickening of the bile duct wall (mean wall thickness, 4.9 mm), and narrowed but usually visible lumen, without vascular invasion (Fig. 9) (Itoh et al. 2009; Kim et al. 2007). According to the location of the strictures, cholangiographic findings in IgG4-SC could be divided into four types (Tokala et al. 2014; Nakazawa et al. 2006). Type 1 includes isolated stricture of the lower common bile duct, and it should be differentiated from chronic pancreatitis, pancreatic carcinoma, and extrahepatic cholangiocarcinoma. This type of IgG4-SC is most commonly associated with AIP, whereas isolated manifestation is extremely rare (Tokala et al. 2014). Type 2 refers to cases with diffusely distributed strictures within intrahepatic and extrahepatic bile ducts, and should be distinguished from PSC. This type is further divided into two subtypes: type 2a, characterized by a narrowing of the intrahepatic bile ducts in association with prestenotic dilation, and type 2b, characterized by strictures of the intrahepatic bile ducts without prestenotic dilation (Nakazawa et al. 2006). Type 3 involves the hilar region and the lower part of the common bile duct (Nakazawa et al. 2006). In

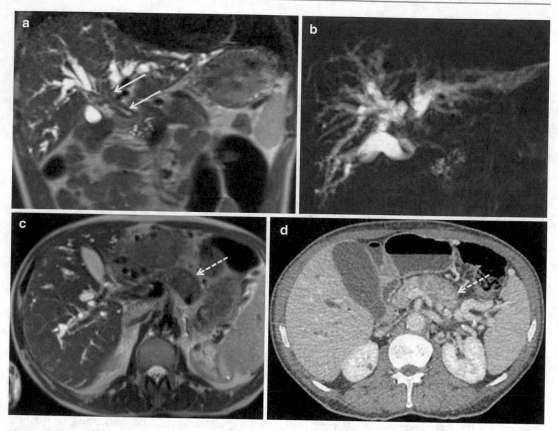

Fig. 9 IgG4-related SC in a 69-year-old male. (**a**) Coronal T2-weighted image shows circumferential wall thickening of common hepatic duct, primary biliary hepatic confluence, and distal parts of both hepatic ducts (*solid arrows*). (**b**) MR cholangiography shows focal stricture in the hilar region with subsequent diffuse biliary dilatation. (**c**) Axial T2-weighted image in the same patient reveals segmental pancreatic enlargement with a slight hypointense rim consistent with pseudocapsule (*dotted arrow*). (**d**) Axial CT examination at the same level as on **C** shows enlargement of pancreatic body with heterogeneous enhancement in portal venous phase, findings highly suggestive of autoimmune pancreatitis (*dotted arrow*)

type 4 strictures are seen only in the hilar region and should be differentiated from hilar cholangiocarcinoma (Nakazawa et al. 2006). While type 1 is almost exclusively seen in association with autoimmune pancreatitis, proximal IgG4-SC including type 2, 3, and 4 may occur either isolated or in association with pancreatitis (Zen et al. 2004). Most patients with isolated IgG4-SC have IgG4-RD in other organs outside the pancreatobiliary system, suggesting that true isolated cholangiopathy is exceptionally rare (Kamisawa et al. 2009).

There are several proposed sets of diagnostic criteria for IgG4-SC, in order to facilitate differential diagnosis from other more common diseases, such as pancreatic adenocarcinoma, PSC, and cholangiocarcinoma (Ohara et al. 2012; Chari et al. 2006). These criteria are based on a combination of clinical, biochemical, radiological, and histomorphological findings, together with multiple organ involvement and response to corticosteroid therapy. In 2012, Japanese authors proposed clinical diagnostic criteria for IgG4-SC (Ohara et al. 2012). According to these recommendations the diagnosis of IgG4-SC is based on the combination of the following four criteria: (1) characteristic biliary imaging findings, (2) elevation of serum IgG4 concentrations, (3) coexistence of IgG4-related diseases apart from those of the biliary tract, and (4) typical histopathological features. Optional criterium is responsiveness to short-term corticosteroid therapy. If characteristic cholangiographic findings are present in association with signs of

IgG4-RD in other organs, the diagnosis of IgG4-SC is straightforward. On the other hand, if characteristic biliary imaging findings are found in combination with elevated serum IgG4 levels, without evidence of other IgG4-RD manifestations, further histopathological confirmation is required. The diagnosis of IgG4-SC is probable if two first criteria are fulfilled together with response to corticosteroid therapy, and possible if only biliary imaging findings and elevated serum IgG4 level are present. Similarly to previously established HISORt criteria for AIP, the HISORt criteria for the diagnosis of IgG4-SC are based on histological findings, imaging, serological examination, other organ involvement, and response to steroid therapy (Chari et al. 2006).

Elevation of serum IgG4 level, with a cutoff value of 135 or 140 mg/dl, is the most sensitive and specific noninvasive examination test for the diagnosis of IgG4-SC (Oseini et al. 2011). It has previously been shown that elevated IgG4 levels were present in approximately 80% of patients with IgG4-SC (Oseini et al. 2011). However, it should be kept in mind that IgG4 may also be elevated in 10% of patients with PSC and in 15% of patients with cholangiocarcinoma (Mendes et al. 2006; Ngwa et al. 2014). The use of twofold higher cutoff value (270 or 280 mg/dl) can increase specificity to more than 90%, but with reduced sensitivity (Oseini et al. 2011).

4.2 Differential Diagnosis

The differential diagnosis between IgG4-SC, hilar cholangiocarcinoma, and extrahepatic cholangiocarcinoma could be very difficult (Sivakumaran et al. 2014). Irregular margins of stenotic area, asymmetric prominent wall thickening with obliteration of the lumen, and abrupt transition between dilated and stenotic bile ducts are findings which favor cholangiocarcinoma over IgG4 cholangiopathy (Itoh et al. 2009; Park et al. 2004). Nevertheless, it can be very hard to find all these slight differences at the site of the stricture. Thus, it is very important to carefully examine all other organs which are frequently involved in IgG4-RD, such as pancreas, kidneys,

and retroperitoneum (Stone et al. 2012). In this regard, pancreatic abnormalities suggestive of autoimmune pancreatitis (diffuse or segmental enlargement, a capsule-like rim around the pancreas, signal intensity abnormalities, abnormal enhancement), retroperitoneal fibrosis, periaortitis, or multiple hypodense kidney lesions strongly suggest the diagnosis of IgG4-SC (Kamisawa et al. 2009). In addition, if elevated serum IgG4 level is present the diagnosis of IgG4-SC is straightforward. However, in the absence of signs of IgG4-RD in other organs, an isolated diagnosis of IgG4-SC can be very challenging (Hart et al. 2013; Matsubayashi et al. 2014). In cases where no definite diagnosis can be made, a short-term (2–4 weeks) treatment with corticosteroids was shown to be helpful, without negative consequences for resectability in case the stricture turns out to be malignant (Moon et al. 2008).

It is of great clinical importance to differentiate IgG4-SC from PSC, since IgG4-SC can be treated with steroids leading to dramatic improvement. Unlike PSC, IgG4-SC often occurs in elderly men (>60 years old), has no clear association with inflammatory bowel disease, and is frequently associated with findings suggestive of autoimmune pancreatitis (Nishino et al. 2007). While in PSC disease progresses slowly with late onset of symptoms, IgG4-SC tends to be more symptomatic at the time of diagnosis. Furthermore, MRCP findings of multiple short band-like strictures affecting whole biliary tree, creating beaded and "pruned-tree" appearance, are diagnostic for PSC (Gardner et al. 2015). On the other hand, long and continuous biliary ductal disease, gallbladder involvement, and biliary wall thickening >2.5 mm are more suggestive of IgG4-SC (Tokala et al. 2014; Gardner et al. 2015). Lymphadenopathy is a nonspecific finding, since it can occur in both IgG4-SC and PSC.

4.3 Treatment of IgG4-Sclerosing Cholangitis

The mainstay of treatment of IgG4-SC is an immunosuppressive therapy with high-dose steroids (prednisone at a dose of 30–40 mg per day), which generally leads to rapid and consistent disease remission (Ghazale et al. 2008; Zen et al. 2016). After successful induction of remission and tapering period of 1 month (typically 5 mg reduced dose each week), steroid therapy is completely withdrawn (Kamisawa et al. 2009). If the disease is refractory to corticosteroids, the diagnosis of IgG4-SC needs to be reevaluated. Disease relapse occurs in approximately 30–50% of patients, either during the reduction of the dose of steroids or after the discontinuation of the therapy, often in the first couple of years (Sandanayake et al. 2009). Increased IgG4 levels and proximal bile duct strictures are known risk factors for disease recurrence (Hart et al. 2013). Relapse usually occurs at the same site as the original disease, but can also involve different parts of biliary tree (Matsubayashi et al. 2014). The treatment of relapse is the same as for initial disease, and includes high-dose steroids (Matsubayashi et al. 2014). In cases where bilirubin levels are high, endoscopic biliary stent placement is required until steroid treatment becomes effective (Sheng et al. 1996).

5 Eosinophilic Cholangitis

Eosinophilic cholangitis is a rare disease characterized by eosinophilic infiltration of the biliary tree in association with peripheral eosinophilia (Sakpal et al. 2010). Clinical presentation is quite nonspecific, since patients usually present with jaundice. The strong association with eosinophilic gastroenteritis can facilitate the diagnosis of this rare entity (Vauthey et al. 2003). Typical histopathological feature is dense transmural eosinophilic infiltration in bile duct walls (Miura et al. 2009). Other findings include thickening of fibromuscular layer and slight fibrosis in the subserosal layer. Characteristic MRI findings in eosinophilic cholangitis include wall thickening of the common bile duct, cystic duct, and gallbladder (Song et al. 1997). Focal stricture of the common hepatic duct at the cystic duct insertion level might also be seen, together with mild narrowing of the proximal common bile duct (Ranson 1990). In addition, diffuse bile duct strictures from the hepatic hilum to the intrahe-

patic ducts have also been reported (Song et al. 1997). Although preoperative diagnosis of eosinophilic cholangitis is very difficult, it should be suspected in patients with jaundice and peripheral eosinophilia, when bile duct wall thickening is present together with involvement of cystic duct and gallbladder. Corticosteroid therapy leads to complete resolution of symptoms and imaging findings (Butler et al. 1985).

6 Recurrent Pyogenic Cholangitis

Recurrent pyogenic cholangitis (RPC) is a chronic, slowly progressive disease featured by recurrent attacks of bacterial cholangitis, hepatolithiasis (HL), and inflammatory biliary strictures, without functional or organic extrahepatic biliary obstruction (Harris et al. 1998; Okuno et al. 1996). RPC occurs with equal frequency among men and women, mostly in the third and fourth decades of life (Tsui et al. 2011). The disease is more common in the rural population, associated with lower socioeconomic status (Tsui et al. 2011).

The high incidence of this disease in Asian countries indicates that environmental factors, especially infection with parasites, such as *Ascaris lumbricoides* and *Clonorchis sinensis*, are involved in the pathogenesis (Leung and Yu 1997). It has been postulated that infestation of the biliary tree with worms leads to biliary epithelial damage and weakens the host immune response making them more vulnerable to sepsis (Stunell et al. 2006). Chronic inflammation promotes fibrotic changes in the bile duct walls and biliary duct stricture development. Strictures are predisposing factors for bile stasis and intrahepatic pigmented stone formation, which is one of the main features of RPC (Leung and Yu 1997). In such an environment, recurrent ascending bacterial infection is common, which worsens biliary strictures, and in severe cases can be the cause of progressive hepatic parenchymal destruction and cirrhosis (Leung and Yu 1997; Stunell et al. 2006). Furthermore, acute attacks of cholangitis can lead to cholangiohepatitis, with multiple hepatic abscesses. Although recurrent pyogenic cholangitis has been initially attributed only to parasitic infestation, similar symptoms and imaging findings can occur in patients without parasitic infection (Tabata and Nakayama 1981). In such cases, the high incidence of positive bile cultures, with most common pathogens being *Escherichia coli*, Klebsiella, Pseudomonas, Proteus species, and anaerobes, favors infection as the main cause of cholangitis (Okuno et al. 1996). Malnutrition or previous cholangiocyte injury makes bile ducts prone to biliary sepsis caused by portal bacteremia. Prolonged inflammation leads to formation of bile duct strictures, subsequent cholestasis, and intrahepatic lithiasis (Okuno et al. 1996). Nevertheless, the exact pathogenesis is still not clear, and remains to be elucidated.

6.1 Diagnosis and Imaging Findings

Patients with recurrent pyogenic cholangitis usually present with fever, right upper quadrant pain, and jaundice (Charcots triad) (Koh et al. 2013). Leukocytosis and moderately elevated bilirubin are common laboratory findings. They usually report previous episodes of undiagnosed similar symptoms, which were not severe enough to cause hospitalization of the patient (Harris et al. 1998). Apart from acute cholangitis, RPC may manifest with biliary colic, acute pancreatitis, and obstructive jaundice (Harris et al. 1998). Patients with postoperative complications, in terms of biliary obstruction and bile stasis, who present with recurrent attacks of cholangitis, should not be diagnosed as recurrent pyogenic cholangitis.

The main imaging findings are dilatation of central intrahepatic bile ducts and intrahepatic lithiasis (Lim et al. 1990; Chau et al. 1987; Chan et al. 1989). Ultrasound examination typically demonstrates dilatation of the large intrahepatic and extrahepatic bile ducts, in combination with little, if any, dilatation of peripheral bile ducts (Lim et al. 1990; Chau et al. 1987). Intrahepatic calculi can be identified in up to 90% of patients,

and if calcified present as single or multiple hyperechogenic lesions, with posterior acoustic shadowing (Fig. 10a) (Chau et al. 1987). Pneumobilia, which is also a frequent finding in RPC, can obscure intrahepatic lithiasis (Lim et al. 1990). Besides initial evaluation, sonography is used for follow-up and is very useful in the timely diagnosis of disease complications (Lim et al. 1990).

Contrast-enhanced CT might fail in visualization of intrahepatic calculi because these gallstones are usually not calcified. Gallstones can be detected on unenhanced CT, since 90% of the stones are hyperdense in comparison to liver parenchyma (Chan et al. 1989). Similarly to ultrasound, CT demonstrates dilatation of large intrahepatic and extrahepatic bile ducts together with lack of visualization of the peripheral bile ducts, which is a characteristic finding for RPC (Koh et al. 2013). Moreover, CT shows slight bile duct wall thickening and increased enhancement, suggestive of acute cholangitis (Koh et al. 2013; Chan et al. 1989). Pneumobilia is easily recognized on CT, and usually is the consequence of previous endoscopic biliary intervention. In patients without clinical history of biliary interventions, pneumobilia occurs as a result of the passage of the calculi through the ampulla, but it can also be caused by gas-forming organisms, such as *Klebsiella pneumonia* or *Clostridium perfringens* (Chan et al. 1989). Ancillary imaging finding is a hepatic parenchymal atrophy, which most commonly occurs in the left lateral and right posterior liver segments (Afagh and Pancu 2004). In addition, segmental or lobar portal vein thrombosis can occur, due to periductal inflammation and portal thrombophlebitis, which then contribute to parenchymal atrophy (Afagh and Pancu 2004). Increased attenuation of affected segments in arterial phase occurs not only in the setting of lobar or segmental portal vein thrombosis, but also during episodes of acute cholangitis.

Similarly to other imaging modalities, MRCP examination shows dilatation of first- and second-order branches of bile ducts, in association with decreased arborization and abrupt tapering of peripheral ducts, resulting in arrowhead

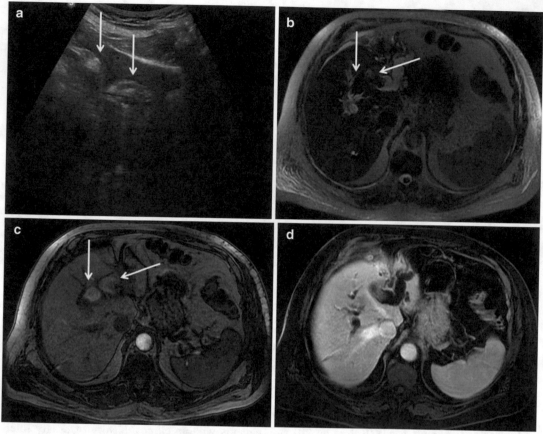

Fig. 10 Intrahepatic lithiasis in 67-year-old male patients with recurrent attacks of cholangitis without prior hepato-biliary surgery and without known parasitic infection. (**a**) Ultrasound examination shows multiple large stones (*solid arrows*) in dilated left hepatic duct. (**b**) Axial T2-weighted image shows large intrahepatic calculi in the left and right hepatic ducts with high signal intensity on T1-weighted image (*solid arrows*) (**c**). Diffuse biliary dilatation is seen on portal venous phase (**d**)

appearance (Park et al. 2001). The distribution of the bile duct dilation is frequently unrelated to the location of calculi. This finding could be explained by the fact that repeated episodes of obstruction and inflammation lead to loss of wall elasticity, with concomitant diffuse bile duct destruction (Park et al. 2001). MRI provides superior depiction of intrahepatic gallstones, which are seen as filling defects in dilated bile ducts on heavily T2-weighted images (Fig. 10b) (Kim et al. 1999). The pigmented stones in RPC typically appear as hyperintense on T1-weighted images (Fig. 10c) (Kim et al. 1999). Bile duct strictures in RPC are usually short (less than 1 cm), and are often missed on CT, but are clearly visible on MRCP (Afagh and Pancu 2004; Jain and Agarwal 2008). The strictures are relative

only to the dilated areas, since their calibers are actually larger than the original normal ducts (Kim et al. 1999). The left lateral segment duct is the most commonly affected, followed by the right posterior segmental duct (Park et al. 2001; Kim et al. 1999). This may be explained by more acute angulation of these ducts and poorer drain-age of bile. In 60% of the cases, stones are also seen in common bile duct and common hepatic duct, which are diffusely dilated, without stric-tures. Moreover, coexisting gallbladder stones are present in 30% of patients (Afagh and Pancu 2004). In these cases, it is very hard to make a differential diagnosis between primary and sec-ondary hepatolithiasis, which refers to a retro-grade migration of stones from the extrahepatic bile ducts. In addition to MRCP, conventional

MR sequences provide insight into parenchymal changes in RPC. Atrophic hepatic segments are usually slightly hypointense on T1-weighted images, with increased signal intensity on T2-weighted images, due to edema and inflammation (Kim et al. 1999). Crowded and dilated bile ducts are a frequent finding in these distorted liver segments (Park et al. 2001; Kim et al. 1999).

6.2 Complications

Long-standing disease is frequently complicated with hepatic abscess or biloma formation. Liver abscess is found in up to 20% of patients, often located in right liver lobe (Kim et al. 1999). The differential diagnosis with biloma is usually not difficult, with rim enhancement supporting the diagnosis of hepatic abscess (Chan et al. 1989). The most important complication of RPC is development of cholangiocarcinoma, which occurs in up to 5% of cases (Chen et al. 1989). Chronic inflammation and mechanical irritation with gallstones are recognized risk factors for cholangiocarcinoma, which has a poor prognosis in the setting of RPC (Chan et al. 1989). One of the main reasons is late diagnosis, since it most frequently develops in segments with high stone burden, where it is obscured by the bile duct and liver parenchymal changes (Al-Sukhni et al. 2008). Recently, Kim et al. have shown that cholangiocarcinoma associated with RPC was found predominantly in segments with atrophy, narrowing, or obliteration of the portal vein (Kim et al. 2006). Therefore, it is very important to examine carefully these regions, and to notice the worsening of bile duct dilatation during follow-up of these patients (Kim et al. 2006). The most common form of cholangiocarcinoma in RPC patients is periductal infiltrating type (Kim et al. 2006). Ancillary findings are lymphadenopathy and increased serum CA 19-9 level.

6.3 Differential Diagnosis

Recurrent pyogenic cholangitis must be differentiated from several other diseases characterized by secondary stone formation. In order to make the diagnosis of RPC, all causes of obstructive cholangiopathy must be excluded. The distinction between RPC and secondary intrahepatic lithiasis is possible when stones are seen in dilated intrahepatic ducts proximal to a stricture (Corcos et al. 2012). It is presumed that these stones are formed in the intrahepatic bile ducts. Caroli disease should also be distinguished from RPC, because of the similar clinical and radiological presentations in both diseases. Unlike RPC, Caroli disease usually appears in childhood (Guy et al. 2002). The changes in Caroli disease are mostly seen in the entire liver, but it can also be lobar or segmental. Imaging findings characteristic for Caroli disease are cystic dilatation of intrahepatic bile ducts, intrahepatic lithiasis, and frequently central dot sign (Guy et al. 2002). On the other hand, RPC is characterized by disproportionate dilatation of the first and second divisions of intrahepatic ducts, reduction of peripheral ducts, pigmented intrahepatic calculi, and parenchymal atrophy of affected segments (Okuno et al. 1996). Liver biopsy with histopathological analysis can provide definitive diagnosis in unclear cases. Differential diagnosis with PSC is usually not difficult, since PSC presents with multiple short segmental strictures of intra- and extrahepatic bile ducts, which are sufficiently different from above-described RPC features (Okuno et al. 1996).

6.4 Treatment of Recurrent Pyogenic Cholangitis

Treatment of recurrent pyogenic cholangitis is complex, and includes a combination of surgery, endoscopic, or percutaneous biliary interventions (Jeyarajah 2004; Van Sonnenberg et al. 1986). In patients with isolated disease in the first-order ducts, surgical biliary drainage or nonoperative ERCP-guided procedures could be chosen, based on surgeon decision and patient's condition (Lam et al. 1978). For patients with intrahepatic lithiasis and strictures in the second-order ducts and smaller ducts, percutaneous transhepatic cholangiographic guided treatment or hepatectomy is indicated (Cheung and Kwok 2005). In the setting of acute cholangitis, decompression of the infected biliary tree is necessary. This can be achieved by percutaneous transhepatic biliary drainage or endoscopic sphincterotomy with biliary stent placement, or by using methods such as percutaneous transhepatic cholangioscopic lithotomy (PTCSL) (Lee et al. 2001).

6.5 Hepatolithiasis

Hepatolithiasis (HL) is defined as the presence of de novo-formed calculi (stone, mud, and/or sludge) within the intrahepatic bile ducts proximal to the common hepatic duct (confluence of the right and left hepatic ducts) (Choi 1989). Intrahepatic lithiasis is the basic pathology of RPC and is the preferred term for this disease in the Japanese literature (Tsui et al. 2011). Although causes and underlying pathophysiology are not clearly understood, it is postulated that complex interaction between nutritional status, bile duct infection, cholestasis, parasites, variation of bile duct, and bile metabolic defect is responsible for changes in primary HL (Attasaranya et al. 2008). Among these factors, cholestasis, infection, and bile metabolic defect are the most important (Attasaranya et al. 2008). Depending on the gallstone composition, primary HL can be classified into three types: calcium bilirubinate stones, cholesterol stones, and mixed stones (Tsui et al. 2011). Clinical manifestations and imaging features are those described for RPC (Okuno et al. 1996). On the other hand, secondary HL refers to a retrograde migration of stones from the extrahepatic ducts and gallbladder, and those liver conditions with secondary stone formation in intrahepatic bile ducts, such as Caroli disease and PSC (Carpenter 1998).

7 Obstructive Cholangiopathy

Biliary obstruction has numerous causes including cholecystitis, biliary stones, surgical anastomotic strictures, tumors, arterial aneurysms, pancreatic disease, and iatrogenic strictures (Lan Cheong Wah et al. 2017). Nevertheless, benign causes of obstruction are much more likely to cause clinical infection than malignant like cholangiocarcinoma and pancreatic carcinoma (Mohammad Alizadeh 2017). Biliary obstruction is followed by bile stasis, which leads to inflammation, superimposed bacterial infection, and, if prolonged, fibrosis and stricture formation (Mohammad Alizadeh 2017). Rarely, if the cause of obstruction is not relieved, secondary biliary cirrhosis can develop as a long-standing complication (Lubikowski et al. 2012).

Patients usually present with right upper quadrant pain, fever, and jaundice (Lan Cheong Wah et al. 2017). Although *Escherichia coli* is the most common pathogen of acute cholangitis, most infections are polymicrobial (Lan Cheong Wah et al. 2017). Echogenic material within involved bile ducts can be seen on US, while CT may display purulent bile as high-density intraductal content (Mohammad Alizadeh 2017). In cases complicated with acute cholangitis, bile duct wall thickening and increased contrast enhancement are also observed on CT (Mohammad Alizadeh 2017). Common complication of ascending cholangitis is formation of hepatic abscesses which are easily identified on US, CT, or MRI (Figs. 11 and 12) (Mohammad Alizadeh 2017). Besides abovementioned findings, the most important diagnostic task in obstructive cholangitis is to identify the cause and level of biliary obstruction, since it determines further therapy.

In addition to intraductal causes of biliary obstruction, long-standing extrinsic obstruction of common bile duct can also be the cause of prolonged bile stasis and changes characteristic for obstructive cholangiopathy (Katabathina et al. 2014). Thus, in patients with cirrhosis and extrahepatic portal vein obstruction, portal biliopathy can develop (Khuroo et al. 2016). This term is related to compressive effect of enlarged collateral vessels on common hepatic and common bile duct (Aguirre et al. 2012). Cholangiography is the preferred modality for diagnosis, with most common abnormalities seen in common bile duct including wall irregularities and localized saccular dilatations (Aguirre et al. 2012). Differential diagnosis is usually not difficult, when MRCP findings are analyzed in association with conventional MR findings (Aguirre et al. 2012).

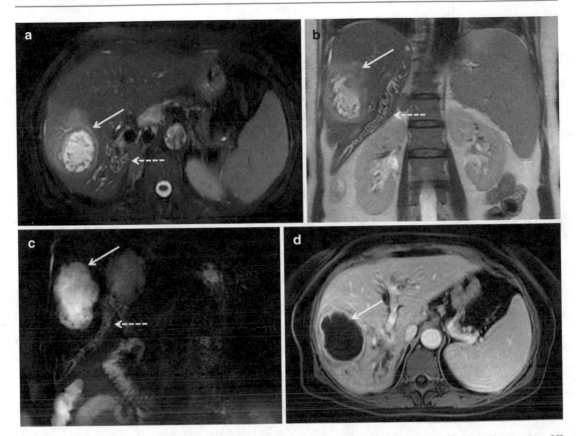

Fig. 11 Obstructive cholangiopathy in 64-year-old women due to right hepatic duct iatrogenic lesion. (**a**) Axial T2-weighted fat-saturated image and coronal T2-weighted image (**b**) show multiple calculi in posterior segment bile ducts (*dotted arrow*), a large hepatic abscess as a complication of ascending cholangitis (*solid arrow*), and hilar lymphadenopathy. (**c**) MRCP in the same patient shows intrahepatic lithiasis in bile duct for segment VI (*dotted arrow*) and hepatic abscess (*solid arrow*). Hyperintense lesion medially to hepatic abscess corresponds to hepatic hemangioma not shown in other images. (**d**) Portal venous axial T1-weighted image shows large necrotic lesion compatible with hepatic abscess (*solid arrow*) and biliary dilatation in segment VI

Recommended therapy includes biliary balloon dilatation and eventually surgery if persistent obstruction is evident (Franceschet et al. 2016).

Heathcote 2006; Cello 1989). Other contributing factors include ischemia, autonomic nerve injury, and direct invasion of bile duct epithelium by HIV (Daly and Padley 1996).

8 AIDS-Related Cholangitis

AIDS-related cholangitis is a rare type of secondary sclerosing cholangitis occurring in patients with human immunodeficiency virus (HIV) infection (Ducreux et al. 1995). Although the exact pathogenesis is not clear, it has been postulated that opportunistic biliary duct infection with pathogens such as cytomegalovirus, *Cryptosporidium parvum*, *Mycobacterium avium* complex, and herpes simplex virus is one of the main causes of this condition (Abdalian and

8.1 Diagnosis and Imaging Findings

Currently, AIDS-related cholangitis is rarely seen due to improved multidrug antiretroviral therapy, usually in patients with advanced disease, and markedly decreased immune function (Ducreux et al. 1995). This condition is also diagnosed in 20% of treated patients with less severe immunosuppression and higher CD4 levels, probably reflecting resistance to first-line antiretroviral

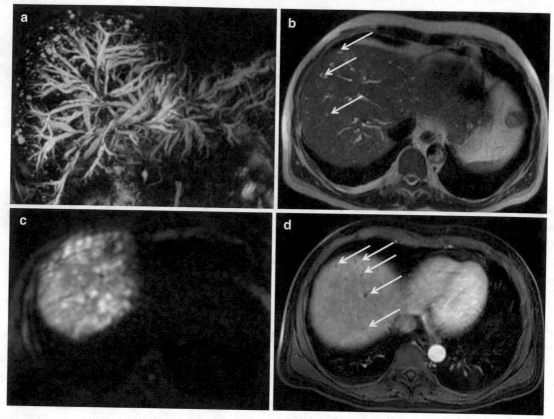

Fig. 12 Obstructive cholangiopathy in a 72-year-old male due to anastomotic stricture after hepaticojejunal anastomosis. (**a**) MRCP shows diffuse biliary dilatation above the level of primary confluence. Multiple small hyperintense lesions are also seen. (**b**) Axial T2-weighted image shows biliary dilatation and multiple hyperintense foci (*solid arrows*) compatible with microabscesses which are better visualized on diffusion-weighted image (**c**) and after contrast administration in arterial phase (*solid arrows*) (**d**)

medications (Abdalian and Heathcote 2006). The patients present with nonspecific clinical features including right upper quadrant pain, which is more severe in the presence of papillary stenosis, diarrhea, hepatomegaly, and weight loss (Devarbhavi et al. 2010). Elevation of serum alkaline phosphatase level, 5–7 times above normal limits, is the key laboratory finding, present in almost all patients (Carucci and Halvorsen 2004). Jaundice, as a result of complete ductal obstruction, is uncommon even in patients with documented cholangiographic abnormalities (Devarbhavi et al. 2010).

Like in all other clinical conditions, where bile duct pathology is suspected, ultrasound examination is the first modality in diagnostic algorithm (Bilgin et al. 2008). In cases where ultrasound evaluation identifies intra- and extra-hepatic dilatation in HIV patients, further investigation with CT or MRI is suggested. CT findings of biliary dilatation in the absence of neoplastic tissue or extrinsic compression indicate HIV-related cholangitis (Catalano et al. 2009). The diagnosis of AIDS cholangiopathy in the past was made by ERCP, which was the gold standard procedure (Abdalian and Heathcote 2006). Four distinct patterns of AIDS-related cholangitis were described according to cholangiographic findings: papillary stenosis (type I, 20% of cases), intrahepatic bile duct strictures alone (type II, 15–20%) or associated with papillary stenosis (type III, 50%), and long extrahepatic bile duct strictures with or without intrahepatic involvement (type IV, 6–15%) (137, 140).

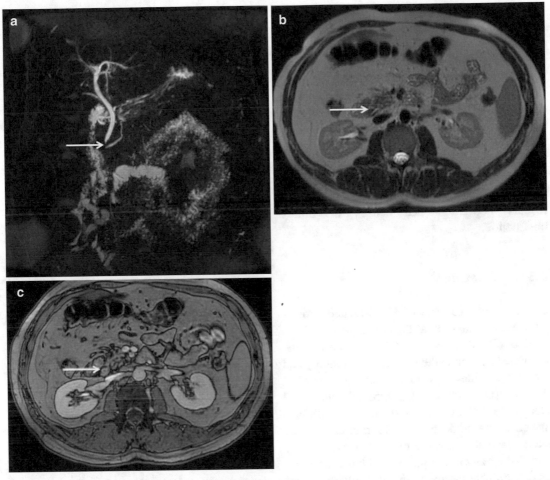

Fig. 13 AIDS-related cholangitis infection in a 48-year-old female. (**a**) MR cholangiography shows a stricture of the distal common bile duct with only slight proximal biliary dilatation (*solid arrow*). (**b**) Axial T2-weighted image reveals papillary stenosis, seen as thickened wall of intra-mural part of common bile duct (*solid arrow*). (**c**) Axial T1-weighted postcontrast out-of-phase image demonstrates increased wall enhancement of distal common bile duct consistent with papillary stenosis (*solid arrow*)

Currently, MRCP, as a noninvasive procedure, has replaced ERCP, and is performed in all patients with clinically suspected AIDS cholangiopathy. The most common cholangiographic finding is papillary stenosis, present in up to 75% of patients (Fig. 13) (Devarbhavi et al. 2010; Tonolini and Bianco 2013). Papillary stenosis in combination with multifocal intrahepatic biliary strictures, creating "beaded" appearance, is the single most common pattern in AIDS cholangitis (Devarbhavi et al. 2010; Vitellas et al. 2002). The fourth and the rarest ERCP pattern refers to long segmental extrahepatic biliary stricture (Tonolini and Bianco 2013).

8.2 Differential Diagnosis

AIDS cholangitis should be differentiated from acute pyogenic cholangitis which is a life-threatening condition (Vitellas et al. 2002). However, besides bile duct dilatation, in patients with acute cholangitis, bile duct wall thickening and increased contrast enhancement are invariably present, suggesting the diagnosis of acute inflammation (Deltenre and Valla 2008). In addition, patchy or wedge-shaped areas of T2-weighted hyperintensity and perfusion abnormalities are associated findings in acute cholangitis (Tonolini and Bianco 2013). Intrahepatic bile duct strictures without identifiable common bile duct abnormalities could be hardly distinguishable from PSC (Northover and Terblanche 1979). However, in appropriate clinical setting, the correct diagnosis is easily made.

Biliary dilatation in HIV patients could be caused by variable other conditions, such as compression of common hepatic duct with enlarged collateral vessels in portal biliopathy, enlarged porta hepatis lymph nodes, or pancreatic tumor (Ducreux et al. 1995). However, cross-sectional imaging with CT and/or MRI in almost all cases reveals abovementioned causes of biliary obstruction.

8.3 Treatment

Conservative treatment of AIDS-related cholangitis with antimicrobial therapy is usually ineffective (Ducreux et al. 1995). Restoring the immune function is the main goal of therapy and could be achieved with modern antiretroviral therapy (Ducreux et al. 1995; Abdalian and Heathcote 2006; Cello 1989). In cases with biliary strictures, endoscopic balloon dilatation and stent placement are the optimal therapy (Daly and Padley 1996). For patients with papillary stenosis sphincterotomy is the therapy of choice (Deltenre and Valla 2008).

9 Ischemic Cholangitis

Ischemic cholangitis is defined as ischemia-induced bile duct injury caused by various conditions (Imam et al. 2013). Since biliary system, unlike hepatic parenchyma, receives its blood supply only from the arterial system, bile ducts are very vulnerable to ischemic injury (Foley et al. 2011). Iatrogenic causes, including liver transplantation (2–19% of patients), hepatic arterial infusion of chemotherapeutic agents, and vessel injury during biliary or pancreatic surgery, are the most common causes of ischemic cholangitis (Imam et al. 2013; Terblanche et al. 1983; Valente et al. 1996). Other less common etiologies include hereditary hemorrhagic telangiectasia, radiotherapy, polyarteritis

nodosa, and atherosclerosis (Imam et al. 2013). Ischemic cholangiopathy predominantly affects the middle third of the common bile duct, followed by the hepatic duct confluence, whereas intrahepatic bile ducts are less commonly involved (Kinner et al. 2012). This particular distribution can partly be explained with the arterial supply to the large bile ducts. Namely, most of the arterial supply for these ducts comes from retroduodenal and retroportal arteries, while a lesser proportion comes from right hepatic artery (Foley et al. 2011). As a result, the middle third of the common bile duct and the biliary confluence are the most vulnerable to ischemic injury (Terblanche et al. 1983).

9.1 Diagnosis and Imaging Findings

The clinical presentations and radiological findings of ischemic cholangitis depend on the stage of disease. In the acute phase, patients present with fever, abdominal pain, jaundice, and sepsis (Gelbmann et al. 2007). Intraluminal filling defects suggestive of biliary casts can be seen on imaging (Kinner et al. 2012). Biliary casts, formed of desquamated epithelium and other bile components, typically show high signal intensity on nonenhanced T1-weighed MR images, similarly to intraductal stones (Kinner et al. 2012). However, difference in their shape usually allows differential diagnosis, as stones are round or oval, while biliary casts have linear or branching pattern. Biliary dilatation is invariably seen in the acute phase, which is probably due to their obstruction by the casts and due to a nonspecific reaction to injury (Imam et al. 2013). In cases of severe ischemic injury, dilated bile ducts are observed on CT and MRI, in association with discontinuity of the wall, suggesting full-thickness necrosis (Gelbmann et al. 2007). Spilling of the bile around damaged bile duct results in the formation of bilomas, which are seen as well-defined fluid collections of low density (Imam et al. 2013). Chronic stage of disease is characterized by fibrous stenosis formation, as part of healing of previous ischemic or necrotic lesions. At this stage, patients present with obstructive

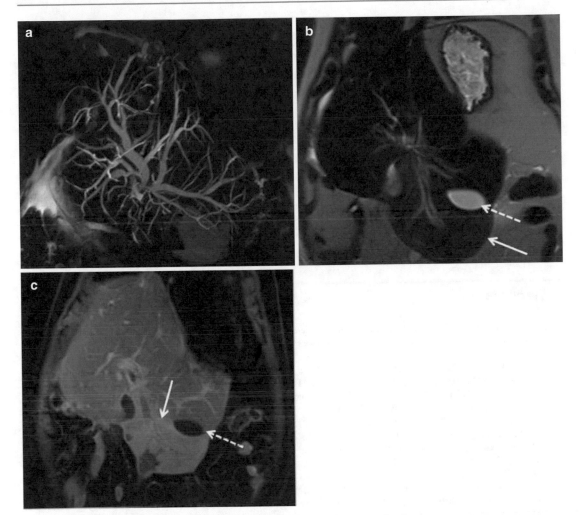

Fig. 14 Ischemic cholangitis due to iatrogenic lesion after cholecystectomy. (**a**) MRCP shows diffuse biliary dilatation due to stricture in the upper part of common hepatic duct. Coronal T2-weighted image (**b**) and T1-weighted in portal venous phase (**c**) show abnormal liver morphology with hypertrophy-atrophy complex and very enlarged left liver lobe with subcapsular moderately hyperintense wedge-shaped lesions corresponding to perfusion abnormalities (*solid arrow*). Focal biliary dilatation and biloma (*dotted arrow*) are also noted

jaundice and laboratory profile of progressive or fluctuating cholestasis (Terblanche et al. 1983). Cholangiographic findings include focal or multiple, segmental bile duct strictures (Fig. 14) (Imam et al. 2013). Clinical course and predominant location of ischemic strictures in the middle third of the common bile duct and the hilar region favor the diagnosis of ischemic cholangitis rather than PSC. Rarely, patients may have fibrotic form of ischemic cholangiopathy as presenting feature, which can be explained by more limited or slowly progressive hepatic arterial injury (Kinner et al. 2012). The correct diagnosis is possible when characteristic imaging findings are present in association with direct or indirect evidence of compromised arterial supply to the liver or bile ducts.

9.2 Treatment of Ischemic Cholangitis

The therapy of ischemic cholangitis depends on each patient's clinical history. If ischemic cholangitis is a complication of liver transplantation, then restoration of arterial flow can be attempted using thrombolytic agents, balloon angioplasty or stenting, and surgical revision with stenting (Valente et al. 1996; Gelbmann et al. 2007). In patients with small artery ischemic injury, since there is no specific curative method, management of complications is of great clinical importance (Imam et al. 2013). Endoscopic procedures are used to remove biliary casts, while percutaneous drainage is useful for biloma and for decompression of dilated bile ducts (Valente et al. 1996). When abovementioned procedures are not sufficient, biliary bypass surgery can be performed for bile duct reconstruction (Gelbmann et al. 2007).

References

Abbas G, Lindor KD (2009) Cholangiocarcinoma in primary sclerosing cholangitis. J Gastrointest Cancer 40:19–25

Abdalian R, Heathcote EJ (2006) Sclerosing cholangitis: a focus on secondary causes. Hepatology 44:1063–1074

Afagh A, Pancu D (2004) Radiologic findings in recurrent pyogenic cholangitis. J Emerg Med 26:343–346

Aguirre DA, Farhadi FA, Rattansingh A et al (2012) Portal biliopathy: imaging manifestations on multidetector computed tomography and magnetic resonance imaging. Clin Imaging 36:126–134

Al-Sukhni W, Gallinger S, Pratzer A et al (2008) Recurrent pyogenic cholangitis with hepatolithiasis: the role of surgical therapy in North America. J Gastrointest Surg 12:496–503

Attasaranya S, Fogel EL, Lehman GA (2008) Choledocholithiasis, ascending cholangitis, and gallstone pancreatitis. Med Clin North Am 92(4):925–960

Azizi L, Raynal M, Cazejust J et al (2012) MR imaging of sclerosing cholangitis. Clin Res Hepatol Gastroenterol 36(2):130–138

Bader TR, Beavers KL, Semelka RC (2003) MR imaging features of primary sclerosing cholangitis: patterns of cirrhosis in relationship to clinical severity of disease. Radiology 226:675–685

Bilgin M, Balci NC, Erdogan A et al (2008) Hepatobiliary and pancreatic MRI and MRCP findings in patients with HIV infection. AJR Am J Roentgenol 191:228–232

Bizzaro N, Covini G, Rosina F et al (2012) Overcoming a "probable" diagnosis in antimitochondrial antibody negative primary biliary cirrhosis: study of 100 sera and review of the literature. Clin Rev Allergy Immunol 42(3):288–297

Bjornsson E, Chari ST, Smyrk TC et al (2007) Immunoglobulin G4-associated cholangitis: description of an emerging clinical entity based on review of the literature. Hepatology (Baltimore, Md) 45(6):1547–1554

Björnsson E, Olsson R, Bergquist A et al (2008) The natural history of small-duct primary sclerosing cholangitis. Gastroenterology 134:975–980

Blachar A, Federle MP, Brancatelli G (2001) Primary biliary cirrhosis: clinical, pathologic, and helical CT findings in 53 patients. Radiology 220(2):329–336

Bonato G, Cristoferi L, Strazzabosco M et al (2015) Malignancies in primary sclerosing cholangitis: a continuing threat. Dig Dis 33(Suppl 2):140–148

Brandsaeter B, Schrumpf E, Bentdal O et al (2005) Recurrent primary sclerosing cholangitis after liver transplantation: a magnetic resonance cholangiography study with analyses of predictive factors. Liver Transplant 11:1361–1369

Butler TW, Feintuch TA, Caine WP Jr (1985) Eosinophilic cholangitis, lymphadenopathy, and peripheral eosinophilia: a case report. Am J Gastroenterol 80:572–574

Campsen J, Zimmerman MA, Trotter JF et al (2008) Clinically recurrent primary sclerosing cholangitis following liver transplantation: a time course. Liver Transpl 14:181–185

Carey EJ, Ali AH, Lindor KD (2015) Primary biliary cirrhosis. Lancet 386(10003):1565–1575

Carpenter HA (1998) Bacterial and parasitic cholangitis. Mayo Clin Proc 73(5):473–478

Carucci LR, Halvorsen RA (2004) Abdominal and pelvic CT in the HIV-positive population. Abdom Imaging 29:631–642

Catalano OA, Sahani DV, Forcione DG et al (2009) Biliary infections: spectrum of imaging findings and management. Radiographics 29:2059–2080

Cello JP (1989) Acquired immunodeficiency syndrome cholangiopathy: spectrum of disease. Am J Med 86:539–546

Chan FL, Man SW, Leong LL et al (1989) Evaluation of recurrent pyogenic cholangitis with CT: analysis of 50 patients. Radiology 170:165–169

Chapman R, Fevery J, Kalloo A et al (2010) Diagnosis and management of primary sclerosing cholangitis. Hepatology 51:660–678

Chari ST, Smyrk TC, Levy MJ et al (2006) Diagnosis of autoimmune pancreatitis: the Mayo Clinic experience. Clin Gastroenterol Hepatol 4(8):1010–1016

Chau EM, Leong LL, Chan FL (1987) Recurrent pyogenic cholangitis: ultrasound evaluation compared with endoscopic retrograde cholangiopancreatography. Clin Radiol 38:79–85

Chen MF, Chen MF, Jan YY, Wang CS et al (1989) Intrahepatic stones associated with cholangiocarcinoma. Am J Gastroenterol 84(4):391–395

Cheung MT, Kwok PCH (2005) Liver resection for intrahepatic stones. Arch Surg 140(10):993–997

Choi TK (1989) Intrahepatic stones. Br J Surg 76(3):213–214

Claessen MM, Vleggaar FP, Tytgat KM et al (2009) High lifetime risk of cancer in primary sclerosing cholangitis. J Hepatol 50:158–164

Cohen SA, Siegel JH, Kasmin FE (1996) Complication of diagnostic and therapeutic ERCP. Abdom Imaging 21:385–394

Corcos G, Monnier Cholley L, Arrivé L (2012) Intrahepatic lithiasis. Clin Res Hepatol Gastroenterol 36(3):197–198

Corpechot C, El Naggar A, Poujol-Robert A et al (2006) Assessment of biliary fibrosis by transient elastography in patients with PBC and PSC. Hepatology 43:1118–1124

Crosignani A, Battezzati PM, Invernizzi P et al (2008) World J Gastroenterol 14:3313–3327

Cullen S, Chapman R (2001) Aetiopathogenesis of primary sclerosing cholangitis. Best Pract Res Clin Gastroenterol 15:577–589

Cullen SN, Chapman RW (2006) The medical management of primary sclerosing cholangitis. Semin Liver Dis 26:52–61

Daly CA, Padley SP (1996) Sonographic prediction of a normal or abnormal ERCP in suspected AIDS related sclerosing cholangitis. Clin Radiol 51:618–621

Dave M, Elmunzer BJ, Dwamena BA et al (2010) Primary sclerosing cholangitis: meta-analysis of diagnostic performance of MR cholangiopancreatography. Radiology 256:387–396

Deltenre P, Valla DC (2008) Ischemic cholangiopathy. Semin Liver Dis 28:235–246

Devarbhavi H, Sebastian T, Seetharamu SM et al (2010) HIV/AIDS cholangiopathy: clinical spectrum, cholangiographic features and outcome in 30 patients. J Gastroenterol Hepatol 25:1656–1660

Ducreux M, Buffet C, Lamy P et al (1995) Diagnosis and prognosis of AIDS-related cholangitis. AIDS 9:875–880

Düşünceli E, Erden A, Erden I et al (2005) Primary sclerosing cholangitis: MR cholangiopancreatography and T2-weighted MR imaging findings. Diagn Interv Radiol 11:213–218

Eksteen B (2016) The gut-liver axis in primary sclerosing cholangitis. Clin Liver Dis 20(1):1–14

European Association for the Study of the Liver (2009) EASL Clinical Practice Guidelines: management of cholestatic liver diseases. J Hepatol 51:237–267

Foley DP, Fernandez LA, Leverson G et al (2011) Biliary complications after liver transplantation from donation after cardiac death donors: an analysis of risk factors and long-term outcomes from a single center. Ann Surg 253:817–825

Franceschet I, Zanetto A, Ferrarese A (2016) Therapeutic approaches for portal biliopathy: a systematic review. World J Gastroenterol 22(45):9909–9920

Gardner CS, Bashir MR, Marin D et al (2015) Diagnostic performance of imaging criteria for distinguishing autoimmune cholangiopathy from primary sclerosing cholangitis and bile duct malignancy. Abdom Imaging 40(8):3052–3061

Gautam M, Cheruvattath R, Balan V (2006) Recurrence of autoimmune liver disease after liver transplantation: a systematic review. Liver Transplant 12:1813–1824

Gelbmann CM, Rummele P, Wimmer M et al (2007) Ischemic-like cholangiopathy with secondary sclerosing cholangitis in critically ill patients. Am J Gastroenterol 102:1221–1229

Ghazale A, Chari ST, Zhang L et al (2008) Immunoglobulin G4-associated cholangitis: clinical profile and response to therapy. Gastroenterology 134(3):706–715

Gossard AA, Angulo P, Lindor KD (2005) Secondary sclerosing cholangitis: a comparison to primary sclerosing cholangitis. Am J Gastroenterol 100:1330–1333

Gotthardt D, Chahoud F, Sauer P (2011) Primary sclerosing cholangitis: diagnostic and therapeutic problems. Dig Dis 29:41–45

Grant AJ, Lalor PF, Salmi M et al (2002) Homing of mucosal lymphocytes to the liver in the pathogenesis of hepatic complications of inflammatory bowel disease. Lancet 359(9301):150–157

Guy F, Cognet F, Dranssart M et al (2002) Caroli's disease: magnetic resonance imaging features. Eur Radiol 12(11):2730–2736

Haliloglu N, Erden A, Erden I (2009) Primary biliary cirrhosis: evaluation with T2-weighted MR imaging and MR cholangiopancreatography. Eur J Radiol 69:523–527

Harris HW, Kumwenda ZL, Chen SM et al (1998) Recurrent pyogenic cholangitis. Am J Surg 176:34–37

Hart PA, Topazian MD, Witzig TE et al (2013) Treatment of relapsing autoimmune pancreatitis with immunomodulators and rituximab: the Mayo Clinic experience. Gut 62(11):1607–1615

Hirschfield GM, Liu X, Xu C et al (2009) Primary biliary cirrhosis associated with HLA, IL12A, and IL12RB2 variants. N Engl J Med 360:2544–2555

Hirschfield G, Heathcote J, Gershwin M (2010) Pathogenesis of cholestatic liver disease and therapeutic approaches. Gastroenterology 139:481–1496

Hirschfield GM, Karlsen TH, Lindor KD et al (2013) Primary sclerosing cholangitis. Lancet 382:1587–1599

Imam MH, Talwalkar JA, Lindor KD (2013) Secondary sclerosing cholangitis: pathogenesis, diagnosis, and management. Clin Liver Dis 17(2):269–277

Ito K, Mitchell DG, Outwater EK et al (1999) Primary sclerosing cholangitis: MR imaging features. Am J Roentgenol 172:1527–1533

Ito K, Mitchell DG, Siegelman ES (2002) Cirrhosis: MR imaging features. Magn Reson Imaging Clin N Am 10(1):75–92

Itoh S, Nagasaka T, Suzuki K et al (2009) Lymphoplasmacytic sclerosing cholangitis: assessment of clinical, CT, and pathological findings. Clin Radiol 64(11):1104–1114

Jain M, Agarwal A (2008) MRCP findings in recurrent pyogenic cholangitis. Eur J Radiol 66:79–83

Jeyarajah DR (2004) Recurrent pyogenic cholangitis. Curr Treat Options Gastroenterol 7:91–98

Jones DE (2007) Pathogenesis of primary biliary cirrhosis. Gut 56(11):1615–1624

Kamisawa T, Shimosegawa T, Okazaki K et al (2009) Standard steroid treatment for autoimmune pancreatitis. Gut 58(11):1504–1507

Kamisawa T, Zen Y, Pillai S et al (2015) IgG4-related disease. Lancet 385:1460–1471

Kaplan MM, Gershwin ME (2005) Primary biliary cirrhosis. N Engl J Med 353:1261–1267

Katabathina VS, Dasyam AK, Dasyam N et al (2014) Adult bile duct strictures: role of MR imaging and MR cholangiopancreatography in characterization. Radiographics 34(3):565–586

Khuroo MS, Rather AA, Khuroo NS (2016) Portal biliopathy. World J Gastroenterol 22(35):7973–7982

Kim MJ, Cha SW, Mitchell DG et al (1999) MR imaging findings in recurrent pyogenic cholangitis. AJR 173:1545–1549

Kim JH, Kim TK, Eun HW et al (2006) CT findings of cholangiocarcinoma associated with recurrent pyogenic cholangitis. AJR 187:1571–1577

Kim JY, Lee JM, Han JK et al (2007) Contrast-enhanced MRI combined with MR cholangiopancreatography for the evaluation of patients with biliary strictures: differentiation of malignant from benign bile duct strictures. J Magn Reson Imaging 26(2): 304–312

Kinner S, Umutlu L, Dechêne A et al (2012) Biliary complications after liver transplantation: addition of T1-weighted images to MR cholangiopancreatography facilitates detection of cast in biliary cast syndrome. Radiology 263:429–436

Kobayashi S, Matsui O, Gabata T et al (2005) MRI findings of primary biliary cirrhosis: correlation with Scheuer histologic staging. Abdom Imaging 30(1):71–76

Koh YX, Chiow AKH, Chok AY et al (2013) Recurrent pyogenic cholangitis: disease characteristics and patterns of recurrence. ISRN Surg 25:536081

Kovač JD, Daković M, Stanisavljević D et al (2012a) Diffusion-weighted MRI versus transient elastography in quantification of liver fibrosis in patients with chronic cholestatic liver diseases. Eur J Radiol 81(10):2500–2506

Kovač JD, Ješić R, Stanisavljević D et al (2012b) Integrative role of MRI in the evaluation of primary biliary cirrhosis. Eur Radiol 22(3):688–694

Kovač JD, Ješić R, Stanisavljević D et al (2013) MR imaging of primary sclerosing cholangitis: additional value of diffusion-weighted imaging and ADC measurement. Acta Radiol 54(3):242–248

Lam SK, Wong KP, Chan PK et al (1978) Recurrent pyogenic cholangitis: a study by endoscopic retrograde cholangiography. Gastroenterology 74(6):1196–1203

Lammert C, Juran BD, Schlicht E et al (2014) Biochemical response to ursodeoxycholic acid predicts survival in a North American cohort of primary biliary cirrhosis patients. J Gastroenterol 49(10):1414–1420

Lan Cheong Wah D, Christophi C, Muralidharan V (2017) Acute cholangitis: current concepts. ANZ J Surg 87(7–8):554–559

Lee SK, Seo DW, Myung SJ et al (2001) Percutaneous transhepatic cholangioscopic treatment for hepatolithiasis: an evaluation of long-term results and risk factors for recurrence. Gastrointest Endosc 53(3):318–323

Leung JW, Yu AS (1997) Hepatolithiasis and biliary parasites. Baillieres Clin Gastroenterol 11:681–706

Lewin M, Vilgrain V, Ozenne V et al (2009) Prevalence of sclerosing cholangitis in adults with autoimmune hepatitis: a prospective magnetic resonance imaging and histological study. Hepatology 50(2):528–537

Lim JH, Ko YT, Lee DH et al (1990) Oriental cholangiohepatitis: sonographic findings in 48 cases. Am J Radiol 155:511–514

Lindor KD, Gershwin ME, Poupon R et al (2009) Primary biliary cirrhosis. Hepatology 50:291–308

Lubikowski J, Chmurowicz T, Post M et al (2012) Liver transplantation as an ultimate step in the management of iatrogenic bile duct injury complicated by secondary biliary cirrhosis. Ann Transplant 17(2):38–34

Ludwig J, Dickson ER, McDonald GS (1978) Staging of chronic nonsuppurative destructive cholangitis (syndrome of primary biliary cirrhosis). Virchows Arch A Pathol Anat Histol 379:103–112

MacQuillan GC, Neuberger J (2003) Liver transplantation for primary biliary cirrhosis. Clin Liver Dis 7(4):941–956

Matsubayashi H, Uesaka K, Sugiura T et al (2014) IgG4-related sclerosing cholangitis without obvious pancreatic lesion: difficulty in differential diagnosis. J Dig Dis 15(7):394–403

Mendes FD, Jorgensen R, Keach J et al (2006) Elevated serum IgG4 concentration in patients with primary sclerosing cholangitis. Am J Gastroenterol 101(9):2070–2075

Miura F, Asano T, Amano H et al (2009) Resected case of eosinophilic cholangiopathy presenting with secondary sclerosing cholangitis. World J Gastroenterol 15:1394–1397

Mohammad Alizadeh AH (2017) Cholangitis: Diagnosis, treatment and prognosis. J Clin Transl Hepatol 28;5(4):404-413

Moon S-H, Kim M-H, Park DH et al (2008) Is a 2-week steroid trial after initial negative investigation for malignancy useful in differentiating autoimmune pancreatitis from pancreatic cancer? A prospective outcome study. Gut 57:1704–1712

Nakazawa T, Ohara H, Sano H et al (2006) Schematic classification of sclerosing cholangitis with autoimmune pancreatitis by cholangiography. Pancreas 32(2):229

Nguyen DL, Juran BD, Lazaridis KN (2010) Primary biliary cirrhosis. Best Pract Res Clin Gastroenterol 24:647–654

Ngwa TN, Law R, Murray D et al (2014) Serum immunoglobulin G4 level is a poor predictor of immunoglobulin G4-related disease. Pancreas 43(5):704–707

Nishino T, Oyama H, Hashimoto E et al (2007) Clinicopathological differentiation between sclerosing cholangitis with autoimmune pancreatitis and primary sclerosing cholangitis. J Gastroenterol 42(7):550–559

Northover JM, Terblanche J (1979) A new look at the arterial supply of the bile duct in man and its surgical implications. Br J Surg 66:379–384

Ohara H, Okazaki K, Tsubouchi H et al (2012) Research committee of IgG4-related diseases; research committee of intractable diseases of liver and biliary tract; Ministry of Health, Labor and Welfare, Japan; Japan Biliary Association. Clinical diagnostic criteria of IgG4-related sclerosing cholangitis 2012. J Hepatobiliary Pancreat Sci 19(5):536–542

Okazaki K, Uchida K, Koyabu M et al (2014) IgG4 cholangiopathy: current concept, diagnosis, and pathogenesis. J Hepatol 61(3):690–695

Okuno WT, Whitman GJ, Chew FS (1996) Recurrent pyogenic cholangitis. AJR 167:484

Oseini AM, Chaiteerakij R, Shire AM et al (2011) Utility of serum immunoglobulin G4 in distinguishing immunoglobulin G4-associated cholangitis from cholangiocarcinoma. Hepatology (Baltimore, Md) 54(3):940–948

Pares A, Caballeria L, Rodes J (2006) Excellent long-term survival in patients with primary biliary cirrhosis and biochemical response to ursodeoxycholic acid. Gastroenterology 130:715–720

Park MS, Yu JS, Kim KW et al (2001) Recurrent pyogenic cholangitis: comparison between MR cholangiography and direct cholangiography. Radiology 220:677–682

Park MS, Kim TK, Kim KW et al (2004) Differentiation of extrahepatic bile duct cholangiocarcinoma from benign stricture: findings at MRCP versus ERCP 1. Radiology 233(1):234–240

Ranson JH (1990) Eosinophilic cholangitis: a self-limited cause of extrahepatic biliary obstruction. Am J Gastroenterol 85:582–585

Reau NS, Jensen DM (2008) Vanishing bile syndrome. Clin Liver Dis 12:203–217

Revelon G, Rashid A, Kawamoto S et al (1999) Primary sclerosing cholangitis: MR imaging findings with pathologic correlation. Am J Roentgenol 173:1037–1042

Rong G, Wang H, Bowlus CL et al (2015) Incidence and risk factors for hepatocellular carcinoma in primary biliary cirrhosis. Clin Rev Allergy Immunol 48(2–3):132–141

Sakpal SV, Shusharina V, Chamberlain RS (2010) Eosinophilic cholangitis and cholangiopathy: a sheep in wolves clothing. HPB Surg 2010:906496

Sandanayake NS, Church NI, Chapman MH et al (2009) Presentation and management of posttreatment relapse in autoimmune pancreatitis/immunoglobulin G4-associated cholangitis. Clin Gastroenterol Hepatol 7(10):1089–1096

Sheng R, Campbell WL, Zajko AB et al (1996) Cholangiographic features of biliary strictures after liver transplantation for primary sclerosing cholangitis: evidence of recurrent disease. AJR Am J Roentgenol 166:1109–1113

Shibuya A, Tanaka K, Miyakawa H et al (2002) Hepatocellular carcinoma and survival in patients with primary biliary cirrhosis. Hepatology 35: 1172–1178

Silveira MG, Talwalkar JA, Lindor KD et al (2010) Recurrent primary biliary cirrhosis after liver transplantation. Am J Transplant 10(4):720–726

Sivakumaran Y, Le Page PA, Becerril-Martinez G et al (2014) IgG4-related sclerosing cholangitis: the cholangiocarcinoma mimic. ANZ J Surg 84(6):486–487

Song HH, Byun JY, Jung SE et al (1997) Eosinophilic cholangitis: US, CT, and cholangiography findings. J Comput Assist Tomogr 21:251–253

Stone JH, Zen Y, Deshpande V (2012) IgG4-related disease. N Engl J Med 366(6):539–551

Stunell H, Buckley O, Geoghegan T et al (2006) Recurrent pyogenic cholangitis due to chronic infestation with Clonorchis sinensis. Eur Radiol 16:2612–2614

Tabata M, Nakayama F (1981) Bacteria and gallstones. Etiological significance. Dig Dis Sci 26(3):218–224

Terayama N, Makimoto KP, Kobayashi S et al (1994) Pathology of the spleen in primary biliary cirrhosis: an autopsy study. Pathol Int 44:753–758

Terblanche J, Allison HF, Northover JM (1983) An ischemic basis for biliary strictures. Surgery 94:52–57

Tischendorf JJ, Hecker H, Krüger M et al (2007) Characterization, outcome, and prognosis in 273 patients with primary sclerosing cholangitis: a single center study. Am J Gastroenterol 102:107–114

Tokala A, Khalili K, Menezes R et al (2014) Comparative MRI analysis of morphologic patterns of bile duct disease in IgG4-related systemic disease versus primary sclerosing cholangitis. Am J Roentgenol 202(3):536–543

Tonolini M, Bianco R (2013) HIV-related/AIDS cholangiopathy: pictorial review with emphasis on MRCP findings and differential diagnosis. Clin Imaging 37(2):219–226

Trivedi PJ, Hirschfield GM (2016) The immunogenetics of autoimmune cholestasis. Clin Liver Dis 20:15–31

Tsui WM, Chan YK, Wong CT et al (2011) Hepatolithiasis and the syndrome of recurrent pyogenic cholangitis: clinical, radiologic and pathologic features. Semin Liver Dis 31:33–48

Valente JF, Alonso MH, Weber FL et al (1996) Late hepatic artery thrombosis in liver allograft recipients is associated with intrahepatic biliary necrosis. Transplantation 61:61–65

Van Sonnenberg E, Casola G, Cubberley DA et al (1986) Oriental cholangiohepatitis: diagnostic imaging and interventional management. AJR 146:327–331

Vauthey JN, Loyer E, Chokshi P et al (2003) Case 57: eosinophilic cholangiopathy. Radiology 227:107–112

Vera A, Moledina S, Gunson B et al (2002) Risk factors for recurrence of primary sclerosing cholangitis of liver allograft. Lancet 360:1943–1944

Vitellas KM, El-Dieb A, Vaswani KK et al (2002) MR cholangiopancreatography in patients with primary sclerosing cholangitis: interobserver variability and comparison with endoscopic retrograde cholangiopancreatography. AJR Am J Roentgenol 179:399–407

Wenzel JS, Donohoe A, Ford KL 3rd et al (2001) Primary biliary cirrhosis: MR imaging findings and description of MR imaging periportal halo sign. AJR Am Roentgenol 176:885–889

Yimam KK, Bowlus CL (2014) Diagnosis and classification of primary sclerosing cholangitis. Autoimmun Rev 13:445–450

Zen Y, Nakanuma Y (2012) IgG4 cholangiopathy. Int J Hepatol 2012:472376

Zen Y, Harada K, Sasaki M et al (2004) IgG4-related sclerosing cholangitis with and without hepatic inflammatory pseudotumor, and sclerosing pancreatitis-associated sclerosing cholangitis: do they belong to a spectrum of sclerosing pancreatitis? Am J Surg Pathol 28(9):1193–1203

Zen Y, Kawakami H, Kim JH (2016) IgG4-related sclerosing cholangitis: all we need to know. J Gastroenterol 51(4):295–312

Printed in the United States
by Baker & Taylor Publisher Services